AF096840

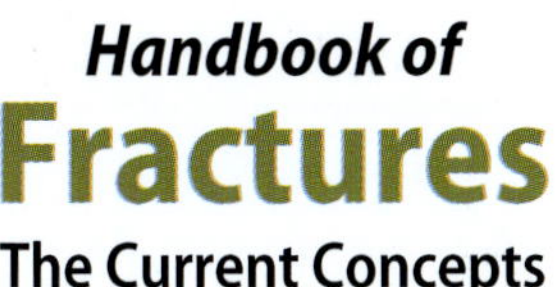
Handbook of
Fractures
The Current Concepts

Handbook of
Fractures
The Current Concepts

Editor-in-Chief

Abdul Ghani
MBBS MS-orthopedics (AIIMS Delhi) MRCS(Edinburgh)
Professor and Head of Unit
Department of Orthopedics
Government Medical College, Jammu
Jammu and Kashmir, India

Editor

Samarth Mittal
MBBS MS-orthopedics (AIIMS Delhi) DNB(Orthopedics) FACS MAMS MIMSA
Additional Professor
Department of Orthopedics
JPN Apex Trauma Centre, AIIMS
New Delhi, India

Forewords

DD Tanna
Mandeep S Dhillon

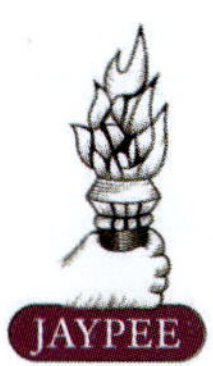

JAYPEE BROTHERS MEDICAL PUBLISHERS
The Health Sciences Publisher
New Delhi | London

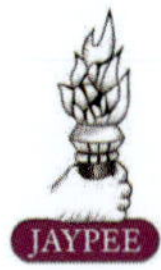

Jaypee Brothers Medical Publishers (P) Ltd

Headquarters
EMCA House
23/23-B, Ansari Road, Daryaganj
New Delhi 110 002, India
Landline: +91-11-23272143, +91-11-23272703
+91-11-23282021, +91-11-23245672
E-mail: jaypee@jaypeebrothers.com

Corporate Office
Jaypee Brothers Medical Publishers (P) Ltd.
4838/24, Ansari Road, Daryaganj
New Delhi 110 002, India
Phone: +91-11-43574357
Fax: +91-11-43574314
E-mail: jaypee@jaypeebrothers.com

Overseas Office
JP Medical Ltd.
83, Victoria Street, London
SW1H 0HW (UK)
Phone: +44-20 3170 8910
E-mail: info@jpmedpub.com

EU GPSR Authorised Representative
Logos Europe, 9 rue Nicolas Poussin
17000, La Rochelle, France
Phone: +33 (0) 6 67 93 73 78
E-mail: Contact@logoseurope.eu

Website: www.jaypeebrothers.com
Website: www.jaypeedigital.com

Inquiries for bulk sales may be solicited at: jaypee@jaypeebrothers.com

***Handbook of Fractures: The Current Concepts* / Abdul Ghani**

First Edition: **2025**
ISBN: 978-93-6616-491-5
Printed in India

DEDICATED TO

The Divine

&

Those We Serve

Contributors

Abhai Singh Bhadwal MBBS
Postgraduate Orthopedics
Resident
Department of Orthopedics
Government Medical College, Jammu
Jammu and Kashmir, India

Abhimanu Kaith MBBS
Postgraduate Resident
Department of Orthopedics
Government Medical College, Jammu
Jammu and Kashmir, India

Abhishek Bral MBBS
Postgraduate Resident
Department of Orthopedics
Government Medical College, Jammu
Jammu and Kashmir, India

Abhishek Mahajan MBBS
Resident
Department of Orthopedics
Government Medical College, Jammu
Jammu and Kashmir, India

Aditya Chaubey MBBS
Postgraduate Resident
Department of Orthopedics
Government Medical College, Jammu
Jammu and Kashmir, India

Agnivesh Tikoo MS(Orthopedics) FNB(Spine Surgery)
Senior Consultant Spine Surgeon
Apollo Hospitals
Navi Mumbai, Maharashtra, India

Akash Narangyal MBBS
Resident
Department of Orthopedics
Government Medical College, Jammu
Jammu and Kashmir, India

Altaf Ahmad Kawoosa
MS(Orthopedics)
Professor and Head
Department of Orthopedics
Government Medical College, Srinagar
Jammu and Kashmir, India

Amandeep Singh Bakshi MBBS MS(Orthopedics)
Professor
Department of Orthopedics
Government Medical College
Patiala, Punjab, India

Aman Koul MBBS
Postgraduate Resident
Department of Orthopedics
Government Medical College, Jammu
Jammu and Kashmir, India

Amarjeet Singh MBBS
MS(Orthopedics) MRCSEd
FASM(TN MGR University)
Senior Clinical Fellow
Department of Trauma and Orthopedics
Homerton University Hospital
London, United Kingdom

Amit Kumar MBBS
MS(Orthopedics)
Consultant
Department of Orthopedics
ESIC Model Hospital, Jammu
Jammu and Kashmir, India

Amit Thakur MS(Orthopedics)
Associate Professor
Department of Orthopedics
All India Institute of Medical Science Vijaypur, Jammu
Jammu and Kashmir, India

Anita Kour MBBS MD(Anesthesia)
Senior Resident
Department of Anesthesiology and Critical Care
Government Medical College, Jammu
Jammu and Kashmir, India

Ankita Khajuria MBBS
Resident
Department of Orthopedics
Government Medical College, Jammu
Jammu and Kashmir, India

Anoop Kumar MBBS
MS(Orthopedics) (CMC Ludhiana)
Professor
Department of Orthopedics
Government Medical College, Jammu
Jammu and Kashmir, India

Apoorva Kabra MBBS(AIIMS) MS(Orthopedics) (AIIMS) MRCS(Glasgow)
Senior Resident
Department of Orthopedics
All India Institute of Medical Sciences
New Delhi, India

Archi Gupta MD(Radiodiagnosis)
Postgraduate Resident
Department of Radiodiagnosis
Government Medical College, Jammu
Jammu and Kashmir, India

Arpan Upadhayay
MS(Orthopedics)
Assistant Professor, SRIMS
Durgapur, West Bengal, India

Aswanikumar Singh Jamedar MBBS Dip(Orthopedics) DNB(Orthoapedics)
Professor
Department of Orthopedics
Ballari Medical College and Research Institute
Ballari, Karnataka, India
Past KOA President

Ayaz Ali Mir MBBS
MS(Orthopedics)
Fellowship Arthroplasty
Fellow Orthopedic Rheumatology
Consultant Orthopedic Surgeon
JK Health Service
Jammu, Jammu and Kashmir, India

Azhar Ud Din MBBS
MS(Orthopedics)
Consultant
Department of Orthopedics
District Hospital Kargil UT
Ladakh, India

Barkat Anwar Shah MBBS
Postgraduate Orthopedics Resident
Department of Orthopedics
Government Medical College, Jammu
Jammu and Kashmir, India

Bhaarath KS MBBS Postgraduate Orthopedics
Resident
Department of Orthopedics
Government Medical College, Jammu
Jammu and Kashmir, India

Bhat Jameel Mohd Jabbar MBBS
Postgraduate Resident
Department of Orthopedics
Government Medical College, Jammu
Jammu and Kashmir, India

Dev Kant MBBS MS(Orthopedics) (AIIMS)
Professor and Unit Head
Department of Orthopedics
SMS Medical College
Jaipur, Rajasthan, India

Dibyendu Biswas MBBS(AMU) MS(Orthopedics) (MAMC, New Delhi) DNB MNAMS
Arthroplasty Fellow
Apollo Hospital, New Delhi, India
Ex-Senior Resident (AIIMS, New Delhi)

Farid Hussain Malik MBBS
MS(Orthopedics)
Assistant Professor
Department of Orthopedics
Government Medical College, Jammu
Jammu and Kashmir, India

Gagandeep Singh Raina MBBS
MS(Orthopedics)
Senior Resident
Department of Orthopedics
Government Medical College, Jammu
Jammu and Kashmir, India

Gurpreet Kour MS(Gynecology and Obstetrics)
Senior Resident
Department of Gynecology and Obstetrics
All India Institute of Medical Science Vijaypur, Jammu
Jammu and Kashmir, India

Harsh Chauhan MBBS
Postgraduate Orthopedics Resident
Department of Orthopedics
Government Medical College, Jammu
Jammu and Kashmir, India

Hayat Khan MBBS
(SKIMS) DNB(Orthopedics) MNAMS(Orthopedics) Fellowship(Upper Extremity) (Basel, Switzerland)
Associate Consultant
Department of Orthopedics
HMG Hospital
Riyadh, Saudi Arabia

Heemanshu Bhat MBBS
Postgraduate Orthopedics Resident
Department of Orthopedics
Government Medical College, Jammu
Jammu and Kashmir, India

Imran Ahmed Hajam MBBS MS
Senior Resident
Department of Orthopedics
All India Institute of Medical Science Vijaypur, Jammu
Jammu and Kashmir, India

Ifzal Ahmed Khan MBBS
Postgraduate Resident
Department of Orthopedics
Government Medical College, Jammu
Jammu and Kashmir, India

Irfan Ahmed Poswal MBBS
Postgraduate Resident
Department of Orthopedics
Government Medical College, Jammu
Jammu and Kashmir, India

Irfan Malik MS(Orthopedics)
Associate Professor
Department of Orthopedics
Government Medical College, Rajouri
Jammu and Kashmir, India

John Mohd MBBS MS(Orthopedics)
Senior Resident
Department of Physical Medicine and Rehabilitation
SKIMS Soura, Srinagar
Jammu and Kashmir, India

Jujhar Singh MBBS(MAMC) MS(Orthopedics) (PGIMER, Chandigarh) DNB MNAMS FACS(USA) FIMSA
Specialist and Senior Consultant
Department of Orthopedics
Dr Baba Saheb Ambedkar Medical College and Hospital
New Delhi, India

Kamal Ji Pandit Dip(Orthopedics) MS(Orthopedics) DNB(Orthopedics)
Senior Resident
Hamdard Institute of Medical Science
New Delhi, India

Kanav Mahajan
Dip(Orthopedics) DNB
Consultant
Department of Orthopedics
Umang Healthcare and Diagnostics
Jammu, Jammu and Kashmir, India

Khalid Muzzafar
MS(Orthopedics) DNB(Orthopedics)
Associate Professor
Department of Orthopedics
Government Medical College
Doda, Jammu and Kashmir, India

Manish Singh MBBS
MS(Orthopedics)
Assistant Professor
Department of Orthopedics
Government Medical College, Jammu
Jammu and Kashmir, India

Meganath V Pawar MBBS
MS(Orthopedic Surgery) (AIIMS, New Delhi)
Professor and Unit Head
Department of Orthopedics
AIIMS Bhubaneswar
Bhubaneswar, Odisha, India

Mohamad Waseem Dar MBBS
Postgraduate Resident
Department of Orthopedics
Government Medical College, Jammu
Jammu and Kashmir, India

Mohammad Farooq Butt
MBBS MS
Associate Professor
Department of Orthopedics
Government Medical College, Jammu
Jammu and Kashmir, India

Mozam Hamid Wani MBBS
Postgraduate Orthopedics Resident
Department of Orthopedics
Government Medical College, Jammu
Jammu and Kashmir, India

Naresh Rana MS(Orthopedics) MBBS
Assistant Professor
Department of Orthopedics
Government Medical College, Rajouri
Jammu and Kashmir, India

Neelam V Ramana Reddy
MBBS MS(Orthopedics) Mch(Orthopedics) (UK)
Chief
Department of Orthopedics
Star Hospital Banjara Hills
Hyderabad, Telangana, India

Neeraj Mahajan
MS(Orthopedics)
Assistant Professor
Department of Orthopedics
Government Medical College, Jammu
Jammu and Kashmir, India

Nishank Mehta MBBS MS
Assistant Professor
Department of Orthopedics
All India Institute of Medical Sciences
New Delhi, India

Nitin Choudhary
MS(Orthopedics)
Senior Resident
Department of Orthopedics
Government Medical College, Jammu
Jammu and Kashmir, India

Nusrat Jabeen MBBS
MS(Anatomy)
Professor
Department of Anatomy
Government Medical College, Jammu
Jammu and Kashmir, India

Omeshwar Singh MBBS
MS(Orthopedics)
Assistant Professor
Department of Orthopedics
MM Medical College and Hospital Kumarhatti
Solan, Himachal Pradesh, India

Pankaj Spolia MBBS
MS(Orthopedics)
Assistant Professor
Department of Orthopedics
MM Institute of Medical Sciences and Research
Ambala, Haryana, India

Pankaj Vir Singh MBBS
MS(Orthopedics)
Senior Resident
Department of Orthopedics
Government Medical College, Jammu
Jammu and Kashmir, India

Pardeep Singh MBBS MS
Assistant Professor
MM Institute of Medical Sciences and Research
Ambala, Haryana, India

Prashant Tank MBBS
MS(Orthopedics)
Senior Resident
Department of Orthopedics
All India Institute of Medical Sciences
New Delhi, India

Pulkit Sharma MBBS
MS(Orthopedics)
Senior Registrar Orthopedics
Department of Orthopedics
Government Medical College,
Jammu
Jammu and Kashmir, India

Rajesh Gupta MBBS
MS(Orthopedics)
Professor and Head
Department of Orthopedics
ASCOMS Jammu
Jammu and Kashmir, India

Rajneesh Garg MS(Orthopedics)
Professor and Head
Department of Orthopedics
Dayanand Medical College and
Hospital
Ludhiana, Punjab, India

Rashid Anjum MBBS
MS(Orthopedics) DNB(Orthopedics)
MNAMS FIPO
Associate Professor
Department of Orthopedics
All India Institute of Medical
Sciences Vijaypur, Jammu
Jammu and Kashmir, India

Ravi Chauhan DNB(Orthopedics)
Consultant
Department of Orthopedics
Sir Ganga Ram City Hospital
New Delhi, India

Rifaaqat Ghani MBBS
Student, Vardhman Mahavir
Medical College
New Delhi, India

Sachin Kudyar MBBS
MS(Orthopedics)
Senior Resident
Department of Orthopedics
Government Medical College,
Jammu
Jammu and Kashmir, India

Sajad Ahmad Wani MBBS
Postgraduate Resident
Department of Orthopedics
Government Medical College,
Jammu
Jammu and Kashmir, India

Sakib Arfee MS(Orthopedics)
Consultant
Department of Orthopedics
Medcard Multispeciality
Hospital
Amritsar, Punjab, India

Samarth Mittal MBBS
MS-orthopedics (AIIMS Delhi)
DNB(Orthopedics) FACS MAMS
MIMSA
Additional Professor
Department of Orthopedics
JPN Apex Trauma Centre, AIIMS
New Delhi, India

Sandeep Kumar
MS(Orthopedics) PGHSC(UK)
Professor and Head
Department of Orthopedics
Hamdard Institute of Medical
Sciences and Research
New Delhi, India

Sanjeev Gupta MBBS
MS(Orthopedics)
Professor and Head
Department of Orthopedics
Government Medical College,
Jammu
Jammu and Kashmir, India

Saransh Bahl MBBS Postgraduate
Orthopedics
Resident
Department of Orthopedics
Government Medical College,
Jammu
Jammu and Kashmir, India

Saravjeet Kour MTech
(Computer Science Engineering)
Assistant Professor
Department of Computer
Science
Mahant Bachittar Singh College
of Engineering and Technology
Jammu, Jammu and Kashmir,
India

Shabir A Dhar MS(Orthopedics)
Associate Professor
Department of Orthopedics
SKIMS Medical College
Srinagar, Jammu and Kashmir,
India

Shafiq Hackla MBBS MS
DNB(Orthopedics) FNB(Sports
Medicine) FASM
Assistant Professor
Department of Orthopedic
Government Medical College,
Jammu
Jammu and Kashmir, India

Shriya Bhat MBBS Postgraduate
General Surgery
Resident
Department of General Surgery
Government Medical College,
Jammu
Jammu and Kashmir, India

Shubam Surmal MBBS
MS(Orthopedics)
Senior Resident
Department of Orthopedics
Government Medical College,
Jammu
Jammu and Kashmir, India

Shubham Pandoh MBBS
MS(Orthopedics)
Senior Resident
Department of Orthopedics
Government Medical College,
Jammu
Jammu and Kashmir, India

Shubhranshu Choudhary
MBBS MS(Orthopedics)
Senior Resident
Department of Orthopedics
IMS and SUM Hospital
Bhubaneswar, Odisha, India

Simran Preet Singh MBBS
MS(Orthopedics) FNB(Arthroplasty)
Arthroplasty Fellow
Department of Orthopedics
Star Hospital Banjara Hills
Hyderabad, Telangana, India

Sonakshi Gupta MBBS
MD(Anesthesia)
Senior Resident
Department of Anesthesiology
and Critical Care
Government Medical College,
Jammu
Jammu and Kashmir, India

Sudhir Kumar Garg MBBS
MS(Orthopedics)
Professor and Head
Department of Orthopedics
Government Medical College
and Hospital
Chandigarh, India

Sukhil Raina MBBS
MS(Orthopedics)
Senior Resident
Department of Orthopedics
Government Medical College,
Jammu
Jammu and Kashmir, India

Sumeet Singh Charak MBBS
MS(Orthopedics)
Assistant Professor
Department of Orthopedics
Government Medical College,
Jammu
Jammu and Kashmir, India

Suraydev Aman Singh
MS(Orthopedics)
Senior Resident
Department of Orthopedics
Government Medical College,
Jammu
Jammu and Kashmir, India

Tahir Afzal MBBS MS
Assistant Professor
Postgraduate Department of
Orthopedics
Government Medical College,
Jammu
Jammu and Kashmir, India

Tanveer Ahmed Bhat
MS(Orthopedics) MBBS
Consultant
Department of Orthopedics
Rajasthan Medical Center
Tohana, Haryana, India

Tejpal Singh MBBS
MS(Orthopedics)
Senior Resident
Department of Orthopedics
Government Medical College,
Udhampur
Jammu and Kashmir, India

Vedant Bajaj MBBS
MS(Orthopedics)
Senior Resident
Department of Orthopedics
Dr Baba Saheb Ambedkar
Medical College and Hospital
New Delhi, India

Vineet Aggarwal MS
DNB(Orthopedics) FNB(Pediatric
Orthopedics)
Professor and Head
Department of Orthopedics
Indira Gandhi Medical College
Shimla, Himachal Pradesh, India

Vipin Sharma MBBS
DNB(Orthopedics)
Dip(Orthopedics) MNAMS Ranawat
Fellow(Arthroplasty) ICMR Fellow
TMH Mumbai(Orthopedic Oncology)
Professor and Head
Department of Orthopedics
Dr Rajendra Prasad Government
Medical College and Hospital
Kangra, Himachal Pradesh, India

Waseem Ahmad Sheikh MBBS
Postgraduate Resident
Department of Orthopedics
Government Medical College,
Jammu
Jammu and Kashmir, India

Yassar Arfat MBBS
Postgraduate Resident
Department of Orthopedics
Government Medical College,
Jammu
Jammu and Kashmir, India

Yassir Mehmood MBBS
Postgraduate Resident
Department of Orthopedics
Government Medical College,
Jammu
Jammu and Kashmir, India

Younis Kamal MS(Orthopedics)
DNB(Orthopedics)
MNMS(Orthopedics) Post Doc
Fellowship in Spine Surgery(Ganga
Hospital)
Associate Professor
Department of Orthopedics
and Spine Surgery, Government
Medical College, Anantnag
Jammu and Kashmir, India

Zubair Ahmad Lone
MS(Orthopedics) MBBS
Assistant Professor
Department of Orthopedics
Government Medical College,
Rajouri
Jammu and Kashmir, India

Shubhanshu Choudhary
MBBS MS(Orthopedics)
Senior Resident
Department of Orthopedics
[illegible] Hospital
[illegible], India

Simran Preet Singh MBBS
[illegible]

Sudhir Kumar Garg MBBS
MS(Orthopedics)
Professor and Head
Department of Orthopedics
[illegible]

Suneet Singh Charak MBBS
MS(Orthopedics)
Assistant Professor
Department of Orthopedics
Government Medical College,
Jammu
Jammu and Kashmir, India

Suraydev Aman Singh
MS(Orthopedics)
Senior Resident
Department of Orthopedics
Government Medical College,
Jammu
Jammu and Kashmir, India

Tahir Afzal MBBS MS
Assistant Professor
Postgraduate Department of
Orthopedics
Government Medical College,
Jammu
Jammu and Kashmir, India

Tanveer Ahmed Bhat
MS(Orthopedics) MBBS
Consultant
Department of Orthopedics
Rajasthan Medical Center
Tohana, Haryana, India

Tejpal Singh MBBS
MS(Orthopedics)
Senior Resident
Department of Orthopedics
Government Medical College,
Udhampur
Jammu and Kashmir, India

Vedant Bajaj MBBS
MS(Orthopedics)
Senior Resident
Department of Orthopedics
Dr Baba Saheb Ambedkar
Medical College and Hospital
New Delhi, India

Vineet Aggarwal MS
DNB(Orthopedics) FNB(Pediatric
Orthopedics)
Professor and Head
Department of Orthopedics
Indira Gandhi Medical College
Shimla, Himachal Pradesh, India

Vipin Sharma MBBS
DNB(Orthopedics)
Dip(Orthopedics) MNAMS Ranawat
Fellow(Arthroplasty) ICMR Fellow
TMH Mumbai(Orthopedic Oncology)
Professor and Head
Department of Orthopedics
Dr Rajendra Prasad Government
Medical College and Hospital
Kangra, Himachal Pradesh, India

Waseem Ahmad Sheikh MBBS
Postgraduate Resident
Department of Orthopedics
Government Medical College,
Jammu
Jammu and Kashmir, India

Yassar Arfat MBBS
Postgraduate Resident
Department of Orthopedics
Government Medical College,
Jammu
Jammu and Kashmir, India

Yassir Mehmood MBBS
Postgraduate Resident
Department of Orthopedics
Government Medical College,
Jammu
Jammu and Kashmir, India

Younis Kamal MS(Orthopedics)
DNB(Orthopedics)
MNAMS(Orthopedics) Post Doc
Fellowship in Spine Surgery(Ganga
Hospital)
Associate Professor
Department of Orthopedics
and Spine Surgery, Government
Medical College, Anantnag
Jammu and Kashmir, India

Zubair Ahmad Lone
MS(Orthopedics) MBBS
Assistant Professor
Department of Orthopedics
Government Medical College,
Rajouri
Jammu and Kashmir, India

Foreword

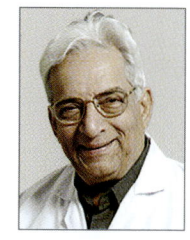

Fractures remain a constant challenge, posing intricate clinical questions and demanding the most current understanding to guide optimal treatment. *"Handbook of Fractures: The Current Concepts"* is a concise and practical resource that brings together the latest advancements, techniques, and insights that shape the management of fractures today.

In a rapidly evolving field, this handbook is an essential reference, helping orthopedic surgeons with a wide spectrum of fracture patterns and treatment options. Designed to be accessible yet thorough, it synthesizes core principles with recent innovations, making it invaluable for orthopedic surgeons at every career stage. Through this book, which is written by two learned orthopedic surgeons (*Dr Abdul Ghani and Dr Samarth Mittal*), readers will find a blend of foundational knowledge and forward-looking practices, equipping them to provide the best care for patients with fracture-related challenges.

DD Tanna MBBS MS(Orthopedics)
Most Experienced Orthopedic Surgeon and Mentor
Ex-Professor
BYL Nair Hospital and Medical College
Expertise in Revision Trauma Surgery, Joint Replacements

Foreword

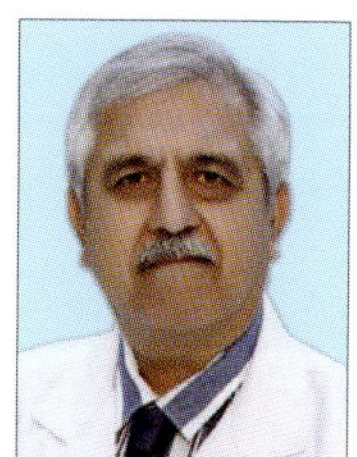

In the ever-increasing word of mechanization and industrialization, the significant increase in incident of orthopedic trauma demands a clear understanding of management of fractures and their complications. This is doubly important at the undergraduate level of medicine, where insights into trauma management are essential, because this is where we lay the foundation of the understanding of this complex situation. Going forward to the postgraduate level, the current book, *Handbook of Fractures: The Current Concepts,* clarifies the perceptions and understanding of orthopedic trauma management in modern times.

This Handbook of Fractures is relevant today, because it starts from the basics like fracture classification and explains and clarifies evaluation of X-rays and goes on to discuss basic science applications. Other chapters then subsequently focus on various individual fractures and explain the intricacies of management at all levels, especially those relevant to the developed world.

With a total of 20 sections, and multiple subsections covering a variety of topics, the unique thing about this orthopedic book is that it looks at varied subjects where trauma can occur and explains about subjects such as tendon injuries and pediatric fractures, in addition to the standard of care in all other complex trauma situations. The book is enriched by the various authors who have contributed chapters and are academic leaders in the field of orthopedic education.

Having written many books, I can fully understand the effort and time that has gone into compiling this volume. The two editors who are surgeons also *(Dr Abdul Ghani and Dr Samarth Mittal)* are to be congratulated for compiling this comprehensive book, which deals into many complex scenarios.

Mandeep S Dhillon MBBS MS (Orthopedics) FAMS FRCS
Director, Orthopedics and Sports Medicine
Fortis Hospital, Mohali, Punjab, India
Chairman, AO Trauma (Asia Pacific)
Founder President, Indian Biological Orthopaedics Society
Past President, Indian Orthopaedic Association
Past President, Indian Arthroplasty Association
Past President, Indian Association for Sports Medicine
Past President, Indian Foot and Ankle Society
Former Professor and Head
Department of Orthopedics
PGIMER, Chandigarh, India

Preface

Fractures represent a significant portion of musculoskeletal injuries encountered in both clinical and emergency settings. As advances in diagnostics, surgical techniques, and postoperative care continue to evolve, it is crucial to synthesize these developments into an accessible, comprehensive reference. *"Handbook of Fractures: The Current Concepts"* seeks to bridge foundational knowledge with the latest insights, offering clinicians, surgeons, and students a practical guide to understanding fracture mechanisms, treatment modalities, and evidence-based management strategies.

This book is structured to cover both fundamental principles and advanced topics across a spectrum of fracture types. Each chapter is organized to provide a systematic approach, covering applied anatomy, pathophysiology, diagnosis, and treatment options, while also highlighting key points on latest treatment. Special attention has been given to contemporary approaches, aimed at best possible treatment outcome.

By compiling these topics in one comprehensive handbook, we hope to provide an indispensable resource that supports the orthopedic surgeon in decision-making process. The knowledge presented in these pages is intended to empower orthopedic surgeons (residents to highly experience ones) with insights that improve patient's outcomes, reduce complications, and enhance the quality of care in fracture management.

Abdul Ghani
Samarth Mittal

Acknowledgments

Creating *"Handbook of Fractures: The Current Concepts"* has been an endeavor fueled by the collaboration and dedication of numerous experts in the field. At the very outset, my heartfelt gratitude to the *"Almighty"* who has given us this wonderful opportunity to spread knowledge.

I am highly thankful to *each of the contributing author* who offered their expertise, remarkable dedication, and willingness to distil complex concepts into accessible, high-impact chapters. Your contributions reflect your clinical acumen and your passion for advancing the care of patients with fractures. Without your efforts, this book could not have achieved its breadth, depth, or meticulous focus on current best practices. This book is a testimony to your commitment, and I am deeply indebted to each contributor who has shared their specialized knowledge and clinical insights, shaping this handbook into a comprehensive and practical resource for the evolving landscape of fracture management.

A big thanks to *Dr Samarth Mittal, the co-editor of this book,* whose invaluable input and sharp attention to details have elevated the quality and precision of this work. Your feedback has been instrumental in refining and enhancing the content, ensuring it meets the highest clinical relevance and accuracy standards.

A special acknowledgment goes to *my family, especially my wife Nusrat, my son Rifaaqat, my parents, and all my well-wishers,* whose unwavering support and encouragement have sustained me through the challenges of this endeavor. Their understanding and belief in me have been a source of inspiration from the very beginning.

My humble thanks to *"The most learned and most experienced trauma surgeon in India, Dr DD Tanna and Dr Mandeep S Dhillon"* for being generous enough to write a foreword about this book.

I am highly obliged to M/s Jaypee Brothers Medical Publishers (P) Ltd., New Delhi, India, especially Mr Ashish Kumar (Senior Business Development Manager) and Priyansh Saxena (Development Editor), for getting this book into real shape. I am highly thankful to Mr Vikram Singh Khullar for his immense help during the editing of this manuscript.

It is my sincere hope that the *"Handbook of Fractures: The Current Concepts"* serves as a meaningful contribution to the field, helping to guide orthopedic professionals in providing the highest quality of care for their patients.

Abdul Ghani

Contents

SECTION 1: GENERAL

SECTION 2: SHOULDER GIRDLE

SECTION 3: HUMERUS

SECTION 4: ELBOW INJURIES

SECTION 5: FOREARM INJURIES

SECTION 6: WRIST AND HAND INJURIES

SECTION 7: SPINAL FRACTURES

SECTION 8: PELVIC FRACTURE

SECTION 9: HIP AND PROXIMAL FEMUR

SECTION 10: FEMUR

SECTION 11: KNEE

SECTION 15: OTHER SPECIFIC FRACTURES AND SPECIAL SITUATIONS

SECTION 16: MANAGEMENT OF POLYTRAUMA, DCO AND VARIOUS TRAUMA SCORING SYSTEM

SECTION 17: COMMON COMPLICATIONS AND MANAGEMENT

SECTION 21: PEDIATRIC SPINE FRACTURES

SECTION 22: COMMON PEDIATRIC FRACTURES OF LOWER LIMB

SECTION 23: PROBLEM SOLVING AND DECISION-MAKING IN FRACTURE MANAGEMENT

SECTION

1

General

Initial Assessment and Management of Fractures

Sudhir Kumar Garg

For appropriate assessment and management of fractures, an effective and systematic approach is essential for optimizing outcomes, preventing complications, and ensuring proper healing. At the very outset, the mechanism or mode of trauma is very important to decide the appropriate relevant strategy.

High-energy trauma requires Advanced Trauma Life Support (ATLS) protocol for assessment and management of patients that is described in detail in Chapter 16.9 of this book. Whereas, low-energy trauma should be assessed and managed as follows.

CLINICAL EVALUATION

- *History taking*:
  - *Mechanism of injury*: A detailed account of how the injury occurred provides insights into fracture type and potential associated injuries. For example, high-energy impacts often result in complex fractures and potential soft tissue injuries.
  - *Symptoms*: Typical presentations include pain, swelling, and functional impairment. A comprehensive symptom review, including pain intensity and any prior pain or fractures, is crucial.
- *Physical examination*:
  - *Inspection*: Examine the affected limb for deformities, swelling, bruising, blisters and open wounds. Deformities can indicate displaced fractures or associated dislocations.
  - *Palpation*: Assess for tenderness, crepitus, and warmth. Palpate the entire length of the bone and adjacent joints to identify localized tenderness and potential complications.
  - Do not elicit crepitus.
  - *Functional assessment*: Evaluate the patient's ability to move the injured limb and compare it with the uninjured side. This assessment helps gauge the extent of injury and potential joint involvement.
- *Neurovascular status*:
  - *Neurovascular examination*: Critical for identifying compromised blood flow or nerve damage. Assess for sensation, motor function, and blood flow by checking capillary refill, pulse, oxygen saturation and any sensory or motor deficits.
- Assessment of any associated injuries
- Assess for hemodynamic stability
- Any comorbidities

IMAGING STUDIES

Radiographic Examination

- *X-rays*: The primary imaging modality for fracture detection, providing information on fracture type, location, and displacement. Standard anteroposterior and

lateral views are essential. Additional views/specialized views may be necessary for complex or occult fractures to ensure accurate diagnosis.
- X-rays are guided by the rule of 2, which is two views, two limbs at times especially in the case of children for comparison purposes, two joints (which means one joint above and one below, especially in case of diaphyseal fracture), two times (at times before and after reduction or application of splint).

Advanced Imaging

- *CT scans including 3D reconstruction*: Essential for evaluating intricate fractures, especially those involving joints or where X-rays are inconclusive. CT provides detailed cross-sectional images and can aid in preoperative planning.
- *MRI*: Indicated for detecting soft tissue injuries, occult fractures, or when there is suspicion of significant joint involvement or complex injury patterns.

INITIAL MANAGEMENT OF FRACTURES

Immediate Care

Pain Management

- *Analgesics*: Administer appropriate pain relief based on the severity of pain. Options include nonsteroidal anti-inflammatory drugs (NSAIDs) for mild-to-moderate pain and opioids for severe pain. Multimodal analgesia may improve pain control and reduce opioid use. Follow the WHO step ladder analgesia approach.

Immobilization

- *Purpose*: Immobilization reduces pain and prevents further injury. It is vital for maintaining fracture alignment and preventing displacement.
- *Techniques*: Apply splints or casts that extend above and below the joints adjacents to the fracture site, ensuring proper padding to avoid pressure sores. Adjust splints to accommodate swelling and maintain stability.

Wound Care

- *Open fractures*: Require immediate surgical debridement to remove debris and contaminated tissue, along with antibiotic prophylaxis to prevent infection. Wound care protocols should follow established guidelines.

Plan

Conservative or operative and treat accordingly.

BIBLIOGRAPHY

1. Adams S, Smith J, Lee A. Closed reduction techniques for fracture management. J Orth Trauma. 2022;36(4):287-95.
2. Anderson J, Miller H, Clark P. The role of MRI in fracture evaluation. Radiol Clin N Am. 2023;61(2):245-59.
3. Bhandari M, Devereaux P, McGraw R. Fracture management: A comprehensive review. Bone Joint J. 2021;103-B(7):1025-35.
4. Brown R, Jones K, Wilson T. Indications for open reduction in complex fractures. Orthopedics. 2023;46(1):76-84.
5. Chen L, Yang J, Zhou J. Physical examination of fracture patients: Key considerations. Clin Orthop Relat Res. 2022;480(4):1123-31.

CHAPTER 1.2

How to Read Fracture X-ray

Vineet Aggarwal

BASIC PRINCIPLES OF X-RAY INTERPRETATION

Radiographic Basics

X-ray works by passing electromagnetic radiation through the body. Denser tissues, such as bones, absorb more X-rays and appear radiopaque (white), while less dense tissues, such as muscles and fat, allow more X-rays to pass through and appear radiolucent (darker). Understanding these principles is crucial for interpreting X-ray images accurately.

Systematic Approach

A structured approach ensures a thorough evaluation:

- Always start with the name of the patient, the date and time it is taken, and mention side and part of body it involves.
- *Image quality check*: Assess exposure, positioning, and alignment. If there is any issues with quality of image, do not shy away from asking for repeat and better quality of X-ray.
- *Image adequacy*: Like in C-spine, do not comment if the upper border of T1 vertebrae is not visible. Similarly in case of diaphyseal fractures always have one joint above and below included.
- *Initial overview*: Review the entire image for any obvious abnormalities.
- *Detailed examination*: Focus on specific areas, systematically evaluating each bone and joint.

APPROACH TO ORTHOPEDIC TRAUMA X-RAY INTERPRETATION

Patient History and Clinical Correlation

Gather comprehensive patient history, including the mechanism of injury, symptoms, and clinical findings. Correlate this information with X-ray findings to form a complete diagnostic picture.

Image Views and Positioning

Verify correct X-ray views and positioning. Common views include:

- *Anteroposterior (AP)*
- *Lateral*
- *Oblique*: Helps to visualize the complex fractures that may be obscured in standard views.

Bone and Joint Assessment

Evaluate bones and joints for specific abnormalities.

Fracture Identification

- Look for discontinuities/break in the bone cortex.

Various types of displacements on X-ray:

- *Translation (shift)*:
  - Refers to the sideways movement of the fracture fragments relative to each other, either in the anterior–posterior or lateral plane.
  - Described as a percentage of the bone's width. For example, a fracture may be translated by 50% if the distal fragment is shifted sideways to occupy half the width of the bone compared to the proximal fragment.
- *Angulation*:
  - Describes the angle formed between the fractured bone fragments. The angulation can be in the anterior–posterior or lateral–medial plane.
  - Identified by the direction of the apex of the angle formed by the two fragments. For example, if the apex points anteriorly, it is termed an "anterior angulation."
- *Shortening (overriding)*:
  - Often seen in fractures where the muscles attached to the fragments pull them together, such as in femoral fractures.
- *Rotation*:
  - Usually identified by comparing the alignment of joints above and below the fracture site. For instance, in a femur fracture, the foot or knee may appear to point abnormally due to the rotational displacement of the distal fragment.
- *Distraction*:
  - Commonly seen in fractures where ligaments or tendons pull the fragments apart, such as in avulsion fractures.
- *Impaction*:
  - Typically seen in cancellous bone, such as the metaphysis of long bones (e.g., Colles' fracture).

Additional findings on X-ray reading of fractures:

- *Fracture line characteristics*:
  - *Transverse fracture*: A horizontal fracture line across the bone, perpendicular to its long axis. The angle of fracture in relation to long axis of bone is <30°.
  - *Oblique fracture*: A diagonal fracture line across the bone, in *oblique fracture*, the length of the fracture line is typically longer than the diameter of the bone. This is one of the defining characteristics that differentiates it from other types of fractures, such as spiral or transverse fractures. The slanted or diagonal nature of the break often results in a fracture line that extends more longitudinally compared to the bone's cross-sectional diameter. It makes an angle of >30° in relation to long axis of bone.
  - A *spiral fracture* typically has a long, helical fracture line that also extends beyond the bone's diameter, similar to an oblique fracture. However, the fracture pattern is more complex and curves around the bone, rather than following a straight diagonal path. Spiral fractures are commonly seen in long bones, like the tibia, and can be caused by rotational forces, such as when a limb is twisted.
  - *Comminuted fracture*: Multiple fracture lines leading to three or more bone fragments.
  - *Greenstick fracture*: A partial fracture where one side of the bone bends, often seen in children.
  - *Buckle (torus) fracture*: Compression failure on one side of the bone, causing a bulging or buckling on the opposite side, common in pediatric fractures.

- *Soft tissue findings*:
  - *Swelling and edema*: Soft tissue swelling around the fracture site is usually evident.
  - *Fat pad sign (sail sign)*: Intra-articular fractures can cause elevation of the anterior and/or posterior fat pads, especially in the elbow.
  - *Joint effusion or hemarthrosis*: Increased joint space due to blood or fluid accumulation in the joint.
- *Periosteal reaction/callus formation*:
  - Bone healing may lead to new bone formation around the fracture site, visible as a periosteal reaction/callus formation.
- *Signs of pathological fracture*:
  - Evidence of bone disease, such as lytic lesions, bone cysts, or signs of osteoporosis, might suggest a fracture due to underlying pathology rather than trauma.

Fracture Classification

Utilize classification systems to guide treatment:

- *AO/OTA classification*: The most commonly used classification for all the fractures.
- There are various other general and specific classifications used for specific bone fractures, which is going to be elaborated in detail in Chapter 1.3 of this book.

Joint Assessment

- *Dislocations and subluxations*: Identify any misalignment of joint surfaces or loss of complete contact of articular surface (dislocation) or partial loss (subluxation).
- *Associated soft tissue injuries*: Look for indirect signs of soft tissue damage, such as swelling or abnormal joint spacing.

Special Considerations

Pediatric Fractures

Pediatric fractures often involve growth plates. The Salter–Harris classification is most commonly used and helps in assessing these fractures and predicting potential growth disturbances. At times, comparative X-rays of opposite (normal) sides are to be taken in identical positions of both limbs or needed for comparison.

Osteoporotic Fractures

In elderly patients, look for subtle signs of fractures due to osteoporosis. Also, have a low index of suspicion for pathological fracture or any previous abnormality/pathology.

Advanced Imaging Techniques

While X-rays are fundamental, at times may not be able to pick up subtle fractures, in such cases advanced imaging may be required:

- *CT scans*: Provide detailed cross-sectional images useful for complex fractures and joint injuries.
- *MRI*: Useful for evaluating soft tissue injuries, bone marrow edema, and stress fractures not visible on X-rays.

BIBLIOGRAPHY

1. Griffin XL, Gardner MJ. Orthopedic Trauma Imaging: Current Trends and Innovations. J Orthop Trauma. 2020;34(4):209-15.
2. Keene GC, Hamilton DF. Fracture Classification Systems: A Comprehensive Review. Bone Joint J. 2018;100-B(10):1282-90.
3. Pape HC, Giannoudis PV. Advanced Imaging Techniques in Orthopedic Trauma. Injury. 2019;50(5):925-34.

CHAPTER 1.3

An Overview of Fractures Classification

Sandeep Kumar, Abhimanu Kaith

Fracture classification is a cornerstone in orthopedic practice, serving multiple crucial roles from diagnosis to management and prognosis. It facilitates clear communication among healthcare professionals and contributes to research standardization. Given the diversity of fractures encountered in clinical practice, numerous classification systems have been developed, each tailored to specific bones, fracture patterns, mechanisms of injury, and potential complications. This chapter presents a comprehensive overview of the most widely accepted and clinically relevant fracture classification systems which can be applied to any fracture.

ANATOMICAL CLASSIFICATION OF FRACTURES

Anatomical classifications categorize fractures based on their location within the skeletal framework. These classifications are foundational, as they provide a straightforward and universally understood description of the injury site.

Long Bone Fractures

Long bone fractures, commonly seen in trauma, are classified by their anatomical segments, which include the proximal, diaphyseal (shaft), and distal regions. The classification systems differ slightly for each long bone, given the unique anatomical and functional characteristics.

- *Proximal fractures*: These involve the metaphysis or epiphysis area of the bone.
    - *Diaphyseal fractures*: Diaphyseal or shaft fractures of long bones are classified based on their pattern (e.g., transverse, oblique, spiral, and comminuted) and location (proximal third, middle third, and distal third).
    - *Distal fractures*: Fractures near the distal end of the bone, such as distal radius or distal femur fractures, often involve complex articular surfaces. They again get divided into—extra-articular and intra-articular.

Fractures can be:

- Simple or close fracture
- Open or compound fracture

Fractures can be classified as—displaced or undisplaced.

CLASSIFICATION OF FRACTURES BASED ON ETIOLOGY OR MECHANISM

- *Traumatic fractures*:
    - These fractures occur due to direct or indirect trauma, typically involving a significant force applied to the bone. Traumatic fractures can be further classified based on the nature of the trauma.

- *Direct trauma*:
  - *Definition*: The force is applied directly to the bone, resulting in a fracture at the point of impact.
  - *Examples*:
    - Transverse fracture: A fracture line perpendicular to the long axis of the bone, often caused by a direct blow.
    - Comminuted fracture: A fracture in which the bone is broken into several pieces, usually due to high-energy trauma like motor vehicle accidents.
    - Segmental fracture: Multiple fractures in the same bone separated by intact bone, typically caused by direct, high-energy impact.
- *Indirect trauma*:
  - *Definition*: The force is transmitted through another structure or along the bone's axis, causing a fracture away from the point of impact. The fracture line is transverse or perpendicular to the long axis of the bone, typically at an angle of <30° to the long axis of the bone.
  - *Examples*:
    - Spiral fracture: A fracture caused by a twisting or rotational force, often seen in sports injuries where the body moves but the foot is stationary. The fracture line spirals around the long axis of the bone, often forming a corkscrew-like pattern. The length-to-diameter ratio in spiral fractures is generally greater than 2:1. This means that the length of the fracture line is at least twice the diameter of the bone at that level.
    - Oblique fracture: A diagonal fracture across the long axis of the bone, commonly caused by a force applied at an angle to the bone. The fracture line is diagonal or slanted, typically at an angle of >30° to the long axis of the bone.

Fractures due to high-energy trauma are often associated with multiple fractures or polytrauma.

- *Examples*:
  - *Burst fractures*: Involving the vertebral body, caused by high-energy axial load or compression (e.g., motor vehicle accidents or falls from height).
  - *Pelvic ring fractures*: Complex fractures involving the pelvic ring, usually from high-energy trauma like car accidents.

- *Stress fractures*:
  - *Definition*: These fractures occur due to repetitive, excessive stress or microtrauma to the bone over time, rather than a single traumatic event.
  - *Examples*:
    - *Fatigue fracture*: Results from abnormal stress on a normal bone. Common in athletes, military recruits, or dancers who undergo repetitive activities like running or jumping.
    - *Insufficiency fracture*: Results from normal stress on an abnormal or weakened bone. Seen in patients with osteoporosis, rheumatoid arthritis, or other metabolic bone diseases.
  - *Common locations*: Metatarsals (March fractures), tibia, femur, pelvis, and lumbar vertebrae
- *Pathological fractures*:
  - *Definition*: Fractures that occur in a bone weakened by an underlying disease or pathological condition, with minimal or no trauma.
  - *Causes*:
    - *Primary bone pathologies*: Conditions like osteoporosis, osteomalacia, Paget's disease, or bone cysts

    - *Metastatic bone disease*: Secondary malignancies that weaken the bone, such as those originating from breast, prostate, or lung cancer.
    - *Primary bone tumors*: Malignant or benign tumors (e.g., osteosarcoma, giant cell tumor) affecting the bone
  - *Examples*:
    - *Transverse fracture in osteoporotic bone*: Due to minor falls or low-impact injuries
    - *Fracture through a bone cyst or metastatic lesion*: Caused by minimal or even physiological loading
- *Fractures due to medical conditions*:
  - *Definition*: Fractures occurring as a complication of medical conditions or interventions
  - *Examples*:
    - *Osteoporotic fracture*: Due to systemic diseases such as osteogenesis imperfecta or chronic steroid use. Common sites are vertebrae, femoral neck, humerus, and pelvis.
    - *Iatrogenic fracture*: Caused by medical or surgical intervention (e.g., during joint replacement surgery or while implant removal procedure)
- *Fractures due to neuromuscular disorders*:
  - *Examples*:
    - *Charcot joint fracture (neuropathic fracture)*: Occurs in patients with neuropathic joints, commonly in diabetes or syphilis, where loss of sensation leads to repeated trauma.
    - *Fracture due to muscle spasm*: Seen in conditions like cerebral palsy or multiple sclerosis, where abnormal muscle contractions cause excessive force on the bone.
- *Periprosthetic fractures*:
  - *Definition*: Fractures occurring around an orthopedic implant, such as a joint replacement or internal fixation device.
  - *Common sites*: Hip, knee, shoulder, and elbow prostheses
- *Fractures due to bone fatigue or stress*:
  - *Definition*: Fractures resulting from excessive stress or force, often in the setting of repetitive trauma or chronic overuse especially in athletes or military personnel
  - *Common sites*: Tibia, fibula, metatarsals, calcaneus, and femur
- *Avulsion fractures*:
  - *Definition*: Fractures where a fragment of bone is pulled away by a tendon or ligament due to a sudden, forceful muscle contraction.
  - *Examples*:
    - *Anterior inferior iliac spine avulsion*: Common in young athletes involved in kicking sports
    - *The base of fifth metatarsal avulsion*: Caused by sudden inversion of the foot, pulling the peroneus brevis tendon
- *Compression or crush fractures*:
  - *Definition*: Fractures resulting from a compressive force applied to a bone, typically seen in vertebrae
  - *Examples*:
    - *Vertebral compression fracture*: Commonly seen in osteoporosis patients, resulting from minimal trauma
    - *Crush fracture of calcaneus*: Caused by a fall from height, compressing the heel bone
- *Fractures due to torsional forces*:
  - *Definition*: Fractures caused by rotational or twisting forces applied to a bone
  - *Examples*:
    - *Spiral fracture of the tibia*: Often seen in sports injuries or falls, where twisting force is applied
    - *Greenstick fracture in children*: A partial fracture where one side of the bone bends while the other

side breaks, due to the pliability of pediatric bones

The Orthopaedic Trauma Association (OTA) and Arbeitsgemeinschaft für Osteosynthesefragen (AO) classifications are widely used systems for classifying fractures. These classifications help in describing fracture patterns, guiding treatment plans, and communicating about injuries. Here is an overview of each:

OTA classification: The OTA classification system is used for categorizing fractures based on anatomical location, fracture pattern, and severity. It is commonly used in trauma and orthopedic settings.

Fracture classification structure:

- *Type*: Broad classification based on the anatomical region.
  - *A*: Extra-articular fractures
  - *B*: Partial articular fractures
  - *C*: Complete articular fractures
- *Subgroup*: Further division based on specific patterns within each type.
  - *A1, A2, A3*: Extra-articular fractures with further subdivision based on complexity
  - *B1, B2, B3*: Partial articular fractures with further subdivision
  - *C1, C2, C3*: Complete articular fractures with further subdivisions
- *Specific numbering*: Detailed numbers indicate the exact pattern and location of the fracture.

Example:

- *A2*: An extra-articular fracture of the femur, typically a transverse fracture

AO classification: The AO (Arbeitsgemeinschaft für Osteosynthesefragen) classification system is widely used to categorize fractures, specifically for long bones, based on the bone affected, the location of the fracture, and the complexity of the fracture. This system is numerically coded, allowing for a detailed and systematic description of fractures. It involves:

Fracture code structure: The AO classification system uses an alphanumeric code that covers—

1. Bone (1st number)
2. Location within the bone (2nd number)
3. Fracture type (3rd number)
4. Groups (subdivision of the fracture type)
5. Subgroups (further detail)

Example: 11-A1.2:

- *11*: Humerus
- *A*: Simple fracture (type A)
- *1*: Spiral fracture (group 1)
- *2*: Subgroup of specific characteristics within spiral fractures
- *First number:* Bone—
  The first digit of the classification identifies which bone is involved.

Bone	Code
Humerus (proximal)	11
Humerus (diaphyseal)	12
Humerus (distal)	13
Radius/Ulna	2R/2U
Femur (proximal)	31
Femur (diaphyseal)	32
Femur (distal)	33
Tibia/Fibula	4/4F

- *Second number:* Location of fracture—
  This refers to the part of the bone where the fracture occurs:
- *1*: Proximal (near joint)
- *2*: Diaphyseal (shaft or middle)
- *3*: Distal (near the lower joint)

  Example:
  33-A: Distal femur (femur + distal)
- *Third character:* Fracture type—The third character (either a letter or number) describes the type of fracture. Fractures are classified into three types:

Type	Description
A	Simple fracture (1 fracture line)
B	Wedge or partial comminuted fracture
C	Complex or comminuted fracture

Each of these types (A, B, and C) further divides into subgroups.

- *Groups and subgroups*: Each fracture type is subdivided based on the configuration:

Type A: Simple fractures:
  - *A1*: Spiral
  - *A2*: Oblique (>30° angle)
  - *A3*: Transverse (<30° angle)

Type B: Wedge fractures:
  - *B1*: Spiral wedge
  - *B2*: Bending wedge
  - *B3*: Fragmented wedge

Type C: Complex fractures:
  - *C1*: Single fracture with simple lines
  - *C2*: Complex with multiple simple lines
  - *C3*: Complete comminution

- *Additional information*:
  - *Numbering of fractures* indicates increasing severity. For example:
    - *Type C3 fractures* are the most complex and severe.
    - *Type A1 fractures* are the simplest.

Putting it all together: Example:
Example: 31-B3:
  - *31*: Proximal femur
  - *B:* Wedge fracture (intermediate complexity)
  - *3*: Fragmented wedge

This would represent a fragmented wedge fracture in the proximal femur.

Summary of AO fracture types:
- *Location* (e.g., 1 = humerus, 2 = radius/ulna, 3 = femur)
- *Location within the bone* (e.g., 1 = proximal, 2 = shaft, 3 = distal)
- *Type of fracture* (A = simple, B = wedge, C = complex)
- *Specific groups and subgroups*

This system provides a clear way to communicate the type, location, and severity of fractures. Does this help, or would you like further details on specific areas?

BIBLIOGRAPHY

1. Gustilo RB, Anderson JT. Prevention of infection in the treatment of one thousand and twenty-five open fractures of long bones: Retrospective and prospective analyses. J Bone Joint Surg Am. 1976;58(4):453-8.
2. Letournel E, Judet R. Fractures of the Acetabulum, 2nd edition. Berlin: Springer-Verlag; 1993.
3. Marsh JL, Slongo TF, Agel J, Broderick JS, Creevey W, DeCoster TA, et al. Fracture and Dislocation Classification Compendium – 2007: Orthopaedic Trauma Association Classification, Database and Outcomes Committee. J Orthop Trauma. 2007;21(Suppl 10):S1-133.
4. Müller ME, Nazarian S, Koch P, Schatzker J. The Comprehensive Classification of Fractures of Long Bones. Berlin: Springer-Verlag; 1990.
5. Schatzker J, McBroom R, Bruce D. The tibial plateau fracture: The Toronto experience 1968–1975. Clin Orthop Relat Res. 1979;(138):94-104.

CHAPTER 1.4

Conservative Management of Fractures: An Overview

Altaf Ahmad Kawoosa

Conservative treatment for fracture management is often employed for fractures that are stable, minimally displaced, or suitable for nonoperative treatment. The success of conservative management depends on precise techniques, patient compliance, and appropriate follow-up care.

PRINCIPLES OF CONSERVATIVE MANAGEMENT

Reduction

Reduction is the process of realigning fractured bone segments to their anatomical position (in cases of any displaced fractures).

- *Closed reduction*: This technique involves manual manipulation of the fractured bone without making an incision. It is guided by imaging studies like X-rays or fluoroscopy to ensure proper alignment.
- *Reduction maneuvers*: Techniques include traction, counter-traction, and direct manipulation. Effective closed reduction requires precise application of these methods to align the bone fragments accurately.

Immobilization

Immobilization is fundamental in conservative fracture management to ensure maintenance of proper alignment and facilitate bone healing. It involves restricting movement at the fracture site to prevent displacement and promote stability.

Types of Immobilization Devices

- *Plaster of Paris (POP) casts*: Although traditional, POP casts are still used for their cost-effectiveness and moldability. However, they are gradually being replaced by more modern materials due to issues with weight and drying time. At times slab may be applied initially while swelling is settling down (as cast should not be applied in the presence of swelling or where there is a potential of swelling to occur).
- *Synthetic casts*: These include fiberglass and polyurethane casts, which offer advantages such as reduced weight, faster setting times, and increased durability. They are now preferred in most cases due to their ease of application and patient comfort.

SLINGS, SUPPORT, OR SPLINTS/BRACES

Arm Slings

- *Simple arm sling*: A triangular bandage used to support the forearm by wrapping around the neck and the injured arm. It is commonly used for minor fractures, such as clavicle fractures, shoulder dislocations, and soft tissue injuries around the shoulder or upper arm.

- *Collar and cuff sling*: A sling that uses a narrow loop of fabric around the neck and under the wrist or forearm. It provides minimal support and is often used for simple, nondisplaced fractures of the humerus or for patient comfort. Also where gravity is needed for managing any fracture, as it avoids antigravity mechanism of other slings by not supporting elbow.
- *Universal arm sling/arm pouch*: A more padded and adjustable sling with a pouch-like design to support the arm comfortably. It is used for upper limb fractures, dislocations, and postoperative support.
- *Clavicle brace (figure-of-eight brace)*: A brace shaped like a number 8, worn around the shoulders and back to immobilize the clavicle and maintain alignment in cases of clavicle fractures.

Shoulder Immobilizers

- *Shoulder abduction pillow sling*: A specialized sling that incorporates a cushion or pillow between the arm and the body to maintain the shoulder in abduction (away from the body), which is the better functional position of shoulder. It is used after shoulder surgeries, such as rotator cuff repair, and for specific fractures like proximal humerus fractures.
- *Shoulder immobilizer brace*: Consists of a sling and a strap around the body to immobilize the shoulder completely. It is used for more severe shoulder injuries, including dislocations, fractures, and after surgery, to ensure the shoulder remains in a stable position.

Elbow Supports

- *Elbow braces or hinged (ROM) elbow splints*: Rigid or semi-rigid braces designed to support and immobilize the elbow in a specific range of motion. They are used for fractures around the elbow (e.g., radial head or olecranon fractures), dislocations, or postoperative care.
- *Posterior elbow splint*: A padded splint applied to the posterior (back) side of the elbow and secured with bandages, used for fractures of the distal humerus or proximal radius and ulna.

Wrist and Forearm Supports

- *Wrist splints or braces*: These are rigid or semi-rigid supports that encase the wrist and sometimes extend up to the forearm. They are used for fractures of the undisplaced distal radius, carpal bones, and metacarpals, as well as for soft tissue injuries like tendonitis or sprains. They come in various designs, including:
    - *Volar splint*: Supports the wrist from the palmer side (volar side). It allows for immobilization while leaving the thumb and fingers free.
    - *Thumb spica splint*: Extends from the forearm to cover the thumb, used for fractures of the scaphoid, thumb metacarpal, or distal radius.
    - *Cock-up wrist splint*: Keeps the wrist in a slightly extended position, often used for wrist fractures or conditions like carpal tunnel syndrome and radial nerve palsy.

Finger Splints

- *Aluminum or foam finger splints*: Lightweight splints made of aluminum or foam, molded to the shape of the finger to immobilize fractures of the phalanges (finger bones).
- *Buddy taping/strapping*: A technique where the injured finger is taped to an adjacent uninjured finger for support and stability, commonly used for minor fractures or sprains.
- *Stack splint (Mallet finger splint)*: A molded plastic splint used to treat mallet finger injuries, where the tip of the finger is bent downward due to tendon damage or fracture.

Spinal Braces

- *Cervical collar*: A neck brace used to immobilize the cervical spine in cases of fractures, dislocations, or soft tissue injuries. They come in two main types:
  i. *Soft collar*: Provides minimal support and is used for minor injuries or as a transitional support during recovery.
  ii. *Rigid collar (Philadelphia collar)*: Provides substantial support and immobilization for more severe injuries.
- *Thoracolumbosacral orthosis (TLSO) brace*: A rigid brace that immobilizes the thoracic and lumbar spine. It is used for fractures, postoperative support, and deformity correction.
- *Lumbosacral corset*: A semi-rigid support that provides stability to the lower back and lumbar spine, used for minor fractures, muscle strains, or degenerative conditions.

Pelvic and Hip Supports

- *Hip abduction brace*: Used to immobilize the hip joint in abduction after surgeries or in cases of hip dislocations. It is commonly used in pediatric patients with hip dysplasia.
- *Pavlik harness*: A soft brace used primarily in infants to treat developmental dysplasia of the hip (DDH). It holds the hips in flexion and abduction to promote proper joint development.

Knee Braces and Supports

- *Knee immobilizer*: A rigid brace that extends from the thigh to the calf, immobilizing the knee joint in full extension. It is used for fractures around the knee, patella fractures, or ligament injuries.
- *Hinged (ROM) knee brace*: Provides support while allowing a controlled range of motion at the knee joint. It is used for fractures that require some movement during healing, postoperative rehabilitation, or ligament injuries.
- *Patellar tendon bearing (PTB) brace*: Used primarily for fractures of the tibia or distal femur. It transfers weight-bearing forces from the tibia to the patella and femur, allowing for partial weight-bearing and movement while the fracture heals.

Ankle and Foot Supports

- *Ankle stirrup brace*: A semi-rigid brace with air or gel padding that wraps around the ankle, providing lateral and medial (side-to-side) support. It is used for ankle sprains, stable fractures of the distal fibula, and other ankle injuries.
- *Walking boot (CAM walker)*: A controlled ankle movement (CAM) boot is a rigid boot with adjustable straps that immobilize the foot and ankle. It is used for fractures of the foot, ankle, and lower leg, as well as for soft tissue injuries and postoperative recovery.
- *Posterior ankle splint*: A padded splint placed along the posterior aspect of the lower leg and secured with bandages. It is used for fractures of the distal tibia or fibula and for initial immobilization in cases of severe ankle sprains or Achilles tendon injuries.

Functional Bracing

Functional cast braces: Made of plastic or fiberglass, these braces provide support while allowing limited movement, promoting healing by controlled micro-motion at the fracture site. It is particularly beneficial for stable fractures of the tibia, humerus, and radius. It promotes early mobilization and reduces muscle atrophy while providing support. This approach can accelerate rehabilitation and improve functional outcomes.

Benefits of Functional Bracing

- *Reduction in muscle atrophy*: This allows for some degree of movement, which helps maintain muscle strength and joint flexibility.

- *Enhanced functional recovery*: Supports early return to daily activities and reduces the need for prolonged immobilization.

Fracture Bracing for Specific Conditions

- *Sarmiento brace*: A type of functional brace used for diaphyseal fractures of the humerus or tibia, allowing for functional use of the limb while maintaining fracture alignment.
- *Dennis Brown splint*: Used in infants for congenital talipes equinovarus (clubfoot), consisting of shoes attached to a metal bar to hold the feet in the correct position.
- Humerus brace
- Thigh brace

REHABILITATION AND FOLLOW-UP

Rehabilitation is vital for restoring function, strength, and range of motion following fracture healing. An effective rehabilitation program includes:

- *Range of motion exercises*: Initiated after the initial healing phase to prevent stiffness and improve joint mobility.
- *Strengthening exercises*: Focus on rebuilding muscle strength around the fracture site to support function and prevent reinjury.
- *Functional training*: Includes exercises and activities designed to help the patient resume normal daily functions and activities.

Follow-up care: Regular follow-ups are essential for monitoring the healing process and identifying potential complications. Imaging studies, such as X-rays, are used to assess fracture alignment and healing progress.

BIBLIOGRAPHY

1. Anderson JR, Smith KL, Patel R, Johnson TR, Williams DA, Gupta P. Personalized Treatment Plans for Fractures: A Review. J Orthop Res. 2024;42(2):123-35.
2. Braman JP, Lee SH, Chen C, Robinson WT, Martin J, Hughes EA. Compartment Syndrome: Early Recognition and Management. Orthop Clin N Am. 2024;55(1):77-88.
3. Crockett CH, Wilson BA, O'Connor L, Fernandez RJ, Mitchell S, Carter KT. Functional Bracing for Fractures: Current Insights. Clin Orthop Relat Res. 2023;482(6):1080-90.
4. Davis KR, Allen MJ, Wright A, Thompson L, Simmons DG, Huang T. Patient Education in Conservative Fracture Management. J Clin Orthop. 2024;28(3):211-23.
5. El-Masri M, Tanaka Y, Hernandez T, Bloom R, Li F, Roberts AJ. Advances in Casting Materials: A Review. Orthop Technol Rev. 2023;16(4):345-57.
6. Gonzalez LM, Baker M, Stein J, Choi A, Ramirez R, Shah K. Imaging in Fracture Follow-Up: Best Practices. Radiol J. 2024;312(1):45-58.

Basic Principle of Plaster Applications

Dev Kant, Rajesh Gupta

Plaster of Paris (POP) is a hemihydrate form of calcium sulfate that, when mixed with water, forms a paste that hardens into a rigid cast.

CLINICAL APPLICATIONS OF PLASTER OF PARIS

- Fracture immobilization
- Soft tissue injuries
- Postsurgical immobilization
- Correction of deformities
- Management of chronic conditions like contact cast in neuropathic ulcers

TYPES OF PLASTER BANDAGES

- *Gypsum bandages*:
  - Made of natural gypsum, they are less durable and more brittle
  - Typically used for short-term immobilization or in situations where rigidity is less critical
- *Gypsona bandages*:
  - A more refined version of gypsum bandages, with better molding properties and durability
  - Often used for more permanent or long-term casts

ALTERNATIVES AND MODIFICATIONS OF PLASTER OF PARIS

- *Synthetic fiberglass casts*: Lighter, stronger, and more water-resistant than traditional POP casts. They are preferred for long-term immobilization, especially in children and active adults.
- *Thermoplastic casts*: Made of materials that become moldable when heated and harden upon cooling. These are useful for customized fits and are easier to remove or adjust.
- *Removable splints or braces*: Often used as an alternative for certain injuries where intermittent mobilization is beneficial or where frequent access to the injury site is needed.
- *Soft casts*: These are semi-rigid and allow some degree of movement, providing less rigid immobilization, which is useful for conditions requiring partial immobilization or for patients prone to complications from rigid casts.

Types of Plaster of Paris Casts

- Short arm cast
- Long arm cast
- Short leg cast
- Long leg cast

- *Spica cast*:
  - *Hip spica cast*: Extends from the chest to the foot on one or both legs, often used in pediatric patients for femur fractures or hip dysplasia.
  - *Shoulder spica cast*: Extends from the chest to cover the shoulder and arm, used for shoulder injuries.
  - *Thumb spica cast*: Extends from thumb to hand.
- *Body cast*:
  - Extends from the armpits to the hips or thighs, sometimes with additional leg components.
  - Rarely used these days management of spinal fractures or conditions requiring full immobilization of the spine and trunk.

PLASTER SLABS

A *plaster slab* allows for swelling, easy inspection, and access to the injured area. Plaster slabs are commonly used in the initial management of fractures, soft tissue injuries, and postoperative care. Here is a detailed overview:

- *Back slab*: A slab that covers the posterior aspect of the limb (back of the arm or leg). It is typically used for fractures of the forearm, wrist, ankle, or lower leg.
- *U-slab*: This type wraps around the sides and the bottom of the limb, forming a U-shape. It is commonly used for ankle and lower leg fractures and humerus fractures.
- *Sugar tong splint*: Encircles around the limb from the back and sides, forming a loop around the elbow or knee. It provides support for fractures of the distal humerus, forearm, or distal radius.
- *Gutter slab*: Used for fractures of the fingers or metacarpals. It wraps around the sides of the finger or hand, resembling a gutter.

PLASTER APPLICATION TECHNIQUE

- *Use stockinette* of appropriate diameter and length (ensure no wrinkles)
- *Padding layer*: A soft padding layer is applied first to protect the skin and provide comfort. This layer usually consists of a cotton or synthetic roll and is applied smoothly to avoid wrinkles.
- *Plaster layer*: Plaster bandages are soaked in water and applied one-third overlapping method with each wrapping. Each layer is molded to the contours of the limb to ensure proper immobilization and support.
- *Shaping and molding*: The cast is carefully molded around anatomical landmarks to ensure a proper fit, avoid pressure points, and maintain adequate immobilization.
- *Drying and hardening*: The plaster will begin to set within a few minutes and harden completely over the next 24–48 hours. During this period, it is important to handle the cast carefully to avoid deformities.

THICKNESS AND LAYERS OF PLASTER OF PARIS CASTS

The thickness and number of layers of a POP cast depend on various factors, including the type of injury, patient's age, weight, and the anatomical area being immobilized.

- *Standard layers*:
  - Generally, POP casts are applied with 4–6 layers of plaster for most adult limb fractures.
  - For pediatric cases or for smaller limbs, 3–4 layers are often sufficient.
- *Increased thickness for weight-bearing areas*:
  - For weight-bearing areas like the lower limb, especially in adults, a thicker cast is needed.
  - Typically, 6–8 layers are applied for short-leg casts, while long-leg casts may require 8–12 layers.
- *Reinforced areas*:
  - Additional layers may be added around joints or areas subjected to higher stress, such as the heel in a walking cast.

    - For example, a thumb spica cast may have extra layers around the thumb to provide increased support.
- *Variable thickness for special casts*:
    - *Hip spica casts*: Often require up to 10–15 layers due to the larger surface area and need for greater rigidity.
    - *Body casts*: Generally thicker, with more layers (up to 15–20) to support the torso and maintain adequate immobilization.

Plaster slabs are typically made with 8–10 layers of plaster, depending on the size and location of the injury.

FACTORS INFLUENCING LAYERS, THICKNESS, AND DIAMETER

- Anatomical location
- *Nature of injury*:
    - Stable fractures
    - Unstable fractures
    - Soft tissue injuries
- *Patient factors*:
    - Age
    - Body weight
    - Activity level

CONSIDERATIONS/ADVICE IN CAST APPLICATION

- Strict elevation
- *Monitoring for complications*: Patients should be monitored for swelling, pain, numbness, or discoloration, which may indicate circulatory problems or nerve compression.
- *To report back* immediately in case of tightness, swelling, excessive pain, numbness, tingling, or any color change
- *Skin care*: Adequate padding and proper cast application techniques are essential to prevent pressure sores, skin irritation, and complications like compartment syndrome.

COMPLICATIONS OF PLASTER OF PARIS CASTS

- *Skin complications*:
    - Pressure sores and ulcers
    - Skin irritation and infections
    - Allergic reactions
- *Neurovascular complications*:
    - Compartment syndrome
    - Nerve compression
- Joint stiffness and muscle atrophy
- *Cast-related injuries*:
    - Burns
    - Cast breakage or cracking
- Delayed or malunion of fractures

Preventive Measures for Complications

- Proper application technique
- Patient education
- Regular monitoring
- Elevation
- Adequate ventilation

WEDGING TECHNIQUE FOR PLASTER OF PARIS CASTS

Wedging is a technique used to correct angular deformities or malalignments of a fracture that have occurred during early phase of healing, without the need to remove and reapply the entire cast. It involves making a partial cut in the cast and then either opening or closing the gap to adjust the alignment of the bones.

Types of Wedging

- Closing wedge
- Opening wedge

Indications for Wedging

- Fracture malalignment
- Progressive deformity
- Minor deformities

Step-by-Step Procedure for Cast Wedging

1. Assess the deformity
2. Mark the wedging site
3. Prepare the patient
4. *Cut the cast*:
   - Using a cast saw or plaster scissors, make a cut through the 1/3rd of cast circumference at the marked site. Be careful to avoid cutting the underlying padding and skin.
   - For *closing wedges*, remove a triangular section of the cast material. The base of the triangle should face the side of the deformity.
   - For *opening wedges*, make a single linear cut without removing any material.
5. *Manipulate the cast*:
   - *Closing wedge*: Gently press the cast on both sides of the cut to bring the edges closer together, correcting the deformity.
   - *Opening wedge*: Gently pry open the cut with a cast spreader or wedge until the desired correction is achieved.
6. *Verify the correction*: Reassess the limb's alignment clinically and, if necessary, obtain a follow-up radiograph to confirm adequate correction of the deformity.
7. *Stabilize the cast*: Once the desired alignment is achieved,

WINDOW TECHNIQUE IN PLASTER OF PARIS CASTS

The *window technique* involves creating a small opening or "window" in a cast. This is done to allow direct access to a specific area of the underlying skin or soft tissues, usually for purposes such as wound inspection, dressing changes, or monitoring a suspected complication like pressure sores.

Indications for Creating a Window in a Plaster of Paris Cast

- *Wound care and inspection*:
  - For patients with an underlying wound, ulcer, or surgical site that needs frequent inspection or dressing changes.
- *Monitoring of complications*:
  - When there is suspicion of a developing pressure sore, infection, or vascular compromise, creating a window allows for regular visual inspection without removing the entire cast.
- *Pain and pressure relief*: If a patient complains of localized pain or pressure under the cast, a window may help relieve pressure over bony prominences or tender areas.
- *Skin grafts or flaps*: In cases where skin grafts or flaps are performed under the cast, a window allows observation of the graft or flap site for signs of viability or complications.

Step-by-Step Procedure for Creating a Window in a Cast

1. *Identify the area for the window*:
   - Determine the precise location for the window based on clinical need, such as the site of a wound or area of concern.
   - Mark the area on the surface of the cast.
2. *Cut the window*:
   - Using a cast saw, carefully cut an opening in the cast, usually a rectangular or circular shape around the marked area.
   - The cut should be deep enough to go through the plaster but should not extend into the underlying padding or skin.

3. *Remove the cut-out section*:
   - Once the window is cut, remove the section of the cast and save it. This piece is often called the "cast plug" and may be replaced later if needed.
4. *Reinforce the edges*:
   - To prevent cracking or further weakening, the edges of the window should be reinforced with additional plaster or a strip of adhesive cast tape.
   - Padding may be added around the window edges to prevent irritation or pressure on the skin.
5. *Replace the cast plug (optional)*: If the window is not needed for ongoing observation or treatment, the saved cast plug can be replaced and secured with plaster or an adhesive bandage to restore the cast's integrity.

Considerations When Creating a Cast Window

- *Size and shape*: The window should be just large enough to achieve its intended purpose (e.g., wound inspection or dressing change) without compromising the overall structural integrity of the cast.
- *Location*: Avoid placing windows over areas that could destabilize the cast, such as near joints or over major weight-bearing areas. Position the window to minimize impact on the cast's strength.
- *Monitoring for complications*: Even with a window, regular monitoring of the patient's symptoms is essential, as complications can still develop elsewhere under the cast.

Potential Complications of the Window Technique

- Weakening of the cast
- Pressure points and skin irritation
- Migration of the cast plug
- Increased risk of infection

Tips for Effective Use of the Window Technique

- Create windows only when absolutely necessary to minimize potential complications.
- *Reinforce properly*: Reinforce the edges of the window and cast to maintain the strength and stability of the cast.
- *Educate the patient*: Instruct patients to avoid inserting objects into the window and to report any changes, such as increased pain, swelling, or drainage.

BIBLIOGRAPHY

1. Harrigan M. Fracture Management: Basic Principles, Immobilization, and Splinting. In: Taylor DA, Sherry SP, Sing RF (Eds). Interventional Critical Care. Cham: Springer; 2021.
2. Schlégl ÁT, Told R, Kardos K, Szőke A, Ujfalusi Z, Maróti P. Evaluation and Comparison of Traditional Plaster and Fiberglass Casts with 3D-Printed PLA and PLA–$CaCO_3$ Composite Splints for Bone-Fracture Management. Polymers (Basel). 2022;14(17):3571.
3. Steele AJ. The Use of Plaster of Paris in Orthopaedics. Open Orthop J. 1893.

CHAPTER 1.6

Basic Principle Operative Management of Fractures

Rajneesh Garg

Surgical treatment is indicated where a particular fracture is not suitable for conservative treatment or where the conservative treatment has failed.

FUNDAMENTAL PRINCIPLES OF OPERATIVE FRACTURE MANAGEMENT

- Anatomical/acceptable reduction
- Stable fixation
- *Early mobilization*: To prevent joint stiffness and muscle atrophy
- *Minimally invasive techniques (wherever possible)*: Techniques such as image-guided, percutaneous fixation and arthroscopy assisted in reducing surgical trauma and facilitated quicker recovery with fewer complications and better functional outcomes compared to traditional open procedures.
- *Infection prevention*: Rigorous infection control practices are vital to prevent surgical site infections (SSI). This includes adherence to sterile techniques, use of prophylactic antibiotics, and careful postoperative wound management.

VARIOUS SURGICAL MODALITIES

Open Reduction and Internal Fixation

Open reduction and internal fixation (ORIF) is employed for fractures that cannot be adequately managed by conservatives or where close reduction does not obtain an acceptable reduction.

Closed Reduction and Internal Fixation

Closed reduction and internal fixation (CRIF) utilizes percutaneous/minimally invasive techniques to reduce fractures without extensive soft tissue dissection.

External Fixation

- *Indications*: Open fractures, extensive soft tissue damage, and fractures requiring temporary stabilization.
- *Techniques*: The most commonly used fixator is tubular/Hofman, however, modern external fixators, including circular and hybrid fixators, and rail fixators (LRS) offer enhanced stability and precision.

The stability after fracture fixation can be:

- *Absolute stability*: Absolute stability aims to achieve near-rigid fixation to prevent any micromovement at the fracture site. This type of stability promotes direct or primary bone healing, characterized by the absence of callus formation. The key techniques include:
    - *Compression plate fixation*: Used for simple fractures, such as transverse or short oblique fractures. The use of dynamic compression plates (DCP) or locking compression plates (LCP) can

bring fracture fragments into direct contact, promoting healing through osteonal remodeling.
  - *Lag screw fixation*: This involves using a screw placed perpendicular to the fracture line, which compresses the fracture fragments together.
  - *Tension band wiring*: Converts tensile forces on the fracture into compressive forces, often used for avulsion fractures (e.g., patella, olecranon)
- *Relative stability*: It allows controlled motion at the fracture site to promote secondary bone healing, which involves callus formation. It is used for fractures where direct bone contact is not achievable like in comminuted fractures. Various techniques include:
  - Intramedullary nailing
  - *Bridge plating*: Used for multifragmentary or comminuted fractures where direct reduction is not feasible.
  - *External fixation with dynamization*: Allows early stabilization with an external fixator, which can later be "dynamized" (adjusted) to allow partial weight-bearing or motion, promoting healing.
- *Biological or minimally invasive osteosynthesis*: This techniques involves relative stability and relative stability, focusing on preserving the fracture's biology by minimizing soft tissue damage during fixation. The primary aim is to preserve blood supply to the fracture site while maintaining adequate stability for healing. Methods include:
  - *Minimally invasive plate osteosynthesis (MIPO)*: Plates are inserted through small incisions away from the fracture site, reducing the risk of periosteal stripping and preserving the blood supply.
  - *Locking plates*: Provide angular stability and do not require the plate to be contoured tightly against the bone, preserving periosteal blood supply.
- *Elastic stability*: It allows controlled deformation under physiological load to promote secondary healing. This is used mainly in pediatric fractures or certain forearm fractures where slight motion helps stimulate healing. Techniques include:
  - *Elastic intramedullary nailing*: Like titanium elastic nail system (TENS) or Nancy nail
- *Hybrid fixation*: Combines different methods of fixation to achieve both absolute and relative stability in different parts of a complex fracture. For example, a combination of a plate and an intramedullary nail can be used in certain periarticular fractures.
- *Bone grafting with fixation*: In cases with significant bone loss or nonunion, bone grafts (autografts, allografts, or bone substitutes) are combined with internal or external fixation methods to achieve stability and promote bone healing.
- *Cerclage wiring*: Used in conjunction with other forms of fixation, such as intramedullary nails or plates, to hold bone fragments together and achieve additional stability.

Various types of plates used for fracture fixation/osteosynthesis:
- Dynamic compression plates
- Limited contact dynamic compression plates (LC-DCP)
- Locking compression plates
- Reconstruction plates
- Anatomical plates for particular areas like clavicle plate, proximal humerus plate, distal humerus plate, olecranon plate, distal radius plate, proximal femur plate, distal femur plate, proximal tibia plate, distal tibia plate, distal fibula plate, calcaneal plate and pelvic plate, etc.

Based on configuration, plates can be:
- Straight plates
- L-plates
- T-shaped plates
- Anatomically contoured plates

- *Tubular plates*: One-third tubular and semitubular plate
- Pelvic reconstruction plates
- Hook plates
- Cobra plate
- J plate pudo plate for HTO

Based on diameter or thickness-based types of plates:
- *Mini-fragment plates*:
  - Usually between 1.5 and 2.7 mm in thickness
  - Used for small bones, such as those in the hand (metacarpals and phalanges) or face (maxillofacial fractures). These plates provide stable fixation without excessive bulk.
- *Small fragment plates*:
  - Typically 3.5 mm in thickness
  - Used for fractures of small-to-medium-sized bones, such as the radius, ulna, clavicle, or fibula. These plates provide a balance between strength and minimal soft tissue irritation.
- *Large fragment plates which can be divided into—(1) narrow DCP and (2) broad DCP*:
  - Usually 4.5 mm in thickness
  - Used for larger bones, like the femur, tibia, or humerus, especially in diaphyseal fractures where substantial mechanical strength is needed.

Plates can also be classified based on biomechanical principles:
- *Compression*: Plates can be used to apply compression across a fracture site, enhancing stability and promoting primary bone healing without the formation of a callus. This is especially useful in transverse fractures.
- *Neutralization*: When fractures are initially reduced and fixed with lag screws, plates can be used to protect (neutralize) the fracture from additional forces (bending, torsion, or shear). The plate does not directly bear the load but supports the construct.
- *Buttressing*: For metaphyseal or intra-articular fractures, plates can be applied to buttress or support the bone fragments and prevent their collapse or displacement under load. This is crucial in fractures where bone fragments are at risk of collapsing, such as tibial plateau fractures, and distal radius.
- *Bridging*: In comminuted fractures where anatomical reduction is not possible, plates act as a bridge, maintaining the length, alignment, and rotation of the bone. The plate spans across the fracture site without disturbing the intermediate fragments, allowing for biological healing.
- *Tension band plates*: Commonly used in **pediatric orthopedics**, it addresses growth plate deformities like **valgus or varus knees** by guiding growth. in fractures it converts tensile forces into compressive forces, enhancing healing
- *External fixator plates*: These plates are designed to be used temporarily as external fixators, usually in situations where soft tissue damage precludes internal fixation.
- *Hybrid plates*: It combines features of locking plates and traditional compression plates to provide both angular stability and load sharing.
- *Distraction plate*: Used across the joint temporarily till fracture healing in case of severely comminuted fracture of the distal radius.

Various intramedullary nails (IM nails):
- *Standard intramedullary interlocking nails*: Designed for diaphyseal fractures in long bones like the femur, tibia, or humerus.
- *Reconstruction nails*: Allow fixation of both diaphyseal and metaphyseal fractures (e.g., femoral shaft and neck fractures)
- *Elastic stable intramedullary nails (ESIN)*: Used mainly in pediatric patients due to their ability to provide adequate stability while allowing some flexibility, promoting bone remodeling.

- Ender nails
- *Rush nails and square nail*: Rarely used (these days) for forearm fractures
- Expandable nails are rarely used.

Specialty nails, e.g.:

- *Gamma nails* are designed for specific fractures, such as those involving the femoral neck and intertrochanter region.
- *Proximal femoral nails (PFN)*: Used for proximal femur fractures like intertrochanteric and subtrochanteric fractures. With variation and designs like PFNA, PFNA 2, Intertan
- *Distal femoral nails (DFN)*: Designed for distal femoral fractures
- *Expert tibial nails*: They have various configurations (proximal or distal locking) depending on the fracture type.
- TTN or tibio-talo-calcaneal nail
- Proximal humerus nails (PHN)
- *Retrograde nails*: Inserted from the distal end of the bone, typically used for fractures near the knee (distal femur). Whereas standard interlocking nails are used in an antegrade fashion.

Principles of nails:

- Load sharing devices
- Minimally invasive
- Biomechanical stronger
- Preservation of soft tissues

Healing characteristics of nailed fractures:

- *Secondary bone healing*: Healing typically occurs with callus formation, which can be advantageous for some fractures.
- *Micro-movement promotion*: Slight motion at the fracture site can stimulate biological healing.
- *Healing time*: Generally faster due to minimal soft tissue disruption and the biological stimulation from micro-movement.

When to choose nails?

- Treating diaphyseal (shaft) fractures of long bones (femur, tibia, humerus)
- The fracture is comminuted, segmental, or has rotational instability.
- When the goal is to allow early weight-bearing and mobilization.

Healing in fractures fixed with plates:

- *Primary bone healing*: Achieved through rigid fixation, often without visible callus formation.
- *Reduced motion*: Rigid fixation eliminates micromotion, which is ideal for fractures requiring absolute stability, such as intra-articular fractures.
- *Healing time*: May be longer, especially if there is significant soft tissue damage or if there is a need for prolonged immobilization.

Plates are used in:

- Treating periarticular or metaphyseal fractures that require precise anatomical reduction.
- Dealing with fractures involving the joint or those with poor bone quality.
- When there is a need for absolute stability with primary bone healing (e.g., intra-articular fractures).
- When there is significant displacement, comminution, or involvement of the fracture near a joint surface.

Plate:

- Load-bearing device
- Greater control over alignment
- Less effective against bending forces

Postoperative care and rehabilitation:
Effective postoperative management is critical for achieving optimal recovery and functional outcomes:

- *Wound care*: Proper wound management involves wound inspection, dressing changes, and patient education to prevent infections and complications.
- *Pain management*: Effective pain control is again crucial for patient comfort and facilitates early mobilization and better rehabilitation. This may include a combination of pharmacologic and regional anesthesia techniques. Treating acute pain aggressively is also important to prevent the development of chronicity of acute pain.

- *Rehabilitation*: A structured rehabilitation program tailored to the fracture type and patient needs is essential for restoring function. Evidence supports early physical therapy as a means to enhance recovery and prevent long-term disabilities.
- *Follow-up*: Regular follow-up visits are necessary to monitor healing, assess fixation stability, and address potential complications. Imaging studies such as X-rays or CT scans are used to evaluate progress of fracture healing and guide further treatment if needed.

MANAGEMENT OF COMPLICATIONS

Complications in operative fracture management can significantly impact outcomes. Key complications include:

- *Neurovascular damage*: If there is such an issue, should be dealt with at the earliest.
- *Joint stiffness*: The goal should be mobilization at the earliest, to prevent such complication.
- Compartment syndrome
- Nonunion and malunion
- Delayed union
- Infection

BIBLIOGRAPHY

1. Adams J, Smith K, Patel R, Chen Y, Rodriguez M, Gupta A. Rehabilitation protocols for fracture recovery: A systematic review. J Orthop Res. 2024;42(1):112-24.
2. Brown L, Wilson H, Martin D, O'Connor P, Zhang X, White T. Advancements in external fixation techniques: A review. Orthop Clin. 2024;55(2):245-59.
3. Cohen J, Ahmed S, Taylor B, Nguyen T, Choi E, Ramirez L. Management of nonunion and malunion in fracture care. Bone Joint J. 2023; 105-B(8):1185-94.
4. Davis M, Thompson R, Lee K, Walker P, Hernandez N, Kim J. Indications for open reduction and internal fixation: A comprehensive review. J Trauma Acute Care Surg. 2024;96(5):712-23.
5. Tazreean R, Nelson G, Twomey R. Early mobilization in enhanced recovery after surgery pathways: current evidence and recent advancements. J Comp Eff Res. 2022;11(2):121-9.

CHAPTER 1.7

Fracture Healing Process and Determinants

Amandeep Singh Bakshi

PHASES OF FRACTURE HEALING

Fracture healing involves three primary overlapping phases:

1. *Inflammatory phase*: This phase begins immediately after the fracture. Hematoma formation at the fracture site acts as a scaffold for the influx of inflammatory cells, including neutrophils, macrophages, and lymphocytes. These cells release proinflammatory cytokines [e.g., interleukin-1 (IL-1), IL-6, and tumor necrosis factor-alpha (TNF-α)] that promote angiogenesis and recruit mesenchymal stem cells (MSCs). The inflammatory response is essential for clearing necrotic tissue and setting the stage for subsequent repair processes. Clinically, this phase is characterized by pain, swelling, and reduced mobility.
2. *Reparative phase*: During this phase, soft callus forms as chondrocytes and fibroblasts increase, creating a cartilaginous matrix that bridges the fracture gap. This phase progresses to hard callus formation through endochondral ossification, where the soft callus is gradually replaced by woven bone. The timing and quality of callus formation depend heavily on mechanical stability. In clinical practice, this phase is when radiographic evidence of callus formation becomes apparent, indicating progression toward healing.
3. *Remodeling phase*: The final phase involves the gradual replacement of immature woven bone with mature lamellar bone, aligning its structure according to Wolff's law. Osteoclasts resorb poorly organized bone, while osteoblasts lay down new bone along lines of mechanical stress. The remodeling phase is critical for restoring the bone's original shape, strength, and function. It can continue for months to years, depending on patient-specific factors and the nature of the fracture **(Figs. 1 and 2)**.

FACTORS INFLUENCING FRACTURE HEALING

Biological Factors

- *Age*: Pediatric patients have a remarkable capacity for bone healing due to the abundance of stem cells and growth factors, while older patients may experience delayed healing due to reduced cellular activity, impaired angiogenesis, and a diminished inflammatory response. Orthopedic strategies may include more aggressive fixation and pharmacological support in older patients.
- *Nutrition*: Adequate intake of calcium, phosphorus, and essential vitamins (D, C, and K) is paramount. Vitamin D enhances calcium absorption and bone mineralization, while vitamin K

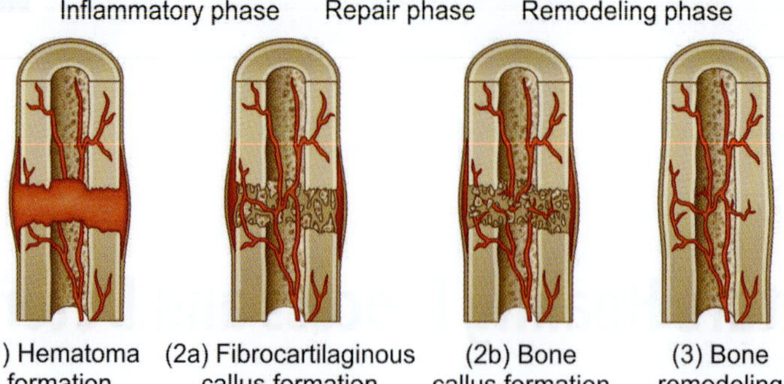

FIG. 1: Stages of secondary bone healing (endochondral ossification). The stages of fracture healing are partially overlapping. (1) Coagulation and acute inflammatory response—initial stabilization, recruitment of inflammatory cells and cytokines. (2) Repair—(a) Revascularization, soft cartilage callus. Chondroblasts derived from MSCs deposit cartilage, mature to chondrocytes that express VEGF, inducing neovascularization; (b) Hard bony callus—hyperproliferative chondrocytes transdifferentiate to osteoblasts and osteocytes, tissue invaded by osteoblasts; (3) Remodeling—deposition of lamellar bone and restoration of preinjury anatomic dimensions.

supports the carboxylation of osteocalcin, crucial for binding calcium in bone tissue. Malnutrition or deficiencies may necessitate dietary supplementation or intravenous administration in cases of severe deficits.

- *Hormonal influence*: Estrogen plays a key role in maintaining bone homeostasis by inhibiting osteoclast activity. Postmenopausal women, who are estrogen-deficient, are at increased risk for delayed union or nonunion. Parathyroid hormone (PTH), particularly in its intermittent form, has an anabolic effect on bone and may be considered as a therapeutic agent to enhance fracture healing in selected patients.
- *Genetic factors*: Genetic predispositions can influence bone density, healing speed, and fracture risk. Understanding these factors can guide personalized treatment strategies.

Mechanical Factors

- *Fracture stability*: Fracture healing is highly dependent on mechanical stability. Absolute stability, achieved through methods such as plate fixation, favors primary bone healing, characterized by direct remodeling without callus formation. Relative stability, obtained through intramedullary nailing or external fixation, promotes secondary healing with visible callus formation. The choice of fixation technique should balance stability needs against the biological environment of the fracture.
- *Mechanical loading*: Weight-bearing and mechanical stimulation are critical modulators of bone healing. Controlled mechanical loading stimulates osteogenic activity via mechano-transduction pathways, enhancing callus formation and maturation. However, excessive or premature loading can lead to nonunion or implant failure. Therefore, the postoperative rehabilitation protocols must be carefully tailored to optimize these mechanical forces.

Systemic and Environmental Factors

- *Smoking*: Nicotine and other toxins found in cigarettes have been shown to reduce perfusion, impair osteoblast function, and decrease collagen synthesis, leading to delayed union or nonunion. Smoking

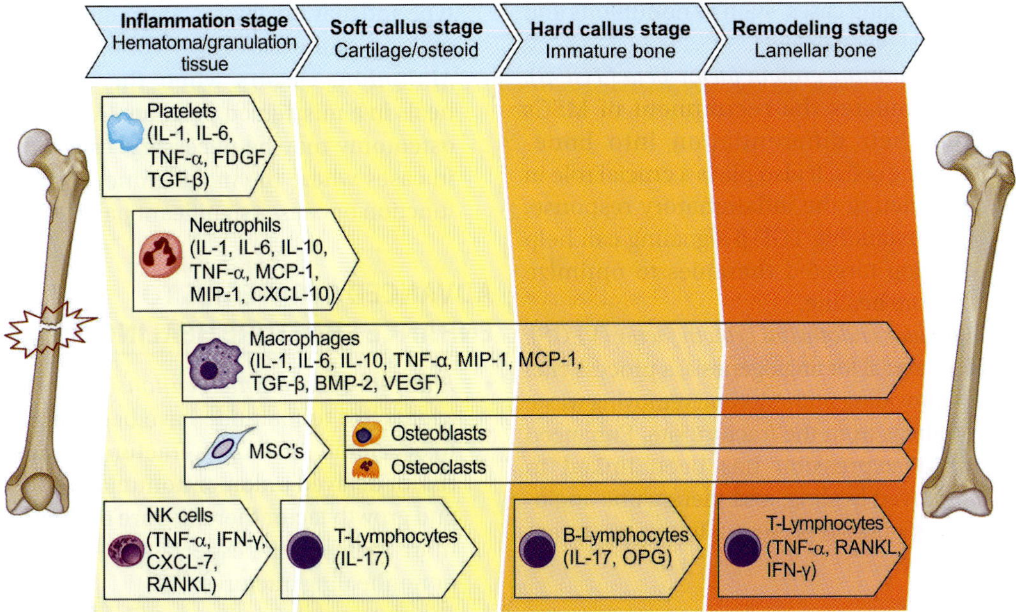

FIG. 2: Immune cells of the fracture healing cascade for each stage of bone healing. The cellular contributions to fracture healing are described. Starting with platelets, a cascade of events that transition the bone from an inflammatory period to a proliferative period noted by soft and hard callus formation and predominated by reparative cells such as osteoblasts and osteoclasts. This phase then transitions to the remodeling phase where the healing site is structurally reinforced. Macrophage, being present throughout the healing cascade, release NO and play an important role throughout all stages of repair. Each stage of bone healing has a different spectrum of immune cells present at the fracture site.

Source: Reproduced with permission. This illustration was adapted by Martin Hofmann (licensed under Creative Commons CC-BY-SA 4.0) using the original illustration from Baht et al. (2018) [licensed under Creative commons CC-BY 4.0 (http://creativecommons.org/licenses/by/4.0/)] and images from Smart Servier Medical Art [licensed under Creative Commons CC-BY-SA 3.0 (https://smart.servier.com/)].

cessation should be strongly advocated in patients undergoing fracture treatment.

- *Medications*: Nonsteroidal anti inflammatory drugs (NSAIDs), commonly used for analgesia, inhibit prostaglandin synthesis, which is crucial for the inflammatory phase of bone healing. Chronic use of corticosteroids can suppress osteoblast differentiation and activity. Conversely, medications like teriparatide (a PTH analog) and bisphosphonates can enhance fracture healing in specific contexts.
- *Comorbid conditions*: Diabetes, osteoporosis, rheumatoid arthritis, and chronic kidney disease are examples of conditions that can adversely affect fracture healing. Diabetic patients, for instance, often exhibit impaired angiogenesis and collagen production, necessitating close monitoring and potentially more aggressive therapeutic interventions.

MOLECULAR AND CELLULAR MECHANISMS IN FRACTURE HEALING

Fracture healing is orchestrated by a complex interplay of growth factors, cytokines, and signaling pathways. Key elements include:

- *Bone morphogenetic proteins (BMPs)*: Particularly BMP-2 and BMP-7, these are potent osteoinductive agents that promote MSC differentiation into osteoblasts and chondrocytes. Clinically, BMPs are used to enhance healing in challenging cases, such as nonunions and critical-sized defects.

- *Transforming growth factor-beta (TGF-β)*: It stimulates the recruitment of MSCs and their differentiation into bone-forming cells. It also plays a crucial role in modulating the inflammatory response. Understanding TGF-β signaling can help develop targeted therapies to optimize fracture healing.
- *Vascular endothelial growth factor (VEGF)*: It is crucial for angiogenesis, a process vital for providing nutrients and removing waste products from the fracture site. Enhanced VEGF expression has been linked to improved healing, and therapeutic angiogenesis may represent a future treatment avenue.

COMPLICATIONS IN FRACTURE HEALING

Orthopedic surgeons must recognize and address complications such as delayed union, nonunion, and malunion:

- *Delayed union*: Defined as slower-than-expected healing. Early identification through clinical and radiological assessment allows for timely intervention, which may include bone grafting, dynamization, or the use of biologics.
- *Nonunion*: Classified as atrophic (biologically inactive) or hypertrophic (biologically active but mechanically unstable). Management strategies depend on the type and may involve restabilization, bone grafting, or the use of BMPs or MSCs.
- *Malunion*: Occurs when the fracture heals in a misaligned position. Corrective osteotomy may be necessary, especially in cases where the malalignment affects function or causes significant pain.

ADVANCED STRATEGIES TO ENHANCE FRACTURE HEALING

- *Pharmacological interventions*: Anabolic agents like teriparatide have been shown to accelerate healing in fractures at high risk of delayed union or nonunion. BMPs and growth factor therapies are becoming more mainstream, especially in complex or nonhealing fractures.
- *Biophysical stimulation*: Techniques such as low-intensity pulsed ultrasound (LIPUS) and electrical stimulation have shown promise in enhancing fracture healing, particularly in cases of delayed union. These modalities stimulate cellular responses that promote bone formation.
- *Stem cell therapy and tissue engineering*: The use of MSCs, combined with scaffolds and growth factors, is an emerging field aimed at improving outcomes in complex fractures. Ongoing research into the optimal cell types, delivery methods, and combination therapies holds promise for future advancements.

BIBLIOGRAPHY

1. Geusens P, Emans PJ, de Jong JJ, van den Bergh J. NSAIDs and fracture healing. Curr Opin Rheumatol. 2023;35(2):139-44.
2. Menger MM, Manuschewski R, Ehnert S, Rollmann MF, Maisenbacher TC, Tobias AL, et al. Radiographic, biomechanical, and histological characterization of femoral fracture healing in aged CD-1 mice. Bioengineering (Basel). 2023;10(275):275-81.
3. Saul D, Menger MM, Ehnert S, Nüssler AK, Histing T, Laschke MW. Bone healing gone wrong: Pathological fracture healing and non-unions—Overview of basic and clinical aspects and systematic review of risk factors. Bioengineering (Basel). 2023;10(1):85.
4. Sheen JR, Mabrouk A, Garla VV. (2023). Fracture Healing Overview. [online] Available from https://www.ncbi.nlm.nih.gov/books/NBK551678/ [Last accessed November, 2024].
5. Uhthoff HK, Garla VV, Kyle RF. Fracture healing and its complications. In: Gustilo RB, Kyle RF, Templeman DC (Eds). Fractures and Dislocations. St. Louis: Mosby; 1993.

SECTION

2

Shoulder Girdle

CHAPTER 2.1

Sternoclavicular Dislocation

Pankaj Spolia

Sternoclavicular joint (SCJ) dislocation is a comparatively infrequent injury, accounting for under 3% of all shoulder girdle injuries.

The SCJ is a diarthrodial saddle-shaped joint framed by the union between the medial end of the clavicle and the manubrium of the sternum, supported by anterior and posterior sternoclavicular ligaments, interclavicular ligament, and costoclavicular ligament. This joint allows limited movements of the clavicle in elevation, descent, protraction, retraction, and rotation, allowing the full range of movement of shoulder blade.

MECHANISM OF INJURY

Sternoclavicular joint dislocation usually occurs by direct trauma to the shoulder or chest, such as a vehicle accident, contact sports, or a fall. Anterior dislocation usually takes place by a force transmitted directly to the anterolateral shoulder, pushing the inner end of the clavicle forward. Posterior dislocation is often caused by a direct blow to the anterior portion of the clavicle or an indirect force propagated from the shoulder, pushing the clavicle backwards. Posterior dislocations are less common but more serious owing to the risk of injury to below structures like the trachea, esophagus, and major arteries and veins.

CLINICAL MANIFESTATIONS

Patients with SCJ dislocation often present with SCJ pain, swelling, tenderness, difficulty in moving the arm, and possible deformity. Anterior dislocation presents as a visible or palpable bulge at the medial end of the clavicle, whereas posterior dislocation is subtle but may be associated with symptoms of compression of mediastinal structures, such as dyspnea, hoarseness, or difficulty swallowing.

DIAGNOSTIC EVALUATION

Imaging

- *X-rays*: This is the first-line imaging; however, due to the complex anatomy, X-rays may not always provide a clear diagnosis on routine anteroposterior (AP) view and additional views like Hobbs view **(Fig. 1)** and serendipity view **(Fig. 2)** should be taken.
- *CT-scan including 3-D reconstruction* ***(Fig. 3)***: The gold standard investigation for diagnosis, CT provides detailed information on the dislocation type, severity and associated injuries **(Fig. 4)**.
- *Magnetic resonance imaging (MRI)*: Important to evaluate soft tissue injuries, including ligamentous or joint injuries.
- *Ultrasound*: Can be used in situations where CT is not available or to confirm findings in real-time.

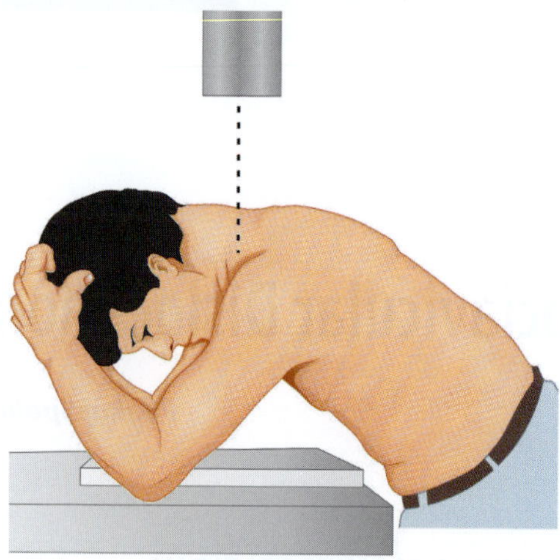

FIG. 1: Hobbs view: Patient position in X-ray assessment of the SCJ suggested by Hobbs.
(SCJ: sternoclavicular joint)

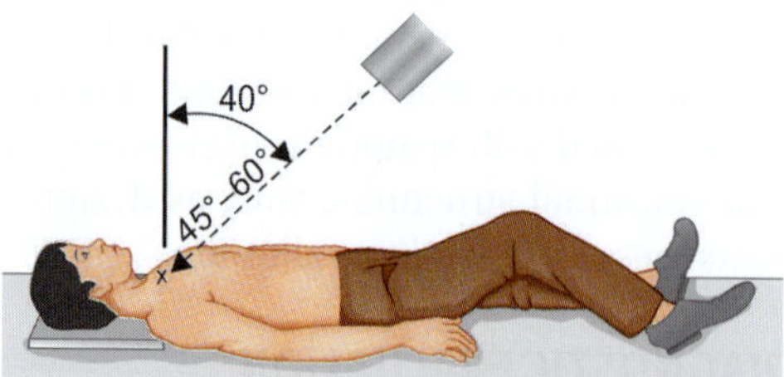

FIG. 2: Serendipity view: Patient position in X-ray assessment of the SCJ. The X-ray beam is angled 40° and vertically directed toward the manubrium.
(SCJ: sternoclavicular joint)

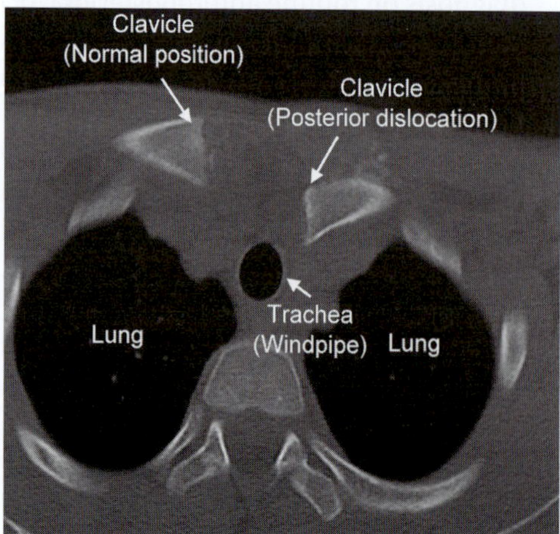

FIG. 3: CT cross-section showing posterior dislocation.

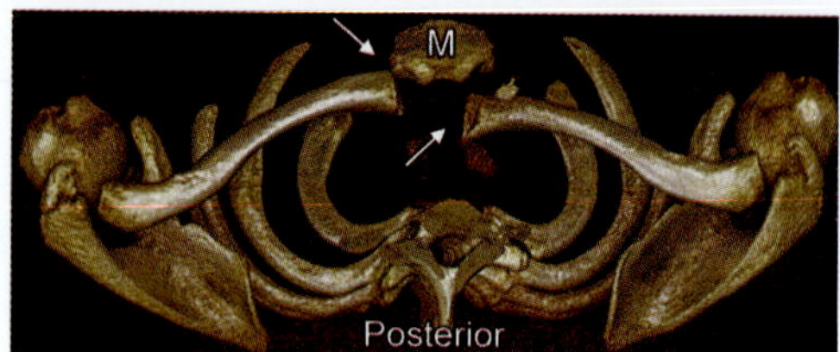

FIG. 4: 3-D CT showing posterior dislocation.

CLASSIFICATION OF STERNOCLAVICULAR JOINT DISLOCATIONS

- Anterior dislocation
- Posterior dislocation

MANAGEMENT AND TREATMENT STRATEGIES

Treatment of SCJ dislocations depends on the type (anterior or posterior), the severity of symptoms, the presence of complications, and the patient's age and activity level.

Anterior Dislocation

- *Nonsurgical management*:
  - *Conservative treatment*: The initial treatment for most anterior SCJ dislocations. This involves immobilizing the affected arm with an arm sling or figure-of-eight bandage for 2–4 weeks, followed by physical therapy to regain movement and strength.
  - *Pain management*: In the acute phase, analgesics like nonsteroidal anti-inflammatory drugs (NSAIDs) relieve pain.
  - *Rehabilitation*: Gradual physiotherapy for shoulder girdle muscle strengthening and joint mobility exercises is advised.
- *Surgical management*:
  - Indications for surgery include persistent pain, instability and functional impairment after conservative management fails, or cosmetic

reasons due to prominent clavicular deformity.
- *Surgical techniques*: Options include open reduction and ligament reconstruction using autografts or allografts. Surgical fixation with screws or plates may be considered, but due to the high mobility of the joint, fixation devices are often avoided.
- *Complications*: Potential complications of surgical management include infection, hardware failure, and redislocation.

Posterior Dislocation

- *Nonsurgical management*:
  - *Closed reduction*: Posterior dislocation often requires immediate reduction because of the risk of mediastinal injury. This is usually done under anesthesia with the patient in the supine position, then applying traction to the arm, and careful anterior pressure to the clavicle **(Figs. 5A to C)**.
  - *Postreduction care*: Immobilization in a sling over 4–6 weeks, with subsequent physiotherapy, is advisable after closed reduction.
- *Surgical management*:
  - *Indications for surgery*: Failed closed reduction, recurrent posterior instability, or associated injuries to mediastinal structures need surgical intervention.
  - *Surgical techniques*:
    - *Open reduction and internal fixation (ORIF)*: ORIF is recommended in cases of persistent instability or failure of reduction. These procedures may include the use of suture anchors, ligament reconstruction, or plates to stabilize the clavicle.
    - *Vascular or mediastinal injury repair*: Complicated posterior dislocation with vascular or airway trauma requires a multidisciplinary approach involving cardiothoracic or vascular surgeons.
  - *Complications*: Surgical treatment carries the chances of infection, nonunion, relentless instability, and damage to adjacent structures.

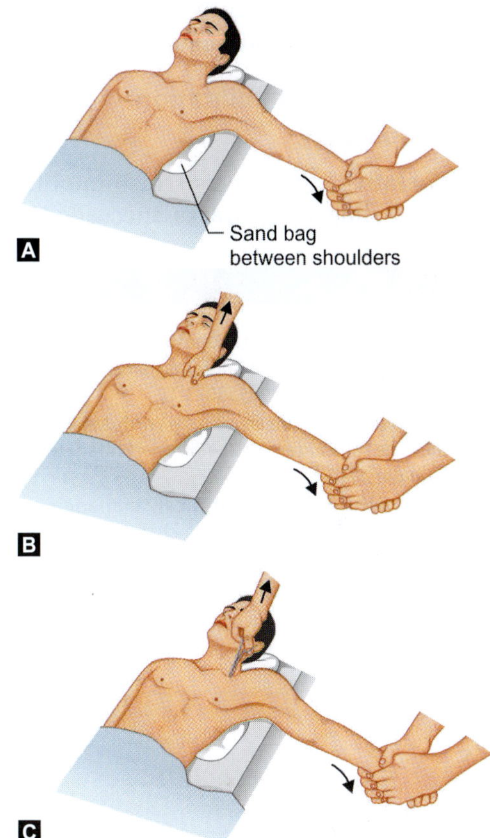

FIGS. 5A TO C: Closed reduction method of SCJ dislocation. (A) Patient is placed in a supine position with a sandbag kept between shoulders. Against the countertraction, traction is put into the abducted and extended position of the arm. Direct pressure on the medial clavicle end reduces the joint in anterior dislocation. (B) The clavicle being lifted upwards manually with digits, and (C) with instruments under sterile conditions, by giving traction and countertraction over the abducted and extended arm.

Recent Advances and Guidelines in Treatment

Newer techniques, such as arthroscopic-assisted reduction and fixation, are being investigated but currently lack sufficient evidence to support wide approval.

Postoperative Rehabilitation and Follow-up

Postoperative care consists of immobilization in a sling for 4–6 weeks, succeeded by a standard rehabilitation program focused on gentle range of motion exercises, advancing to strengthening exercises after 6–8 weeks. Follow-up imaging is beneficial to ensure stability and assess for issues such as recurrence or hardware failure.

BIBLIOGRAPHY

1. Inman VT, Saunders JB, Abbott LC. Observations of the function of the shoulder joint. 1944. Clin Orthop Relat Res. 1996;(330):3-12.
2. Rockwood CA Jr, Matsen FA III, Wirth MA, Lippitt SB. The Shoulder, 4th edition. Philadelphia: Saunders; 2017.
3. Sohn HS, Shin SJ. Surgical management of sternoclavicular joint dislocation and medial clavicular fractures. Clin Orthop Surg. 2020;12(1):18-26.
4. Morell DJ, Thyagarajan DS. Sternoclavicular joint dislocation and its management: A review of the literature. World J Orthop. 2016;18;7(2):244-50.
5. Wirth MA. Current treatment of acute and chronic sternoclavicular joint dislocations. J Bone Joint Surg Am. 2018;100(20):1811-8.

Clavicle Fracture

Abhishek Mahajan

Clavicle fractures are 2.6% of all fractures and 44–66% of fractures around the shoulder girdle.

Midclavicular fracture is one of the common injuries of the skeleton, representing 3–5% of all fractures and 45% of shoulder injuries.

MECHANISM OF INJURY

The clavicle can be injured either by direct or indirect trauma.

Typical Fracture Patterns

Middle third fractures: These account for approximately 70–80% of all clavicle fractures. They typically occur due to the lack of muscular or ligamentous support in this region and are often transverse or oblique. They may be displaced or nondisplaced, depending on the severity of the injury.

Lateral third fractures: These represent 15–30% of clavicle fractures and are often associated with injuries to the coracoclavicular ligaments. These fractures can be either stable or unstable, depending on the extent of ligamentous injury.

Medial third fractures: These are rare, accounting for only 5% of clavicle fractures. They are often the result of high-energy trauma and may be associated with injuries to the sternoclavicular joint.

RADIOGRAPHIC EVALUATION

Evaluation of Middle-third Clavicle Fractures

An anteroposterior view and a 45° cephalic tilt view are required.

Evaluation of Acromioclavicular Joint and Distal Clavicle

Anteroposterior oblique stress film with the patient standing and 10-pound weights suspended from each wrist should be sufficient to diagnose an unstable distal clavicle fracture.

CLASSIFICATION

- *Allman classification*:
  - *Group I*: Midshaft fractures (middle third, most common type)
  - *Group II*: Lateral (distal) fractures which is further divided into—
    - *Type I*: Fracture lateral to the coracoclavicular ligaments (nondisplaced)
    - *Type II*: Fracture medial to the coracoclavicular ligaments (displaced), type II again get divided into:
      a. IIA: Coniod and trapeziod attached to distal segment
      b. Coniod torn, trapeziod attached to the distal fragement

- *Type III*: Fracture into the acromioclavicular joint
- *Group III*: Medial (proximal) fractures, less common and often associated with high-energy trauma.

Other classifications are:
- AO/OTA classification
- Neer's classification
- Edinburgh's classification
- Robinson's classification

TREATMENT

Conservative Management

Conservative management remains a cornerstone for treating most of clavicle fractures, particularly those that are nondisplaced or minimally displaced.

- *Indications for conservative management*:
  - Middle-third fractures with <2 cm of shortening and no comminution
  - Lateral third fractures without significant displacement or disruption of the coracoclavicular ligaments
  - Medial third fractures without associated thoracic or neurovascular injuries
- *Conservative treatment protocols*:
  - In the conservative stream, various braces are introduced to immobilize the mid-third clavicle especially the commercial figure of eight braces and most commonly shoulder arm pouch or sling is used **(Fig. 1)**.
  - Early initiation of shoulder range-of-motion exercises is recommended as soon as pain allows, typically within 1–2 weeks for minimally displaced fractures, with progressive strengthening exercises commencing around 6–8 weeks.

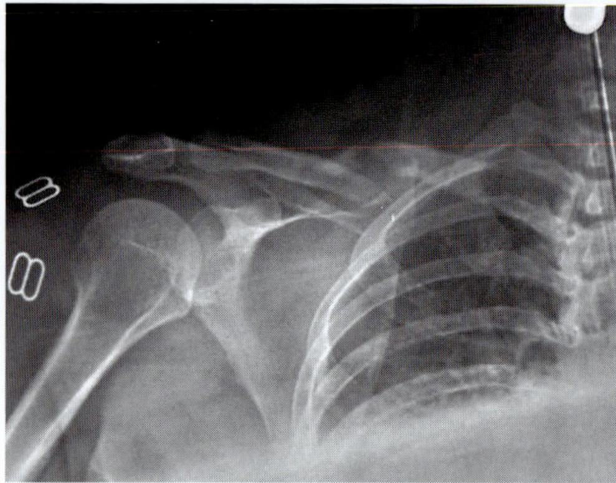

FIG. 1: Clavicle fracture was managed conservatively.

Complications of conservative treatment:
- *Malunion*: Shortening or angulation occurs as a common complication of displaced clavicular fractures. Significant shortening especially >3 cm can be associated with a lack of full strength in the shoulder girdle and pain as well.
- *Delayed union and nonunion*: Studies report high union rates (90–95%) for nonsurgically managed minimally displaced middle-third fractures. However, up to 30% of displaced fractures treated nonoperatively may develop significant malunion, nonunion, or functional deficits, particularly in active young adults.
- *Neurovascular sequelae*: Neurovascular sequelae can occur in both united and nonunited fractures. Abundant callus or fracture deformity may narrow the costoclavicular space. It can cause compression of neurovascular structures and produce symptoms.

Surgical Management

Recent literature advocates for a more selective surgical approach, particularly for fractures with substantial displacement or high-risk features. Surgical fixation has been associated with improved functional outcomes, earlier return to activity, and reduced rates of nonunion in selected patients.

- *Relative indications for surgical management*:
  - Displaced middle-third fractures with greater than 2 cm shortening or comminution
  - Fractures with a "Z-shaped" deformity or significant angulation
  - Open fractures or impending open fractures or fractures with associated neurovascular compromise

- Displaced lateral third fractures, particularly those involving the coracoclavicular ligament complex
- Bilateral clavicle fractures or fractures in polytrauma patients where early mobility is advantageous
- High-demand patients, including athletes, laborers, or those requiring an early return to function
- *Associated injuries*:
  - Vascular injury
  - Progressive neurological deficit
  - Ipsilateral upper extremity injuries
  - Floating shoulder
  - Bilateral clavicular fractures
- *Patient factors*:
  - Polytrauma with requirement for early upper extremity weight bearing
  - Patient motivation for rapid return of function (sports persons)

- *Surgical techniques*:
  - *Plate fixation*: Superior plating **(Fig. 2)** or anteroinferior plating **(Fig. 3)** remains the gold standard for middle-third fractures. Anatomically contoured plates with locking options provide rigid fixation while minimizing soft tissue irritation. Recent innovations in plate design, such as low-profile plates, have reduced the risk of hardware prominence and soft tissue complications.
  - *Intramedullary fixation*: Suitable for simple, noncomminuted fractures, intramedullary devices, such as intramedullary nail **(Fig. 4)**, titanium elastic nails **(Fig. 5)**, or screw rods offer a less invasive option with minimal soft tissue disruption. However, they may be associated with a higher risk of hardware migration or

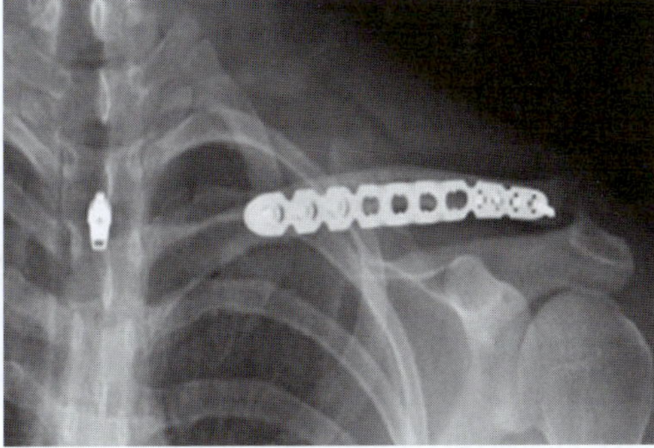

FIG. 3: Fracture of middle-third clavicle managed with anterior plating.

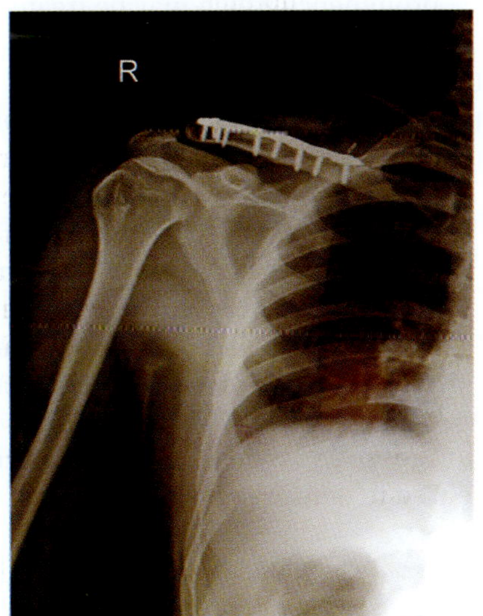

FIG. 2: Fracture of middle-third clavicle managed with superior plating.

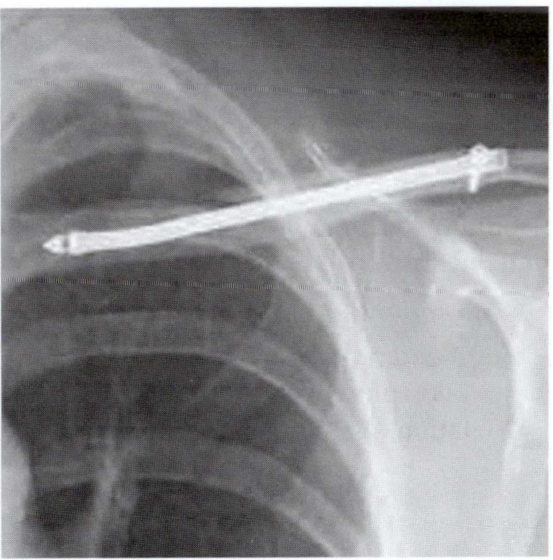

FIG. 4: Fracture shaft of clavicle managed with intramedullary nailing.

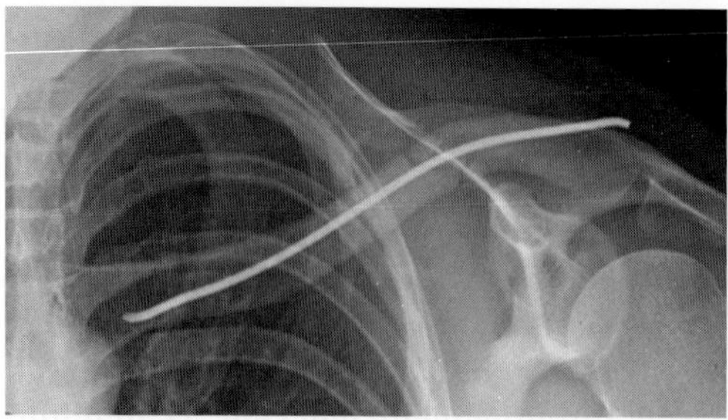

FIG. 5: Fracture shaft of clavicle managed with TENS nail.

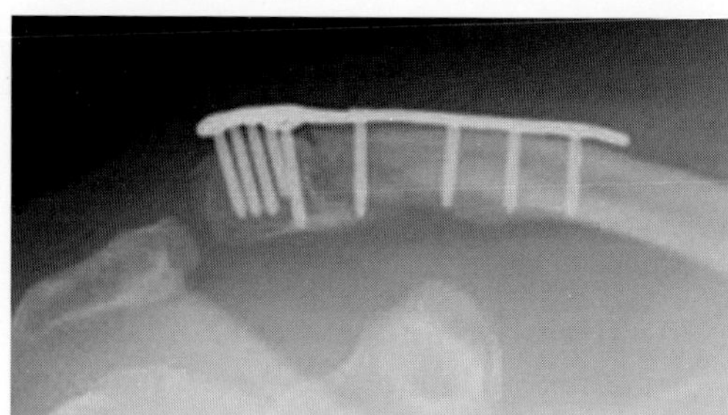

FIG. 7: Fracture lateral end clavicle managed with locking plates.

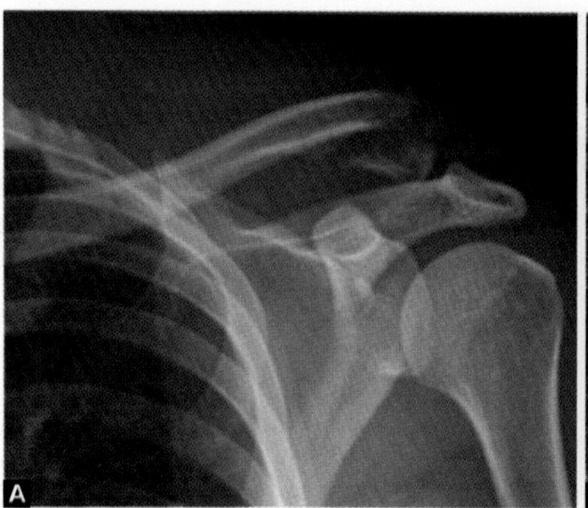

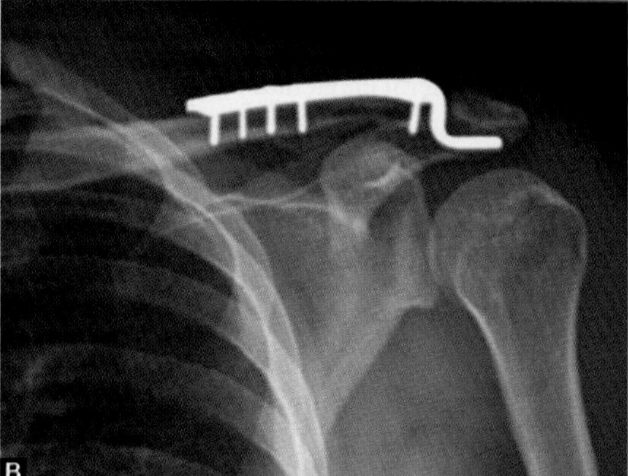

FIGS. 6A AND B: Fracture lateral end clavicle managed with hook plating.

failure, particularly in case of severe comminution.

Lateral end fractures: These require specialized techniques, such as hook plates **(Figs. 6A and B)**, special lateral end locking plates **(Fig. 7)**, or coracoclavicular suture augmentation, to manage ligamentous instability and maintain acromioclavicular joint integrity.

Complications of surgical treatment:
- *Hardware problems*:
    - Like plate loosening, plate angulation, plate breakage and hardware prominence which may be treated by replating
- Infection
- Hypertrophic scar
- Delayed union and nonunion

Outcomes of surgical management: Meta-analyses and randomized controlled trials (RCTs) consistently show that surgical management of displaced middle-third fractures results in faster recovery times, better functional outcomes, and lower rates of nonunion and symptomatic malunion compared to conservative treatment.

BIBLIOGRAPHY

1. American Academy of Orthopaedic Surgeons. (2022). Treatment of clavicle fractures: Evidence-based clinical practice guideline. [online] Available from https://www.aaos.org/globalassets/quality-and-practice-resources/clavicle-fractures/clavicle-fractures-cpg.pdf [Last accessed November, 2024].
2. Canadian Orthopaedic Trauma Society. Nonoperative treatment compared with plate fixation of displaced midshaft clavicular fractures: A multicenter, randomized clinical trial. J Bone Joint Surg Am. 2007;89:1-10.
3. Lu M, Qiu H, Liu Y, Dong J, Jiang L. Intramedullary fixation versus plate fixation in the treatment of midshaft clavicle fractures: a meta-analysis of randomized controlled trials. Front Surg. 2023;10:1194050.
4. Smekal V, Irenberger A, Struve P, Wambacher M, Krappinger D, Kralinger FS. Elastic stable intramedullary nailing versus nonoperative treatment of displaced midshaft clavicular fractures: A randomized controlled trial. J Orthop Trauma. 2009;23(2):106-12.
5. Van der Meijden OA, Houwert RM, Hulsmans M, Wijdicks FJ, Dijkgraaf MG, Meylaerts SA, et al. Operative treatment of dislocated midshaft clavicular fractures: plate or intramedullary nail fixation? A randomized controlled trial. J Bone Joint Surg Am. 2015;97(8):613-9.

CHAPTER 2.3

Acromioclavicular Joint Dislocation

Abhishek Bral, Anoop Kumar

Injuries to the acromioclavicular (AC) joint are common, particularly among athletes and people participating in high-impact sports. It is more common in male as compared to females and the male:female ratio is 5:1.

Acromioclavicular joint is important for maintaining stability and range of motion of the shoulder girdle. To stabilize the joint there are:

- *Static stabilizers*:
    - *Acromioclavicular ligaments*: Provide horizontal stability by resisting anterior–posterior displacement
    - *Coracoclavicular ligaments (conoid and trapezoid)*: Offer vertical stability, preventing superior displacement of the clavicle
    - *Joint capsule*: Surrounds the joint, contributing to overall stability
- *Dynamic stabilizers*:
    - *Deltoid and trapezius muscles*: Maintain joint congruence during upper limb movements

Mechanisms of injury often involve a direct blow to the shoulder or a fall onto the acromion.

CLASSIFICATION OF ACROMIO-CLAVICULAR JOINT INJURIES

The Tossy classification categorizes AC joint dislocations into three grades, which was subsequently expanded by Rockwood et al. to include an additional three types as shown in **Figures 1A to F**. The Rockwood classification **(Table 1)** is widely regarded as the gold standard for classifying AC joint injuries, providing a practical framework for clinical decision-making.

CLINICAL EVALUATION

Tenderness over the AC joint, prominence or step-off deformity of the distal clavicle, and pain exacerbated by cross-arm adduction or resisted horizontal adduction.

IMAGING STUDIES

- *Radiographs*: Standard anteroposterior (AP) view **(Fig. 2)**, axillary view, cross-body adduction view (Alexander view/ modified Y view), and Zanca views (cephalic angled obliqued view 10–15°) are critical for assessing AC joint alignment and determining injury grade.
- *Modified axillary view* is taken when the axillary view is impossible, like in polytrauma patients. It is taken in senna position. The abduction angle between the trunk and upper limb required is about 30° as opposed to the axillary view which is 70–90°.
- *Weighted/stress views* in which 5 kg weight suspended to both wrists help in unmasking AC joint dislocation but many

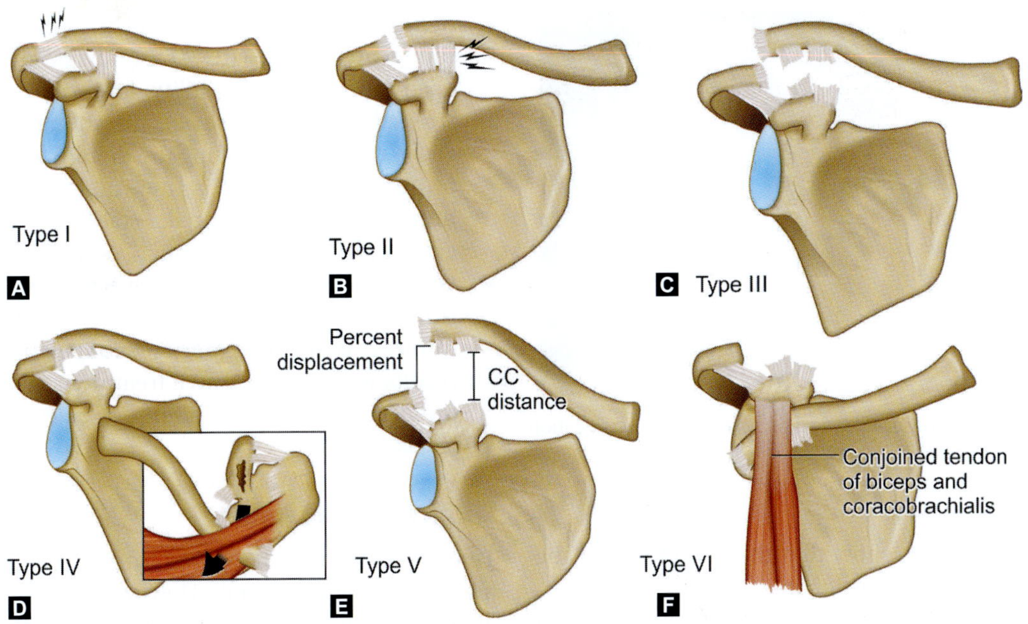

FIGS. 1A TO F: Rockwood classification of acromioclavicular joint (ACJ) dislocation.

TABLE 1: Rockwood classification of AC joint dislocation.

Type	AC joint ligament	AC joint capsule	CC ligament	AC joint displacement	Deltopectoral fascia
I	Sprained	Intact	Intact	None	Intact
II	Torn	Disrupted	Intact	50% AC subluxation	Intact
III	Torn	Disrupted	Torn	100% AC superior dislocation	Intact
IV	Torn	Disrupted	Torn	• 100% AC posterior dislocation • Posterior displacement of the distal clavicle into or through the trapezius muscle	Disrupted
V	Torn	Disrupted	Torn	• 100–300% AC superior dislocation • Complete detachment of deltoid and trapezius muscle from their clavicular insertion	Disrupted
VI	Torn	Disrupted	Torn	• 100% AC inferior dislocation • Inferior displacement of the distal clavicle into a subacromial or subcoracoid position	Disrupted

(AC: acromioclavicular; CC: coracoclavicular)

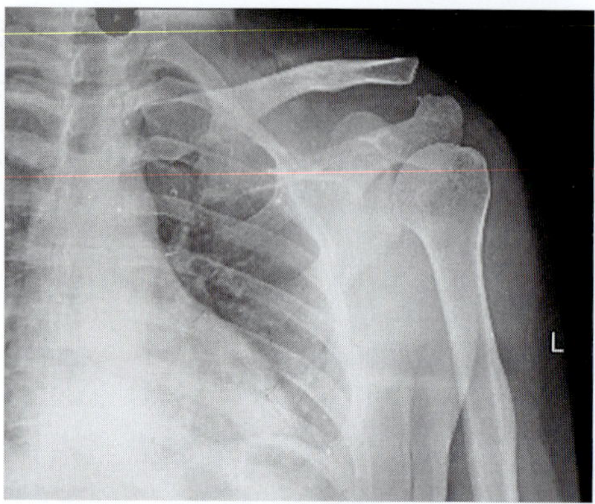

FIG. 2: X-ray of acromioclavicular joint (ACJ) dislocation left shoulder.

studies show that the usefulness of this view is questionable.

- So far, no functional radiographic techniques have been developed to quantify horizontal instability in acute AC joint dislocations. Horizontal instability of the distal clavicle in these acute injuries often indicates the need for surgical intervention. Dynamic axillary radiologic assessment could identify unstable injuries that might have been overlooked and could be important in determining the need for surgical stabilization of the AC joint.

MANAGEMENT OF ACROMIOCLAVICULAR JOINT INJURIES

Management strategies are tailored to the type and severity of injury, patient activity level, and specific functional demands. The choice between nonoperative and operative treatment largely depends on these factors.

Nonoperative Management

Indications: Type I, type II, and some type III injuries, particularly in nonathletes or low-demand patients.

- Sling is used for 1–3 weeks to alleviate pain and inflammation.
- *Rehabilitation*: Initially, early passive range of motion (ROM) exercises are used to maintain flexibility, followed by strengthening exercises for the shoulder girdle muscles, including the deltoid and trapezius. Emphasis is then placed on proprioception and scapular stabilization exercises to restore function.
- *Outcomes*: Most patients with type I and II injuries, as well as some with type III injuries, typically experience excellent results with nonoperative treatment and often return to their preinjury activity levels.

Surgical Management

Type IV-VI injuries have traditionally been managed through surgery. However, there is ongoing debate regarding the best approach for treating type III injuries. The AC joint ligaments generally lose their ability to heal after 3 weeks postinjury. As a result, AC joint dislocations are typically classified as acute if they occur within 3 weeks and chronic if they persist beyond 6 weeks.

Surgical modalities for treating acute AC joint dislocation:

- *Stabilization with metallic devices*:
  - Bosworth screw (historically used)
  - Minimal invasive K wire fixation, but can lead to migration or breakage of wires **(Fig. 3)**.
  - *Hook plate* ***(Fig. 4)***: To prevent potential subacromial impingement related to the hook plate, it should be removed within 3 months. Doing so might reduce postoperative pain and complications compared to suspensory device fixations, though the latter generally results in better shoulder function scores.
- *Suspensory devices*: They are minimally invasive; hardware does not need to be removed.
  - Cortical fixation devices (Endobutton, Tightrope)

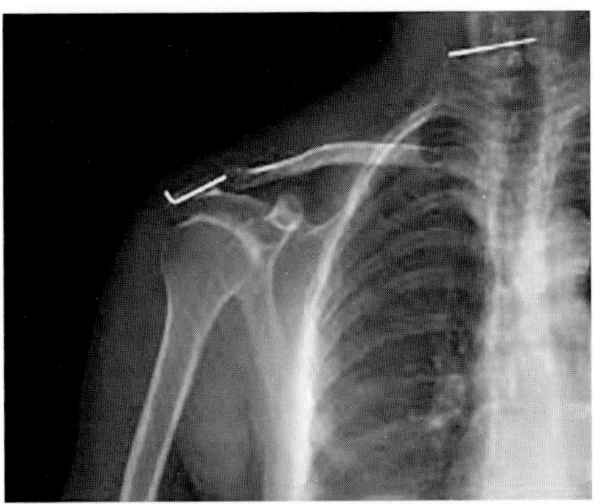

FIG. 3: Breakage and migration of wire.

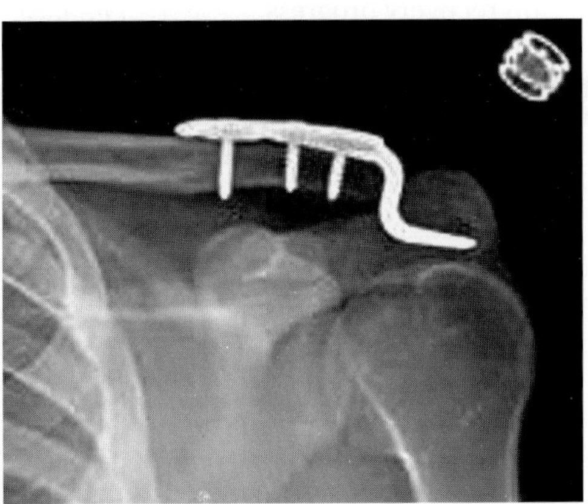

FIG. 4: Hook plate for treatment of acromioclavicular joint (ACJ) dislocation.

In a tightrope system **(Fig. 5)**, the four-strand continuous loop of No. 5 FiberWire interlaced between two titanium buttons provides strong mechanical fixation while the coracoclavicular and acromioclavicular ligament disruptions heal.

- *ACCR (anatomical coracoclavicular ligament reconstruction) with allograft*: The anatomic coracoclavicular reconstruction (ACCR) restores stability to the AC joint by reconstructing the CC and AC ligaments. In this surgical technique, allograft or autograft tissue is used as a biological graft, and a suture or tape is used as a nonbiological method of fixation.

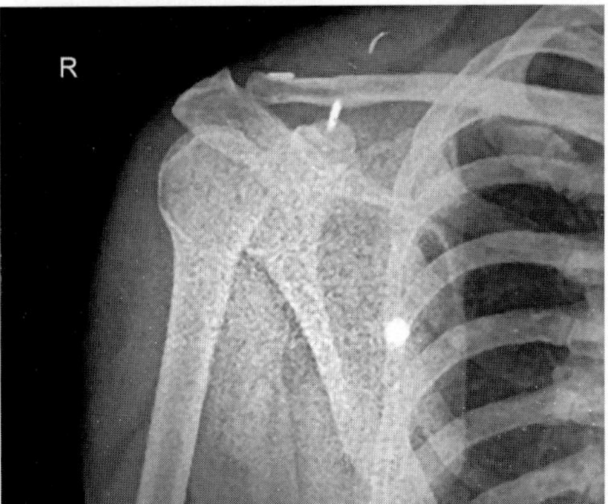

FIG. 5: X-ray of acromioclavicular joint (ACJ) dislocation treated with Endobutton.

CHRONIC ACROMIOCLAVICULAR JOINT DISLOCATION

Biological capabilities are compromised in chronic cases. Therefore, mechanical stabilization of the dislocated joint alone without the use of biological augmentation may be insufficient.

- *Ligament and tendon transfers*: Modified Weaver–Dunn procedure in which transposition of the coracoacromial (CA) ligament to the distal clavicle along with numerous changes to the original technique such as additional augmentation (e.g., sutures, screws, suspensory button devices, and plates) and fixation techniques (e.g., bone chip from the acromion) is used.
- *Synthetic ligaments*: Numerous synthetic materials such as carbon fiber, polytetrafluoroethylene, and polyethylene terephthalate have been used as artificial ligaments for the treatment of chronic AC joint dislocations but can cause foreign body reactions.
- *Dynamic fixation with conjoined tendons*: In order to avoid harvesting

the CA ligament with the possibility of weakening the coracoacromial arc, the idea of utilizing the short head of the biceps was first introduced in 1942. However, clinical results are not yet available for this technique and CA ligament harvesting again poses the risk for anterosuperior migration of the humeral head.

- *Reconstruction with allografts and autografts*: Although allografts and autografts such as palmaris longus, flexor carpi radialis, peroneus longus, and tibialis anterior tendons have been utilized for the treatment of AC joint dislocations, hamstring tendons are most commonly used.

Postoperative rehabilitation is important for optimizing outcomes:

- *Early phase (0–6 weeks)*: Immobilization with a sling, followed by passive ROM exercises to prevent stiffness and promote healing.
- *Intermediate phase (6–12 weeks)*: Gradual progression to active-assisted and active exercises, focusing on strength, proprioception, and dynamic stabilization.
- *Late phase (12+ weeks)*: Functional training, sport-specific exercises, and a gradual return to preinjury activity levels. Full return to contact sports or heavy labor may take up to 6 months, depending on recovery progress.

BIBLIOGRAPHY

1. Chillemi C, Franceschini V, Dei Giudici L, Alibardi A, Salate Santone F, Ramos Alday LJ, et al. Epidemiology of isolated acromioclavicular joint dislocation. Emerg Med Int. 2013;2013(1):171609.
2. Flint JH, Wade AM, Giuliani J, Rue JP. Defining the terms acute and chronic in orthopaedic sports injuries: a systematic review. Am J Sports Med. 2014;42(1):235-41.
3. Haugaard KB, Bak K, Ryberg D, Muharemovic O, Hölmich P, Barfod KW. The ISAKOS subclassification of Rockwood type III AC joint dislocations in a stable type A and an unstable type B is not clinically relevant. Knee Surg Sports Traumatol Arthrosc. 2024;32(7):1821-9.
4. Heers G, Hedtmann A. Correlation of ultrasonographic findings to Tossy's and Rockwood's classification of acromioclavicular joint injuries. Ultrasound Med Biol. 2005;31(6):725-32.
5. Monig SP, Burger C, Helling HJ, Prokop A, Rehm KE. Treatment of complete AC joint dislocation: present indications and surgical techniques with biodegradable cords. Int J Sports Med. 1999;20(8):560-2.

CHAPTER 2.4

Scapula Fracture

Saransh Bahl

Scapula fractures are relatively uncommon, constituting only 0.4–0.9% of all fractures and approximately 3–5% of fractures involving the shoulder girdle. These injuries most often result from high-energy trauma and are frequently seen in polytrauma patients. Scapula fractures are typically unilateral, with bilateral or open fractures being exceedingly rare. These injuries are more common in men, accounting for about 72% of total cases, with a mean age of 44 years.

MECHANISMS OF INJURY

Scapula fractures generally occur due to direct trauma or indirect mechanisms that impose extreme stress on the bone. The common mechanisms include:

- Direct trauma
- Fall from height
- *Impact of the humeral head*: In some cases, the humeral head can dislocate or be driven forcefully against the scapula during a shoulder dislocation, causing fractures of the scapular processes or glenoid rim.
- *Muscle contracture*: Violent muscle contractions, such as those seen during electrical injuries or epileptic seizures, may result in scapular fractures.
- *Avulsion fractures*: The coracoid process may sustain avulsion fractures due to the pull of the coracoclavicular (CC) ligament, particularly in cases of acromioclavicular (AC) joint dislocations.

Associated Injuries

Due to the high-energy nature of the trauma that often leads to scapula fractures, they are frequently associated with other injuries. These may include:

- Rib fractures
- *Thoracic and lung injuries*: Such as pneumothorax, hemothorax, or lung contusions can occur alongside scapular fractures.
- *Injuries to the shoulder girdle*: These include clavicular fractures, AC joint dislocations, and soft tissue injuries such as rotator cuff tears.
- *Head injuries*: Traumatic brain injuries are often seen in polytrauma patients with scapular fractures.
- *Vascular and nerve injuries*: Approximately 10% of scapula fractures involve injuries to major blood vessels, including the subclavian, axillary, and brachial arteries. Brachial plexus injuries are also possible.

IMAGING AND DIAGNOSTIC METHODS

Accurate diagnosis of scapula fractures requires a combination of clinical evaluation and imaging studies. Key imaging modalities include:

- *Radiographs*:
    - *Chest radiograph*: Particularly useful in polytrauma patients, it helps assess

scapulothoracic dissociation by visualizing both scapulae in relation to the spine.
- ◦ *Neer I projection (true AP view)*: This view is ideal for evaluating the glenohumeral joint and assessing glenoid displacement relative to the lateral scapular border **(Fig. 1)**.
- ◦ *Neer II projection (Y-view)*: A true lateral view of the scapula, useful for assessing fractures of the scapular body, lateral border, and fragment overlap.
- ◦ *AP view*: Provides a detailed view of the shoulder girdle, including the clavicle and scapula.
- *CT scans*:
  - ◦ *2D-CT*: Mainly used to assess the glenoid articular surface, especially in fractures involving the glenoid fossa or coracoid base.
  - ◦ *3D-CT reconstructions*: Provides a detailed understanding of the fracture pattern, especially for complex fractures of the scapular body and neck **(Fig. 1)**.

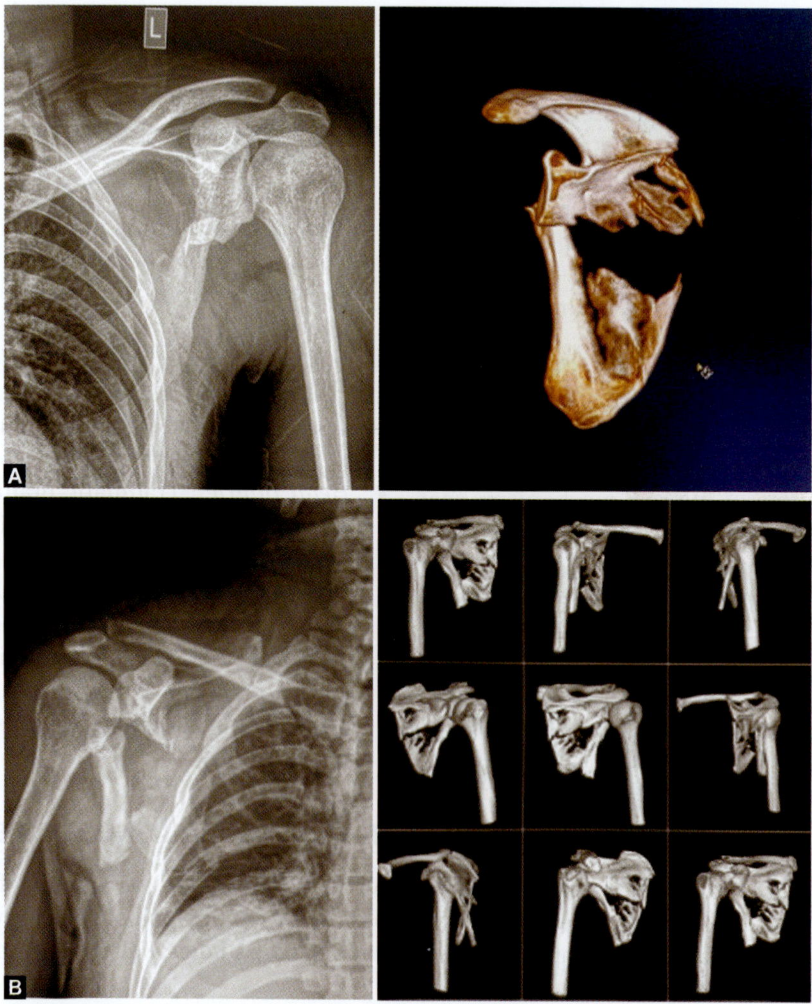

FIGS. 1A AND B: Radiographs and CT scans of (A) extra-articular and (B) intra-articular fractures of scapula.

CLASSIFICATION OF SCAPULA FRACTURES

Several classification systems are used to categorize scapular fractures, each with its specific focus:

- *Anatomical classification*:
  - *Process fractures*: Fractures of the superior border, acromion, or coracoid process
  - *Body fractures*: Anatomical and biomechanical body fractures
  - *Neck fractures*: Anatomical and surgical neck fractures
  - *Glenoid fractures*: Involve fractures of the superior, anterior, inferior, or posterior glenoid rim
  - *Combined fractures*: Involve fractures of multiple regions of the scapula **(Fig. 2)**
- *Ideberg classification (specific to glenoid fractures)*:
  - *Type I*: Anterior glenoid rim fractures
  - *Type II*: Inferior glenoid fractures involving the neck
  - *Type III*: Superior glenoid fractures extending into the coracoid
  - *Type IV*: Horizontal fractures involving both the scapular neck and body
  - *Type V*: Combined fractures of the glenoid and neck **(Figs. 3A to E)**

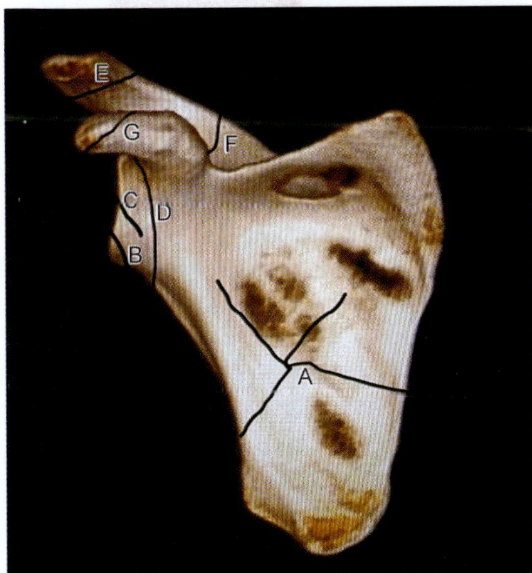

FIG. 2: Anatomical classification of scapula fractures showing fractures of A—body, B and C—glenoid, D—neck, E—acromion, F—scapular spine, and G—coracoid process.

Other classification:

- *Euler and Rüedi classification*: Based on the Müller/AO classification
- AO/OTA (Orthopaedic Trauma Association) system

TREATMENT OF SCAPULA FRACTURES

Nonoperative Treatment

Most scapula fractures, especially those that are minimally displaced, can be treated nonoperatively. The key principles include:

- *Pain management and immobilization*: The patient is typically immobilized in a sling for about 2 weeks.
- *Early mobilization*: Passive range-of-motion exercises are initiated early, aiming for full passive mobility within 1 month post-injury. Active motion exercises are started after the second month.
- *Muscle strengthening*: Strengthening of the rotator cuff and parascapular muscles begins in the third month.

Potential disadvantages of nonoperative treatment include scapular deformity and glenohumeral joint instability.

Operative Treatment

- *Intra-articular fractures*:
  - Articular step-off greater than 4–5 mm
  - Involvement of >20% of the glenoid surface
  - Unstable glenohumeral articulation despite closed reduction
- *Extra-articular fractures*:
  - Glenopolar angle <20° **(Fig. 4)**
  - Lateral border offset greater than 20 mm
  - Angulation greater than 45°
  - Translation of >100%

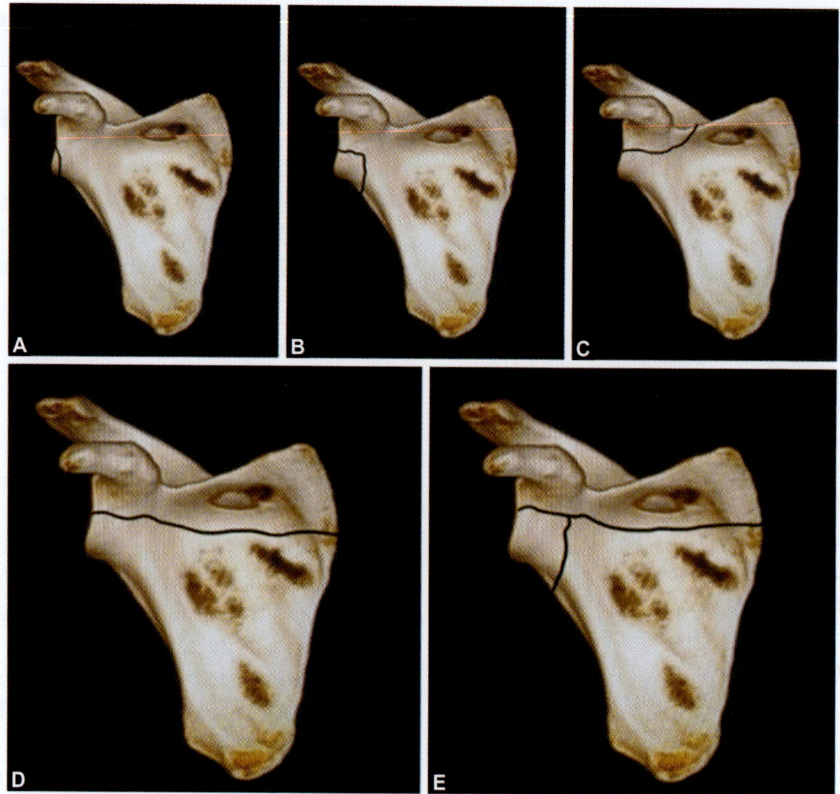

FIGS. 3A TO E: Illustration showing Ideberg classification of glenoid fractures. (A) *Type I*: Anterior glenoid rim fractures, (B) *Type II*: Inferior glenoid fractures involving the neck, (C) *Type III*: Superior glenoid fractures extending into the coracoid, (D) *Type IV*: Horizontal fractures involving both the scapular neck and body, (E) *Type V*: Combined fractures of the glenoid and neck.

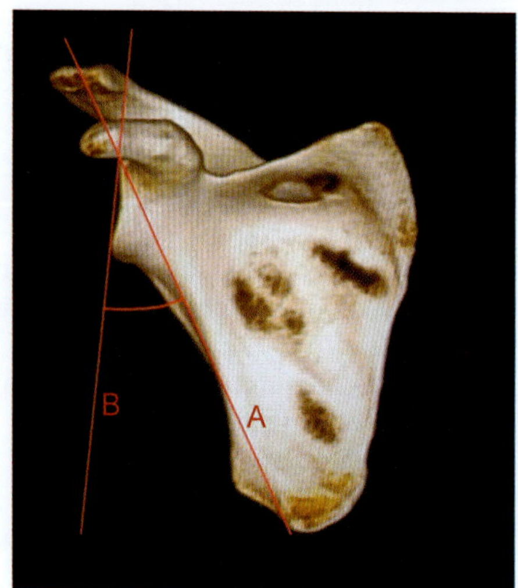

FIG. 4: Glenopolar angle of scapula.

Surgical Approaches

- *Judet posterior approach*: Provides excellent exposure of the infraspinous fossa, lateral and medial borders of the scapula, and the posterior glenoid
- *Anterior deltopectoral approach*: Useful for fractures of the anteroinferior rim of the glenoid and coracoid
- *Extended Judet approach*: Allows treatment of associated clavicular fractures or AC dislocations
- *Posterosuperior approach*: Indicated for isolated fractures of the posterior glenoid or scapular spine
- *Dupont-Evrard posterolateral approach*: Direct access to the lateral scapular border

Operative Management

Fixed by small and mini implants, including 3.5- or 2.7-mm cortical screws, 3.5- or 2.7-mm reconstruction plates, a 3.5-mm semitubular plate, a 3.5-mm T-plate, or a 2.7-mm L- or T-shaped plate, anatomically shaped plates, designed specifically for the scapula **(Fig. 5)**.

Postoperative Protocol

- *Passive range-of-motion exercises*: First postoperative day and continue for about 6 weeks using a CPM machine.
- *Active range-of-motion exercises*: 4–5 weeks postoperatively, depending on the extent of the surgical approach and the presence of other injuries.
- Range of motion is assessed at 6 weeks and, if unsatisfactory, the shoulder is examined under general anesthesia and careful manipulation is performed if necessary.
- Active resistance exercises may be started after about 8 weeks of surgery.
- Full range of motion activities are started around 3 months postoperatively.

MANAGEMENT OF FRACTURES OF SPECIFIC PARTS OF THE SCAPULA

Acromion and Lateral Scapular Spine Fractures

- *Undisplaced fractures*: Treated conservatively with sling immobilization for 3 weeks followed by passive mobilization.
- *Displaced fractures*: If there is a reduction in the subacromial space or impingement on the rotator cuff, open reduction and internal fixation (ORIF) may be necessary.

Coracoid Process Fractures

The management of coracoid process fractures depends on the location and degree of displacement. According to the Ogawa classification:

- *Type I*: Involves fractures at the base of the coracoid. These fractures, particularly if displaced, may require surgical fixation to restore stability to the shoulder girdle.
- *Type II*: Avulsion fractures of the coracoid tip typically occur with AC dislocation and can often be managed nonoperatively.

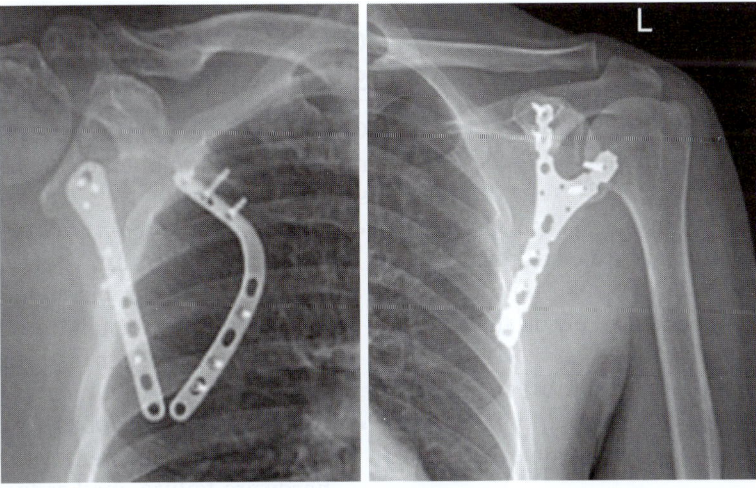

FIG. 5: Radiographs of scapula fractures fixed using plates and screws.

Scapular Neck Fractures

- *Anatomical neck fractures*: Rare, and often treated conservatively unless significant displacement is present
- *Surgical neck fractures*: Often require surgical intervention if there is associated ligament rupture or clavicular displacement

Glenoid Fractures

Glenoid fractures are often complex and may involve significant displacement of the articular surface. Surgical fixation is indicated when the joint surface is disrupted, and stability cannot be achieved through nonoperative means.

COMBINED FRACTURES AND SPECIAL CASES

Floating Shoulder

A floating shoulder occurs when a scapular neck fracture is associated with a clavicular fracture. This injury results in shoulder girdle instability, and operative fixation of the clavicle and scapula is typically recommended to ensure early rehabilitation and reduce the risk of malunion.

Scapulothoracic Dissociation

This is a rare but severe injury that results from violent lateral traction on the scapula, causing massive soft tissue damage, including the avulsion of the scapula from the thorax. Scapulothoracic dissociation is often associated with neurovascular injuries, and the prognosis depends largely on the extent of the assocaited injuries.

Treatment for scapulothoracic dissociation is complex and tailored to the extent of the damage. It typically involves multiple steps:

1. *Initial management*: Based on the Advanced Trauma Life Support (ATLS) protocol
2. Vascular repair
3. Neurological assessment (especially brachial plexuses) and treatment
4. *Orthopedic management*:
   - *Fracture fixation*: If there are associated fractures (e.g., clavicle or scapula), they may require surgical fixation, especially in cases of severe displacement or instability.
   - *Stabilization of the shoulder girdle*: Reconstructing the shoulder girdle function is important for restoring arm mobility. This might include repairing the clavicle or scapula if dislocated.
   - In cases of severe destruction of the shoulder joint or irreparable damage, reconstructive surgeries or even amputation may be considered in the worst scenarios.

Prognosis

The outcome of scapulothoracic dissociation largely depends on the severity of the injury, particularly the extent of vascular and nerve damage. Early recognition and treatment, especially of vascular injuries, improve limb survival, but neurological recovery can be limited in severe cases.

COMPLICATIONS OF SCAPULA FRACTURES

Complications can arise from both nonoperative and operative management of scapula fractures:

- *Nonoperative complications*: These include malunion, delayed union, nonunion, and chronic shoulder pain due to deformity or instability. In addition, nerve injuries such as suprascapular nerve palsy may occur.
- *Operative complications*: Complications of surgery include neurovascular injury, hardware failure, mail reduction, screw perforation, and postoperative issues such as infection, hematoma, or implant failure.

BIBLIOGRAPHY

1. Ada JR, Miller ME. Scapula fractures. Analysis of 113 cases. Clin Orthop Rel Res. 1991;269:174-80.
2. Adam FF. Surgical treatment of displaced fractures of the glenoid cavity. Inter Orthop. 2002;26: 150-3.
3. Althausen PL, Lee MA, Finkemeier CG. Scapulothoracic dissociation: Diagnosis and treatment. Clin Orthop Relat Res. 2003;416: 237-44.
4. Anavian J, Wijdicks CA, Schroder LK, Vang S, Cole PA. Surgery for scapula process fractures: good outcome in 26 patients. Acta Orthop. 2009;80(3):344-50.
5. Baldwin KD, Ohman-Strickland P, Mehta S, Hume E. Scapular fractures: A marker for concomitant injury? A retrospective review of data in the national trauma database. J Trauma. 2008;65(2):430-5.
6. Bartoníček J, Fricˇ V. Scapular body fractures: Results of the operative treatment. Inter Orthop. 2011;35:747-53.
7. Bestard EA, Schvene HR, Bestard EH. Glenoplasty in the management of recurrent shoulder dislocation. Contemp Orthop. 1986;12:47-55.
8. Cameron SE. Arthroscopic reduction and internal fixation of an anterior glenoid fracture. Arthroscopy. 1998;14:743-6.
9. Coimbra R, Conroy C, Tominaga GT, Bansal V, Schwartz A. Causes of scapula fractures differ from other shoulder injuries in occupants seriously injured during motor vehicle crashes. Injury. 2010;41(2):151-5.
10. Cole PA, Gauger EM, Schroder LK. Management of scapular fractures. J Am Acad Orthop Surg. 2012;20:130-41.

SECTION

3

Humerus

CHAPTER 3.1

Shoulder Dislocation

Hayat Khan

The shoulder is the most common dislocating joint of the body. It is not a true ball and socket joint and the geometry is often compared with the golf-ball model. The inherently unstable nature of the joint makes it dependent on the anterior and posterior restraints (both static and dynamic). And the nature of force makes it traumatic or atraumatic.

TRAUMATIC DISLOCATION

Anterior Dislocation

It occurs most commonly due to a fall on an abducted, externally rotated shoulder.

Diagnosis

- *Clinical:* Anteriorly palpable shoulder with empty glenoid (Hamilton ruler test), painful attempted movements with arm in the abduction and external rotation. Usually, patient holds it when presenting to an emergency.
- *X-ray:* Anteroposterior (AP) view of the shoulder will usually show an overlap of the humeral head over the glenoid.

  In normal X-rays, the glenohumeral joint can be seen with clear space **(Figs. 1A to C)**.

Other views are:
- True AP **(Fig. 2)**
- Scapular Y view **(Fig. 3)**
- Axillary view **(Figs. 4A and B)**

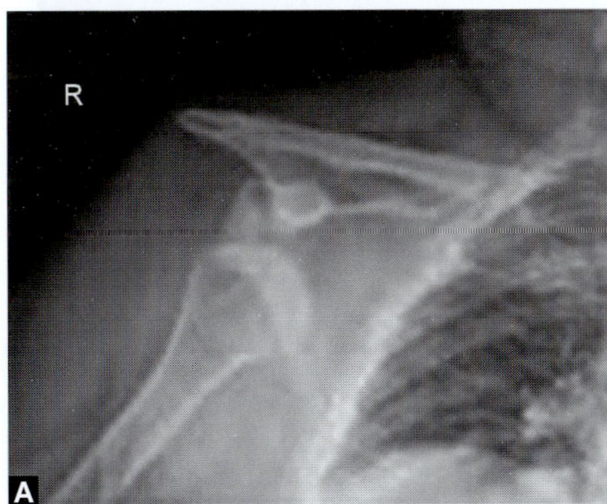

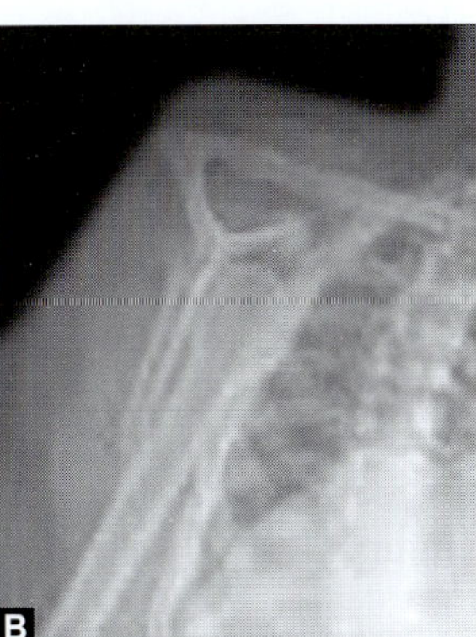

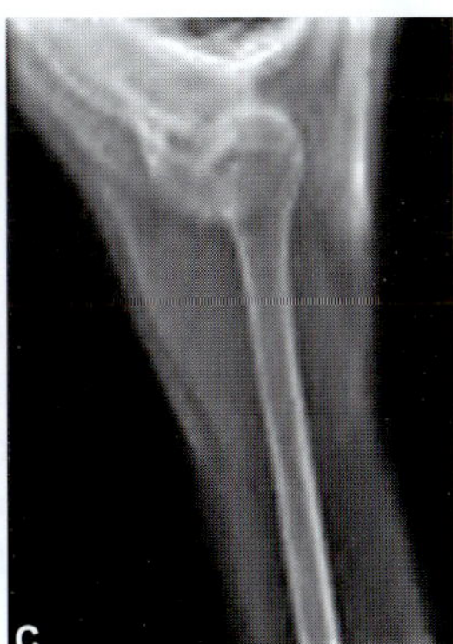

FIGS. 1A TO C: X-rays showing (A) anteroposterior (AP); (B) scapular Y view; and (C) axillary view.

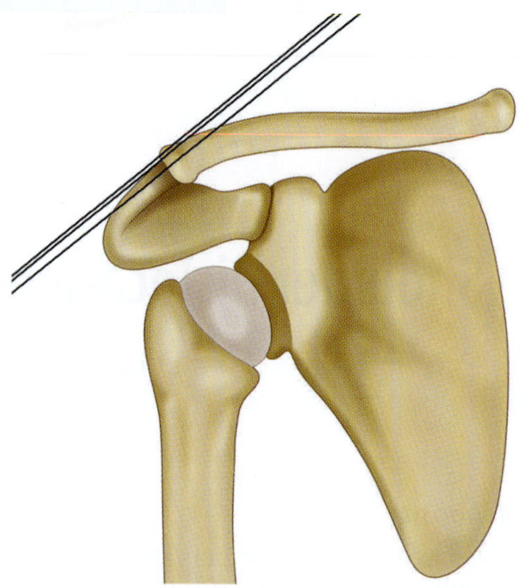

FIG. 2: True anteroposterior (AP) view—45°. Angulated to lateral side to get the beam in line with the scapula. Patient may be sitting, lying, or standing.

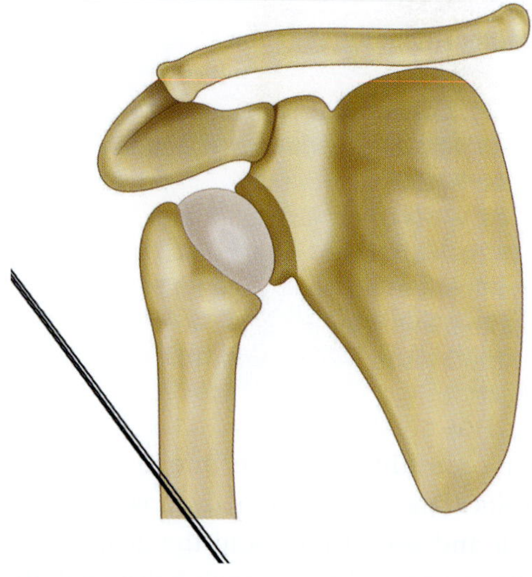

FIG. 3: Beam aimed with 10° caudal tilt with affected shoulder against X-ray plate. Scapular Y view (lateral view).

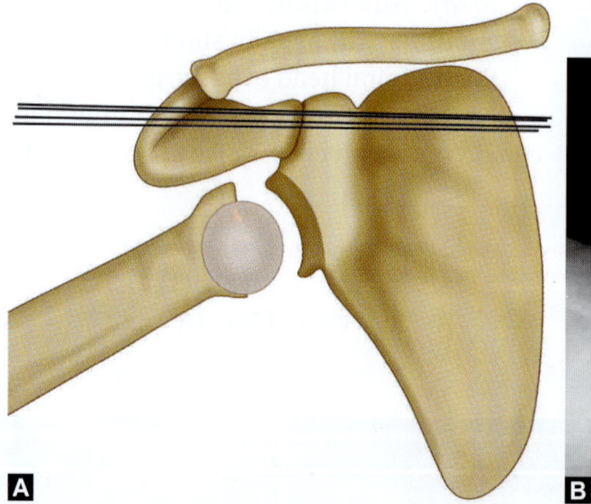

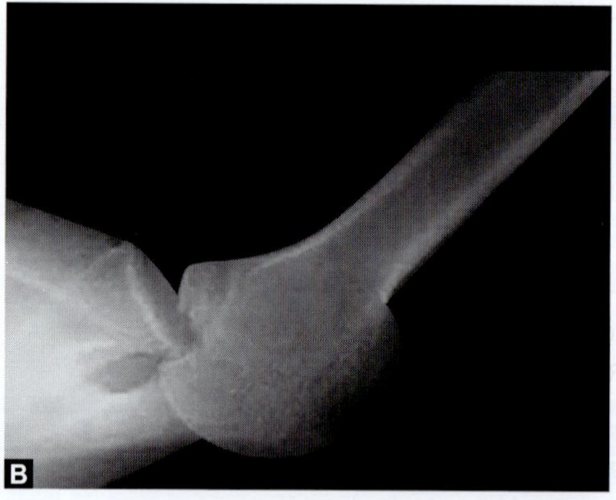

FIGS. 4A AND B: Axillary view: To see the relation of humeral head with glenoid and Hill–Sach lesion.

- *Computed tomography (CT) scan:* CT scan is a must in cases of fracture-dislocations
- *Magnetic resonance imaging (MRI):* Visualizes the labrum, cartilage, Hill-Sachs and rotator cuff injuries

Associated Injuries

- Greater tuberosity fracture **(Figs. 5A and B)**
- Bankart lesion [anterior labrum and inferior glenohumeral ligament (IGHL)]
- Humeral avulsion glenohumeral ligament (HAGL)
    - Associated with a high recurrence rate
    - Indication for open repair
- Glenoid labral articular defect
- Anterior labral periosteal sleeve avulsion
- Bony Bankart anterior labrum and IGHL
- Hill–Sachs defect (80% cases)

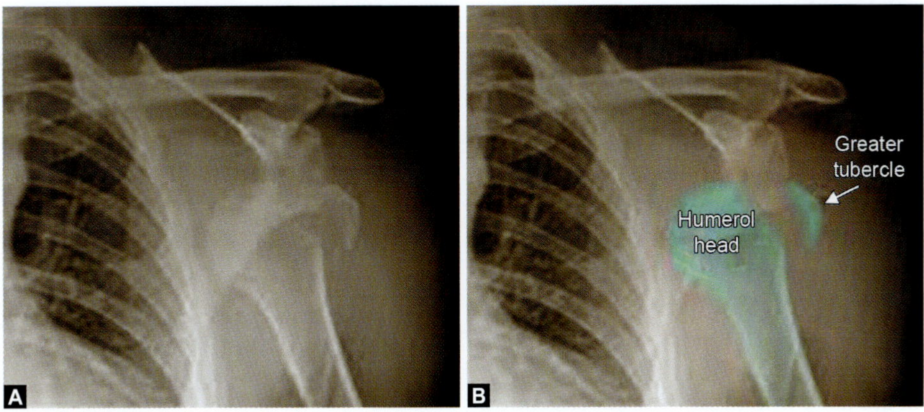

FIGS. 5A AND B: Shoulder dislocation associated with greater tuberosity fracture.

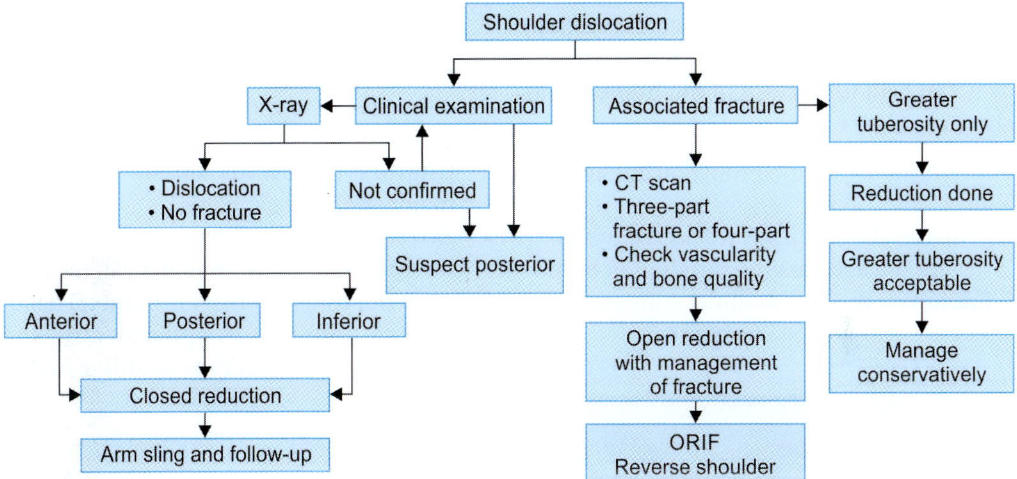

FLOWCHART 1: Treatment algorithm for shoulder dislocation with or without fractures.
(ORIF: open reduction and internal fixation)

- Rotator cuff tears (should be ruled out if age >40 years and 80% cases occur above age 60 years.)
- The axillary nerve in jury (neuropraxia)

Treatment

Closed reduction is the treatment of choice, but never ever try reduction without having seen the X-rays. At times, there may be fracture dislocation, mostly undisplaced fracture, and the close reduction can completely displace an undisplaced fracture that can have a significant negative impact on the eventual outcome. An algorithm-based approach is given in **Flowchart 1**.

Multiple maneuvers for close reduction are available.

Master the most commonly used Kocher's maneuver.

- *Kocher's method:* It is done by flexing the elbow first then adducting and externally rotating the shoulder to unlock it, followed by flexion abduction and internal rotation.
- *Traction/Countertraction method*: Traction is applied to the affected arm while the assistant gives the countertraction with a cloth through the axilla.

- *Milch technique:* External rotation is done while abducting the arm. The head is guided to the glenoid with the other hand.
- *Stimson method:* It is not so famous. Prone the patient and apply weight to the affected shoulder through the arm.
- *Vertical traction method:* Apply vertical traction to the affected shoulder. Externally rotate the head and guide it with the other hand. It can be used in chest trauma patients.

All are used with promising success rates.

Make sure that the patient has full muscle relaxation preferably under short general anesthesia (GA) and under image-intensifier guidance. However, avoid forceful rotation, especially in old age osteoporotic patients, as it can lead to fracture of the humerus, as shown in **Figure 6**.

Postreduction: Confirm reduction by checking X-rays.

An arm sling for a few weeks is advised.

More the age, less the duration of immobilization, to prevent shoulder stiffness.

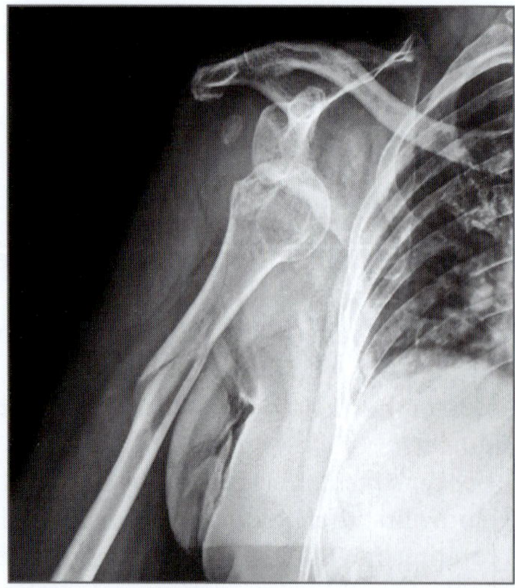

FIG. 6: An example of fracture humerus after an attempted before forceful reduction of dislocation.

Open Reduction

Irreducible anterior shoulder dislocations are rare usually due to interposed soft tissue or associated fractures.

Approach: Deltopectoral approach

Posterior Shoulder Dislocation

Incidence: These injuries amount to 10% of shoulder dislocations, often missed by primary care and emergency physicians (80% missed on initial examination).

Mechanism of Injury

The shoulder is in adduction, internal rotation, and flexion.

- *Indirect trauma*: Electric shock and convulsions are the two main causes of posterior dislocation, possibly due to forceful contraction of the internal rotators (latissmus dorsi, pectoralis major, and subscapularis).
- *Direct trauma:* Direct application of the force to the anterior shoulder can result in posterior translation of the humeral head.

(Please note that in epilepsy also, the most common dislocation is still anterior dislocation)

Diagnosis

- *Clinical examination*:
    - Flattening of the anterior axillary fold (very difficult to appreciate)
    - Posteriorly palpable head around the glenoid as compared to the other side (again, difficult to interpret)
    - Lack of external rotation is the key physical examination finding in fixed posterior dislocations.
- *Radiology*:
    - *AP shoulder:* The typical *bulb* sign is pathognomic but not always present.
    - *Axillary view:* Shows a posterior dislocated head with reverse Hill-Sachs lesion.

- *CT scan confirms dislocation:* Can measure the percentage of reverse Hill-Sachs lesion and also see any associated fracture.

Treatment

Closed reduction: Apply traction in 90° of arm abduction.

Open reduction: If closed, reduction fails.

Approach: Posterior Judet approach

Inferior Shoulder Dislocation (Luxatio Erecta)

Inferior shoulder dislocation is caused by hyperabduction injury (between 100° and 160°). The head of the humerus is levered against the acromion causing the inferior dislocation.

Clinical Examination

- Salute position of the shoulder with arm in abduction and forward elevation
- Diminished pulses or absent pulses.
- *Radiology*:
    - *X-rays:* Shoulder AP view is usually diagnostic with inferior humeral head (dislocated) and upward direction of the shaft.

Treatment

- Traction-countertraction method
- Arm sling as in other shoulder dislocations
- Check vascularity.

DISLOCATION OF SHOULDER WITH FRACTURE

Fracture dislocations are often seen in elderly patients with osteoporotic bones.

Closed reduction is often difficult and should not be tried, as the traction forces are not transmitted to the head directly. Meanwhile, it can create a displaced fracture in an undisplaced fracture **(Fig. 7)**.

CT scan helps to assess the fracture pattern and to decide on the definitive treatment.

Such cases are often treated with open reduction and internal fixation or hemiarthoplasty or reverse shoulder arthroplasty (if bone quality is poor or communication).

Postreduction management: For rehabilitation and follow-up after reduction please refer to the **Flowchart 2**.

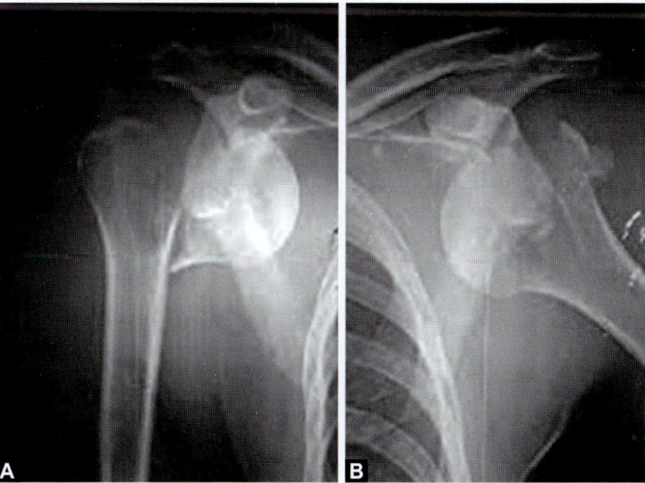

FIGS. 7A AND B: Fracture dislocation of shoulder.

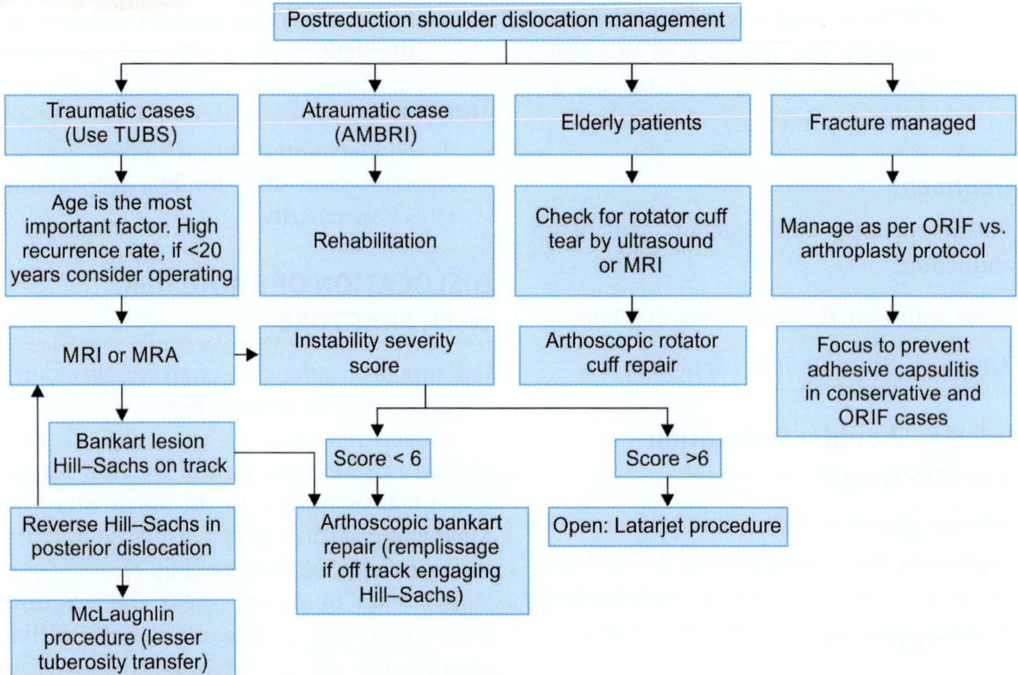

FLOWCHART 2: Treatment algorithm for shoulder dislocation management, postreduction.

(AMBRI: atraumatic, multidirectional, bilateral, rehabilitation, inferior capsular shift; MRA: magnetic resonance angiography; MRI: magnetic resonance imaging; TUBS: traumatic, unilateral, Bankart lesion, surgery)

BIBLIOGRAPHY

1. De Laat EA, Visser CP, Coene LN, Pahlplatz PV, Tavy DL. Nerve lesions in primary shoulder dislocations and humeral neck fractures. A prospective clinical and EMG study. J Bone Joint Surg Br. 1994;76(3):381-3.
2. Dodson CC, Cordasco FA. Anterior glenohumeral joint dislocations. Orthop Clin North Am. 2008;39(4):507-18.
3. Dyrna FGE, Ludwig M, Imhoff AB, Martetschläger F. Off-track Hill-Sachs lesions predispose to recurrence after nonoperative management of first-time anterior shoulder dislocations. Knee Surg Sports Traumatol Arthrosc. 2021;29(7):2289-96.
4. Gottlieb M, Holladay D, Peksa GD. Point-of-care ultrasound for diagnosing shoulder dislocation: A systematic review and meta-analysis. Am J Emerg Med. 2019;37(4):757-61.
5. Polyzois I, Dattani R, Gupta R, Levy O, Narvani AA. Traumatic first-time shoulder dislocation: Surgery vs non-operative treatment. Arch Bone Jt Surg. 2016;4(2):104-8.
6. Simank HG, Dauer G, Schneider S, Loew M. Incidence of rotator cuff tears in shoulder dislocations and results of therapy in older patients. Arch Orthop Trauma Surg. 2006;126(4):235-40.

Proximal Humerus Fracture

Hayat Khan

The fractures of the anatomical neck, surgical neck, greater tuberosity, and lesser tuberosity are included in the proximal humerus fractures.

EPIDEMIOLOGY

They can occur in combination or in isolation. They constitute nearly 6% of all adult fractures and are third most common fractures in the elderly. The risk factors include osteopenia or osteoporosis (female gender).

ATTACHMENTS

Table 1 shows the attachments and the deforming forces acting upon the proximal humerus.

The involvement of one or more fracture lines (segments) usually determines the final deformity pattern.

- Blood supply to the humeral head
- Anterior humeral circumflex artery
- Posterior humeral circumflex artery. (Newer data is in favor of the posterior humeral circumflex artery.)
- *Nerve supply:* The axillary nerve is the main nerve supply. It lies proximal to the inferior capsule and is at risk of anterior dislocations.

TABLE 1: Deforming forces.

Segment involved	Displacement	Deforming force
Greater tuberosity	Displaced superiorly and posteriorly	Supraspinatus External rotators
Lesser tuberosity	Displaced medially	Subscapularis
Shaft	Displaced medially	• Pectoralis major • Latissimus dorsi
Deltoid tuberosity (depending upon the fracture)	Abducted	• Lateral fibers of deltoid are abductors • Anterior fibers cause forward flexion

DIAGNOSIS

- *X-rays* in anteroposterior (AP) and axial (or velpeau) views are usually enough for the initial diagnosis. It helps in classifying the proximal humerus fractures and to make the treatment plan regarding the type of fracture.
- *CT scan* provides more information regarding the fracture pattern and helps

in preoperative planning. It is mostly used in type 3 and type 4 fractures and to rule out any glenoid fracture in fracture dislocations.
- *MRI* is rarely used to assess the soft-tissue components like rotator cuff tears.

CLASSIFICATION

Neer's Classification

One-part Fracture

One-part fracture is when the fracture is present between any of the segments but is neither displaced nor angulated. 70–80% of the proximal humerus fractures fall in this category.

Please note that displacement of <1 cm and angulation of <45° is regarded as undisplaced/minimally displaced and is considered as one (single part) as per Neer's criteria.

Two-part Fractures

The fracture line involves 2–4 segments and one part is displaced, i.e., >45° and/or >1 cm.

These account for around 15–20% of fractures.

Examples:
- Surgical neck fractures (most common)/ anatomic neck fractures (less common)
- *Greater tuberosity fracture:* Mostly associated with anterior shoulder dislocation.
- Isolated lesser tuberosity fractures are uncommon.

Three-part Fractures

The fracture line involves three to four parts and two parts are displaced (>1 cm and > 45°).

These fractures account for 5% of proximal humerus fractures.

Greater tuberosity and shaft are displaced with respect to lesser tuberosity and articular surface (more common pattern) or lesser tuberosity and shaft are displaced with respect to the greater tuberosity and articular surface **(Fig. 1)**.

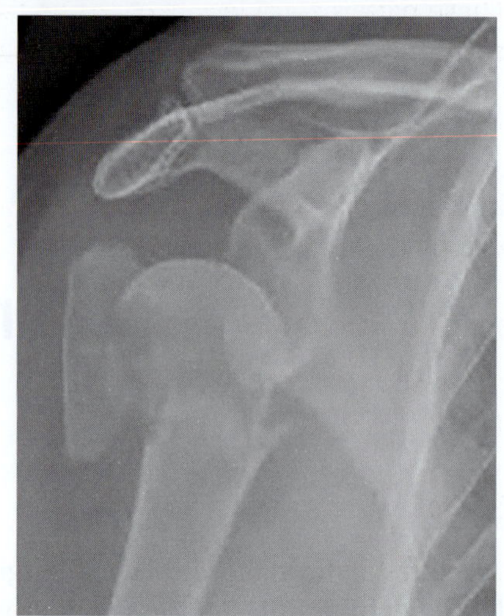

FIG. 1: Three-part fracture of the proximal humerus.

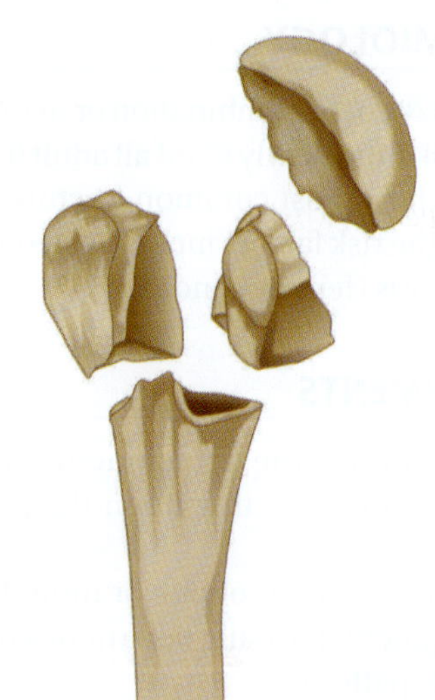

FIG. 2: Four-part fracture pattern.
Source: Dr Hayat Khan.

Four-part Fractures

Fracture involves four segments **(Fig. 2)**.

Three parts are displaced (i.e., >1 cm and >45°) with respect to the 4th part.

These patterns are less likely to be fixed owing to the low vascularity of the articular segment and are prone to osteonecrosis. Please note that due to comminution and different fracture patterns, it becomes difficult to differentiate between type 3 and type 4 fractures and a CT scan is advised in such cases.

Other Classifications

AO classification of proximal humerus fractures.

TREATMENT

One-part Fracture

Conservation management:
- Cuff and collar sling/arm sling
- *Close follow-up:* Check for displacement.

Two-part Fractures

Conservative or operative treatment depends on the fracture displacement.

Operative treatment: Closed reduction with percutaneous pinning (CRPP) is used in selective cases. Complications include musculocutaneous nerve injury, biceps tendon injury with anterior pins, and axillary nerve injury with lateral pins **(Fig. 3)**.
- ORIF PHILOS: The proximal humerus interlocking osteosynthesis (PHILOS) **(Fig. 4)**.

Three-part Fractures

Treatment depends on bone stock and vascularity **(Table 2)**.

Open reduction and internal fixation (ORIF) with a locked plate is typically performed when there is adequate vascularity and bone stock to support the procedure. Locked plates provide stable fixation, particularly in cases where the bone quality is poor or there is a risk of poor healing, such as in osteoporotic bones **(Table 2 and Box 1)**.

Approach: Deltopectoral approach.

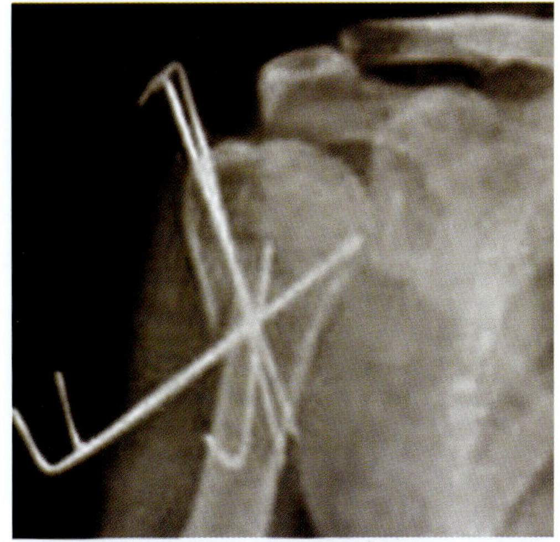

FIG. 3: Percutaneous fixation with K wires.

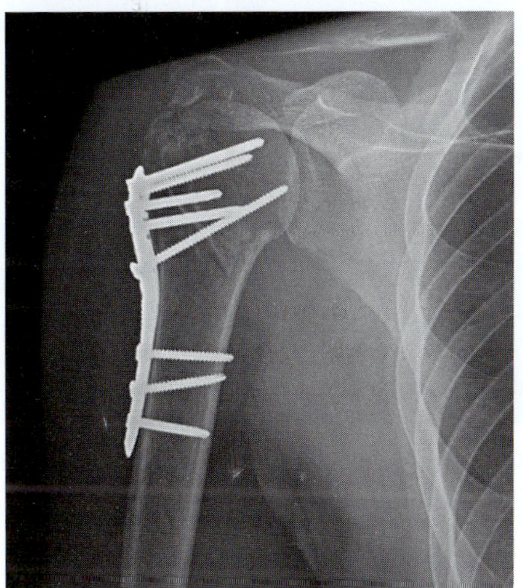

FIG. 4: Fracture fixation with proximal humerus interlocking osteosynthesis (PHILOS).

TABLE 2: Treatment options depending on bone stock and vascularity.

Bone stock	Vascularity	Treatment
Good	Good	ORIF
Good	Not promising	Consider ORIF
Not good	Good	Consider ORIF
Poor	Poor	Arthroplasty

(ORIF: open reduction and internal fixation)

BOX 1 Vascularity predictors.

Vascularity prediction:
- Short medial calcar (< 8 mm)
- Disrupted medial hinge
- Fracture type
- Head angulation > 45°
- Tuberosity displacement
- Head split.

Source: Hertel R, Hempfing A, Stiehler M, Leunig M. Predictors of humeral head ischemia after intracapsular fracture of the proximal humerus. J Shoulder Elbow Surg. 2004;13(4):427-33

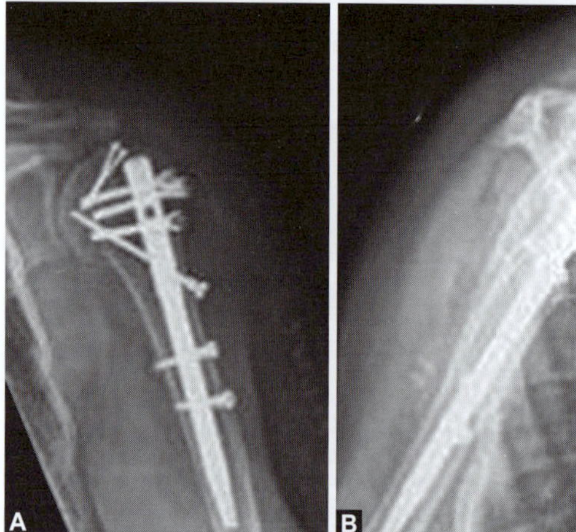

FIGS. 5A AND B: Fracture fixation done with intramedullary (IM) nail.

Four-part Fractures

- Minimally displaced fractures in low-demand patients are managed nonoperatively.
- Displaced valgus fractures with good vascularity are managed with ORIF.
- Younger patients with poor vascularity are treated with hemiarthroplasty
- Other options include multilocking nail, again depends upon the bone quality and amount of displacement **(Figs. 5A and B)**.
- Older patients with poor vascularity need reverse shoulder arthroplasty (RSA). Tuberosity repair can be added to enhance external rotation **(Fig. 6)**.

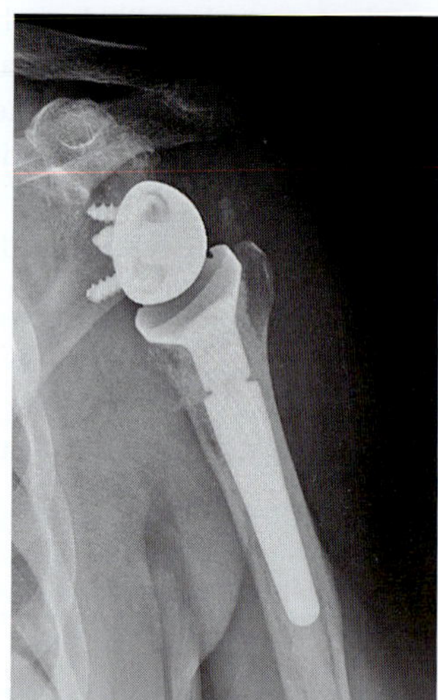

FIG. 6: Reverse shoulder arthroplasty in an elderly female.

COMPLICATIONS OF PROXIMAL HUMERAL FRACTURES

The complications involved are as follows:
- *Malunion:* Results in varus collapse causing restricted abduction and impingement. Tuberosity malunions are more difficult to correct, they may also cause external rotation restriction (posterior) or impingement (superior).
- *Nonunion*: It is caused mostly in surgical neck fractures and unstable fractures.

  Treat with ORIF with bone grafting/ hemi or reverse shoulder arthroplasty.
- *Osteonecrosis [avascular necrosis (AVN)]:* Total or partial damage to the humeral head.

  Generally, well tolerated if anatomy is restored.
- *Post-traumatic arthritis:* Hardware-related problems in operated cases; cut out/screw penetration into the joint
- *Neurovascular injury*: Infection in operated cases (rare as compared to other

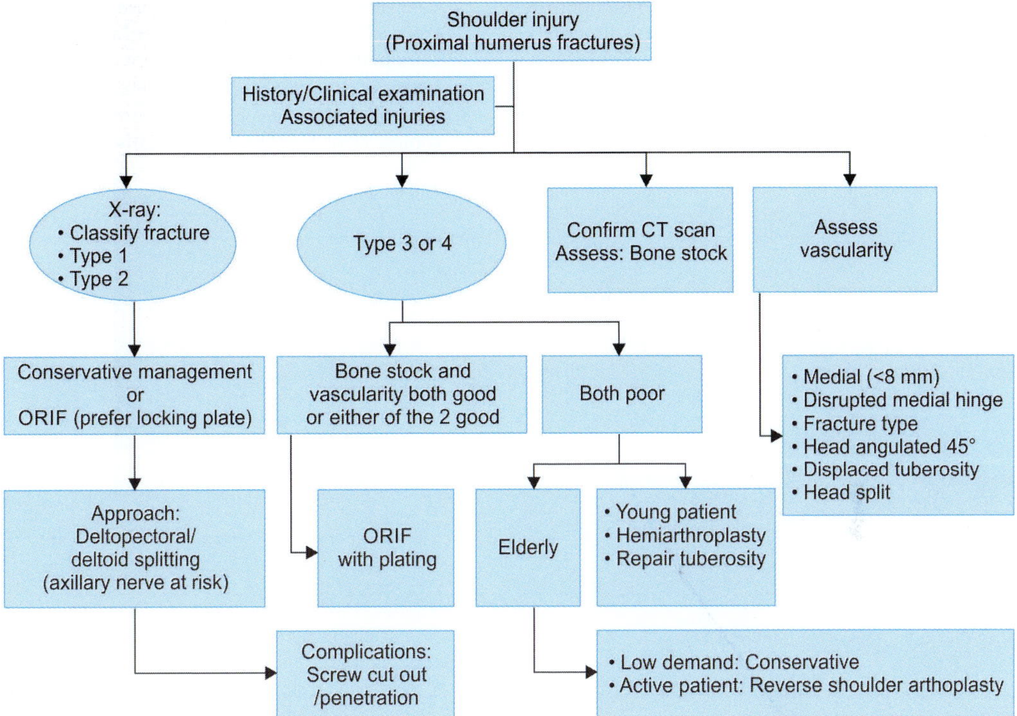

FLOWCHART 1: Treatment algorithm for proximal humerus fractures.
(ORIF: open reduction and internal fixation)

joints); often with axillary commensal (*Propionibacterium acnes*).

The treatment algorithm for the management of proximal humerus fractures is helpful in management **(Flowchart 1)**.

REHABILITATION

Counseling the patient regarding the fracture pattern and the treatment options is one of the important factors to determine the functional outcome.

- *Early period:* Arm sling, pain management, and guided movements including passive assisted movements
- *Late period:* Stretching and strengthening exercises should be started once the signs of clinical and radiological healing are present.

BIBLIOGRAPHY

1. Aiyer A, Varacallo M, Boateng H, Reid JS. Humeral shaft fracture with ipsilateral anterior shoulder dislocation and posterior elbow dislocation: A case report and review of the literature. JBJS Case Connect. 2014;4(3):e77.
2. Court-Brown CM, Caesar B. Epidemiology of adult fractures: A review. Injury. 2006;37(8):691-7.
3. Donnally III CJ, DiPompeo CM, Varacallo M. In: StatPearls [Internet]. Treasure Island (FL): StatPearls Publishing. Available from: https://www.ncbi.nlm.nih.gov/books/NBK448171/ [Last accessed November, 2024].
4. Kim SH, Szabo RM, Marder RA. Epidemiology of humerus fractures in the United States: Nationwide emergency department sample, 2008. Arthritis Care Res (Hoboken). 2012;64(3):407-14.
5. Porter JL, Varacallo M. Osteoporosis. In: StatPearls [Internet]. Treasure Island (FL): StatPearls Publishing. Available from: https://www.ncbi.nlm.nih.gov/books/NBK441901/ [Last accessed November, 2024].

6. Varacallo M, Davis DD, Pizzutillo P. Osteoporosis in Spinal Cord Injuries. In: StatPearls [Internet]. Treasure Island (FL): StatPearls Publishing. Available from: https://www.ncbi.nlm.nih.gov/books/NBK526109/ [Last accessed November, 2024].
7. Varacallo MA, Fox EJ, Paul EM, Hassenbein SE, Warlow PM. Patients' response toward an automated orthopedic osteoporosis intervention program. Geriatr Orthop Surg Rehabil. 2013;4(3):89-98.
8. Varacallo MA, Fox EJ. Osteoporosis and its complications. Med Clin North Am. 2014;98(4):817-31.

Greater Tuberosity Fracture

Hayat Khan

The greater tuberosity is located laterally on the proximal humerus and serves as the insertion site for the supraspinatus, infraspinatus, and teres minor tendons.

MECHANISM OF INJURY

Greater tuberosity fractures are often associated with direct trauma to the shoulder, such as a fall onto an outstretched arm or they may occur in conjunction with anterior shoulder dislocations. In younger, active individuals, these fractures typically result from high-energy mechanisms. In contrast, elderly patients, particularly those with osteoporotic bone, often sustain these fractures from low-energy trauma.

CLASSIFICATION OF GREATER TUBEROSITY FRACTURES

The classification of greater tuberosity fractures has traditionally been based on the degree of displacement and fragment size, guiding treatment decisions.

- *Nondisplaced fractures:* Displacement < 5 mm
- *Minimally displaced fractures:* Displacement between 5 and 10 mm
- *Displaced fractures:* Greater than 10 mm of displacement, usually indicating a need for surgical intervention.

Recent studies have suggested that even fractures with displacement as low as 3–5 mm can result in poor functional outcomes if left untreated, particularly in active patients.

TREATMENT

The treatment of greater tuberosity fractures is influenced by several factors, including:

- Degree of displacement
- Patient age and activity level
- Bone quality
- *Associated injuries:* Rotator cuff tears, shoulder dislocations, or other soft-tissue injuries often accompany greater tuberosity fractures, complicating treatment.
- *Patient expectations and comorbidities:* Elderly or low-demand patients may benefit from more conservative treatment **(Flowchart 1)**.

Nonoperative Management

Nonoperative treatment remains the standard of care for nondisplaced or minimally displaced fractures (displacement < 5 mm). These fractures are typically stable, and conservative management allows for predictable healing with good functional outcomes in selected patients **(Figs. 1A and B)**.

Principles of Nonoperative Management

- The initial phase involves 2–4 weeks of immobilization in a sling or shoulder immobilizer.
- After 2–4 weeks, depending on pain and radiographic evidence of stability,

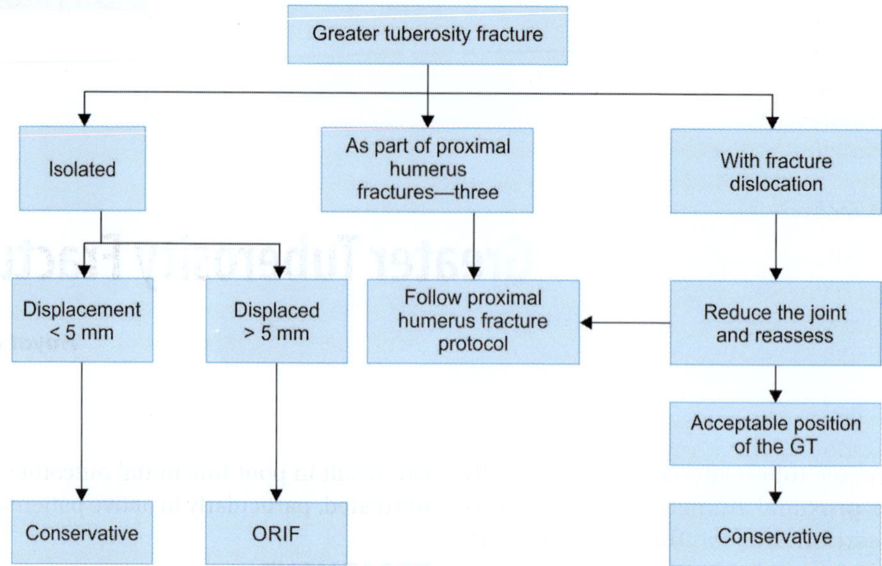

FLOWCHART 1: Treatment algorithm for greater tuberosity fractures.
(GT: greater tuberosity; ORIF: open reduction and internal fixation)

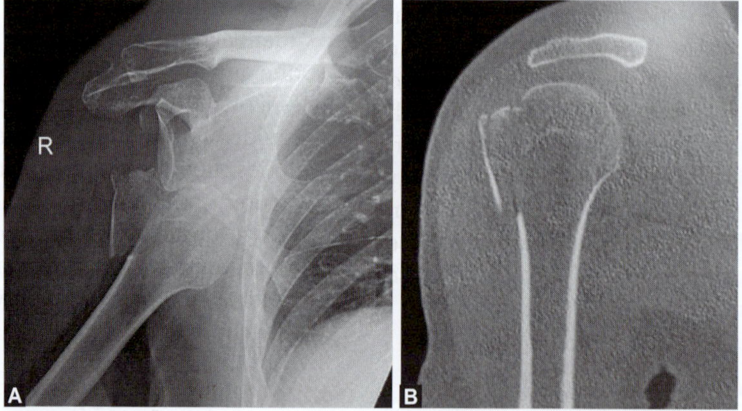

FIGS. 1A AND B: Greater tuberosity fracture before and after the reduction of shoulder dislocation.

passive range-of-motion (ROM) exercises are initiated to prevent joint stiffness. Gentle exercises focus on maintaining mobility without stressing the fracture site.

- By 4–6 weeks, once clinical and radiographic signs of healing are evident, active ROM exercises are introduced. Strengthening of the rotator cuff and periscapular muscles typically begins at 6–8 weeks.

Operative Management

Indications for surgery are:

- Displacement greater than 5 mm, particularly when exceeding 10 mm
- Presence of rotator cuff tears or other soft-tissue injuries
- Progressive displacement or nonunion following conservative treatment
- High-demand patients (e.g., athletes and manual laborers) with functional requirements

- In cases where conservative treatment fails (e.g., persistent pain, loss of function, or secondary displacement), surgery may be required to restore normal anatomy and function.

Surgical Techniques

Various surgical techniques are as follows:

- *Open reduction and internal fixation (ORIF):* ORIF remains the gold standard for displaced greater tuberosity fractures. The procedure typically involves anatomic reduction of the fracture fragment followed by fixation with screws, plates, or suture anchors. ORIF ensures stable fixation, allowing for early rehabilitation and reduced risk of malunion **(Figs. 2A to C)**.
- *Arthroscopic-assisted fixation:* Arthroscopy provides excellent visualization of the rotator cuff and allows for precise fracture reduction. Suture anchors are frequently used for fixation. Arthroscopy is especially useful in managing concomitant rotator cuff pathology **(Figs. 3A to D)**.
- *Percutaneous fixation:* For minimally displaced fractures or fractures in osteoporotic bone, percutaneous fixation with K wires or cannulated screws may be an option **(Figs. 4A and B)**. This technique is less invasive but requires careful patient selection, as the risk of instability is higher and there is a risk of wire loosening and redisplacement.
- *Hemiarthroplasty or preferably reverse shoulder arthroplasty (RSA)*: In elderly patients with osteoporotic bone or comminuted fractures, RSA may be considered. This option is typically reserved for complex fracture patterns or cases with rotator cuff arthropathy, where restoring function through traditional fixation may not be possible. RSA has shown promise in elderly patients with poor bone quality and high functional demands.

Postoperative Rehabilitation

A rehabilitation protocol typically includes:

- A brief period of immobilization (2–3 weeks) to protect the surgical repair
- Early passive ROM exercises to prevent stiffness
- Gradual strengthening exercises targeting the rotator cuff and scapular stabilizers, typically beginning at 6–8 weeks postoperatively
- Full functional recovery, including a return to sport or labor, is expected at around 3–6 months, depending on fracture severity and patient compliance with rehabilitation.

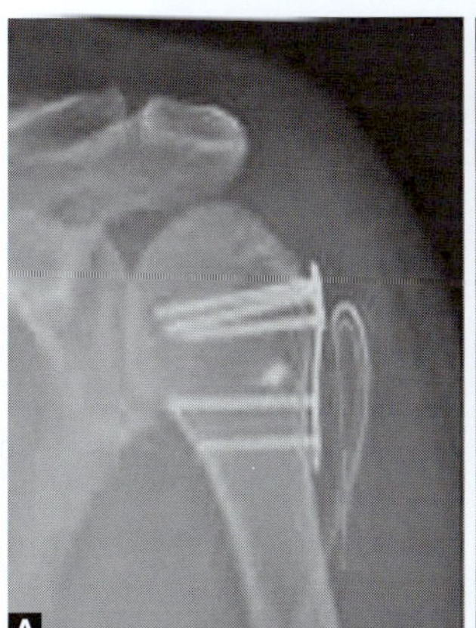

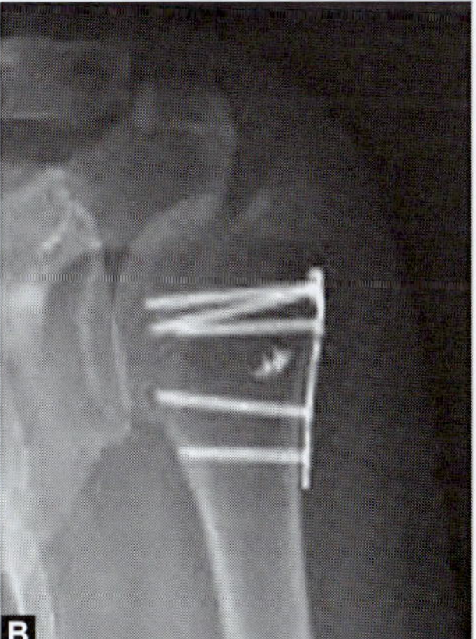

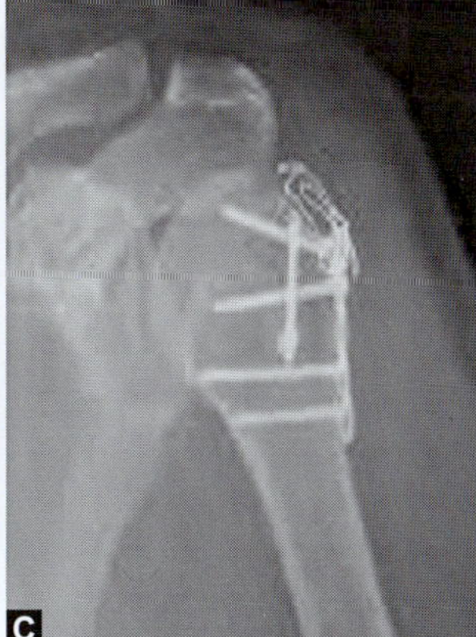

FIGS. 2A TO C: Fracture fixation with plate and screws.

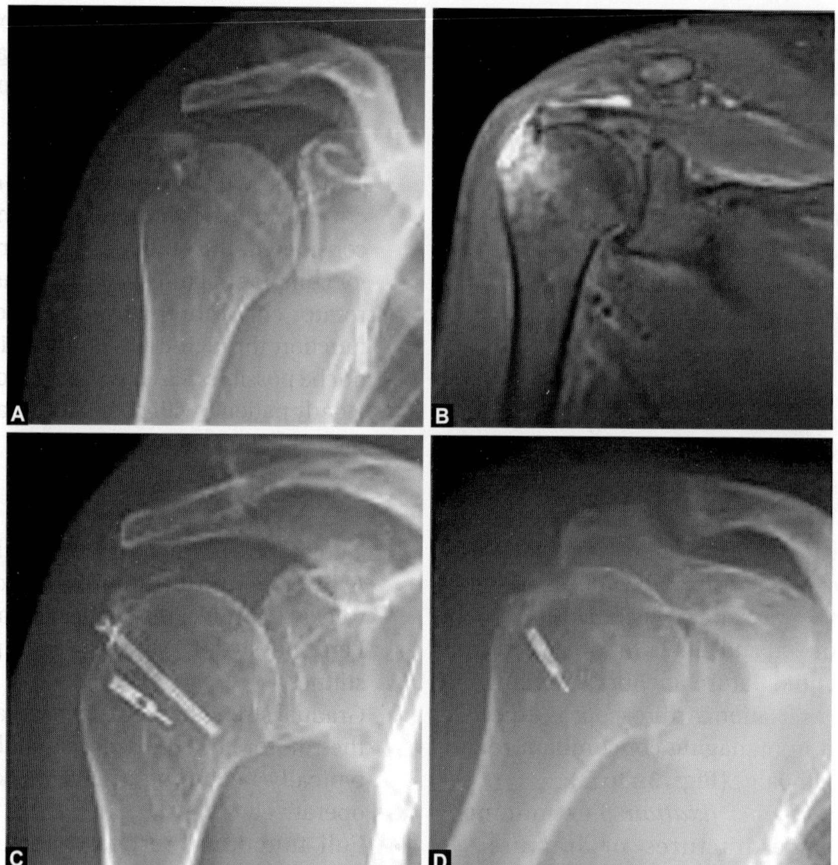

FIGS. 3A TO D: Fracture fixation with arthroscopy-assisted screws and anchors.

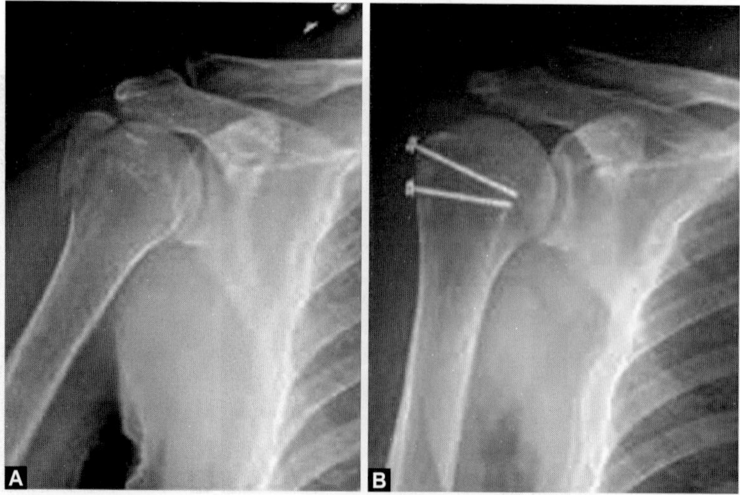

FIGS. 4A AND B: Fracture fixation with percutaneous cannulated screws.

COMPLICATIONS

The complications include:

- Nonunion or malunion
- Post-traumatic stiffness
- Rotator cuff dysfunction
- *Hardware failure:* Surgical fixation hardware, such as screws or plates, may become loose or cause irritation, necessitating revision surgery or hardware removal.
- *Infection:* As with any surgical procedure, infection is a potential risk, particularly in open fractures or patients with comorbidities like diabetes.

BIBLIOGRAPHY

1. Grubhofer F, Wieser K, Meyer DC, Catanzaro S, Schürholz K, Gerber C. Management of fractures of the proximal humerus: Shoulder expert group consensus statement. J Shoulder Elbow Surg. 2016;25(10):1740-50.
2. Park JS, Park JW, Kim YS, Kim MS, Oh JH. Non-displaced and minimally displaced isolated greater tuberosity fractures were treated non-operatively in patients younger than 50. J Shoulder Elbow Surg. 2019;28(5):982-9.
3. Platzer P, Kutscha-Lissberg F, Lehr S, Vecsei V, Gaebler C. The influence of displacement on shoulder function in patients with minimally displaced fractures of the greater tuberosity. Injury. 2005;36(10):1185-9.
4. Rouleau DM, Balg F, Dahan P, Petit Y. Fractures of the greater tuberosity of the humerus: A clinical and radiological review. J Shoulder Elbow Surg. 2011;20(3):538-44.

CHAPTER 3.4

Fracture Shaft of Humerus

Sumeet Singh Charak

EPIDEMIOLOGY

Incidence:
- Represents 3–5% of all fractures; 20% of humeral fractures involve the shaft.
- 60% of this fracture occurs in patients over 50 years old; bimodal distribution with high-energy trauma in younger patients (peak in third decade) and low-energy falls in elderly osteopenic patients.
- 70% occur in men under 50 years and 70% in women over 50 years.
- 30% of this fracture occurs in the proximal third, 60% in the middle third (most common), and 10% in the distal third of the humeral shaft.
- Contributing factors include previous fractures, smoking (in men), advanced age, and osteoporosis.

MECHANISM OF INJURY

The mechanism of injury is given as follows:
- Ground-level falls (60%) are the most common cause.
- Motor vehicle accidents (30%) are the second most common cause.
- Proximal fractures often result from falls onto an outstretched hand.
- Middle fractures can result from direct blows or torsional forces.
- Distal fractures usually result from falls onto a flexed elbow.

ASSOCIATED INJURIES

Associated injuries are as follows:
- *Floating elbow:* Fracture of the humeral shaft with proximal to middle radius and ulna fractures; more common in pediatric patients.
- *Ipsilateral shoulder dislocation:* Typically posterior

ANATOMY

The anatomy upper arm is illustrated in **Figure 1**.

CLASSIFICATION

The major systems of classification are given as follows:
- *Arbeitsgemeinschaft für Osteosynthesefragen (AO)/Orthopedic Trauma Association (OTA) classification*: It is based on bone number, fracture location, and pattern (simple, wedge, and complex) **(Fig. 2)**.
- *Other classification*:
    - Garnavos classification
    - *Holstein-Lewis fracture:* It is spiral fracture of the distal humeral shaft, often associated with radial nerve neuropraxia **(Fig. 3)**.

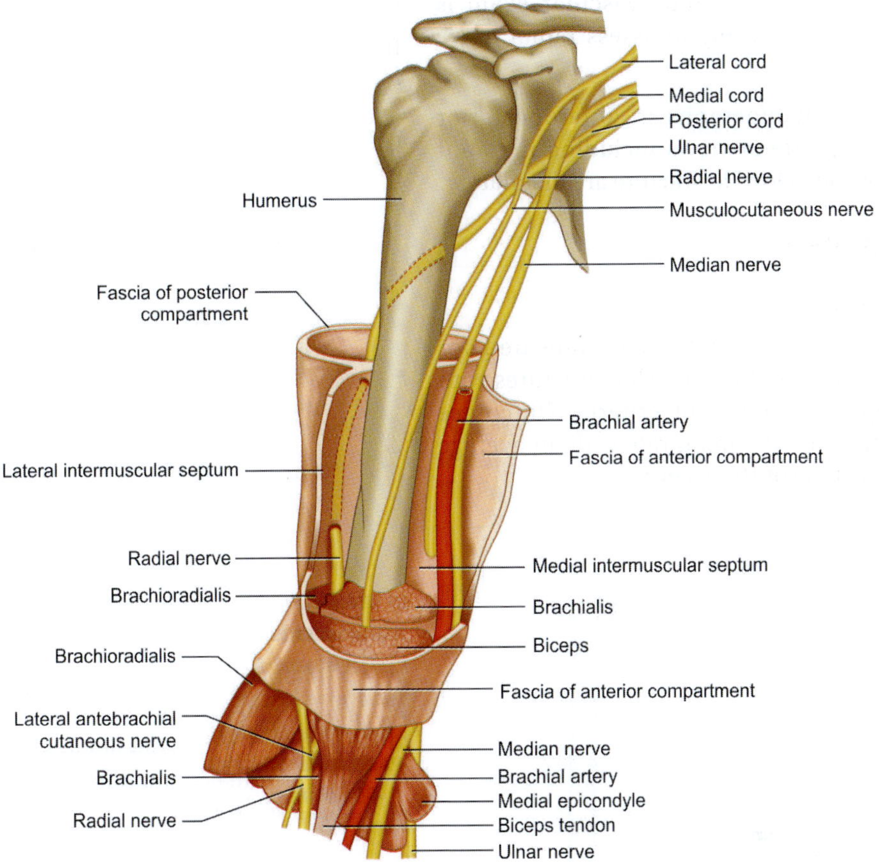

Lateral cord
Medial cord
Posterior cord
Ulnar nerve
Radial nerve
Musculocutaneous nerve
Median nerve
Humerus
Fascia of posterior compartment
Brachial artery
Fascia of anterior compartment
Lateral intermuscular septum
Radial nerve
Medial intermuscular septum
Brachioradialis
Brachialis
Biceps
Brachioradialis
Fascia of anterior compartment
Lateral antebrachial cutaneous nerve
Median nerve
Brachialis
Brachial artery
Medial epicondyle
Radial nerve
Biceps tendon
Ulnar nerve

FIG. 1: The neurovascular anatomy of upper arm.

12-A1
12-A2
12-A3
12-B1
12-B2
12-B3
12-C1
12-C2
12-C3

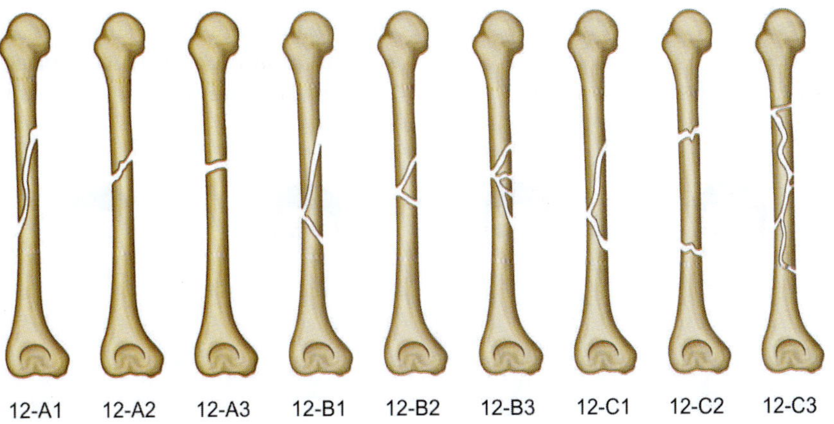

FIG. 2: Arbeitsgemeinschaft für Osteosynthesefragen (AO)/Orthopedic Trauma Association (OTA) classification of diaphyseal humerus.

Physical exam: A neurovascular exam is essential, especially to assess radial nerve function.

Imaging: Radiographs in anteroposterior (AP) and lateral views including the joint above and below the fracture are mandatory.

TREATMENT

Nonoperative Treatment

Nonoperative treatment is indicated for the majority of humeral shaft fractures with acceptable alignment criteria. Outcomes include a 93.5% union rate with an average healing time of 10.7 weeks.

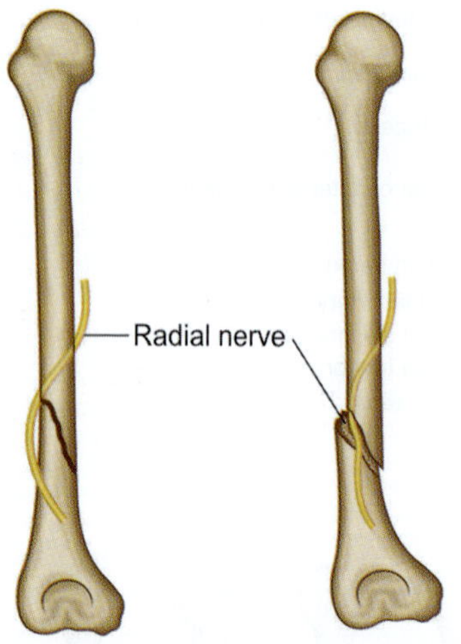

FIG. 3: The Holstein–Lewis fracture.

Techniques

The techniques include:

- *Coaptation splint and functional bracing*:
  - Coaptation Splint/U slab
  - Used until swelling resolves
  - Proper application extends up to the axilla and over the shoulder.
  - Common deformities include varus and extension.
  - A valgus mold is applied to counteract varus displacement.
- *Hanging arm cast* **(Figs. 4A to D)**:
  - Indicated in the initial phase when there is an overriding of bones in transverse fractures.
  - A sling should not be used to allow gravity-assisted fracture reduction.
- Weekly radiographs are required for the first 3 weeks to ensure that reduction is maintained, then every 3–4 weeks thereafter.

Criteria for acceptable alignment include:

- Anterior angulation < 20°
- Varus or valgus angulation < 30°
- Rotational malalignment < 30°
- Shortening < 3 cm

Operative Treatment

Open reduction internal fixation with plating is the gold standard in most shafts of humerus fracture in case it needs surgery.

- Commonly uses narrow or broad 4.5 mm dynamic compression plates or limited

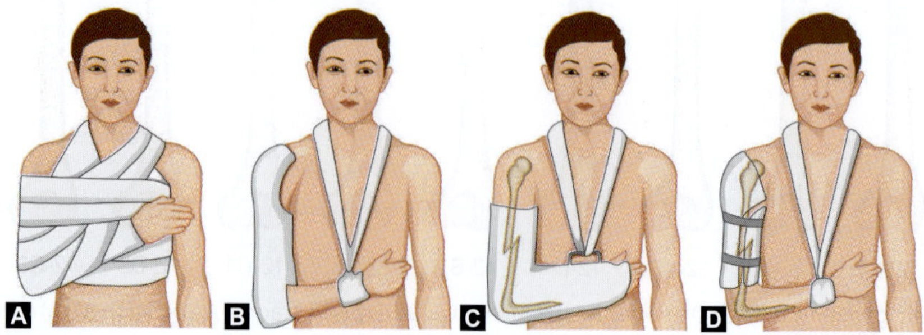

FIGS. 4A TO D: Different modalities of nonoperative treatment. (A) Velpeau bandage; (B) U slab; (C) Hanging cast; and (D) Functional brace.

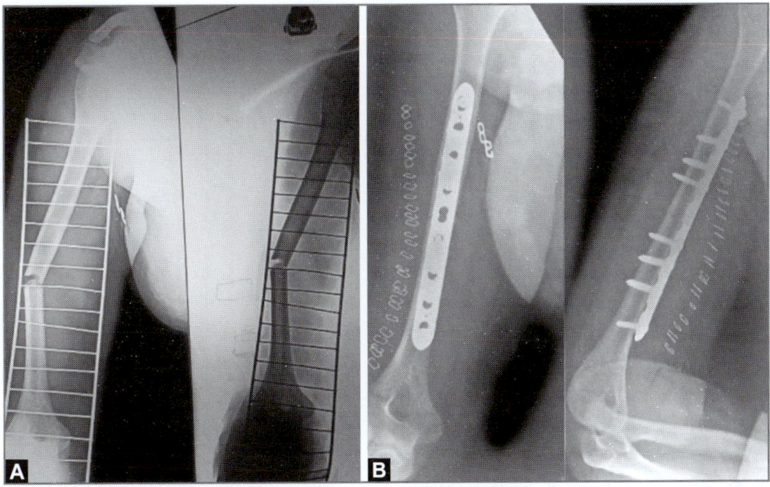

FIGS. 5A AND B: Preoperative and postoperative X-rays of humerus shaft fracture fixed with 4.5 mm narrow plate.

contact dynamic compression plates with 4 screws or 8 cortices on each side

- Absolute stability is achieved with a lag screw or compression plating in simple patterns.
- Bone defects up to 3 cm may be managed with shortening, while larger defects (>3 cm) often require grafting **(Figs. 5A and B)**.

For the metaphyseal distal part of the extra-articular humerus fracture, posterolateral metaphyseal/J plate is used **(Figs. 6A to C)**.

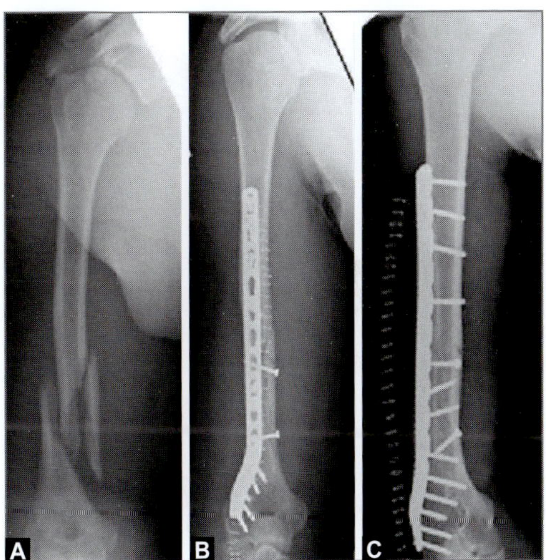

FIGS. 6A TO C: Preoperative and postoperative X-rays of distal extra-articular humerus shaft fracture fixed with 4.5 mm narrow metaphyseal/J plate.

Intramedullary Nailing

Intramedullary nailing (IMN) is suitable for segmental, osteoporotic, and pathologic fractures. It offers the advantage of being minimally invasive but may increase shoulder impingement risk, iatrogenic distal humerus fracture in tight humerus canal, and nonunion if there is any distraction left over. IMN can be performed in antegrade or retrograde mode **(Figs. 7A to C)**.

External Fixation

External fixation is used for high-energy, comminuted, or open fractures. It can be used provisionally or definitively **(Fig. 8)**.

- *Proximal pins*:
  - These are inserted on the anterolateral surface of the proximal humerus.
  - Mini-open approach with dissection of the bone is used to avoid axillary nerve injury.
- *Distal pins*:
  - These are placed on the lateral aspect of the distal fragment with a mini-open approach to avoid radial nerve injury.

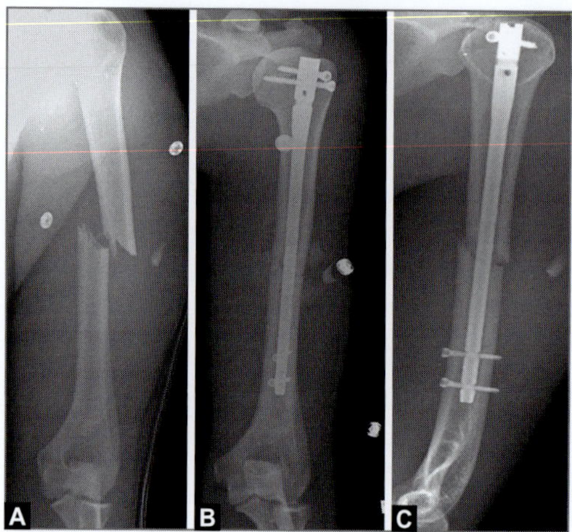

FIGS. 7A TO C: Preoperative and postoperative X-rays of humerus shaft fracture fixed with antegrade intramedullary interlocking nail.

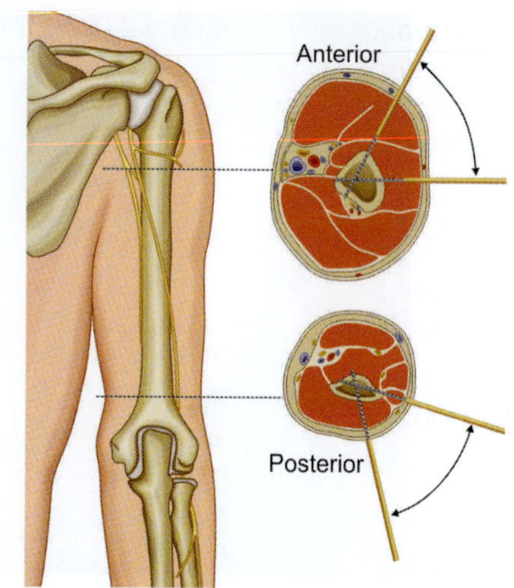

FIG. 8: Safe zones of pin placement on the lateral aspect of proximal and distal aspect of the humerus.

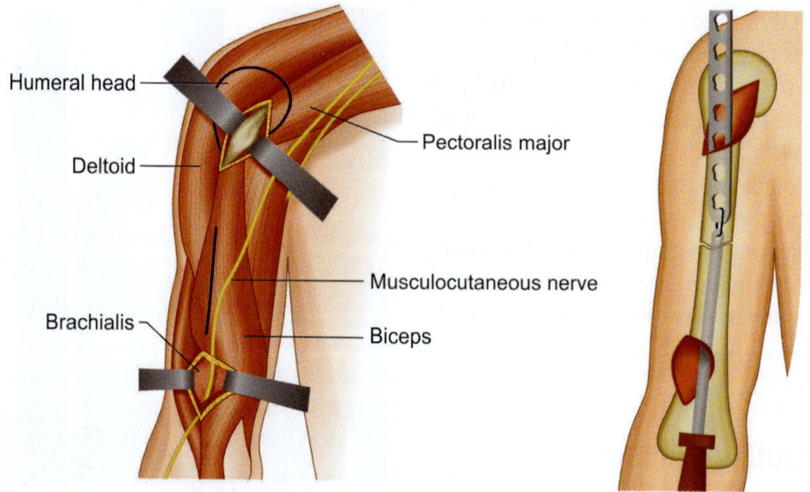

FIG. 9: Anterior approach for minimally invasive plate osteosynthesis of humerus diaphysis.

- ◦ The most distal pin is positioned just proximal to the olecranon fossa, with cortical surface visualization before pin insertion.

COMMONLY USED APPROACHES FOR OPEN REDUCTION INTERNAL FIXATION

- *Anterolateral approach*:
    - Used for fractures from the proximal third to the middle third of the humeral shaft
    - A distal extension of the deltopectoral approach, performed in a supine or beach chair position with the arm abducted at 45–60°.
- *Posterior approach*: It is used for distal to middle-third shaft fractures and can be extensile to expose the humeral shaft from the olecranon fossa to the junction of the proximal and middle thirds.
- *Minimally invasive plate osteosynthesis/ anterior bridge plating* **(Fig. 9)**: Involves proximal and distal incisions through

an anterolateral approach, followed by the creation of an extra periosteal tunnel for plate positioning under fluoroscopic guidance.

COMPLICATIONS

- Nonunion
- Malunion

RADIAL NERVE PALSY

Incidence

- *Overall:* 12.3% (range 8–15%), with a higher incidence in distal third fractures (22%)
- Neuropraxia is most common in closed fractures; neurotmesis is more common in open fractures.
- Iatrogenic radial nerve palsy is most frequent following ORIF via anterolateral (20%) or posterior approaches (11%).
- Average spontaneous recovery begins at 7 weeks, with full recovery around 6 months.

Risk Factors

- *Location:* Distal third (56.9%) > middle third (41.5%) > proximal third (1.5%)
- *Fracture type:* Transverse (21.2%) > spiral (19.8%) > oblique (8.4%) > comminuted (6.8%)
- Open fractures

Treatment

- *Observation:* Initial management in closed fractures; approximately, 77.2% recover spontaneously, with 85–90% of those recovering within 3 months.
- *Nerve conduction study (NCS)/ electromyography (EMG)*: These are recommended around 6–8 weeks to assess nerve damage and monitor recovery.

Surgical Exploration

- Indicated for open fractures with radial nerve palsy and closed fractures that fail to improve in 4–6 months, or fibrillations seen on EMG.
- May require debridement, removal of incarcerated fragments, nerve grafting, or transfers
- Outcomes depend on radial nerve status at exploration
- Nerve in continuity (62.7%), lacerated (26.8%), and incarcerated (10.5%)

Timing of Exploration

- *Early (within 3 weeks):* ~90% recovery
- *Late (8 weeks or more):* ~68% recovery

Tendon Transfers

- *Indications:* Persistent radial nerve palsy
- Common transfers include pronator teres (PT) to extensor carpi radialis brevis (ECRB) (wrist extension), flexor carpi radialis (FCR)/flexor carpi ulnaris (FCU) to extensor digitorum communis (EDC) (finger extension), and palmaris longus (PL) to extensor pollicis longus (EPL) (thumb extension).

OUTCOMES

The following are the outcomes:

- *Overall recovery rate:* 88.6%
- *Primary nerve palsy recovery:* 88.2%
- *Iatrogenic/secondary nerve palsy recovery:* 93.9%
- *Predictable recovery pattern:* Brachioradialis and extensor carpi radialis longus recover first; extensor pollicis longus and extensor indicis proprius recover last.

BIBLIOGRAPHY

1. Devers BN, Lebus GF, Mir HR. Incidence and functional outcomes of malunion of nonoperatively treated humeral shaft fractures. Am J Orthop (Belle Mead NJ). 2015;44(11):E434-7.
2. Hegeman EM, Polmear M, Scanaliato JP, Nesti L, Dunn JC. Incidence and management of radial nerve palsies in humeral shaft fractures: A systematic review. Cureus. 2020;12(11):e11490.
3. Papasoulis E, Drosos GI, Ververidis AN, Verettas DA. Functional bracing of humeral shaft fractures. A review of clinical studies. Injury. 2010;41(7): e21-7.
4. Rockwood CA, Green DP, Bucholz R W, Heckman JD. Rockwood and Green's Fractures in Adults. Philadelphia: Lippincott Williams & Wilkins; 2014.
5. Sarmiento A, Zagorski JB, Zych GA, Latta LL, Capps CA. Functional bracing for the treatment of fractures of the humeral diaphysis. J Bone Joint Surg Am. 2000;82(4):478-86.
6. Zhao JG, Wang J, Wang C, Kan SL. Intramedullary nail versus plate fixation for humeral shaft fractures: A systematic review of overlapping meta-analyses. Medicine (Baltimore). 2015;94(11):e599.

CHAPTER 3.5

Distal Humerus Fracture

Sanjeev Gupta

- Distal humerus fractures have bimodal distribution concerning age and gender.
- Peaks of incidence are in young males and in older females.
- Most distal humerus fractures are intra-articular, involving both columns.

MECHANISM OF INJURY

Distal humerus fractures may be caused by trauma due to fall on the elbow, which is flexed >90° leading to force driving ulna against trochlea.

Axis and angulations are illustrated in **Figures 1A to C**.

- The lateral column (including capitellum) curves anteriorly into flexion with the center of rotation.
- The medial column is in line with the humeral shaft.
- The spoon-shaped trochlea lies centrally and is angulated in a slight flexion of around 25°.
- The distal humerus articular surface is aligned 35–40° anteriorly and 3–8° internally rotated.

CLASSIFICATION

Multiple classification systems exist with a wide array of possible fracture patterns and complexity.

- The Arbeitsgemeinschaft für Osteosynthesefragen (AO)/Orthopedic Trauma Association (OTA) classification is illustrated in **Figure 2**.
    - *13-A:* Extra-articular fractures
    - *13-B:* Partial articular fractures
    - *13-C:* Complete articular fractures
- Other classification systems include:
    - Jupiter and Mehne classification is based on the column and ties arch concept of elbow stability. It is useful for preoperative planning.
    - Mehne and Matta's classification is based on fracture line configurations

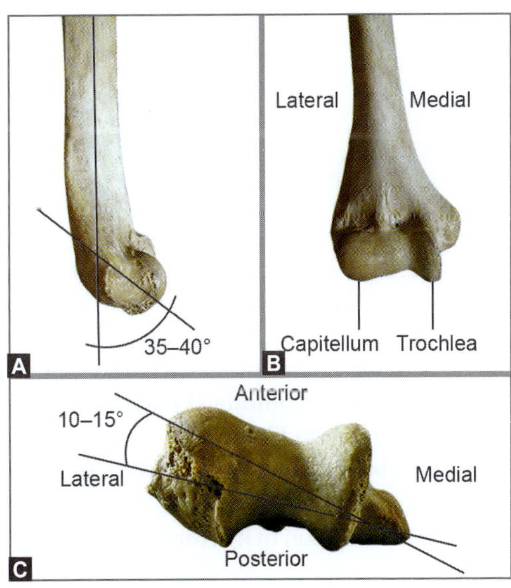

FIGS. 1A TO C: (A) Distal humerus articular surface is aligned 35–40° anteriorly; (B) spoon-shaped trochlea; and (C) distal humerus articular surface is aligned 3–8° internally rotated.

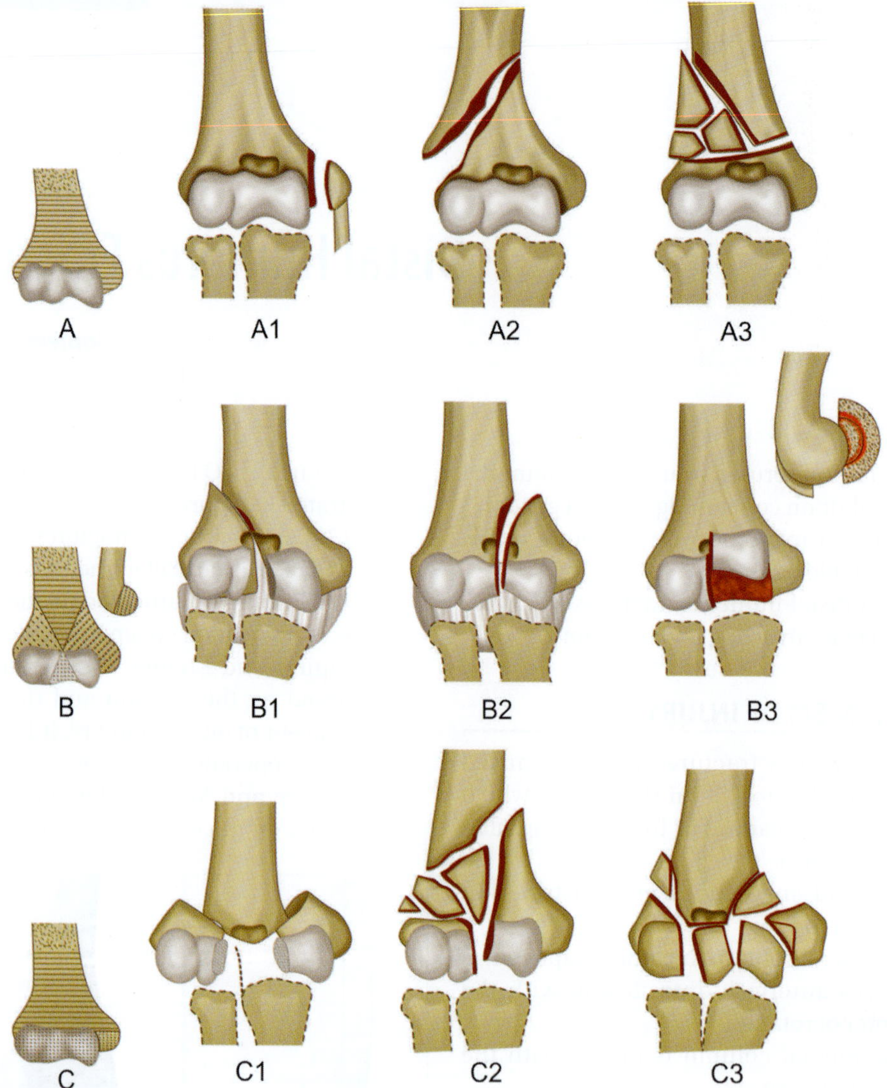

FIG. 2: AO classification of distal end humerus fractures.

into high and low T, Y, H, and medial and lateral Lambda (λ) fractures. It is illustrated in **Figure 3**.

- Riseborough and Radin classification is based on displacement, rotation, and comminution of fracture fragments.

RADIOGRAPHIC WORKUP

The following radiographic work must be done.

- Standard anteroposterior (AP) and lateral views for diagnosis. At times, it is better to have traction views and provisional reduction of fracture. After reduction, doing an X-ray and computed tomography (CT) scan to define fracture is advisable.
- CT scan is a must for proper evaluation of classification and preoperative planning **(Figs. 4A to D)**.

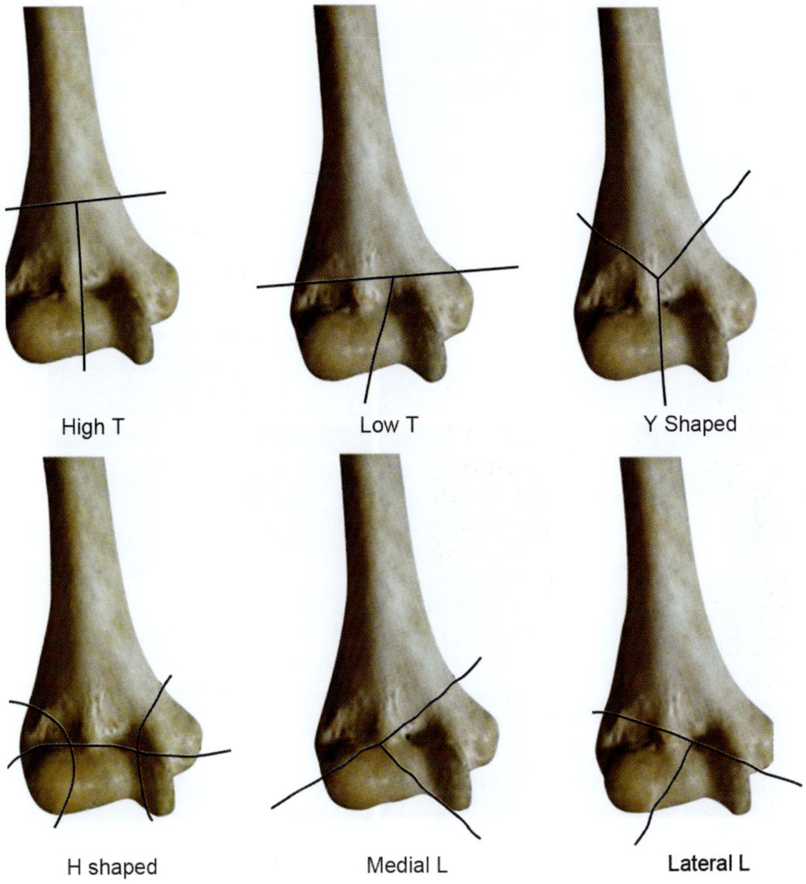

FIG. 3: Mehne and Matta classification.

TREATMENT

Nonoperative Management

Nonoperative treatment is rarely used and is typically reserved for stable, nondisplaced fractures, or patients who are poor surgical candidates due to advanced age or comorbidities. Management involves immobilization with a cast or splint, followed by a structured rehabilitation program. Although conservative treatment can achieve reasonable outcomes in select cases, studies indicate that it often results in suboptimal functional recovery and increased risk of complications like stiffness and nonunion, especially for complex fractures.

Surgical Treatment is the Treatment of Choice

Aim of surgery: Anatomical reduction of fracture fragments is done to restore articular congruity and correct alignment of the metaphysis with stable fixation to allow range of motion as early as possible.

Various modalaties used for fixation include:

Open Reduction and Internal Fixation

Open reduction and internal fixation (ORIF) remains the standard of care for most displaced distal humerus fractures. Intercondylar articular restoration with screw and dual plate fixation for columns is preferred **(Figs. 5A and B)**.

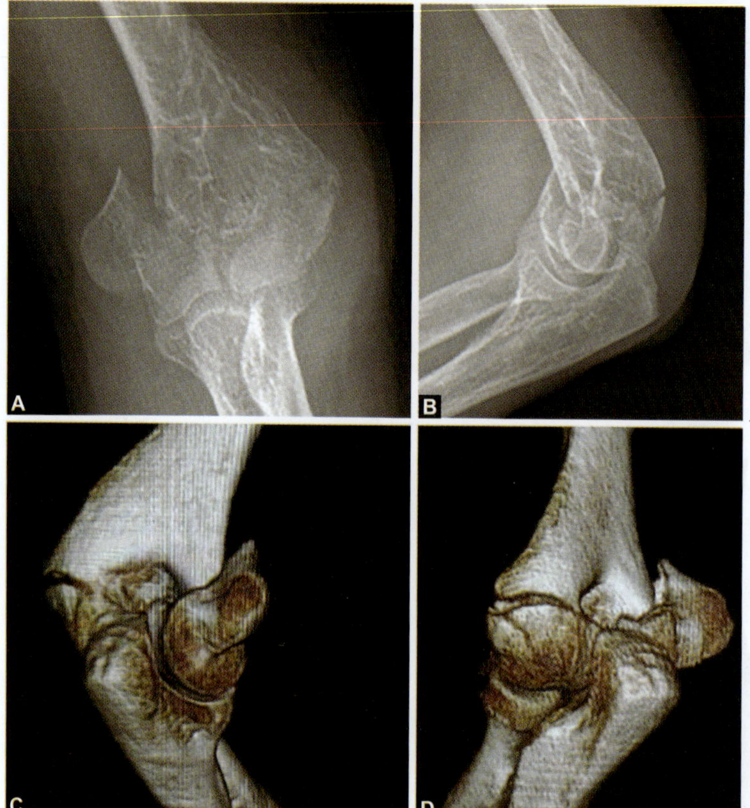

FIGS. 4A TO D: X-ray and computed tomography (CT) scan evaluation after reduction to better define fracture.

- The dual plate fixation can be a 90–90 construct or a 180° parallel construct.
- After anatomical reduction, interfragmentary compression is achieved by lag screw followed by:
  - *Standard plating technique (90–90 construct):* One plate is placed medially, and another plate is placed posterolaterally at an orthogonal angle.
  - *180° parallel construct:* Direct medial and lateral plating—biomechanically sound and recent studies confirm stable fixation with a high rate of union.

The surgical approach is determined by the fracture configuration:

- *Olecranon osteotomy approach:* This is preferred for complex intra-articular fractures, providing excellent visualization of the articular surface and facilitating precise reduction. However, complications such as nonunion at the osteotomy site or hardware irritation can occur.
- *Triceps-sparing approaches:* These are increasingly favored as they avoid disrupting the extensor mechanism, reducing postoperative morbidity. Studies comparing triceps-splitting versus triceps-sparing approaches have shown comparable outcomes in terms of fracture healing and elbow function, but the latter offers reduced complication rates.

Total Elbow Arthroplasty

Total elbow arthroplasty (TEA) **(Figs. 6A and B)** is considered for elderly patients with severely comminuted fractures that are unsuitable for ORIF. It provides immediate

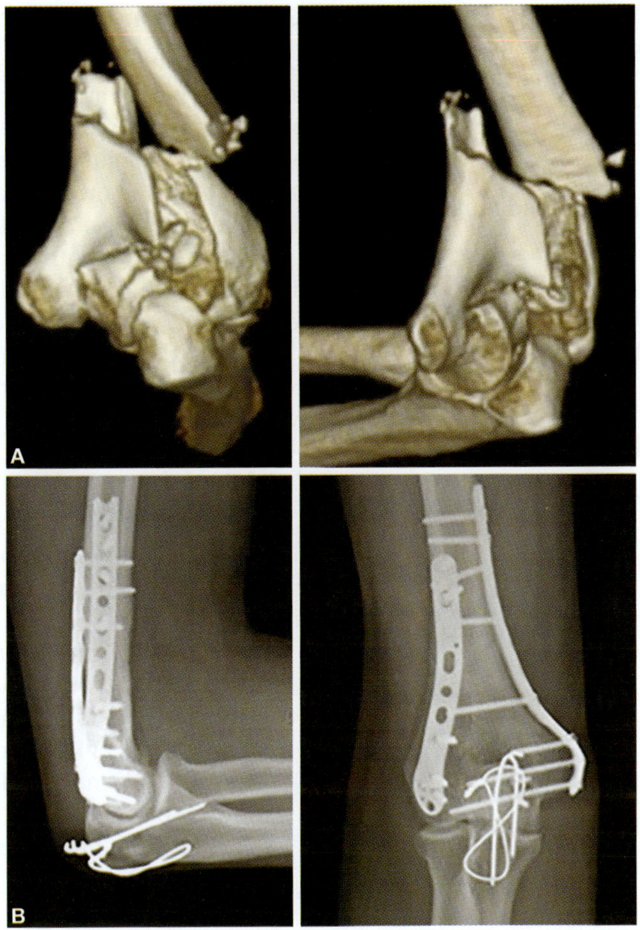

FIGS. 5A AND B: Screw and dual plate fixation for columns.

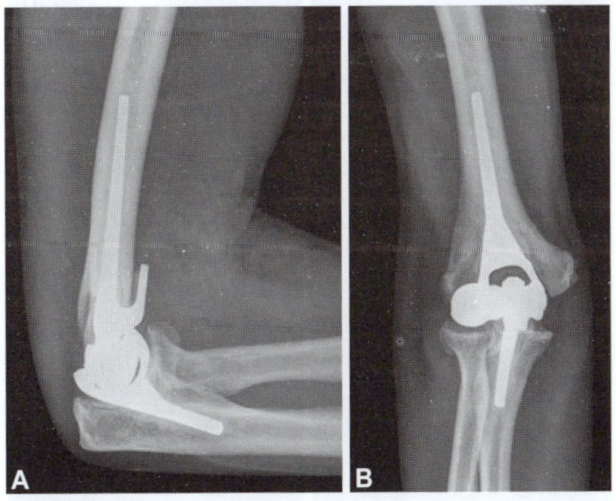

FIGS. 6A AND B: Total elbow arthroplasty.

stability and pain relief, with good short-to-mid-term outcomes. However, TEA is associated with significant limitations, such as restricted weight-bearing capacity and potential long-term complications like aseptic loosening or implant failure. Current evidence supports its use primarily in low-demand patients or as a salvage procedure after failed fixation.

Distal Humerus Hemiarthroplasty

A distal humerus hemiarthroplasty (rare) is an emerging option for fractures that cannot be reconstructed adequately. This procedure involves replacing only the distal articular surface, preserving the native joint mechanics. Early results are promising, suggesting that hemiarthroplasty may provide a viable alternative to TEA in younger, more active patients. However, long-term outcomes and comparative studies with traditional methods are still needed.

MEDIAL EPICONDYLE, LATERAL EPICONDYLE, AND CONDYLE FRACTURES

Medial Epicondylar Fractures

Medial epicondylar fractures of the distal humerus are relatively uncommon, accounting for approximately 10–20% of all elbow fractures.

Management

- *Nonoperative treatment:* Undisplaced or minimally displaced fractures can be managed with immobilization and physical therapy. Immobilization in a long arm cast should be done in the 1st week with the elbow flexed to 90°. It is followed by a protected exercise program including active range of motion exercises.
- *Operative treatment:* Indications for surgical referral and operative management of medial epicondyle fractures include
  - Displaced fractures
  - Comminuted fractures
  - Open fractures
  - Incarcerated intra-articular fragments
  - Valgus instability
  - Intra-articular fragment entrapment (occurs in 5–18% of cases)

Operative Techniques

Open reduction and internal fixation with a screw and washer construct, Kirschner wires (K-wires), sutures, and tension band techniques can be done. K-wires are the most common option for fragmented fractures in children, a posterior-medial approach is preferred.

Lateral Epicondylar Fractures

Lateral epicondylar fractures in adults are rare injuries, typically arising from direct trauma or valgus forces applied to the elbow. They often occur in conjunction with more complex injuries of the elbow, such as dislocations or ligament tears **(Figs. 7A and B)**.

In cases where the lateral collateral ligament (LCL) is involved, the elbow may feel unstable when subjected to varus stress

Potential damage to the radial nerve could cause weakness or numbness in the wrist and hand.

Treatment

The treatment of lateral epicondylar fractures depends on the degree of displacement, elbow stability, and the presence of associated injuries.

- *Nonoperative management*: Indicated in nondisplaced or minimally displaced fractures (<2 mm) and stable elbow without signs of ligamentous disruption. Immobilization in a long-arm above elbow splint or cast for 3–4 weeks, followed by gradual mobilization to avoid stiffness is done. Active range of motion

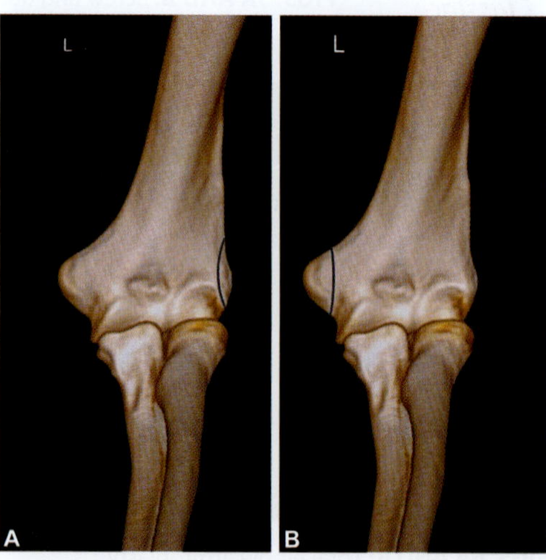

FIGS. 7A AND B: Illustration showing lateral epicondyle and medial epicondyle fractures. (A) Lateral epicondyle fracture and (B) Medial epicondyle fracture.

exercises can be initiated once fracture union is confirmed radiographically.

- *Operative management*

Indications include:
  - Displaced fractures (>2 mm)
  - Instability due to lateral collateral ligament injury
  - Open fractures or fractures associated with elbow dislocations

Surgical Technique

Open reduction and internal fixation using screws, plates, or K-wires may be used to stabilize the fracture. Repair of the lateral collateral ligament is required if there is instability of the elbow.

Condylar Fractures

Condylar fractures of the distal humerus, which involve the medial or lateral condyle, represent a subset of distal humerus fractures. These are more common in the pediatric population than in adults.

Lateral condylar fractures are more common than medial condylar fractures, given the exposure of the lateral aspect of the elbow during falls.

Classification

The most common is Milch classification **(Figs. 8A and B)**.

- *Milch type I*:
  - The fracture line is lateral to the trochlear groove and does not involve the trochlea.
  - This type is considered more stable as the articular surface is less involved.
- *Milch type II*:
  - The fracture line extends into the trochlea, making it an intra-articular fracture.
  - These fractures are more unstable and require more aggressive intervention due to the loss of joint congruity.

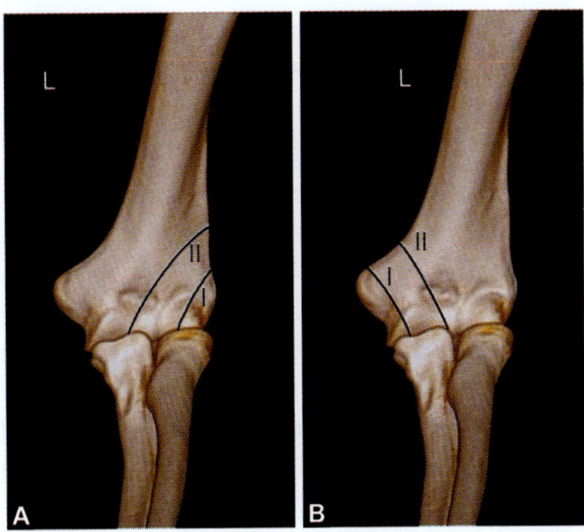

FIGS. 8A AND B: Lateral and medial condylar fractures with type I and II Milch-type fractures. (A) Lateral condyle fractures and (B) Medial condyle fractures.

Treatment

- *Nonoperative treatment*:
  - Indicated in nondisplaced or minimally displaced fractures.
  - Immobilization in a cast or splint, typically for 4–6 weeks.
  - Early motion exercises are initiated as soon as the fracture shows signs of healing to prevent stiffness.
- *Surgical treatment*:
  - Indicated for displaced fractures, fractures with articular involvement, or those associated with neurovascular compromise.
  - Goal of surgery is anatomical reduction and stable fixation to allow early mobilization.
  - ORIF using plates and screws is done to stabilize the fracture fragments and restore joint congruity.
  - *Total elbow arthroplasty:* In elderly patients with severe comminution or poor bone quality.

Post-surgery, early mobilization is encouraged to reduce the risk of joint stiffness, a common complication following elbow fractures.

Medial condyle fractures are less frequent but involve the same principles.

Postoperative Rehabilitation

Early mobilization is crucial to prevent joint stiffness and promote functional recovery. The rehabilitation protocol generally begins with passive and assisted active range-of-motion exercises, progressing to active strengthening as healing permits. Close follow-up with serial radiographs is essential to monitor fracture healing and ensure the integrity of the fixation.

MANAGEMENT OF COMPLICATIONS

Common Complications

- *Post-operative stiffness:* This can be due to
  - Capsular contracture
  - Arthrofibrosis
  - Prominent implants
  - Intra or extraarticular deformity

Treatment: Elbow arthrolysis

- *Implant failure:* Despite osteosynthesis protected by the short period of immobilization, it can occur due to,
  - Unstable fixation
  - Over stripping of periosteum
  - Osteoporosis
  - Smoking or alcoholic habits

Treatment: Stable internal fixation with compression and bone graft may be required.

- *Ulnar nerve dysfunction:* Ulnar nerve management is a particular concern during surgery. Usually transient, tingling paresthesia and weakness in the zone of distribution of the ulnar nerve are present. Those not improving with time need intervention with various options including in-situ decompression, anterior transposition, or subcutaneous transposition, depending on the fracture pattern and surgical approach. Meta-analyses suggest that transposition may reduce the risk of postoperative ulnar neuropathy, though it is not without risks.
- Radial nerve palsy can be iatrogenic due to long lateral column plating.
- *Nonunion:* It occurs usually at the supracondylar level. Risk factors include:
  - Inadequate fixation and/or immobilization in the early postoperative period
  - Metaphyseal comminution and bone loss

Treatment: Autogenous bone grafting

- *Heterotopic ossification*:
  - Associated traumatic brain injury
  - Delayed fixation
  - Forced passive stretching or massaging

Postoperative rehabilitation should be active with self-assisted stretching exercises and never include passive manipulation.

BIBLIOGRAPHY

1. Chen RC, Harris DJ, Leduc S, Borrelli JJ Jr, Tornetta P 3rd, Ricci WM. Is ulnar nerve transposition beneficial during open reduction internal fixation of distal humerus fractures? J Orthop Trauma. 2010;24(7):391-4.
2. Coles CP, Barei DP, Nork SE, Taitsman LA, Hanel DP, Henley MB. The olecranon osteotomy: A six-year experience in the treatment of intraarticular fractures of the distal humerus. J Orthop Trauma. 2006;20(3):164-71.
3. McKee MD, Wilson TL, Winston L, Schemitsch EH, Richards RR. Functional outcome following surgical treatment of intra-articular distal humeral fractures through a posterior approach. J Bone Joint Surg Am. 2000;82(12):1701-7.
4. Mehlhoff TL, Bennett JB. Distal humeral fractures: Fixation versus arthroplasty. J Shoulder Elbow Surg. 2011;20(2 Suppl):S97-106.
5. Shearin JW, Chapman TR, Miller A, Ilyas AM. Ulnar nerve management with distal humerus fracture fixation: A meta-analysis. Hand Clin. 2018;34(1):97-103.
6. Zlotolow DA, Catalano LW III, Barron OA, Glickel SZ. Surgical exposures of the humerus. J Am Acad Orthop Surg. 2006;14(13):754-65.

Coronal Shear (Capitellum and Trochlea) Fractures

Zubair Ahmad Lone, Tanveer Ahmed Bhat, Mohammad Farooq Butt

The capitellum and trochlea are involved in the coronal shear injuries of the distal humerus. These injuries are rare, complex, and challenging; comprising around 1% of all elbow fractures. Patients of any age group may be involved; however, in elderly people, the fractures tend to be more comminuted. Association with radial head fractures and ligamentous injuries of the elbow is common.

PATHOMECHANICS

Classically, high-energy trauma in young males and low-velocity falls in elderly females lead to these injuries. Most of these are a result of a fall on to an outstretched hand (FOOSH).

Two mechanisms have been described:
In the first, a FOOSH creates a direct axial load through the radial head, producing shear forces at the capitellar-trochlear area, which eventually causes a coronal shear fracture of the capitellum, trochlea, or both **(Fig. 1A)**.

The second mechanism describes an initial failure of the lateral collateral ligament (LCL) secondary to a FOOSH, which leads to a transient posterolateral subluxation of the radial head **(Fig. 1B)**. During the spontaneous reduction of the radial head, a shear force transmitted through the radial head produces a coronal shear fracture **(Fig. 1C)**. This pathomechanics also explains the high incidence of associated

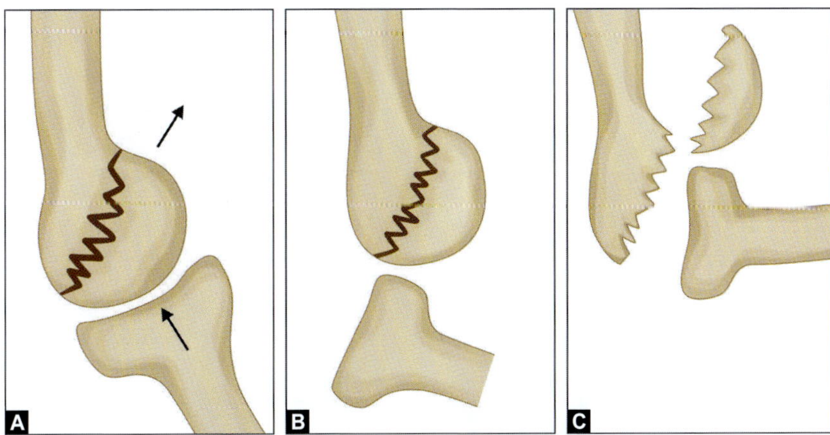

FIGS. 1A TO C: Mechanisms of injury as elucidated by Faber et al. (2004). (A) FOOSH injury creating a shear force at the capitello-trochlear area by a direct axial load through the radial head; (B) due to the failure of the lateral collateral ligament (LCL), a transient subluxation of radial occurs; and (C) the radial head while relocating into its place creates a fracture.

radial head fractures and lateral collateral injury, in these fractures.

CLASSIFICATION

The classification for these fractures in the AO/OTA system labels them as 13B3 fractures and subdivides these into three types:

1. 13B3.1: Capitellum fracture
2. 13B3.2: Trochlea fracture
3. 13B3.3: Both capitellum and trochlea fracture

The Modified Dubberley Classification is the most helpful for a surgeon with respect to planning and decision on approach, fixation, and choice of implant **(Fig. 2)**.

Four types of fractures are described in this classification, each with sub-types labeled as "A" or "B" on the basis of the absence or presence of posterior comminution respectively.

Type 1 fracture is a fracture of the capitellum and may extend up to the lateral trochlear ridge. Type 2 fracture is a single chunk, capitello-trochlear fracture. Coronal

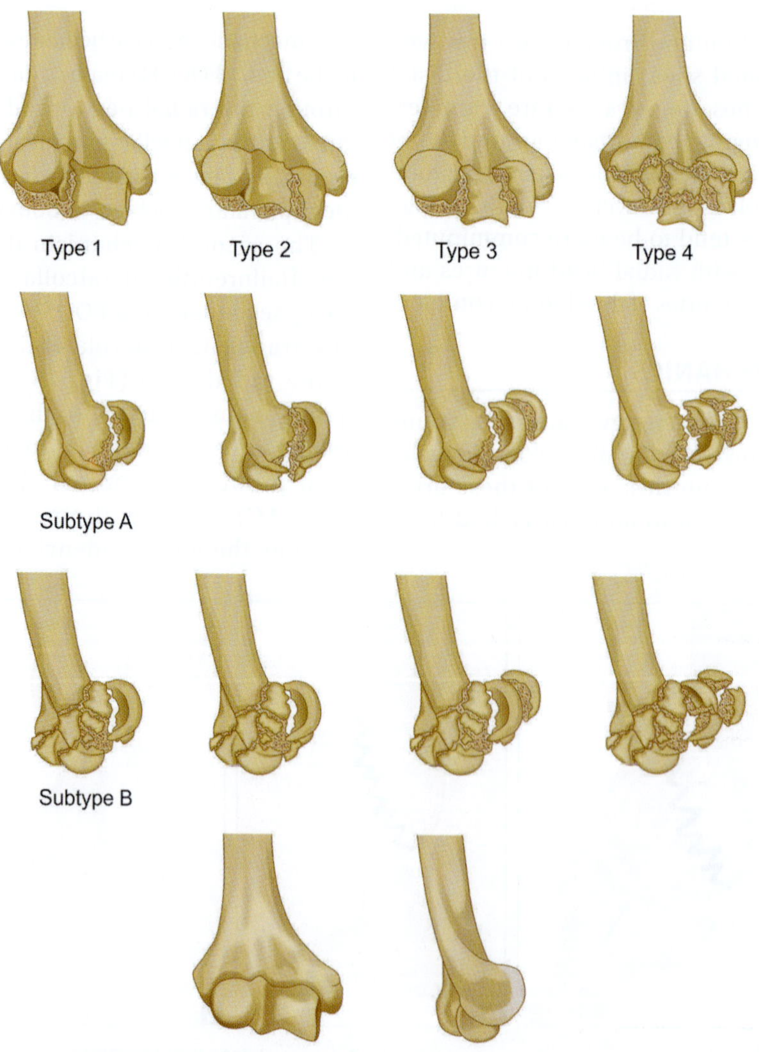

FIG. 2: Modified Dubberly classification for coronal shear fractures of the distal humerus.
Source: Watson et al. (2020).

shear injury, with isolated fracture fragments of capitellum and trochlea, is labeled as a type 3 fracture. In a type 4 fracture, there is marked comminution of the capitello-trochlear area, because of the multitude of axial and sagittal plane fractures.

Bryan and Morrey have propounded another classification, which described three variants of coronal shear fractures on the basis of size and comminution.

CLINICAL EVALUATION

Though it is difficult to rule out ligamentous injuries immediately because of pain, but a fair idea is obtained after examination of the elbow under anesthesia. Associated injuries like radial head fractures, coronoid fractures, epicondyle fractures, and Essex-Lopresti lesions need to be ruled out.

RADIOLOGICAL EVALUATION

Plain radiographs may reveal a coronal shear fracture on standard lateral and anteroposterior views of the elbow **(Figs. 3A and B)**. A radio-capitellar (Coyle's) view is useful in these injuries **(Fig. 3C)**. Sometimes, a "half-moon sign" may be appreciated in a capitellum fracture. Also, "double or triple arc signs" may be seen on a lateral radiograph, suggesting the involvement of trochlea and the possibility of more than one fragment. However, these are not sufficient enough for drafting a management plan.

A computed tomography (CT) scan is imperative, especially a 3D reconstruction, in order to assess the extent of trochlear involvement, posterior comminution, and number of fracture fragments, which helps a surgeon draft a meticulous preoperative plan and avoid any surprises intraoperatively **(Figs. 4A to E)**. The use of magnetic resonance imaging (MRI) has been documented for pregnant females with suspected coronal shear injuries and for evaluation of any associated ligamentous injury; however, the latter is not routine, as clinical assessment under anesthesia is enough for diagnosis.

TREATMENT

Conservative treatment in these fractures is only reserved for elderly patients with cognitive impairment, chronic physical ailments, and patients unfit for surgery.

The gold standard is surgical fixation to aid early rehabilitation for optimal outcomes. The surgical planning is tailored according to the type of fracture classified according

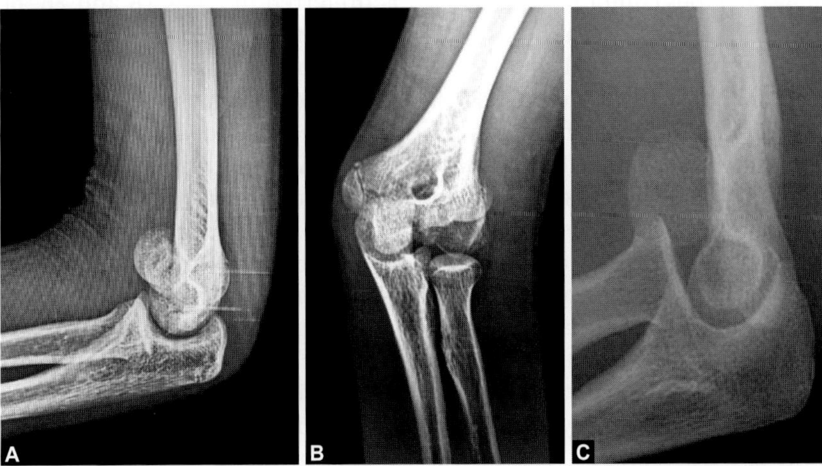

FIGS. 3A TO C: Radiographs reveal coronal shear fractures of the distal humerus. (A) Lateral view (B) anteroposterior view; and (C) Coyle's view.

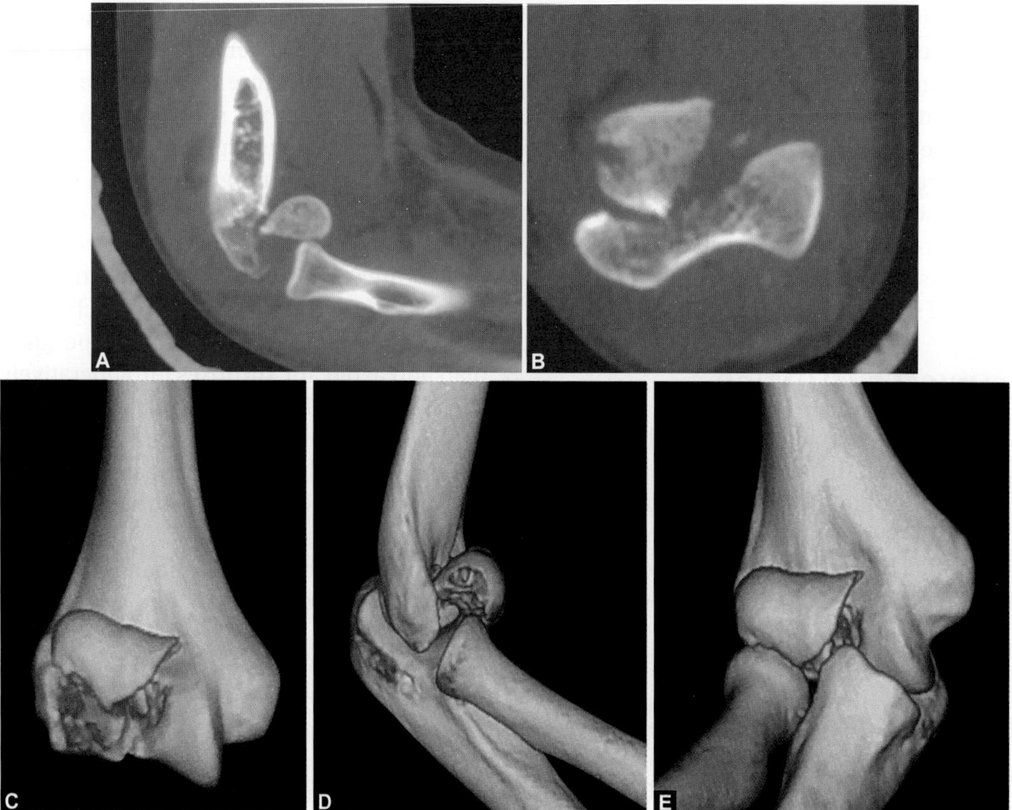

FIGS. 4A TO E: Computer tomography along with 3D cuts demonstrating a coronal shear injury in a patient with a single chunk capitello–trochlear fragment.

to modified Dubberley classification, size of the fragment, and presence of an associated fracture or ligamentous compromise.

Most type 1 and 2 fractures are approached through a lateral or anterolateral approach for open reduction **(Figs. 5A and B)**. Type 1A and 2A fractures do not have posterior comminution and are amenable to fixation by headless or Herbert screws, which may be placed either in anterior to posterior direction or back to front. In a few unstable fractures with compromised anterior periosteal hinge, it is prudent to add an anterior antiglide plate. However, in types 1B and 2B, there hardly is any potential hold posteriorly when fixed using screws and hence, a posterior-lateral locking plate is needed to create a support through with locking screws can be placed to hold the fracture. Hence, a lateral approach, utilizing the Kocher's or Kaplan's interval, is preferred in types 1B and 2B, because if needed, the approach may be extended and a posterolateral plate may be placed through the same approach, which is not possible with an isolated anterolateral approach. Type 3A fractures are present with two fragments, one from the capitellum and the other from the trochlea.

The fixation of both the fracture fragments is performed through two approaches, one lateral and the other medial. The medial approach utilizes the interval between brachialis and pronator teres **(Figs. 6A to C)**. For fracture types 3B and 4, an attempt should be made for fixation, by combining various fixation techniques and if needed an arthroplasty may be performed.

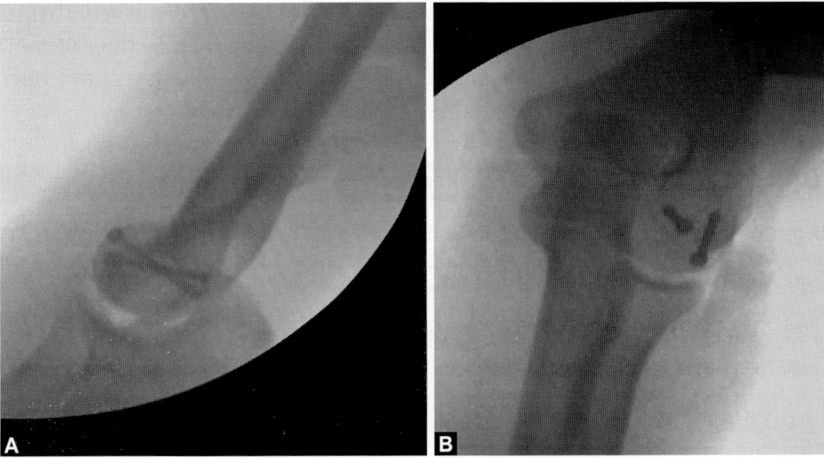

FIGS. 5A AND B: A type 2 Dubberley coronal shear fracture managed by open reduction and internal fixation using Herbert scores in anterior-to-posterior direction utilizing a lateral approach to the elbow.

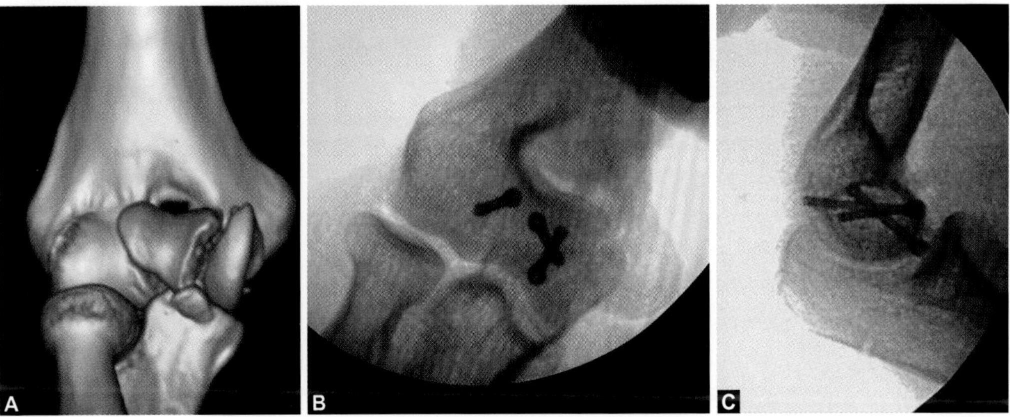

FIGS. 6A TO C: Coronal shear injury with a two-part trochlea fracture fixed using Herbert screws utilizing an anteromedial approach to the elbow.

A triceps sparing or an olecranon osteotomy approach may be required. Triceps-sparing approaches may include a para tricipital or a para olecranon approach. The advantage of this approach is that if fixation is not possible, a hemiarthroplasty or a total elbow arthroplasty can be performed through the same approach. However, it is imperative to repair the elbow collaterals, so that early elbow movements can be started. The advantage of the olecranon osteotomy approach is that the medial and the lateral collateral ligaments are preserved, however, for proper visualization of the anterior fragments an additional lateral window is needed.

In order to achieve the best possible results, it is imperative to appropriately manage the associated injuries. Radial head fractures and lateral collateral injuries are associated commonly. Due attention should be given to the fixation or replacement of the radial head, as needed, depending upon the fracture type. Also, if on the table, clinical assessment under anesthesia reveals a ligamentous compromise, it must be dealt with properly by repairing the collateral ligaments using suture anchors.

There are reports of managing small osteochondral fragments with absorbable sutures, which are passed through small tunnels created by Kirschner wires (K-wires). Also, biodegradable darts have been used to fix such fractures.

BIBLIOGRAPHY

1. Dubberley JH, Faber KJ, Macdermid JC, Patterson SD, King GJ. Outcome after open reduction and internal fixation of capitellar and trochlear fractures. J Bone Joint Surg Am. 2006;88(1):46-54.
2. Faber KJ. Coronal shear fractures of the distal humerus: The capitellum and trochlea. Hand Clin. 2004;20(4):455-64.
3. McKee MD, Jupiter JB, Bamberger HB. Coronal shear fractures of the distal end of the humerus. J Bone Joint Surg Am. 1996;78(1):49-54.
4. O'Driscoll SW. Coronal plane fractures of the distal humerus: Capitellum and trochlea. In: Bucholz RW, Heckman JD, Court-Brown CM (Eds). Rockwood and Green's Fractures in Adults. 7th edition. Philadelphia: Lippincott Williams & Wilkins; 2010. pp. 965-72.
5. Ring D, Jupiter JB. Fracture of the distal humerus including capitellar and trochlear fractures. In: Browner BD, Jupiter JB, Levine AM, Trafton PG (Eds). Skeletal Trauma: Basic Science, Management, and Reconstruction, 3rd edition. Philadelphia: W.B. Saunders; 2003. pp. 1485-510.
6. Watson JJ, Bellringer S, Phadnis J. Coronal shear fractures of the distal humerus: Current concepts and surgical techniques. Shoulder Elbow. 2020;12(2):124135.

SECTION

4

Elbow Injuries

Elbow Dislocation

Kanav Mahajan, Amit Kumar

Elbow dislocation is the second most common large joint dislocation in adults and is most common in children.

The elbow joint is stabilized by:

- *Static stabilizers*:
  - Primary stabilizers:
    - Ulnohumeral joint
    - Anterior bundle of medial collateral ligament (MCL)
    - Lateral collateral ligament (LCL) complex
  - Secondary:
    - Radiocapitellar joint
    - Joint capsule
    - Origins of flexor and extensor tendons
- Dynamic stabilizers:
  - Anconeus
  - Brachialis
  - Triceps

CLASSIFICATION

The elbow dislocation is of two types:

1. Simple dislocation—dislocation without fracture
2. Complex dislocation—dislocation with associated fracture

The most common fracture associated with elbow dislocation in adults is radial head fracture, although coronoid process fracture is also common **(Figs. 1A and B)**. When all of these occur together in a severe posterior elbow dislocation, it is known as the terrible triad of the elbow.

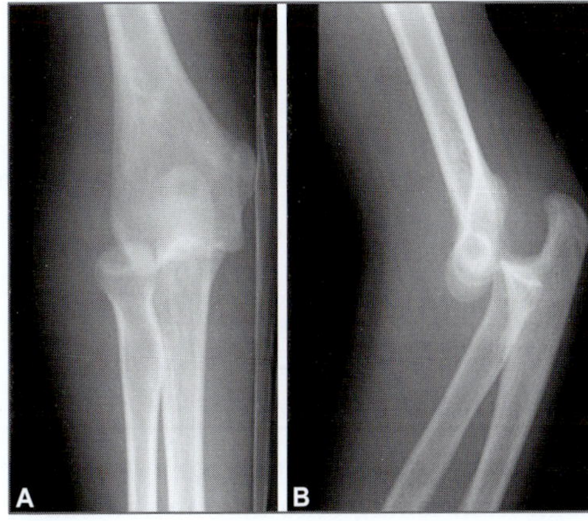

FIGS. 1A AND B: X-ray showing (A) anteroposterior (AP) and (B) lateral view with elbow dislocation.

The most common associated fracture in children is medial epicondyle fracture.

The elbow dislocation is also classified based on the location of the olecranon relative to the humerus **(Fig. 2)**:

- Posterior:
  - Posterolateral (80%, most common)
  - Posteromedial (20%)
- Anterior
- Lateral
- Medial
- Divergent

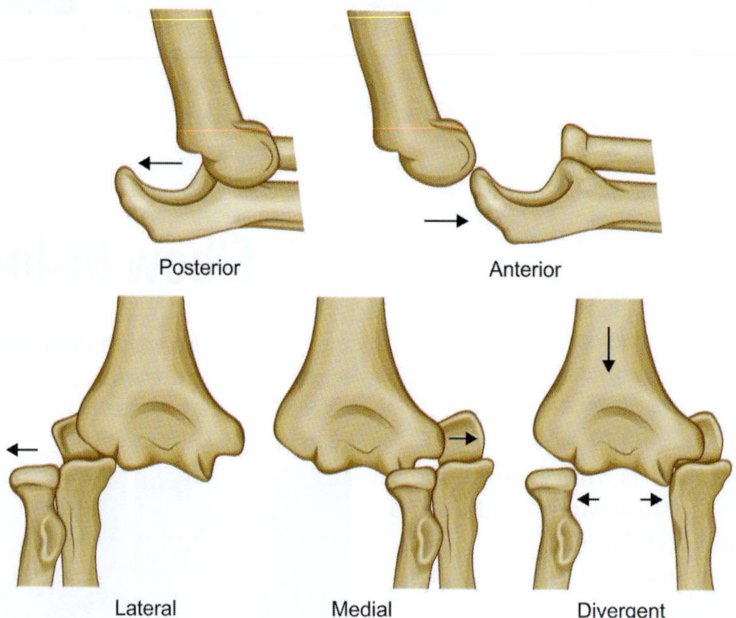

FIG. 2: Types of elbow dislocation.

MECHANISM OF INJURY CAUSING ELBOW INSTABILITY

Posterior elbow dislocations typically result from falling onto an outstretched or extended arm, either with hyperextension or a posterolateral rotatory mechanism. For posterior elbow dislocation, the forces involved in causing elbow dislocation include axial compression, valgus stress, and supination.

Anterior elbow dislocations usually involve a fall on a flexed elbow, with an anterior-directed force on the proximal ulna.

CLINICAL PRESENTATION

The clinical presentations are as follows:

- Three-bony-point relationship of the joint is lost.
- Tenting of skin on the posterior aspect of the elbow joint is seen.
- Neurovascular assessment and documentation should always be done in elbow dislocation, because associated brachial artery, ulnar nerve, and median nerve injuries are commonly seen.

IMAGING

- *Radiographs:* Anteroposterior (AP), lateral, and oblique views should be advised.
- A computed tomography (CT) scan may be required to rule out other associated fractures.
- Magnetic resonance imaging (MRI) may be needed to assess the ligamentous injury at the elbow joint.

TREATMENT

Nonoperative Treatment

Closed reduction is the mainstay of treatment.

There are several techniques or methods used for closed reduction of an elbow dislocation, typically performed under sedation or anesthesia to minimize pain and allow for muscle relaxation.

Here are the commonly used methods for closed reduction:

Traction-countertraction Method

- *Procedure:* This is one of the most widely used methods. The patient is typically made to either lie flat on their back or sit upright.
    - A provider holds the upper arm (humerus) to provide countertraction, while another provider applies traction on the forearm (pulling it gently but firmly).
    - Any translation mediolateral needs to be corrected first.
    - While applying traction, the elbow is flexed to about 45–90°, and a gentle anterior (forward) force is applied to the olecranon (the bony part of the elbow) to reduce the dislocation.
- *Use:* Commonly used for simple posterior elbow dislocations.

Milch Technique

- *Procedure:* This method involves abducting (moving the arm out to the side) and externally rotating the shoulder.
    - The elbow is gradually flexed while applying pressure to guide the radial head and humeral head back into place.
- *Use:* It is mostly used for posterior or posterolateral dislocations. This technique is particularly favored in pediatric patients.

Leverage or Flexion Technique

- *Procedure:* This method is used when the elbow is in full extension (stuck straight).
    - The elbow is flexed slowly, applying downward pressure on the distal humerus while supporting the proximal forearm.
    - Gradual flexion helps guide the joint back into its normal position.
- *Use:* Primarily for simple dislocations (without fractures).

Prone or Gravity-assisted Technique

- *Procedure:* The patient lies prone (face down) on a table with the arm hanging over the edge.
    - Weights or gentle traction are applied to the hanging forearm, using gravity to assist in the reduction.
    - Manual manipulation may be done as needed.
- *Use:* Particularly useful for muscular patients where traction might be difficult manually, or in a posterior dislocation.

Interlocking Hands Technique

- *Procedure:* The provider grips the patient's forearm with both hands in an interlocking position, with one hand above and one hand below the elbow joint.
    - Gentle traction is applied while flexing the elbow and manipulating the joint into proper alignment.
- *Use:* This technique offers better control and stability during reduction.

Hanging Arm Technique (Modified Stimson Method)

- *Procedure:* This is similar to the gravity-assisted method. The patient lies prone with the dislocated arm hanging off the side of the bed.
    - Weights (typically 5–10 lbs) are attached to the wrist, and over time, the weight gradually reduces the dislocation.
- *Use:* This is particularly helpful when other methods are unsuccessful, as it uses a more passive approach relying on gravity.

Postreduction Carc

- Once reduction is achieved, stability of the joint is confirmed by checking the range of motion and obtaining postreduction X-rays to rule out fractures or incomplete reduction.
- The elbow is usually immobilized in a sling or splint for a short period (often 1–2 weeks), followed by rehabilitation to restore range of motion and strength.

Operative Treatment

- Surgical management is required only in certain conditions.
- For complex dislocations, open reduction and internal fixation (ORIF) of fractures and reconstruction of the torn capsuloligamentous structure are done.
- The surgical approach selected for dislocation depends on the type of dislocation, pattern of instability, and severity of soft-tissue injury.

Indications for open reduction:
- Unstable elbow dislocation
- Unreduced elbow by closed attempt
- Delayed and neglected cases
- Associated fractures
- Terrible-triad injury
- Open injuries
- Dislocation with neurovascular injury

Operative Options

Operative options include the following:
- Open reduction and internal fixation with ligament repair in unstable elbow dislocation
- Open reduction with joint capsule release and dynamic hinged fixator in neglected elbow dislocations
- Fixation or repair of coronoid fracture and radial head fracture

The approach to elbow joint depends on the location of the injury:
- Kocher approach is used to fix the LCL complex injury, coronoid fracture, capitellum fracture, and/or radial head fractures.
- Medial approach used to fix the MCL injury, and/or comminuted coronoid fractures.
  Always identify, isolate, and protect the ulnar nerve in the medial approach.
- The posterior approach is used for chronic elbow dislocations. It is the most extensive and versatile approach.

COMPLICATIONS

The complications involved are as follows:
- Stiffness is seen in cases with prolonged immobilization.
- Ulnar nerve injury is seen in simple elbow dislocations and median nerve injury is seen in complex elbow dislocations.
- Vascular injury, i.e., brachial artery injury is seen rarely.
- Volkmann contracture results due to massive soft-tissue swelling resulting in increased intracompartment pressure.
- Instability or recurrent dislocation is seen in complex dislocations, i.e., terrible-triad injury.
- Arthrosis
- Heterotopic/myositis ossificans occurs due to multiple reduction attempts, severe soft-tissue injury, oil bandage massages, and in presence of associated fractures.
  - Usually seen anteriorly between the brachialis muscle and anterior capsule; posteriorly it is seen between the triceps and posterior capsule.

BIBLIOGRAPHY

1. Bridgeforth GM, Cherf J. Lippincott's Primary Care Musculoskeletal Radiology. Philadelphia: Lippincott Williams & Wilkins; 2011.
2. Dines, Lorich DG, Helfet DL. Solutions for Complex Upper Extremity Trauma. New York: Thieme; 2008.
3. Hyvönen H, Korhonen L, Hannonen J, Serlo W, Sinikumpu J. Recent trends in children's elbow dislocation with or without a concomitant fracture. BMC Musculoskelet Disord. 2019;20(1):294.
4. Marincek B, Dondelinger RF. Emergency Radiology: Imaging and Intervention. Berlin, Heidelberg: Springer; 2006.
5. Meyn MA Jr, Quigley TB. Reduction of posterior dislocation of the elbow by traction on the dangling arm. Clin Orthop Relat Res. 1974;(103):106-8.
6. Parvin RW. Closed reduction of common shoulder and elbow dislocations without anesthesia. AMA Arch Surg. 1957;75(6):972-5.

Radial Head and Neck Fracture

Waseem Ahmad Sheikh

Radial head and neck fractures are relatively common injuries, and while the majority involve the radial head, around 15–20% specifically affect the radial neck.

APPLIED ANATOMY

About one-third diameter of radial head is nonarticular and is often devoid of articular cartilage.

Mechanism of Injury and Pathophysiology

- These fractures typically occur following axial loading of the radial head during a fall on an outstretched hand.
- High-energy trauma, such as road traffic accidents, may also involve ligamentous injuries or dislocations, complicating management.

ASSOCIATED INJURIES

- Tears of medial and lateral collateral ligaments
- Other associated injuries are elbow dislocations, fractures of olecranon, capitellum, coronoid, and proximal ulna.

CLASSIFICATION SYSTEMS

The major classification systems are:

- Mason classification **(Figs. 1A to D)**:
    - *Type I:* Nondisplaced or minimally displaced (<2 mm) fractures
    - *Type II:* Displaced fractures with displacement (>2 mm)
    - *Type III:* Comminuted fractures
    - *Type IV:* Fractures with associated elbow dislocation
- *Broberg-Morrey classification:* It focuses on the degree of articular surface involvement and the elbow stability, providing further insight into the prognosis and surgical decision-making.

CLINICAL EVALUATION

- A lateral epicondyle tenderness may indicate an associated lateral collateral ligament (LCL) injury, while a comparable medial epicondyle tenderness indicates a medial collateral ligament (MCL) injury.
- Neurovascular examination is crucial to exclude posterior interosseous nerve or brachial artery injuries.

Imaging Studies

- Standard anteroposterior and lateral radiographs of the elbow should be obtained.
- Greenspan view **(Figs. 2A and B)**, also known as the radial head-capitellum view, with the tube angled at 45° cephalad toward the radial head, provides visualization of radiocapitellar articulation.

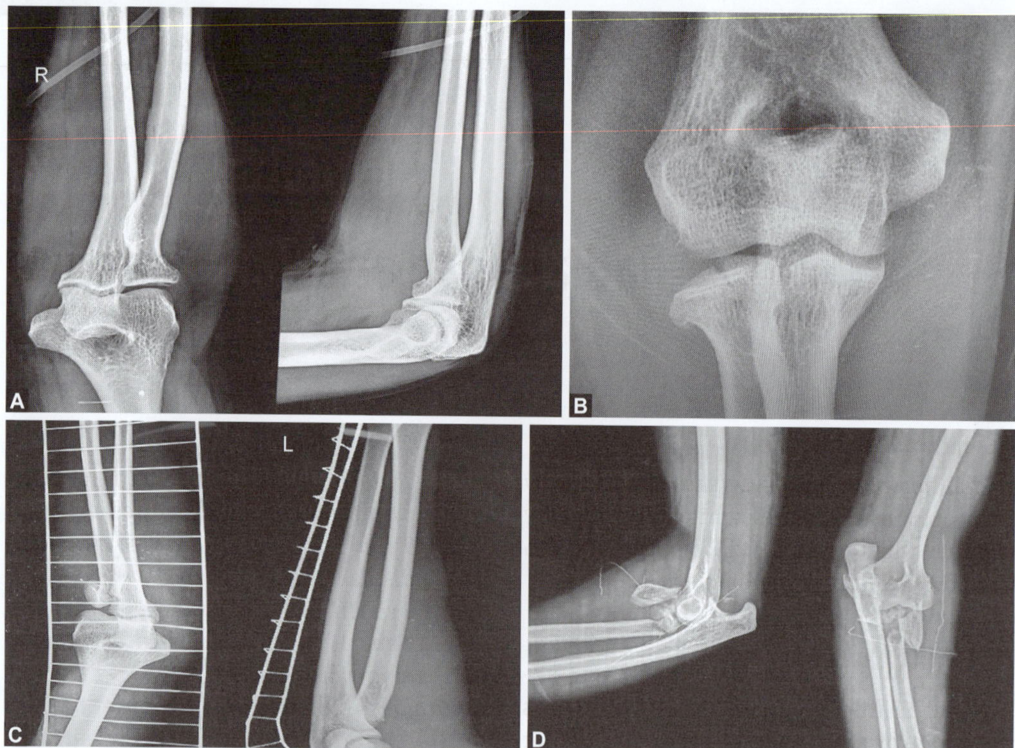

FIGS. 1A TO D: (A) Mason type I; (B) Mason type II; (C) Mason type III; and (D) Mason type IV.

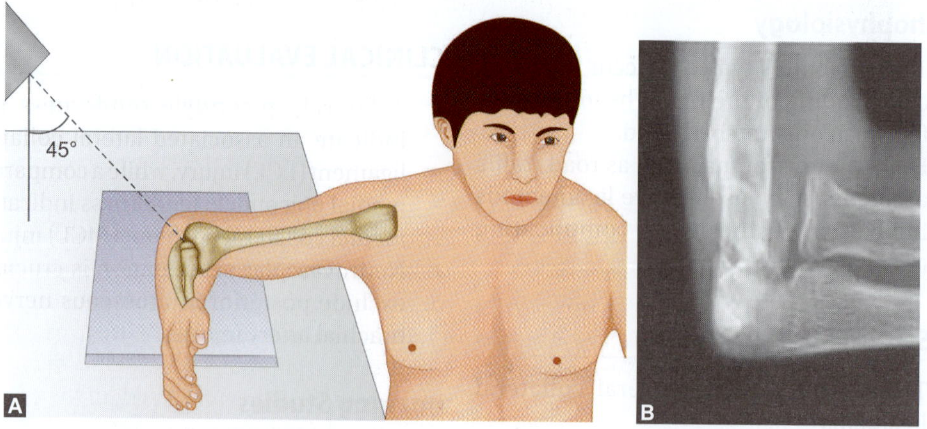

FIGS. 2A AND B: Greenspan view.

- Nondisplaced fractures may not be readily appreciable on radiographs. In such cases, diagnosis is based on anterior fat pad displacement by hemarthrosis (positive fat pad sign) **(Figs. 3A and B)**, combined with tenderness over the radial head.
- *Computed tomography (CT) scan* is indicated for complex fractures, to look for comminution and displacement, and guide surgical planning.

MANAGEMENT STRATEGIES

Nonoperative Management

Nonoperative management is indicated in the case of *Mason type I and type II fractures* without significant displacement or mechanical block to motion.

Short-term immobilization in a sling or a splint for 5–7 days, with early active range of motion exercises, is recommended. Prolonged immobilization is avoided in order to reduce the risk of joint stiffness.

Surgical Management

Surgery is indicated for fractures with significant displacement, comminution, instability, or fractures presenting with block to motion. Various surgical modalities include:

- Open reduction and internal fixation (ORIF) **(Figs. 4 and 5)**.
  - Preferred for displaced fractures with large, constructible fragments.
  - Techniques involve mini-fragment screws, headless compression screws, or low-profile plates.
  - The "safe zone" for placement of screws, determined intraoperatively, is crucial. It is advisable to place the plate 10° anterior to the mid-axial line, keeping the forearm in a neutral position during surgery.

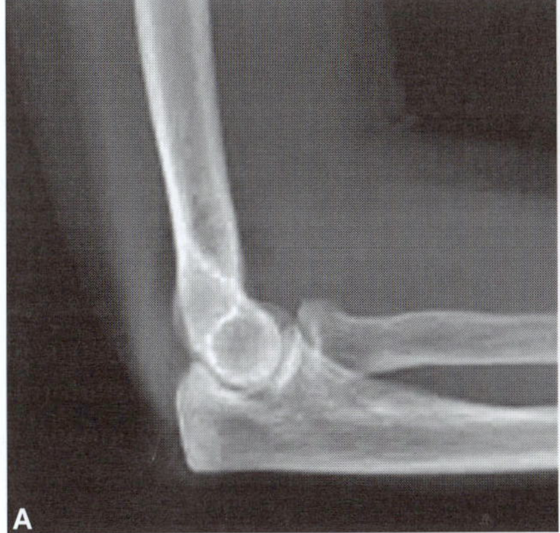

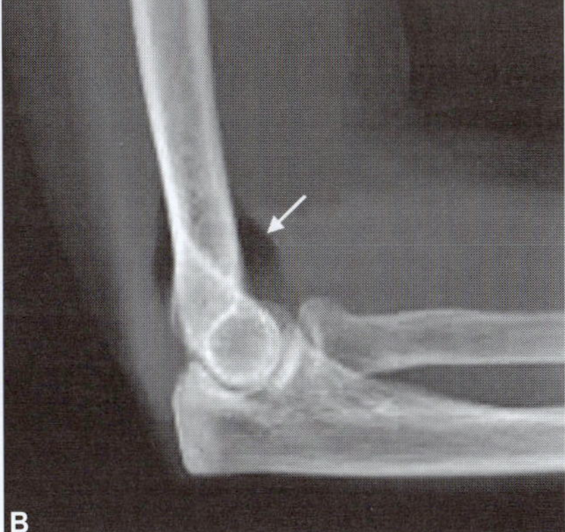

FIGS. 3A AND B: Raised fat pads (arrow).

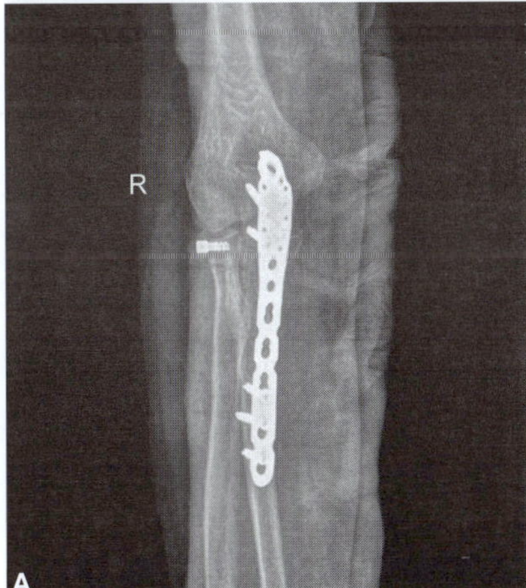

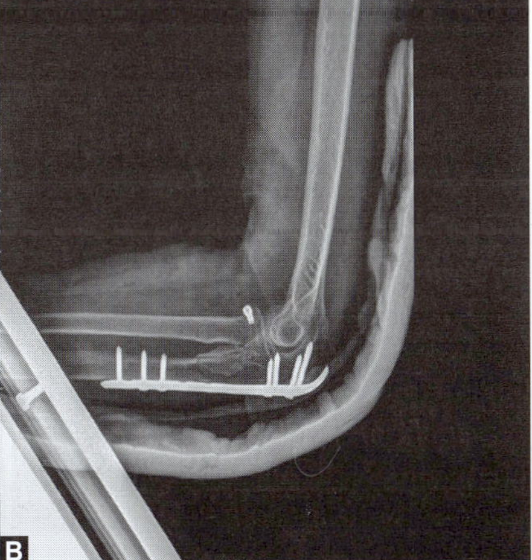

FIGS. 4A AND B: Fixation of radial head fracture with Herbert screws.

- Radial head arthroplasty **(Figs. 6A and B)**:
  - Used in case of severely comminuted, nonreconstructable fractures (Mason type III) and in fractures presenting with elbow instability (Mason type IV).
  - An appropriate size prosthesis is crucial; overstuffing the joint is to be avoided in order to reduce the risk of radiocapitellar arthritis and limited range of motion.
- Radial head excision **(Figs. 7A and B)**:
  - It is rarely recommended due to its potential to destabilize the elbow, particularly in younger or active patients.
  - It is considered in cases with severe comminution where reconstruction is not possible, provided the ligamentous structures are intact, and there is no instability.

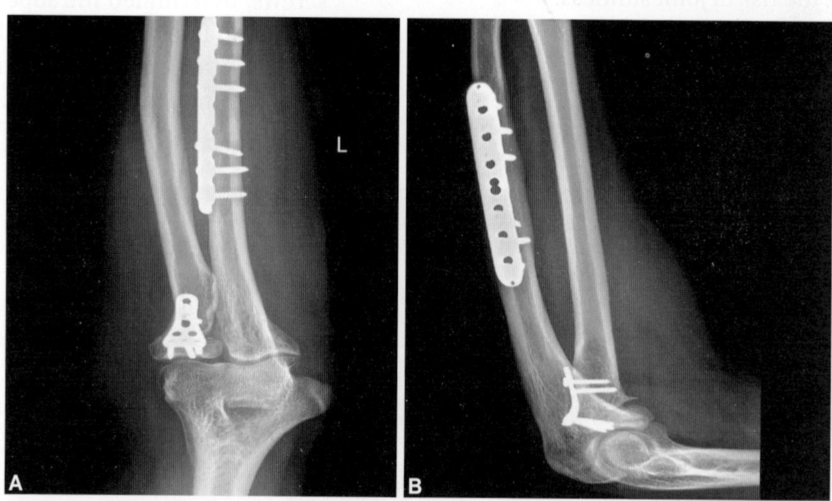

FIGS. 5A AND B: Radial head plating.

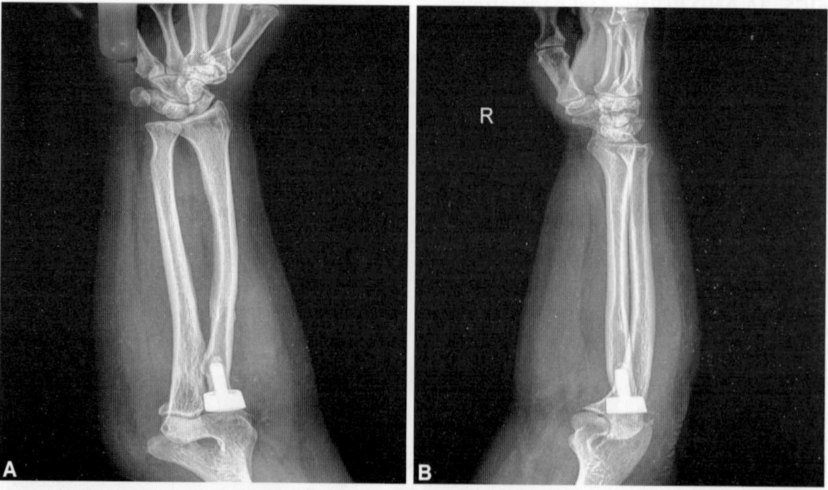

FIGS. 6A AND B: Radial head arthroplasty.

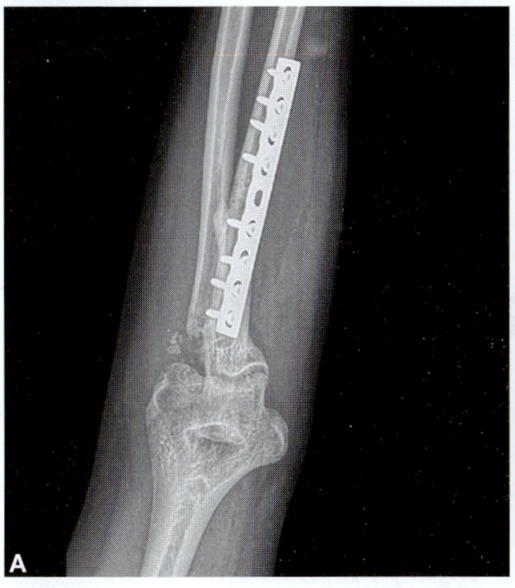
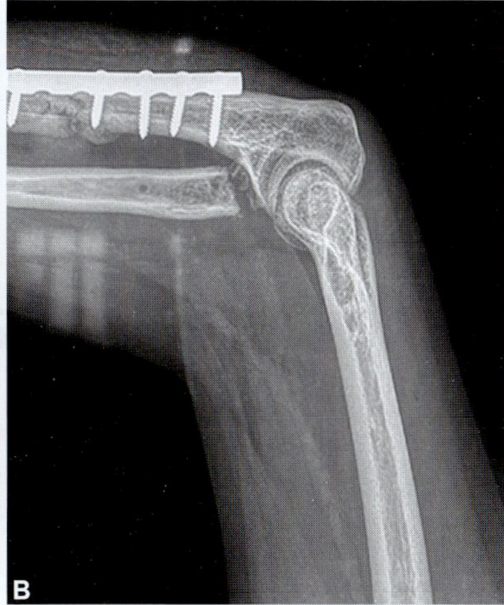

FIGS. 7A AND B: Radial head excision.

- Excision is more favorable in low-demand patients with isolated fractures.

COMPLICATIONS

The complications that may be caused are as follows:

- Elbow stiffness
- Nonunion or malunion
- Post-traumatic osteoarthritis
- Heterotopic ossification
- Hardware complications
- Complex regional pain syndrome
- Chronic instability

RECENT ADVANCES AND GUIDELINES

- *Orthopaedic Trauma Association (OTA) Consensus (2023 Update):* It emphasizes radial head preservation over excision. ORIF is recommended where feasible; arthroplasty is preferred for nonreconstructable comminuted fractures.
- *European Society of Sports Traumatology, Knee Surgery and Arthroscopy (ESSKA) Guidelines (2023):* Support early functional rehabilitation following ORIF or arthroplasty. Suggest considering prophylaxis against heterotopic ossification in high-risk patients.
- *Patient-specific instrumentation (PSI) and 3D printing:* Emerging technologies are enhancing surgical precision in complex cases, enabling custom solutions tailored to individual anatomical variations.

BIBLIOGRAPHY

1. Broberg MA, Morrey BF. Results of delayed excision of the radial head after fracture. J Bone Joint Surg Am. 1986;68(5):669-74.
2. Duckworth AD, Clement ND, Jenkins PJ, Aitken SA, Court-Brown CM, McQueen MM, et al. The epidemiology of radial head and neck fractures. J Hand Surg Am. 2012;37(1):112-9.
3. Hotchkiss RN. Displaced fractures of the radial head: Internal fixation or excision? J Am Acad Orthop Surg. 1997;5(1):1-10.
4. Jensen SL, Olsen BS, Søjbjerg JO. Elbow joint stability following experimental radial head excision and lateral collateral ligament rupture: A biomechanical study. J Shoulder Elbow Surg. 1999;8(5):452-6.
5. Morrey BF, Sanchez-Sotelo J. The Elbow and its Disorders, 4th edition. Philadelphia: Saunders; 2009.
6. O'Driscoll SW, Jupiter JB, Cohen MS, Ring D, McKee MD. Difficult elbow fractures: Pearls and pitfalls. Instr Course Lect. 2003;52:113-34.
7. Ring D, Quintero J, Jupiter JB. Open reduction and internal fixation of fractures of the radial head. J Bone Joint Surg Am. 2002;84(10):1811-5.

CHAPTER 4.3

Coronoid Process Fracture and Terrible Triad

Shubham Pandoh, Sonakshi Gupta

CORONOID PROCESS

- The coronoid process is an important structure for the concentric alignment of the elbow joint.
- The anterior bundle of the medial collateral ligament (MCL), brachialis tendon, and anterior capsule attach to it.
- It acts as an anterior buttress to the ulna-humeral joint and helps to resist varus stress; therefore, helps in preventing posterior subluxation or dislocation of the elbow.

Fractures of the coronoid process constitute about 10–15% of elbow fractures. They are frequently associated with complex elbow dislocations (terrible triad injuries), radial head fractures, and capsuloligamentous injuries.

Injury Mechanism

Fall on outstretched hand:
- Axial loading
- Posterolateral rotatory loading
- Posteromedial loading

Classification

Regan and Morrey Classification

The Regan and Morrey classification of the coronoid process is given in **Figure 1**.

The percentage of coronoid process involvement on the lateral radiographic view of the elbow serves as the basis for the Regan and Morrey classification.

Limitation: This classification does not allow for the recognition of anteromedial facet fragments.

Type I	Coronoid TIP	No instability
Type II	< 50% height	Instability
Type III	> 50% height	Posterior instability

• Modification

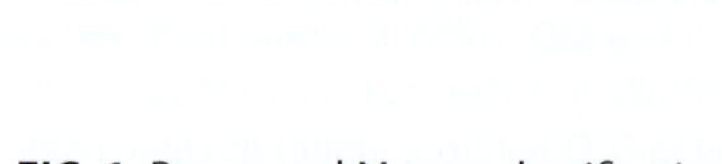

Class A	Isolated fracture
Class B	Fracture dislocation

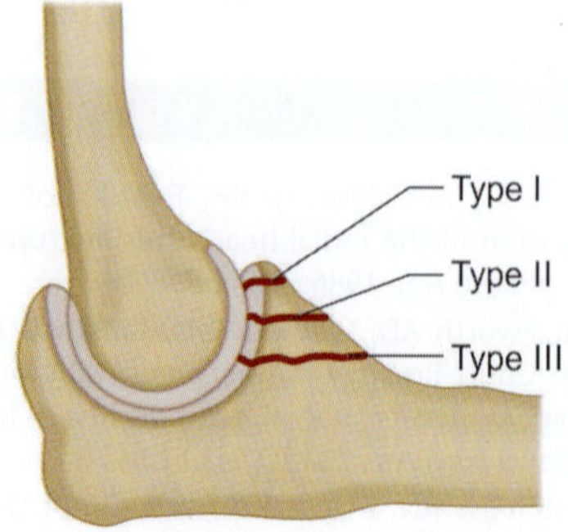

FIG. 1: Regan and Morrey classification.

O'Driscoll Classification

O'Driscoll suggested categorization according to the anatomic location, degree of coronoid fracture, comminution, stability of ulnohumeral joint, and related injuries **(Fig. 2 and Table 1)**.

Imaging Studies

- Radiographs of the elbow—anteroposterior, lateral, and oblique views
- Computed tomography (CT) including 3D reconstruction.
- Magnetic resonance imaging (MRI), if ligamentous injury is suspected.

Treatment

Nonoperative Treatment

Indications:

- Type 1 fractures
- Small, nondisplaced type 2 fractures

Immobilization in a splint or hinged brace for 10–14 days followed by early mobilization.

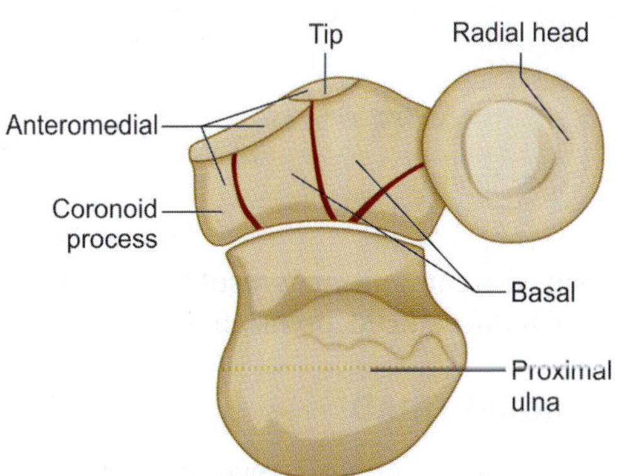

FIG. 2: Showing different parts of coronoid process.

Operative Treatment

The goals are anatomic restoration and joint stability.

Indications:

- Displaced fractures, particularly type 3 fractures
- Type 2 or 3 fractures with significant instability
- Concomitant injuries like radial head fractures or ligament injuries

Surgical Approaches

The choice of surgical approach should cater to specific fracture patterns and associated injuries **(Table 2)**.

Fixation Techniques

The fixation techniques are given in **Table 3**.

Emerging Techniques

- Arthroscopic-assisted fixation
- 3D printed patient-specific implants

These techniques allow precise reduction and fixation with less soft-tissue disruption, fast recovery, and reduced postoperative pain.

Rehabilitation Protocol

The aim is to restore range of motion (ROM), strength, and stability.

The protocol is given in **Table 4**.

Complications

- *Early complications*:
  - Neurovascular (posterior interosseous nerve and brachial artery)

TABLE 1: O'Driscoll classification.

Type I Coronoid tip	*Subtype 1:* < 2 mm coronoid process	Terrible triad
	Subtype 2: > 2 mm coronoid process	Valgus posterolateral rotatory instability
Type II Anteromedial fracture	*Subtype 1:* Anteromedial rim	Varus posteromedial rotatory instability
	Subtype 2: Rim + tip	
	Subtype 3: Rim + tubercle +/– tip	Lateral collateral ligament tear
Type III Basal fracture	*Subtype 1:* Body + base	Fractures of radial head, proximal ulna, and concomitant ligament injuries
	Subtype 2: Transolecranon + base	

TABLE 2: Surgical approaches.

Indications	Operative procedure
Type 1, 2, and 3 with persistent elbow instability	ORIF with medial approach
Posteromedial rotatory instability	ORIF with medial approach
Fracture dislocation of olecranon	ORIF with posterior approach
Terrible triad of elbow	ORIF with posterior approach/lateral approach
Isolated coronoid fracture	ORIF with anterior approach

TABLE 3: Fixation techniques.

Techniques	Indications
Suture anchor **(Fig. 3A)**	Small tip fractures
Screw fixation **(Fig. 3B)**	Large fragments (type 2 and 3 fractures)
Plate fixation **(Fig. 3C)**	Basal fractures or comminuted fractures
Hinged external fixation	Poor bone quality and difficult revision cases

TABLE 4: Rehabilitation protocol.

Phase 1	Passive motion initiation within the first week postoperatively
Phase 2	Active motion by the third week
Phase 3	Functional bracing + targeted physical therapy exercises

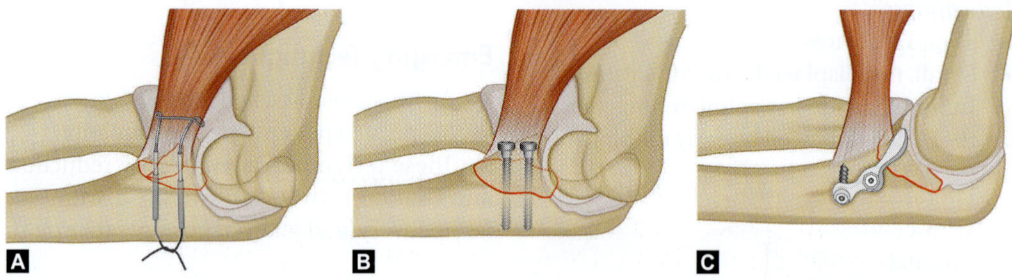

FIGS. 3A TO C: (A) Anchor suture; (B) screw fixation; and (C) plate fixation.

- Recurrent dislocation
- Internal fixation failure

• *Late complications*:
  - Heterotopic ossification
  - Stiffness
  - Post-traumatic arthritis

Prognosis

The prognosis of coronoid process fractures is directly proportional to the severity of the fracture, related injuries, and the adequacy of the treatment. Early and appropriate management typically leads to favorable outcomes, with good to excellent functional recovery in most cases. However, fractures associated with complex elbow instability or delayed treatment may result in persistent pain, reduced ROM, or instability.

TERRIBLE TRIAD

Hotchkiss, in the year 1996, described the term terrible triad of the elbow.

The terrible triad of the elbow refers to a complex injury pattern characterized by the simultaneous presence of three components: Posterior dislocation of the elbow, radial head fracture, and fracture of the coronoid process of the ulna.

There is substantial soft-tissue injury with capsuloligamentous disruption. The lateral ulnar collateral ligament (LUCL) is particularly injured **(Fig. 4)**.

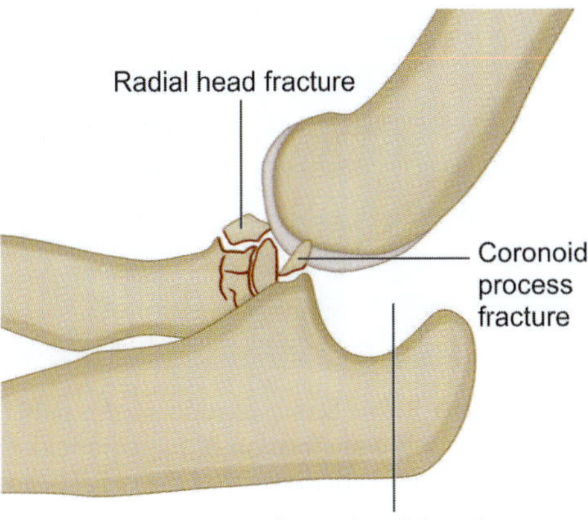

FIG. 4: Terrible traid.

Injury Mechanism

Fall on outstretched hand:
- Axial loading
- Posterolateral rotatory loading
- Posteromedial loading

Investigations

- *X-rays of the elbow*: Anteroposterior lateral and oblique views **(Figs. 5 and 6)**
- CT including 3D reconstruction **(Fig. 7)**
- MRI to evaluate ligamentous injury

Attention to neurovascular status is crucial due to the proximity of ulnar and median nerves.

Treatment

Nonoperative Treatment

Indications:
- Stable elbow joints after reduction
- Nondisplaced fractures
    - Mason type 1 radial head
    - Regan–Morrey type 1 coronoid
- Patients with low functional demand

Closed reduction is done followed by immobilization for a brief period followed by early ROM.

Operative Management

Indications:
- Unstable radial head fracture

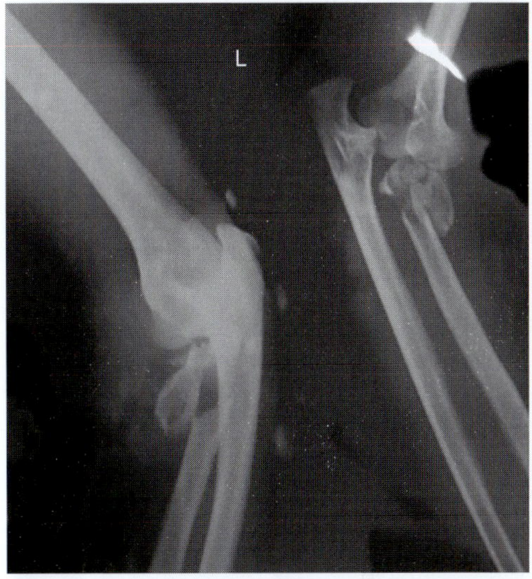

FIG. 5: X-rays anteroposterior (AP) and lateral views of elbow joint.

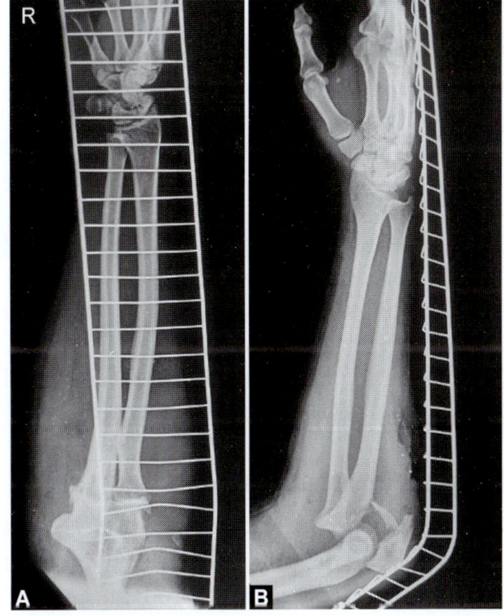

FIGS. 6A AND B: X-rays with anteroposterior (AP) and lateral views of elbow joint with forearm.

- Type 3 coronoid fracture
- Associated elbow dislocation

Early fixation, particularly within the first 2 weeks after injury significantly reduces the risk of residual instability and post-traumatic arthritis.

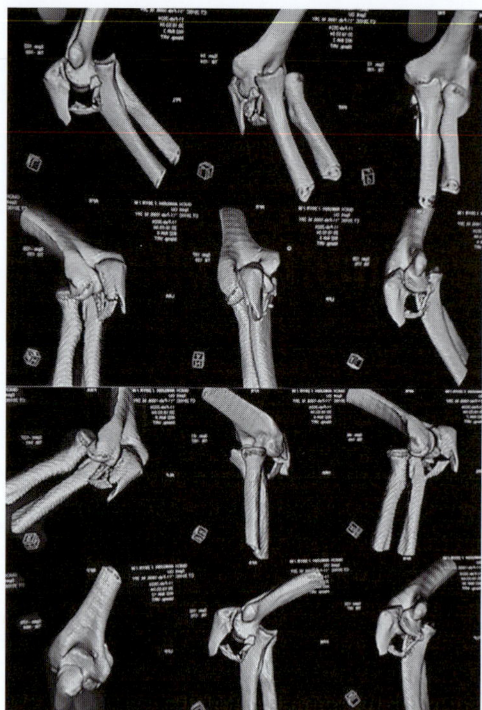

FIG. 7: Noncontrast computed tomography (NCCT) of elbow joint with 3D reconstruction.

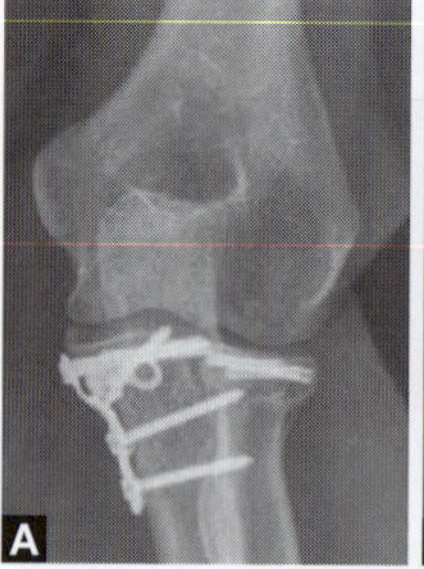

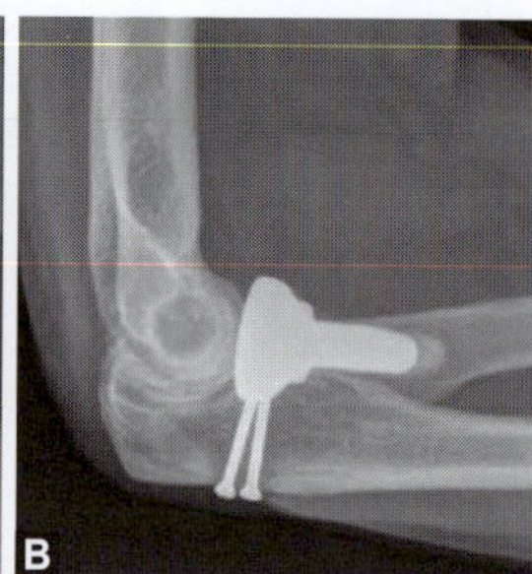

FIGS. 8A AND B: (A) Screw fixation of the radial head + screw and plate fixation of the coronoid + ligament repair; (B) Replacement of the radial head + screw fixation of the coronoid + ligament repair.

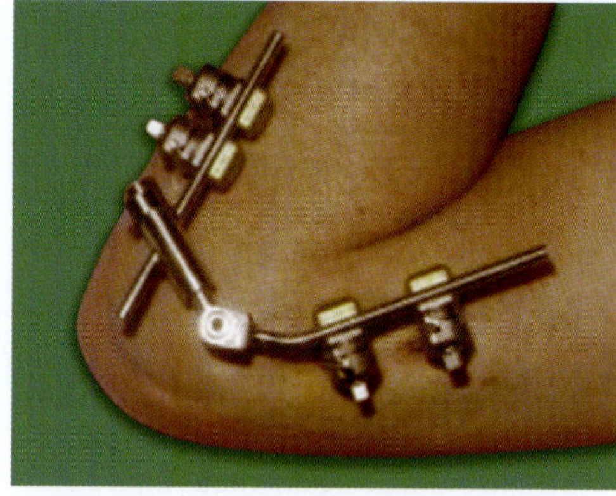

FIG. 9: A hinged/static external fixator.

Sequence of fixation:
1. Mobilization of fragments of radial head and coronoid fracture fixation
2. Fixation of radial head/neck or radial head replacement
3. Reattachment of origin of lateral collateral ligament (LCL) to the lateral epicondyle

Surgical Approaches

- *Lateral approach (Kocher approach):* It is used when the radial head has to be fixed or replaced and for LUCL repair.
- *Medial approach (Hotchkiss approach):* It is used when coronoid fixation is required or when MCL repair is necessary.

Repair of lateral and medial collateral ligament **(Figs. 8A and B)**:
- Repair of LUCL using suture anchors is preferred.
- Repair of medial collateral ligament should be done when there is evidence of persistent medial instability, even after lateral ligament repair.

A hinged/static external fixator is used when joint stability is not sufficient **(Fig. 9)**.

It is indicated in cases of poor bone quality and difficult revision cases.

Postoperative Rehabilitation

Position of immobilization: If MCL is intact and LCL has been repaired, then keep the elbow at 90° flexion/full pronation.

If MCL and LCL both have been repaired, then the splint is in a neutral position.

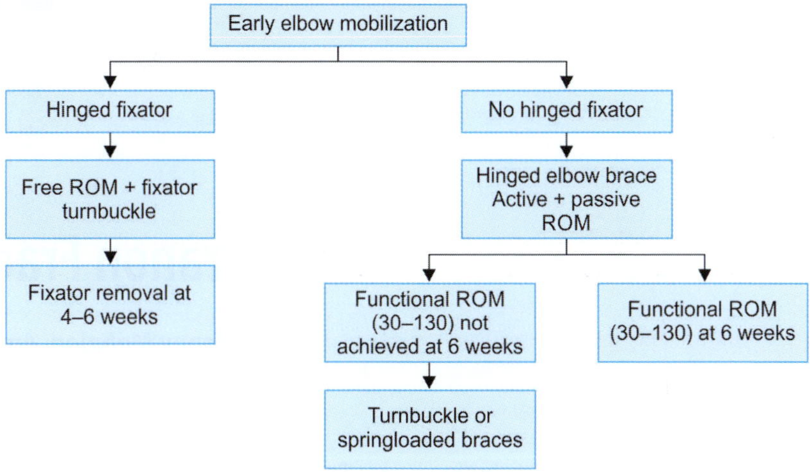

FLOWCHART 1: Early elbow mobilization.

If LCL is intact and MCL has been repaired, then keep the elbow at 90° flexion and full supination.

Range of Motion

The ROM is shown in **Flowchart 1**:

- *Begin ROM:* Within 7-10 days postsurgery
- *Stable arc of motion:* Intraoperatively determined
    - A hinged elbow brace should be used to control ROM and prevent varus and valgus stress
- Functional physical therapy exercises

Emerging Techniques

Emerging techniques include arthroscopic-assisted fixation.

Complications

- Stiffness
- Residual instability
- Post-traumatic arthrosis
- Heterotopic ossification

Outcome

The prognosis of the terrible triad of the elbow is based on multiple factors like the severity of the initial injury, the adequacy of surgical repair, and the effectiveness of the rehabilitation program. Recent studies suggest that early, stable fixation combined with a carefully planned rehabilitation protocol can yield satisfactory results in most patients, with good functional outcomes and a low rate of complications.

BIBLIOGRAPHY

1. Bozon O, Chrosciany S, Loisel M, Dellestable A, Gubbiotti L, Dumartinet-Gibaud R, et al. Terrible triad injury of the elbow: A historical perspective. Int Orthop. 2022;46(10):2265-72.
2. Bhashyam AR, Chen N. Arthroscopic-Assisted Fracture Fixation About the Elbow. Hand Clin. 2023;39(4):587-95.
3. de Klerk HH, Ring D, Boerboom L, van der Bekerom MPJ, Doonberg JN. Coronoid fractures and traumatic elbow instability. JSES Int. 2023;7(6):2587-93.
4. Harding P, Rasekaba T, Romero L, Hollan AE. Early mobilisation for elbow fractures in adults. Cochrane Database Syst Rev. 2011:CD008130.
5. Thayer MK, Swenson AK, Hackett DJ, Hsu JE. Classifications in brief: Regan-Morrey Classification of Coronoid fractures. Clin Orthop Relat Res. 2018;476(7):1540-3.
6. Zhang Y, et al. 3D-printed implants in elbow fracture management. J Orthop Sci. 2023;42:94-112..

CHAPTER 4.4

Olecranon Fracture

Kanav Mahajan, Amit Kumar

Olecranon fractures have bimodal distribution. They are caused by:

- High-energy trauma in young population
- Low-energy trauma/simple falls in the elderly population

MECHANISM OF INJURY

The mechanism of injury is given in **Box 1**.

CLINICAL FINDINGS

- The inability to extend the elbow against gravity suggests a displaced fracture and loss of the triceps extensor mechanism.
- Rarely, ulnar nerve injury is also seen that can result in long-term sensory and motor impairment in the hand.
- Associated injuries of the coronoid process, radial head, or proximal radioulnar joint may be seen.

IMAGING

- Anteroposterior and lateral views are advised.
- True lateral view is required to access fracture extent, severity, comminution, and articular surface involvement.
- A computed tomography (CT) scan may be needed in severe comminution and articular fractures.

BOX 1 Mechanism of injury.

- *Direct*: Direct blow to the olecranon—comminuted fracture
- *Indirect*: Fall on outstretched hand (FOOSH)—transverse fracture or oblique fracture (more common)
- *Avulsion fracture:* Triceps bony avulsion fracture
- *Stress fracture:* Throwers, athletes, and gymnasts

CLASSIFICATION

Mayo Classification

Mayo classification is based on displacement, communication, and stability **(Fig. 1 and Table 1)**.

Schatzker Classification

Schatzker classification is based on fracture pattern **(Fig. 2 and Table 2)**.

TREATMENT

The goals of treatment are:

- Articular restoration of joint
- Stability of elbow joint
- Early mobilization of the joint to avoid stiffness and other complications
- Preservation of the extensor mechanism

Nonoperative Treatment

Indications:

- Undisplaced fractures with intact extensor mechanism
- Low-demand patients
- Elderly patients unfit for operative intervention

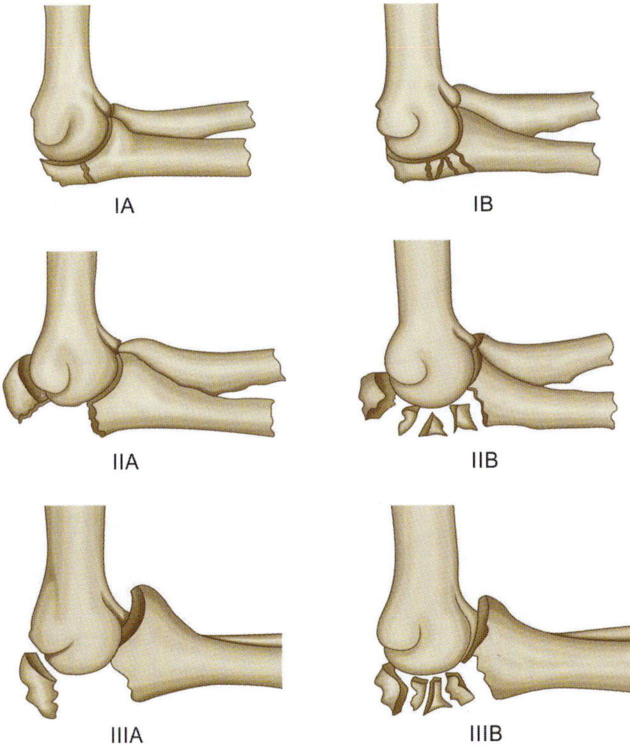

FIG. 1: Mayo classification.

TABLE 1: Mayo classification.

Type	Fracture pattern
A	Transverse fracture
B	Transverse impacted fracture
C	Oblique fracture
D	Comminuted fracture
E	Oblique distal fracture (extra articular)
F	Fracture dislocation

Nonoperative treatment involves immobilization in 45–90° flexion with above elbow plaster of Paris (POP) slab/cast for 3 weeks followed by gradual range of motion exercises.

Operative

Indications:
- Displaced (>2 mm) and comminuted fractures
- Open fractures
- Articular incongruity

Options for operative treatment:
- *Tension band wiring (TBW)* ***(Figs. 3A to D)***: This is the most common form of surgical treatment, *especially in transversely displaced fractures with good bone quality.*
  - *Principle:* It counteracts the tensile forces at the fracture site and converts them into compressive forces at the fracture site during elbow flexion.
  - A single knot or double knot can be used to achieve the desired compression at the fracture site.
- *Intramedullary screw fixation* ***(Figs. 4A and B)***:
  - 6.5 mm cancellous screws or intramedullary Kirschner wires (K-wires) can be used for fixation of fracture fragments alone or in combination with TBW.
  - Used in simple fractures or fractures without any comminution

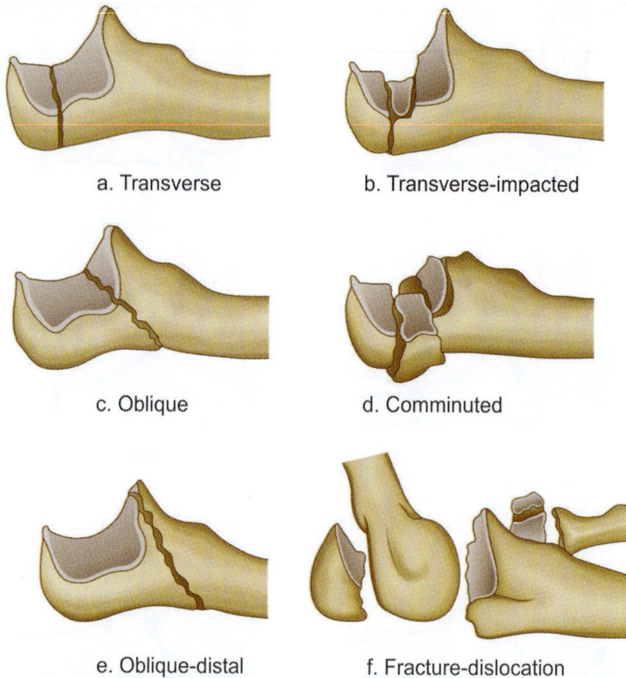

FIG. 2: Schatzker classification.

TABLE 2: Schatzker classification.

Type I Undisplaced	• Noncomminuted • Comminuted
Type II Displaced (stable)	• Noncomminuted • Comminuted
Type III Unstable	• Noncomminuted • Comminuted

- *Plate and screws fixation* (**Fig. 5**):
  - Indications:
    - Comminuted fractures
    - Osteoporotic bones
    - Unstable fractures
    - Fracture dislocations
    - Monteggia fractures
    - Fractures that extend distal to the coronoid
- *Excision of the fragment with triceps resuturing to distal fragment*:
  - Indications:
    - Severely comminuted fractures
    - Osteoporotic bones
    - Nonunion of fracture
    - Low-demand patients
  - Contraindications:
    - In fracture-dislocations
    - Associated radial head fracture
    - Unstable elbow

  It can be done in fractures with <50% articular surface involvement.
- *Anchor suture fixation:* Used for chip and avulsion fractures of olecranon

Postoperative Care

- The posterior removable splint or above elbow plaster slab can be used postoperatively for 7–10 days with the elbow at 90° of flexion and the wrist in the neutral position.
- Immobilization is then followed by gradual range of motion exercises as tolerated by the patient.
- Active range of motion and strengthening exercises begin approximately 6–8 weeks postoperatively.

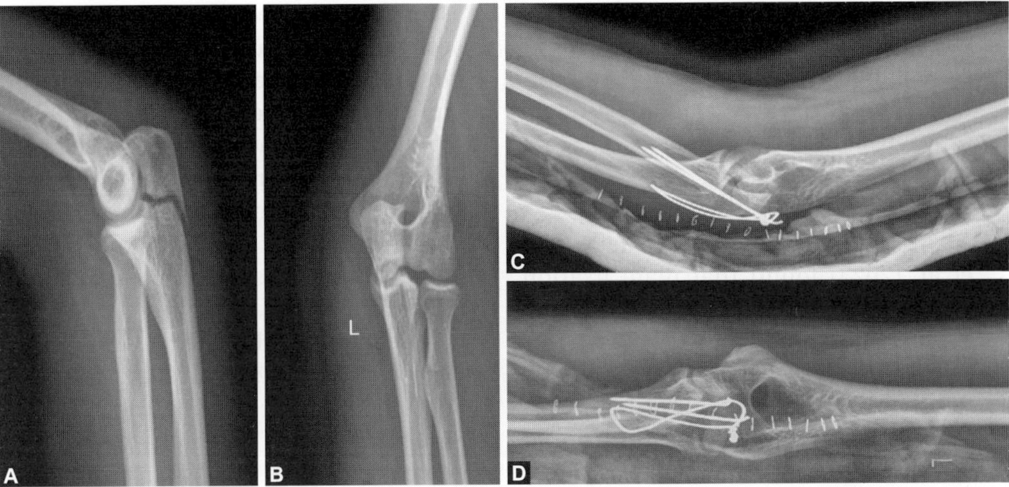

FIGS. 3A TO D: Tension band wiring (TBW). (A and B) X-ray showing transverse fracture of olecranon (L); (C and D) X-ray showing fracture fixed with TBW done with a single loop.

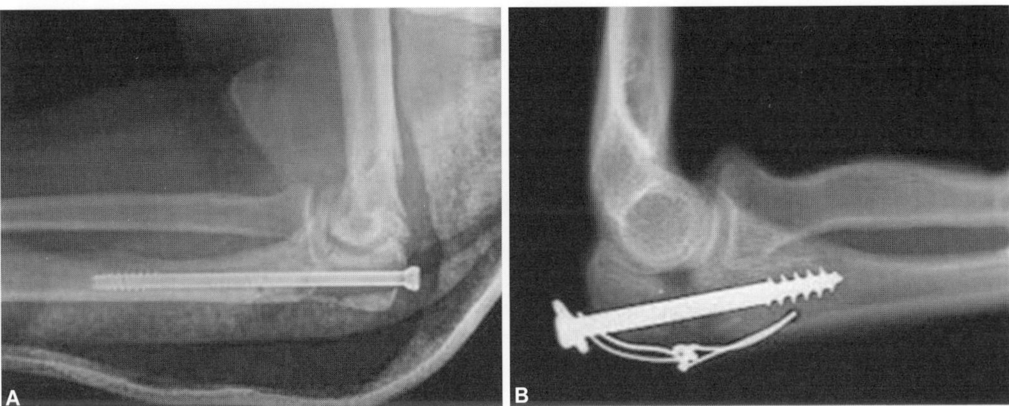

FIGS. 4A AND B: Intramedullary screw fixation. (A) X-ray showing fracture fixed with cannulated cancellous screw; (B) X-ray showing fracture fixed with tension band wiring (TBW) principle using a screw.

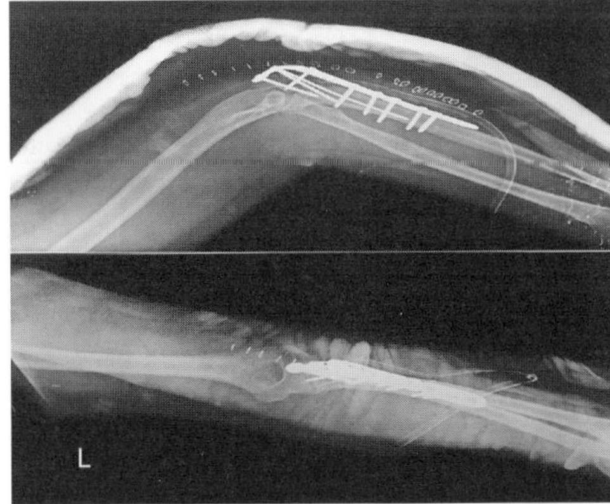

FIG. 5: X-ray showing fracture fixed with olecranon plating.

- Patients may return to work involving sporting activities and vigorous use of the extremity at 3–4 months post-operatively.

Common complications following olecranon fracture surgery include:

- *Hardware irritation:* It is particularly common with TBW. Early removal may be necessary if symptomatic.
- *Nonunion and malunion:* These are rare but may occur with inadequate fixation or in osteoporotic bone.
- *Infection:* Risk factors include open fractures and poor soft-tissue condition.

- *Post-traumatic osteoarthritis:* Associated with intra-articular incongruity or comminution
- *Ulnar nerve injury:* Due to surgical exposure or hardware irritation

Evidence from Recent Studies

- A systematic review by Duckworth et al. (2023) found that plate fixation provides better functional outcomes and lower reoperation rates than TBW for comminuted fractures.
- Randomized trials comparing intramedullary fixation with traditional methods show favorable results for patient satisfaction and reduced hardware-related complications (Hussain et al., 2022).
- In 2021, Rantalaiho et al. also found no differences between TBW and plate fixation for displaced unstable olecranon fractures with respect to clinical or patient-rated outcome measures.
- In 2022, Hongfei et al. reported similar results in a retrospective comparison of TBW with plating.
- Guidelines from the Orthopaedic Trauma Association (2024) advocate for early mobilization protocols and patient-specific fixation methods to optimize outcomes.

BIBLIOGRAPHY

1. Baecher N, Edwards S. Olecranon fractures. J Hand Surg Am. 2013;38(3):593-604.
2. Browner BD, Jupiter JB, Levine AM, Trafton PG (Eds). Skeletal Trauma: Fractures, Dislocations, Ligamentous Injuries. Philadelphia: WB Saunders; 1992. p. 1137.
3. Bucholz RW, Heckman JD, Court-Brown CM, Rockwood CA, Green DP (Eds). Rockwood and Green's fractures in Adults, 6th edition. Philadelphia: Lippincott Williams & Wilkins; 2006.
4. Chen MJ, Campbell ST, Finlay AK, Duckworth AD, Bishop JA, Gardner MJ. Surgical and nonoperative management of olecranon fractures in the elderly: A systematic review and meta-analysis. J Orthop Trauma. 2021;35(1):10-6.
5. Duckworth AD, Clement ND, Court-Brown CM, McQueen MM. Plate fixation versus tension-band wiring for olecranon fractures: A randomized clinical trial. J Bone Jt Surg. 2023;105:112-3.
6. Hussain S, Rasheed R, Khan N. Intramedullary screw fixation of olecranon fractures: A comparative study. J Orthop Res. 2022.
7. Qi H, Li Z, Lu Y, Ma T, Ji S, Du B, et al. Comparison of clinical outcomes of three internal fixation techniques in the treatment of olecranon fractures. A retrospective clinical study. BMC Musculoskelet Disord. 2022;23(1):521.
8. Rantalaiho IK, Miikkulainen AE, Laaksonen IE, Äärimaa VO, Laimi KA. Treatment of displaced olecranon fractures: a systemic review. Scand J Surg. 2021;110(1):13-21.

SECTION

5

Forearm Injuries

CHAPTER 5.1

Both Bone Forearm Fracture

Sukhil Raina, Heemanshu Bhat

Forearm fractures in adults are commonly caused by trauma such as falls, motor vehicle accidents, or direct impacts. Isolated radial fractures often also result from falls on an outstretched hand.

APPLIED ANATOMY

- *Radius:* It is primarily responsible for transmitting forces from the wrist to the forearm. It articulates with the ulna at both proximal and distal radioulnar joints, which are critical for forearm rotation.
- *Ulna:* The proximal end of the ulna forms the elbow's hinge joint with the humerus. It serves as the stabilizing structure of the forearm while the radius moves around it during rotation.
- *Interosseous membrane:* The interosseous membrane stabilizes the two bones, aids in load distribution across the forearm, and contributes to the function of the distal radioulnar joint.

CLASSIFICATION OF FOREARM FRACTURES

Anatomical Classification

- *Isolated radius or ulna fractures:* These fractures involve only one bone.
- Both bone fractures involving both radius and ulna **(Fig. 1A)**
- Both isolated fractures and both bone fractures can be further classified based on location like—proximal, middle, and distal third fracture.
- *Monteggia fractures:* These are fractures of the proximal third of the ulna with dislocation of the radial head. These injuries are associated with significant soft-tissue damage and require prompt reduction and fixation to avoid chronic instability **(Fig. 1B)**.
- *Galeazzi fractures:* It is a fracture of the distal third of the radius with dislocation or subluxation of the distal radioulnar joint. This injury pattern necessitates anatomical reduction to prevent chronic joint dysfunction **(Fig. 1C)**.
- *Nightstick fracture:* It is mostly distal third of ulna fracture caused by direct trauma while the patient is trying to protect himself/herself during any direct assault on the forearm **(Fig. 2)**.

Arbeitsgemeinschaft Für Osteosynthesefragen/Orthopaedic Trauma Association Classification

The Arbeitsgemeinschaft für Osteosynthese-fragen/Orthopaedic Trauma Association (AO/OTA) classification is given in **Figure 3**.

- Type A (simple fracture)
- Type B (wedge fracture)
- Type C (multi-fragmentary/complex fracture)

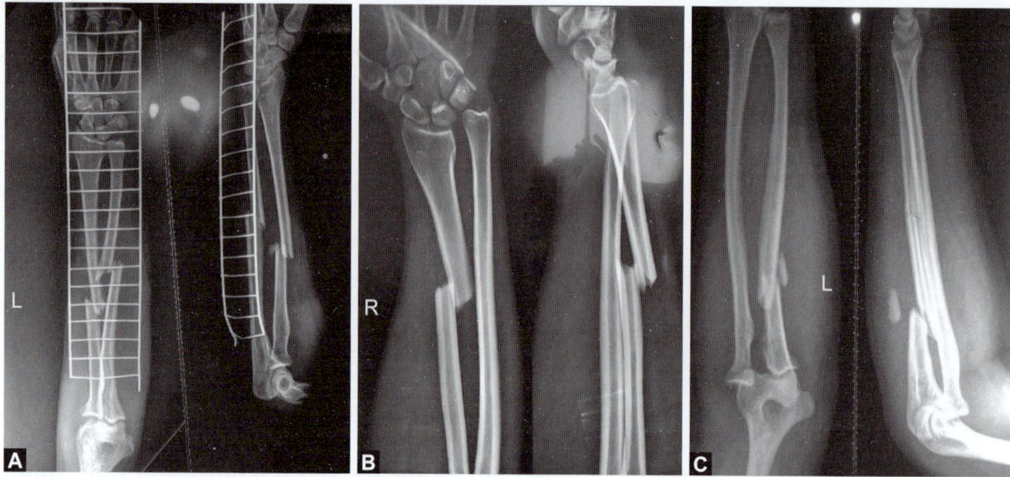

FIG. 1A TO C: (A) Fracture of both bones of the forearm; (B) Monteggia fracture; and (C) Galeazzi fracture.

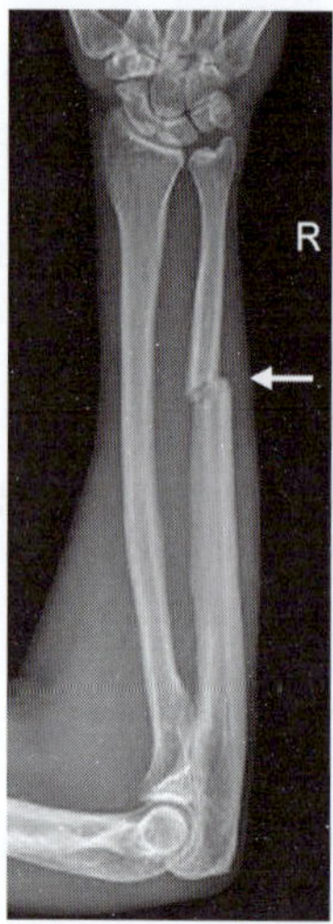

FIG. 2: Nightstick fracture.

PRINCIPLES OF MANAGEMENT

A thorough neurovascular examination and suspecting and ruling out compartment syndrome are essential.

Radiological Evaluation

Radiographs: Standard anteroposterior (AP) and lateral radiographs are essential to evaluate fracture type, displacement, and involvement of adjacent joints. Radiographs of one joint proximal to the fracture and one joint distal to the fracture must also be taken.

NONSURGICAL MANAGEMENT

Nonsurgical management is appropriate for only fractures that are stable, undisplaced, or in patients with significant comorbidities where surgical risk outweighs the benefits.

Procedure: A long-arm cast or splint is applied for 4–8 weeks and then converted to a functional below-elbow cast, depending on fracture stability and healing rates. The functional below-elbow cast allows the elbow range of motion while restricting supination and pronation of the forearm. During immobilization, regular radiographic evaluation is necessary to ensure maintenance of reduction.

SURGICAL MANAGEMENT

Surgical management is the treatment of choice:

- *Open reduction and internal fixation (ORIF):* ORIF with plating is the standard of care for most displaced fractures of the radius, ulna, or both. Dynamic compression plates (DCPs) are preferred in two-part fracture patterns as they produce absolute fracture stability **(Fig. 4)**. The goal of DCPs is cortical opposition and compression at the fracture site. Locking compression

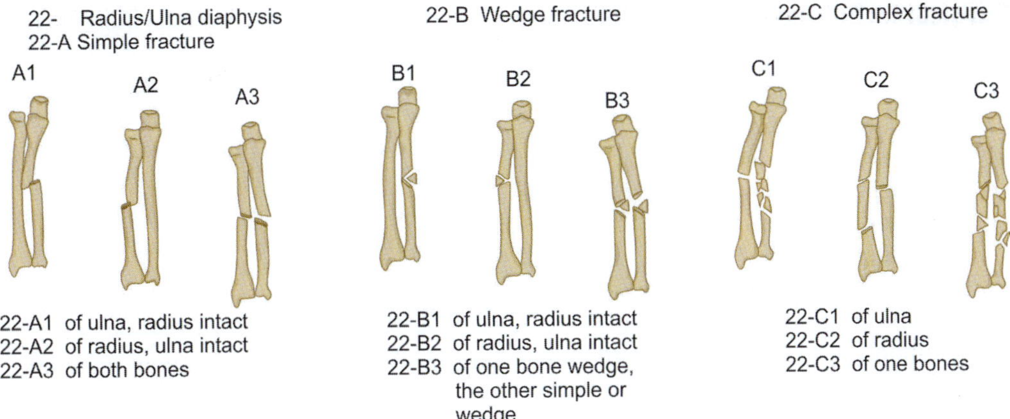

FIG. 3: Arbeitsgemeinschaft für Osteosynthesefragen/Orthopaedic Trauma Association (AO/OTA) classification.

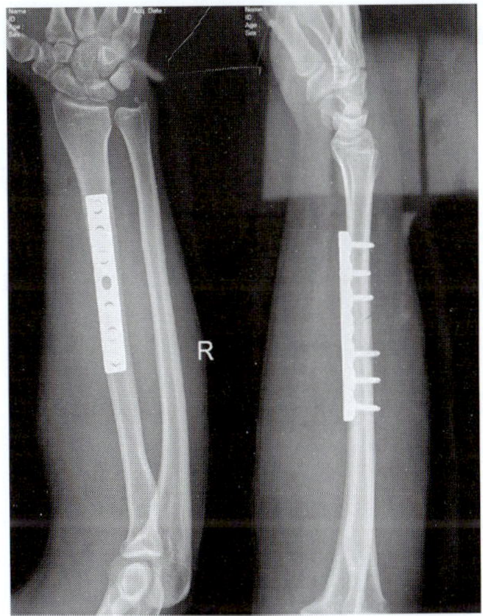

FIG. 4: Galeazzi fracture managed by ORIF with plating (dynamic compression plating).

(ORIF: open reduction and internal fixation)

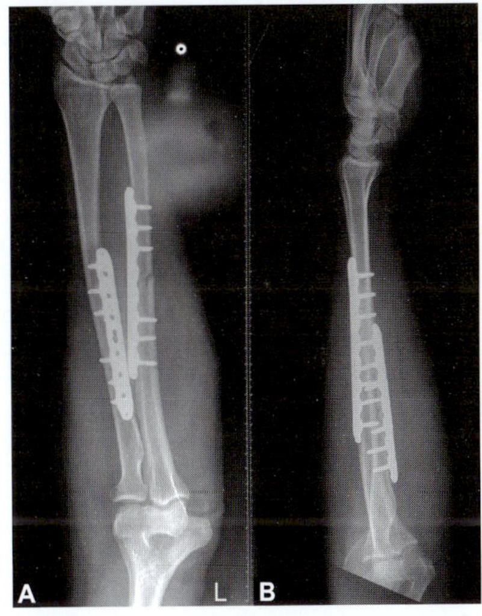

FIGS. 5A AND B: Fracture of both bones of forearm managed by ORIF with plating.

(ORIF: open reduction and internal fixation)

plates (LCPs) are favored in osteoporotic bone for superior fixation properties. Restoration of the radial bow is the most important variable in achieving a good functional outcome **(Figs. 5A and B)**. At least six cortices or three screws fixation need to be on either side of the fracture

- *Intramedullary nailing:* This technique is less common for forearm fractures but may be indicated in selected cases, such as segmental fractures and open injuries. Intramedullary nails provide less rotational control compared to plates.
- *External fixation:* Typically used for open fractures with extensive soft-tissue injury or when immediate internal fixation is contraindicated (Gustilo IIIB and C). External fixators provide temporary stabilization while allowing access for wound management.

Surgical Techniques and Considerations

Approaches: Surgical approaches should be tailored to fracture location and type. Common surgical approaches are:

- *Henry approach:* The Volar Henry approach is commonly used for middle third and distal third radius fractures (including Galeazzi fractures) and even for the proximal third of fractured radius.
- *Thompson approach:* This approach is commonly used for proximal third radius fractures. The posterior interosseous nerve must be protected during this approach by keeping the forearm pronated during dissection.

Reduction techniques: Anatomical reduction of the fracture is critical. Reduction of the radial head in case of Monteggia fractures and distal ulna in case of Galeazzi fracture must be confirmed intraoperatively under fluoroscopy. The use of intraoperative fluoroscopy ensures proper alignment, length, and rotation of the radius and ulna.

COMPLICATIONS

The most common complications include:

- Compartment syndrome
- Infection
- Nonunion or delayed union
- Malunion

BIBLIOGRAPHY

1. Adams JE. Forearm Instability: Anatomy, biomechanics, and treatment options. J Hand Surg Am. 2017;42(1):47-52.
2. Bot AG, Doornberg JN, Lindenhovius AL, Ring D, Goslings JC, van Dijk CN. Long-term outcomes of fractures of both bones of the forearm. J Bone Joint Surg Am. 2011;93(6):527-32.
3. Droll KP, Perna P, Potter J, Harniman E, Schemitsch EH, McKee MD. Outcomes following plate fixation of fractures of both bones of the forearm in adults. J Bone Joint Surg Am. 2007;89(12):2619-24.
4. George AV, Lawton JN. Management of complications of forearm fractures. Hand Clin. 2015;31(2):217-33.
5. Kalyani BS, Fisher BE, Roberts CS, Giannoudis PV. Compartment syndrome of the forearm: A systematic review. J Hand Surg Am. 2011;36(3):535-43.

Monteggia Fracture

Sukhil Raina, Shriya Bhat

A Monteggia fracture is defined as a fracture of the ulna (typically in the proximal third) combined with a dislocation of the radial head.

HISTORY AND EPIDEMIOLOGY

First described by Giovanni Monteggia in 1814, this fracture pattern still remains clinically significant today. It is relatively uncommon, representing <5% of forearm fractures in adults and <1% in the general population. Monteggia fractures are more common in children than adults, especially around the age of 4–10 years, and occur in adults predominantly due to high-energy trauma.

MECHANISM OF INJURY

Monteggia fractures are typically caused by a fall on an outstretched hand, often with the forearm in a hyperpronated position. High-energy trauma such as road traffic accidents or sports injuries can also produce this fracture. The mechanism involves a combination of axial load and rotational force on the ulna, resulting in fracture, while the radial head is driven out of its anatomical alignment.

CLASSIFICATION

Bado Classification

The most widely used classification system for Monteggia fractures is the Bado classification, which is based on the direction of the radial head dislocation:

- *Type I:* Anterior dislocation of the radial head with a fracture of the proximal ulna (most common type)
- *Type II:* Posterior dislocation of the radial head
- *Type III:* Lateral dislocation of the radial head
- *Type IV:* Anterior dislocation with fractures of both the radius and ulna

CLINICAL EVALUATION

Check for the potential nerve involvement, particularly the posterior interosseous nerve (PIN), which may cause weakness in thumb and finger extension.

TREATMENT

Nonoperative Management

Nonoperative management is rarely indicated, typically reserved for pediatric patients with minimally displaced fractures where the radial head remains stable.

In these cases, the fracture can be treated with *immobilization* in a long-arm cast, with the forearm in supination and the elbow at 90° of flexion. Close follow-up with serial radiographs is mandatory to monitor for any displacement or subluxation of the radial head during the healing process.

Surgical Management

In adults, surgical management is the gold standard for treating Monteggia fractures, especially when there is a radial head dislocation. Surgery aims to achieve anatomical reduction of the ulna, restore stability to the radial head, and address any soft-tissue or neurovascular injuries.

Surgical Techniques

The primary surgical treatment for Monteggia fractures *involves open reduction and internal fixation (ORIF)* of the ulna. Fixing the ulna with plates and screws after restoration of length and normal ulnar bow often results in the spontaneous reduction of the radial head due to the restoration of anatomical alignment. Beware of plastic deformation of ulna (straightening of normal bow).

- *Ulnar reduction*:
    - *Posterior approach:* This is commonly used for Bado type II fractures and involves direct visualization and reduction of the ulna.
    - *Anterior approach:* More appropriate for Bado type I fractures, where the radial head dislocation is anterior.

      A stable fixation of the ulna is crucial. Plates and screws are preferred as they allow rigid stabilization, facilitating early mobilization.
- *Radial head reduction:* Once the ulna is stabilized, the radial head typically reduces spontaneously. However, in cases where it does not, a direct approach may be required to reposition the radial head manually.

MANAGEMENT OF SOFT-TISSUE AND NEUROVASCULAR INJURIES

Careful attention is given to the soft tissues, and the PIN, which is vulnerable in these injuries. Nerve function must be assessed pre-and postoperatively, with exploration if necessary in cases of neuro-deficit.

POSTSURGICAL IMMOBILIZATION

Following ORIF, the elbow is typically immobilized in a long-arm splint or cast for approximately 3–6 weeks, depending on the fracture stability and patient factors. The forearm is maintained in supination to promote radial head stability, and the elbow is flexed at around 90°.

COMPLICATIONS AND THEIR MANAGEMENT

Potential complications include:

- *Missed diagnosis*: Monteggia fractures are often missed on initial presentation, particularly in cases where the radial head dislocation is subtle. Delayed diagnosis increases the risk of complications such as chronic radial head instability and decreased elbow function. In missed cases, revision surgery may be necessary, often involving corrective osteotomy of the ulna and soft-tissue reconstruction.
- *Recurrent instability*:
    - *Radial head subluxation may occur* if not properly addressed during surgery. Radial head dislocations may recur if the ulnar fracture is not properly aligned. In such cases, revision surgery with the reassessment of the radial head alignment and possible ligamentous reconstruction is required.
- *Posterior interosseous nerve palsy* typically resolves but may require surgical decompression in persistent cases.
- *Elbow stiffness* can be minimized with early mobilization and adherence to physiotherapy protocols.
- *Nonunion or malunion* may occur if proper healing of the ulna does not occur, revision surgery with bone grafting or refixation may be required.

BIBLIOGRAPHY

1. Carbone A, Moracci C, Gumina S. Surgical treatment and functional outcomes of Monteggia fractures: A long-term follow-up study. J Orthop Surg Res. 2020;15(1):96.
2. Maripuri SN, Ganesan S, Sriharsha K, Ashfaq M. Current management of Monteggia fracture-dislocations: A review. Orthop Trauma. 2021;35(1):29-35.
3. Ring D, Jupiter JB, Waters PM. Monteggia fractures in children and adults. J Am Acad Orthop Surg. 1998;6(4):215-24.
4. Ruchelsman DE, Christoforou D, Jupiter JB. Monteggia Fractures in Adults. J Bone Joint Surg Am. 2013;95(12):1152-60.

Galeazzi Fracture and DRUJ Injuries

Sukhil Raina, Vipin Sharma

Galeazzi fractures, named after the Italian surgeon Riccardo Galeazzi, represent a complex injury pattern involving a fracture of the distal third of the radius combined with disruption of the distal radioulnar joint (DRUJ). This injury accounts for approximately 3–7% of all forearm fractures and commonly results from high-energy trauma, such as falls on an outstretched hand (FOOSH) or motor vehicle accidents.

Galeazzi fractures are called as "fractures of necessity" because they almost always require surgical intervention for successful outcomes.

Physical Signs: There may be obvious displacement of the radius, and in more subtle cases, palpation of the DRUJ may reveal tenderness, instability, or a palpable subluxation.

The "piano key" test, in which the ulnar head is pressed like a piano key to check for abnormal movement, may help assess instability.

Signs of DRUJ injury on radiographs include **(Figs. 1A to C)**:

- Ulnar styloid fracture
- On an anteroposterior (AP) view, there is a widening of DRUJ.
- On the lateral view, there is the dorsal or volar displacement of the distal ulna.
- Radial shortening (>5 mm)

PRINCIPLES OF MANAGEMENT

The primary goal in the treatment of Galeazzi fractures is to restore normal

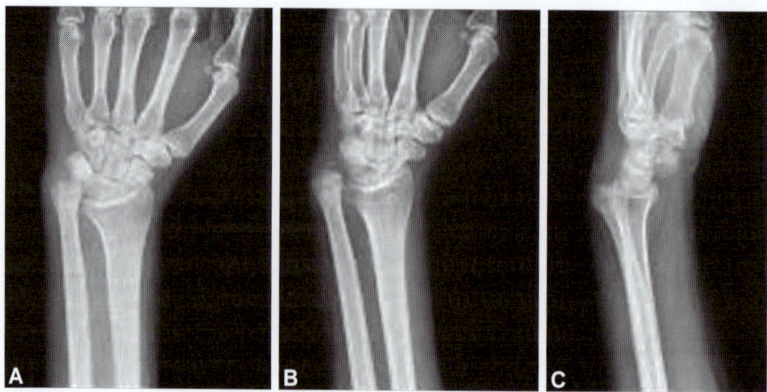

FIGS. 1A TO C: Signs of distal radioulnar joint (DRUJ) injury on radiographs.

anatomic alignment of the radius and secure stable reduction of the DRUJ. Due to the unstable nature of these injuries, nonsurgical management generally results in poor outcomes, with high rates of residual instability and deformity. Therefore, surgical intervention remains the gold standard.

Surgical Management

The cornerstone of surgical management for Galeazzi fractures is open reduction and internal fixation (ORIF) of the radial fracture. The rationale behind ORIF is to restore the anatomical alignment of the radius, which indirectly stabilizes the DRUJ.

Accurate reduction and fixation of the radial fracture are critical. Intraoperative fluoroscopy is used to confirm the correct alignment.

Addressing Distal Radioulnar Joint

Once the radius has been anatomically reduced and fixed, attention is turned to the DRUJ. Restoration of the radius's length, rotation, and alignment typically results in a spontaneous reduction of the DRUJ. However, persistent DRUJ instability must be addressed.

- *DRUJ testing:* After fixation of the radius, the DRUJ should be tested for stability intraoperatively. This is done by examining the forearm in supination and pronation and checking for abnormal movement or subluxation of the ulnar head.
- *DRUJ stabilization:* If the DRUJ remains unstable after radius fixation, several options are available:
  - *Temporary Kirschner wires (K-wire) fixation:* In cases of persistent instability, a percutaneous K-wire may be used to temporarily pin the ulnar head to the radius, preventing movement while soft-tissues heal.
  - *Repair of soft-tissue structures:* In some cases, the triangular fibrocartilage complex (TFCC) or other soft tissues may require direct repair to stabilize the DRUJ.
  - *Ulnar shortening osteotomy:* In rare instances where DRUJ instability is related to ulnar variance, an ulnar shortening procedure may be considered.

Postoperative Care

The goals are to maintain stability while promoting early mobilization to prevent stiffness.

Immobilization:

- *Short-term immobilization:* A long-arm splint or cast is typically applied for 4–6 weeks postoperatively to protect the surgical repair and maintain DRUJ stability. The forearm is placed in a position of neutral-to-slight supination, which maximizes DRUJ stability.
- *Removal of K-wires:* If K-wire fixation was used, it is usually removed after 4–6 weeks, once soft tissues have sufficiently healed.

COMPLICATIONS AND LONG-TERM OUTCOMES

The most common complications following Galeazzi fractures involve residual DRUJ instability, nonunion, and restricted forearm rotation. Early identification of complications through postoperative radiographic evaluation and clinical follow-up is essential for timely intervention.

- *Malunion and nonunion:* Proper fixation techniques and vigilant follow-up reduce the risk of these complications, though delayed union or nonunion may necessitate additional surgical intervention.
- *Chronic DRUJ instability:* Persistent DRUJ instability may require further procedures, such as TFCC reconstruction or ulnar head resection.
- *Stiffness and loss of motion:* Aggressive rehabilitation protocols, including physical therapy, can minimize these risks.

ISOLATED DISTAL RADIOULNAR JOINT DISLOCATION AND SUBLUXATION

Isolated distal radioulnar joint dislocation or subluxation is a rare but significant injury that involves disruption of the joint between the distal radius and ulna, without an associated fracture of the radius. The DRUJ is essential for both pronation and supination of the forearm, and improper management of these injuries can result in chronic instability, reduced range of motion, and pain.

Applied anatomy of the DRUJ:

- The DRUJ is formed by the ulnar head, which articulates with the sigmoid notch of the distal radius.
- *Stabilizing structures:* The primary stabilizers of the DRUJ are the TFCC, the pronator quadratus muscle, and various ligaments (such as the palmar and dorsal radioulnar ligaments).

Mechanism of Injury

Isolated DRUJ dislocation typically occurs due to high-energy trauma or a FOOSH. The force of the fall often results in a hyperpronated or hyper-supinated forearm, disrupting the ligamentous stability of the DRUJ. Recurrent or chronic subluxation can result from repetitive microtrauma, such as in athletes or workers performing repetitive forearm motions.

Types of Distal Radioulnar Joint Dislocations

Isolated DRUJ injuries are classified based on the direction of ulnar head displacement:

- *Dorsal dislocation:* The ulnar head dislocates posteriorly relative to the radius. This is the most common type of DRUJ dislocation and is often caused by forced pronation.
- *Volar dislocation:* The ulnar head dislocates anteriorly. This less common injury occurs with forced supination.
- *Subluxation:* In cases of subluxation, the ulnar head partially displaces but does not completely lose contact with the radius. This injury may result from repetitive strain rather than a single traumatic event.

Clinical Evaluation

Tenderness over the ulnar head and sigmoid notch of the radius should be checked. Dorsal or volar prominence of the ulnar head may be noted in dislocations.

- *Piano key test:* The "piano key" sign is positive when the ulnar head exhibits excessive mobility and instability when pressed dorsally, resembling a piano key.
- *Grip strength:* Weakness in grip strength is commonly observed due to the instability of the wrist.

IMAGING

- *Plain radiographs:* Standard AP and lateral wrist radiographs are essential. Lateral views often show the dislocation clearly, especially in dorsal dislocations where the ulnar head is displaced posteriorly.
- *Stress radiographs:* These can be useful for identifying subtle subluxations or instability, particularly under pronation or supination stresses.
- *Computed tomography (CT):* CT scans provide superior visualization of the DRUJ and are particularly helpful in detecting subtle subluxations, evaluating the congruency of the joint, and planning surgical intervention.
- *Magnetic resonance imaging (MRI):* MRI is primarily used to assess the integrity of soft tissues, particularly the TFCC, which is often injured in these cases.

Nonsurgical Management

Nonoperative treatment is considered in cases of acute, reducible DRUJ dislocations without associated fractures or significant soft tissue injury. The success of nonsurgical management relies heavily on early detection, stable reduction, and appropriate immobilization.

Closed Reduction

In most cases, isolated DRUJ dislocations can be reduced through closed manipulation:

- *Technique*:
  - For dorsal dislocations, gentle supination of the forearm while applying pressure to the dorsally dislocated ulnar head is typically successful.
  - For volar dislocations, pronation is applied with simultaneous pressure on the volar ulnar head.
- *Postreduction imaging:* After reduction, radiographs (strict AP and lateral view) are essential to confirm joint congruency and stability.

Immobilization

Following successful closed reduction, immobilization is required to allow the soft tissues to heal:

- *Positioning:* The forearm is immobilized in a long-arm cast, typically in supination for dorsal dislocations and in pronation for volar dislocations.
- *Duration:* Immobilization is maintained for approximately 4–6 weeks, with regular follow-up to ensure that the reduction remains stable and healing progresses without complications.

Surgical Management

Surgical intervention is indicated in cases of:

- Irreducible dislocation
- Chronic instability
- Significant damage to the TFCC or other stabilizing structures that require surgical repair

Surgical Techniques

- *ORIF:* The ulnar head is reduced, and any interposed soft tissue is cleared.
- *TFCC repair:* TFCC tears are common in DRUJ dislocations and often require surgical repair, particularly in athletes or individuals requiring high-demand wrist function. Arthroscopic or open repair techniques can be used, depending on the extent of the tear.
- *Stabilization procedures:* In cases of chronic instability, ligamentous reconstruction or tendon transfers (e.g., using the flexor carpi ulnaris tendon) may be employed to restore DRUJ stability.

Postoperative Care

Immobilization: Post-operatively, the forearm is typically immobilized in a splint or cast for 4–6 weeks to protect the surgical repair. The positioning of immobilization depends on the direction of instability (supination for dorsal dislocations and pronation for volar dislocations).

Complications and Long-term Outcomes

Complications following isolated DRUJ dislocation include:

- *Chronic instability:* In cases where the DRUJ remains unstable, patients may experience recurrent subluxation or dislocation, leading to chronic pain and functional limitations.
- *Post-traumatic arthritis*: Untreated or recurrent instability can lead to degenerative changes within the DRUJ, resulting in pain and stiffness.
- *Loss of forearm rotation:* Inadequate rehabilitation or prolonged immobilization may result in stiffness and reduced pronation/supination.

BIBLIOGRAPHY

1. Knirk JL, Jupiter JB. Management of distal radioulnar joint instability. J Hand Surg Am. 2019;44(5):400-10.
2. Mohan AT, Carter N, MacDermid JC, Faber KJ, King GJ. Triangular fibrocartilage complex tears in distal radioulnar joint injuries: Evaluation and management. Hand Clin. 2021;37(1):113-23.
3. Saini P, Kumar R, Jindal N, Lal M. Current concepts in management of Galeazzi fractures. J Clin Orthop Trauma. 2020;11(4):631-7.
4. Wong TT, Ip SP, Fung BK, Wong WM. Outcomes and complications of open reduction and internal fixation for Galeazzi fractures: A retrospective study. J Orthop Surg Res. 2019;14(1):413.
5. Zlatkin MB, Shaffer BS, Moore TM, Small KM, Banks KP. Distal radioulnar joint injuries: Current concepts. Radiol Clin North Am. 2023;61(1):139-53.

Distal Radius, Radial and Ulnar Styloid Process Fracture

Azhar Ud Din

DISTAL RADIUS FRACTURE

Distal radius fractures are one of the most common upper limb injuries making up for 8–15% of all bony injuries in adults.

Abraham Colles, in 1814, defined Colles' fracture as an injury occurring within 2–3 cm of the articular surface of the distal radius with its characteristic displacements 80 years before the advent of X-rays **(Fig. 1)**.

Applied Anatomy

The most important two characteristics of the articular surface of the distal radius are that it tilts around 21° in the anteroposterior (AP) plane and 5–11° in the lateral plane. The distal radius transfers around 80% of the axial load at the wrist.

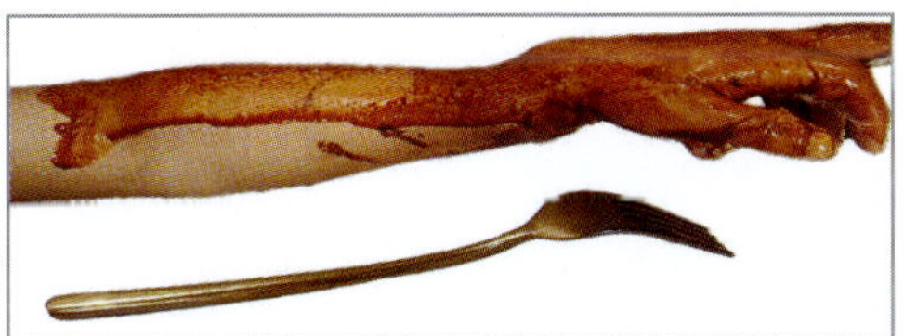

FIG. 1: Dinner fork deformity seen in dorsally displaced distal radius fracture.

Mechanism of Injury

The most common cause is a fall on an outstretched hand in the elderly population with the wrist in dorsiflexion. The form and severity of the fracture depend on the position of the wrist at the moment of hitting the ground. In younger patients, it happens usually due to high-velocity injury.

Diagnostic Evaluation

X-rays: It needs true posteroanterior (PA), true lateral, and oblique or scaphoid views to rule out any associated fracture as well **(Table 1)**.

Computed tomography (CT): It provides detailed information especially when there are high-velocity injuries with intra-articular extension.

TABLE 1: Normal radiographic relationship.

Parameter	X-ray	Normal range	Acceptable limit
Radial inclination	PA	23° (13–30°)	<5° change
Radial height	PA	11 mm (8–18 mm)	<5 mm shortening
Volar tilt	Lateral	11° (0–28°)	Dorsal angulation <5° or within 20° of the contralateral side
Ulnar variance	PA	± 2 mm	

(PA: posteroanterior)

Classification

Fernandez Classification

It is classified based on the mechanism of injury into the following five types:

- *Type I:* Metaphyseal bending fracture (Colles' and Smith's fracture)
- *Type II:* Shearing fractures requiring open reduction and internal fixation (ORIF) with buttress plating (volar or dorsal Barton fractures)
- *Type III:* Compression of the distal articular joint surface with significant interosseous ligament injury.
- *Type IV:* Avulsion fractures or radiocarpal fracture–dislocation
- *Type V:* Combined fractures (1, 2, 3, and 4) with significant soft-tissue involvement owing to high-velocity energy injury

Frykman Classification

Odd numbers are without ulnar styloid fractures and even numbers are with ulnar styloid fractures **(Table 2)**.

Cooney Classification

- *Type I:* Extra-articular and undisplaced
- *Type II:* Extra-articular displaced
- *Type III:* Intra-articular and undisplaced
- *Type IV:* Intra-articular and displaced

Eponyms

Eponyms and their description are given in **Table 3**.

Management and Treatment Strategies

The management and treatment strategies are given in **Flowchart 1**.

TABLE 2: Ulnar styloid fractures and distal radius.

	Ulnar styloid fracture	
Distal radius fracture	**Yes**	**No**
Extra-articular	1	2
Intra-articular involving radiocarpal joint	3	4
Intra-articular involving DRUJ	5	6
Intra-articular involving both radiocarpal joint and DRUJ	7	8

(DRUJ: distal radioulnar joint)

TABLE 3: Different eponyms.

Eponym	Description
Colles' fracture	Low-energy extra-articular distal radius fracture, dorsally displaced
Smith's fracture	Low-energy extra-articular distal radius fracture, volarly displaced
Volar Barton fracture	Fracture-dislocation of radiocarpal joint with intra-articular fracture involving the volar lip
Dorsal Barton fracture	Fracture-dislocation of radiocarpal joint with intra-articular fracture involving the dorsal lip
Chauffeur's fracture	Radial styloid fracture
Die-punch fracture	Depressed fracture of the lunate fossa of the articular surface of the distal radius

Management depends upon the answer to the following questions:

- Is the fracture displaced or undisplaced?
- Is it intra or extra-articular?
- Is it reducible or irreducible?
- Is it stable or unstable? (Fracture comminution)

Nonoperative Treatment

It consists of 4–6 weeks of well-molded below elbow pop or fiber cast as shown in **Figures 2A and B** with weekly follow-up with X-rays for the first 3 weeks.

Indications:

- All undisplaced fractures
- Displaced extra-articular fractures that are reducible and stable
- In some low-demand patients >65 years of age with unstable fractures (when some degree of malunion may be tolerated)

Surgery

Indications:

- *Irreducible and unstable fractures*: Dorsal tilt >20°, dorsal comminution, intra-articular fractures, and associated ulnar styloid fracture
- Bilateral distal end radius fractures
- Compound fractures
- Distal end radius fractures with polytrauma
- Secondary displacement after casting
- Associated neurovascular or tendon injury

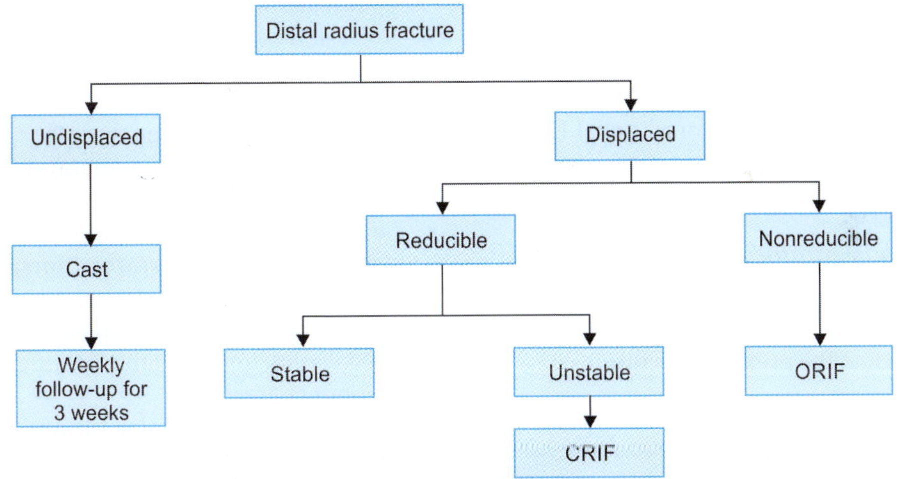

FLOWCHART 1: Management and treatment strategies.
(CRIF: closed reduction and internal fixation; ORIF: open reduction and internal fixation)

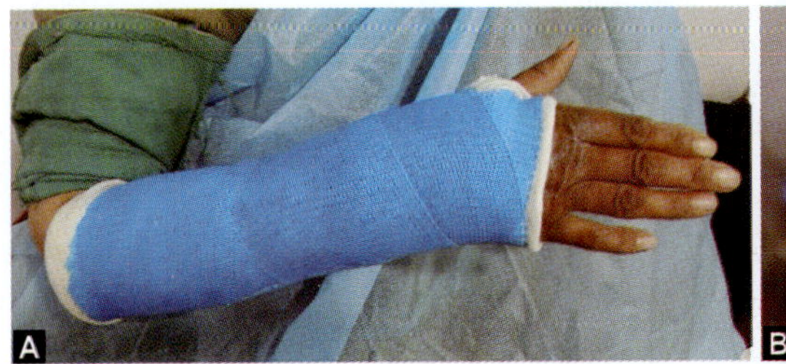

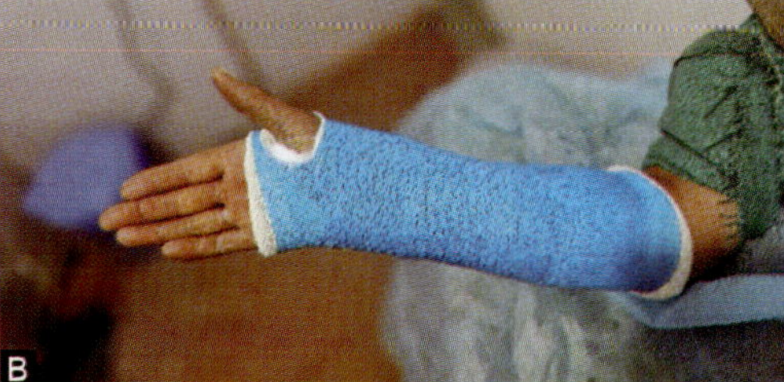

FIGS. 2A AND B: Below elbow fiber or Colles' cast.

Surgery for distal end radius fractures consists of:

- *Percutaneous pinning*: Extrafocal or intrafocal Kirschner wiring (K-wiring)
- *External fixation:* Spanning or nonspanning external fixators, Joshi's external stabilization system (JESS), Ilizarov, etc.
- *Internal fixation:* Volar or dorsal locking distal radius plates
- *Hybrid fixation:* Fixators along with plates or K-wires
- Distraction/joint spanning plating in severely osteoporotic and comminuted fracture and plate needs subsequent removal and mobilization of the wrist.

Indications for closed reduction and internal fixation (CRIF) with K-wires: Extra-articular fracture with stable volar cortex.

Extrafocal Percutaneous Pinning

- Pure trans-styloid radial
- Trans-styloid and dorsal radial **(Figs. 3A and B)**
- Trans-styloid and ulnoradial pinning

Kapandji Intrafocal Technique

K-wires are placed dorsally into the fracture and used as reduction tools until they are driven into the proximal fracture.

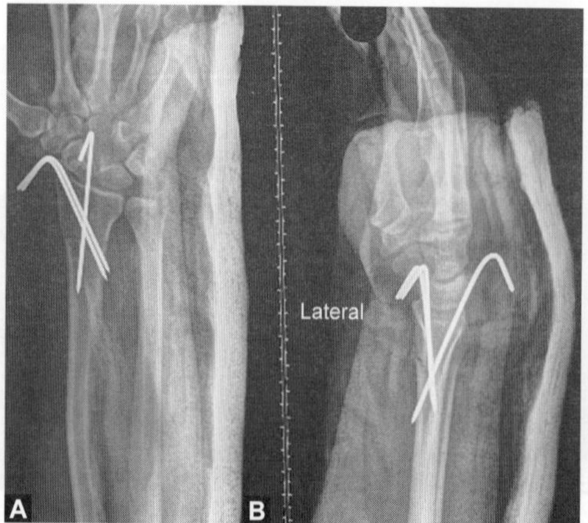

FIGS. 3A AND B: Extrafocal percutaneous pinning with K-wires (trans-styloid and dorsal radial).

Complications specific to this treatment:

- Radial sensory nerve injury
- Pin tract infections

External fixator relies on ligamentotaxis to maintain reduction.

Indications:

- Compound fractures
- Fractures that are highly comminuted
- Polytrauma patients who are unable to undergo a lengthy procedure

Open Reduction and Internal Fixation with Volar, or Dorsal, or Combined Approaches

Indications:

- Radiographic findings indicating instability (prereduction radiographs are best predictor of stability.)
- Dorsal angulation >5° or >20° of contralateral distal radius
- Volar or dorsal comminution
- Displaced intra-articular fractures > 2 mm
- Radial shortening > 5 mm
- Associated ulnar fracture
- Associated ulnar styloid fractures do not require fixation
- Severe osteoporosis
- Articular margin fractures (dorsal and volar Barton's fractures)
- Comminuted and displaced extra-articular fractures (Smith's fractures)
- Die-punch fractures
- Progressive loss of volar tilt and radial length following closed reduction and casting

Various types of plates used to treat distal radius fracture include:

- *Volar locking plates*:
    - These are used for both simple and complex fractures, especially intra-articular fractures and osteoporotic bones.
    - Many volar plates have locking screws **(Figs. 4A and B)**, which provide angular stability and prevent screw loosening. There are variable locking plates available as well to have flexibility in inserting screws.

- *Dorsal plates*:
  - These are less commonly used now, but may still be required for specific dorsal fracture patterns.
  - Higher risk of tendon irritation or rupture, especially of the extensor tendons
  - Applied on the dorsal aspect of the distal radius or those with significant dorsal comminution
- *Fragment-specific plates*:
  - Tailored fixation for individual fragments in highly comminuted fractures; can be applied in multiple planes
  - Complex, comminuted fractures where traditional plates may not offer adequate stability
  - Usually consist of small, low-profile plates that target individual fracture fragments.
- *Radial styloid plates*: Isolated radial styloid fractures or fractures with major radial styloid involvement
- *Bridge plates*:
  - These plates span across the fracture and immobilize the wrist, often extending to the second or third metacarpal.
  - These are used for severely comminuted fractures where conventional plates can not achieve adequate fixation.
  - These require a second surgery for plate removal after fracture healing, as it temporarily immobilizes the wrist.
- *Nonlocking plates*:
  - Standard plates with nonlocking screws
  - Used for simple, noncomminuted fractures in good bone quality
- *Rim plate:* Used for distalmost fractures only **(Figs. 5A to C)**, as this plate can be placed distal to watershed area, whereas other plates are not supposed to be used distal to watershed area as that can lead to flexor tendon attrition and subsequent pain and rupture

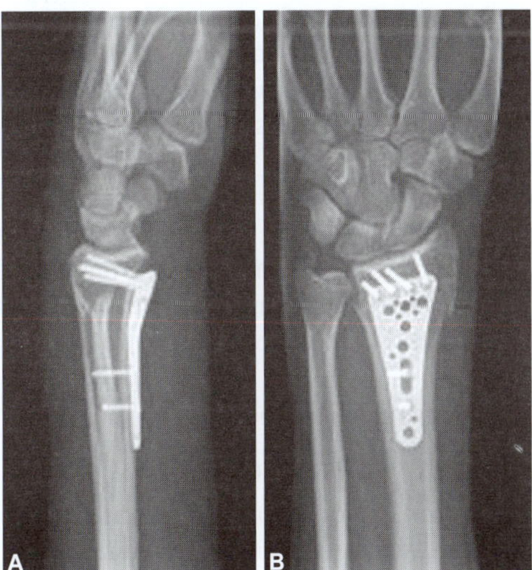

FIGS. 4A AND B: Distal radius volar locking plate.

Complications

Surgical interventions carry risks such as:

- Median nerve neuropathy (carpal tunnel syndrome)
- Infection
- Malunion
- Persistent instability
- Screw penetration into the radiocarpal joint

Recent Advances in Treatment

- *Intramedullary nailing of the distal radius* of various designs is available and indicated for either extra-articular or simple intraarticular distal radius fractures.
- *Intramedullary cage constructs:* The distal radius cage system consists of an expandable implant that is placed into the medullary canal of the distal radius thereby providing a scaffold on which fracture fragments can be held using specific screws. The implant is made of a nickel–titanium alloy, indicated for either extra-articular or simple intra-articular distal radius fractures.

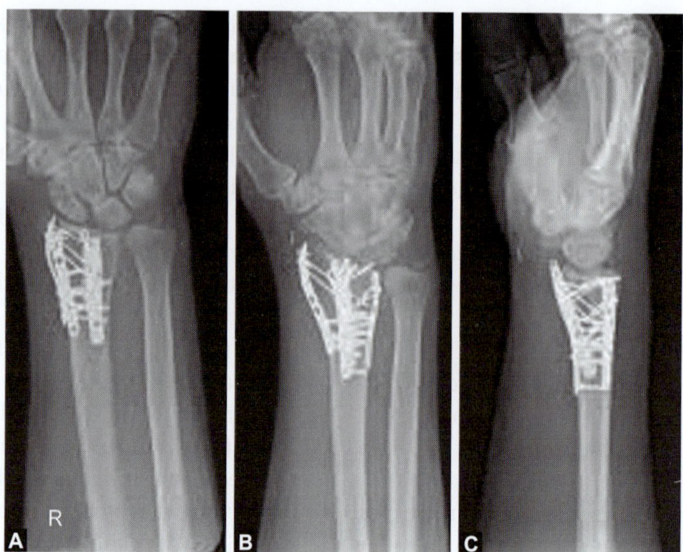

FIGS. 5A TO C: Distal radius rim plates.

- *Polyether etherketone (PEEK) volar locking plate:* Indicated for extra- and intra-articular fractures. Salient features of the implant are:
  - Modulus of elasticity similar to bone
  - Improved visualization of fracture reduction and bone healing
  - No risk of cold welding between screws and plate
  - Low artifact interference with magnetic resonance imaging (MRI) and CT imaging

RADIAL STYLOID PROCESS FRACTURES

Fractures of the radial styloid process, commonly known as chauffeur's fractures, typically result from axial loading or high-energy trauma and are characterized by injury at the distal end of the radius. Historically, these fractures were suffered by drivers (1950–1990) who would have to start their cars using a hand crank. Seldom when these cranks backfired, it would forcefully strike the back of the wrist of the driver causing this fracture.

Classification of Radial Styloid Fractures

- *Isolated radial styloid fracture:* These involve the fracture of the styloid process without significant disruption to the surrounding joints or ligaments.
- *Comminuted fracture:* These involve fragmentation of the radial styloid and are usually associated with higher-energy trauma.
- *Intra-articular fractures:* These extend into the radiocarpal joint and are often associated with cartilage and ligament damage, especially scapholunate ligament injury.
- *Associated ligamentous injuries:* These frequently occur with scapholunate dissociation or triangular fibrocartilage complex (TFCC) injuries, necessitating special considerations during treatment.

Management Strategies

Nonoperative Management

Indications: Nondisplaced or minimally displaced fractures without carpal instability or ligamentous damage.

Immobilization: Short arm cast or wrist splint for 4–6 weeks, followed by a gradual return to wrist motion and strengthening exercises.

Surgical Management

Indications for surgery:

- Displacement > 2 mm
- Involvement of the articular surface
- Associated scapholunate ligament injury
- Carpal instability
- Failure of conservative treatment

Fixation techniques:

- *ORIF:* The gold standard for treating displaced or intra-articular radial styloid fractures, ORIF allows direct visualization and anatomical reduction of the fracture. Screws, plates, or K-wires are used depending on the fracture pattern.
    - *Plates and screws:* Low-profile plates designed for the distal radius have been refined, allowing for more precise fixation with minimal soft-tissue disruption. These plates provide rigid fixation, ensuring early mobilization and reducing the risk of post-traumatic arthritis.
    - *K-wires:* In cases where less invasive stabilization is needed, percutaneous pinning with K-wires can be an effective option, especially in noncomminuted fractures.
- *Arthroscopic-assisted fixation:* Arthroscopy offers the advantage of direct visualization of intra-articular fractures and associated ligamentous injuries, such as scapholunate tears. Recent studies have demonstrated that arthroscopy improves outcomes in radial styloid fractures by ensuring more precise reduction and enabling concurrent ligament repair.
- *Fragment-specific fixation:* Newer techniques focus on addressing the radial styloid fragment independently from the rest of the radius, preserving soft tissue and allowing for a more anatomical reduction of the fracture. This approach is useful in cases of complex, comminuted fractures.

Complications

The most common complications associated with radial styloid fractures include:

- Post-traumatic arthritis
- *Carpal instability:* Especially when associated with scapholunate ligament injuries
- *Nonunion or malunion:* Though uncommon with modern fixation techniques, these complications can lead to chronic pain and reduced wrist function.

ULNAR STYLOID PROCESS

The ulnar styloid process (USP) is located at the distal end of the ulna and is part of TFCC, a structure crucial for distal radioulnar joint (DRUJ) stability. The USP serves as an attachment point for several key structures:

- *Ulnar collateral ligament (UCL):* Provides medial stability to the wrist
- *Dorsal and volar radioulnar ligaments:* Maintain DRUJ stability
- *TFCC proper:* Acts as a cushion between the ulnar head and carpal bones, contributing to wrist stability

Due to its involvement in wrist stabilization, even small fractures or avulsions of the USP can lead to functional impairment, pain, and instability. Accurate assessment of the extent of injury and the impact on surrounding structures is critical in guiding management.

Ulnar styloid fractures are typically classified based on the location of the fracture and its involvement with the DRUJ and TFCC.

- *Type 1:* Tip fractures
    - These fractures occur at the distal tip of the USP, often resulting from avulsion of the TFCC or UCL While these fractures may not significantly impact DRUJ stability, they can contribute

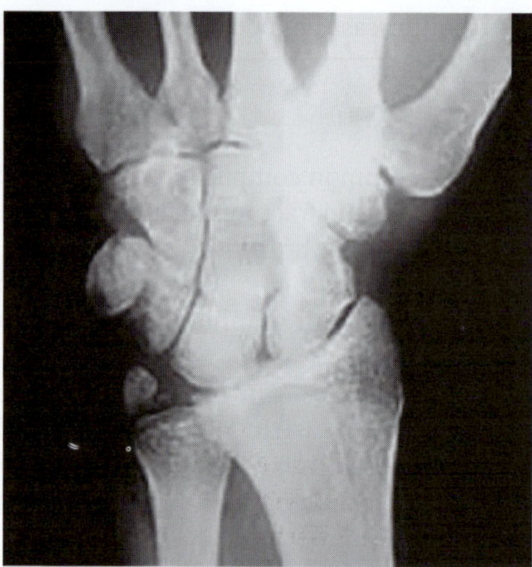

FIG. 6: Ulnar styloid base fracture.

to TFCC dysfunction, particularly if displacement is present.

- *Type 2:* Base fractures
    - These fractures occur at the base of the USP **(Fig. 6)**, near the DRUJ. Base fractures are more likely to disrupt DRUJ stability and are associated with TFCC injuries. They carry a higher risk of long-term instability and dysfunction compared to tip fractures.

Management of Ulnar Styloid Fractures

Nonsurgical Management

Nonsurgical management is typically indicated for:

- Minimally displaced fractures
- Fractures without DRUJ instability
- Isolated tip fractures with minimal soft-tissue injury

The mainstay of conservative treatment is the immobilization of the wrist with a short arm cast or splint, typically worn for 4–6 weeks, followed by physical therapy to restore wrist motion and strength. Serial radiographs may be taken during follow-up to monitor fracture healing and assess for any signs of DRUJ instability.

Surgical Management

The most common indications for surgical management include:

- Displaced base fractures of the USP
- Persistent DRUJ instability despite conservative treatment
- TFCC injury requiring surgical repair

Surgical options for managing USP fractures include:

- ORIF using screws, wires, or small plates
- *TFCC repair or reconstruction:* In cases where the ulnar styloid fracture is associated with a significant TFCC injury, direct repair of the TFCC may be necessary. This can be performed using arthroscopic or open techniques based on operating surgeons training and experience.

Complications

Common complications include:

- Nonunion or malunion
- DRUJ instability

BIBLIOGRAPHY

1. Caldwell RA, Shorten PL, Morrell NT. Common upper extremity fracture eponyms: A look into what they really mean. J Hand Surg Am. 2019;44(4):331-4.
2. Factor S, Atlan F, Pritsch T, Rumack N, Golden E, Dadia S. In-hospital production of 3D-printed casts for non-displaced wrist and hand fractures. SICOT J. 2022;8:20.
3. Karl JW, Olson PR, Rosenwasser MP. The epidemiology of upper extremity fractures in the United States, 2009. J Orthop Trauma. 2015;29(8):e242-4.
4. Loisel F, Bourgeois M, Rondot T, Nallet J, Boeckstins M, Rochet S, et al. Treatment goals for distal radius fractures in 2018: Recommendations and practical advice. Eur J Orthop Surg Traumatol. 2018;28(8):1465-8.
5. Mauck BM, Swigler CW. Evidence-based review of distal radius fractures. Orthop Clin North Am. 2018;49(2):211-22.
6. Meena S, Sharma P, Sambharia AK, Dawar A. Fractures of distal radius: An overview. J Family Med Prim Care. 2014;3(4):325-32.
7. Naranje SM, Erali RA, Warner WC, Sawyer JR, Kelly DM. Epidemiology of pediatric fractures presenting to emergency departments in the United States. J Pediatr Orthop. 2016;36(4):e45-8.

SECTION

6

Wrist and Hand Injuries

Scaphoid Fracture

Younis Kamal

SCAPHOID FRACTURE

Scaphoid fractures remain one of the most complex and clinically significant injuries in orthopedic trauma due to their high risk of complications, including nonunion and avascular necrosis (AVN). Accounting for 60–70% of all carpal fractures, the scaphoid is pivotal to wrist function, acting as the primary stabilizer between the proximal and distal carpal rows.

Applied Anatomy of the Scaphoid

The scaphoid spans both the proximal and distal carpal rows, with key articulations to the radius, lunate, trapezium, and trapezoid. This strategic positioning makes it critical for wrist kinematics, with any disruption in scaphoid integrity severely impairing wrist motion and grip strength.

Vascular Supply

The scaphoid's vascularity presents one of the primary challenges in fracture management. The bone's blood supply is largely retrograde, with the majority of the vascular input entering through the distal pole and progressing toward the proximal pole. This pattern renders the proximal third particularly susceptible to ischemia following a fracture, especially in displaced or comminuted cases.

- *Dorsal branches of the radial artery:* These supply 80% of the scaphoid, entering distally and traveling proximally.
- *Palmar branches of the radial artery:* These supply the distal pole, which has better healing potential compared to the proximal segments.

Mechanisms of Injury and Epidemiology

The most common mechanism of injury for scaphoid fractures is a fall onto an outstretched hand (FOOSH) with the wrist in hyperextension, radial deviation, and pronation. This mechanism transfers significant axial load through the carpus, concentrating stress on the scaphoid. The demographic most affected are young, active males aged 15–40, often involved in sports or high-energy activities.

Fracture Locations

The scaphoid can fracture at different anatomic locations, each with distinct implications for healing and treatment strategies:

- *Distal pole fractures:* Least common (~10%), typically heal well due to the robust blood supply
- *Waist fractures:* The most frequent (~65%), with an intermediate risk of nonunion due to its proximity to the scaphoid's blood supply watershed **(Figs. 1A and B)**.

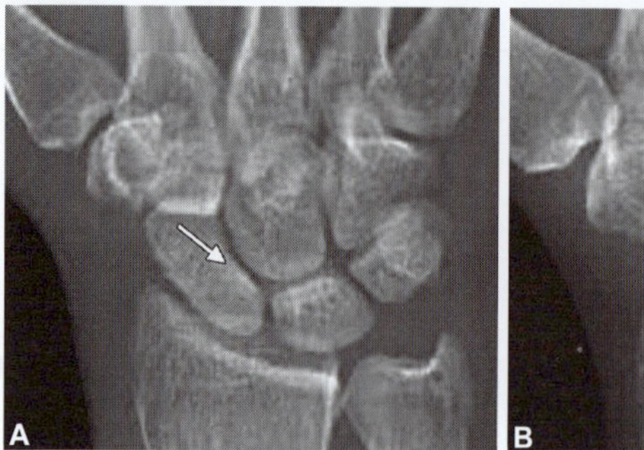
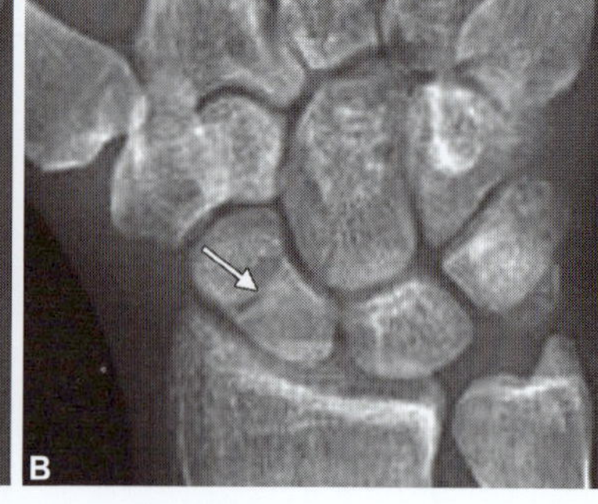

FIGS. 1A AND B: X-rays showing scaphoid waist fracture.

- *Proximal pole fractures:* Represent 15–20% of cases, with the highest risk of nonunion and AVN due to the tenuous blood supply.

Clinical Evaluation

While the classic signs of a scaphoid fracture are well-known, they can often be subtle, especially in the acute setting. High suspicion is essential when evaluating patients with wrist trauma, particularly young adults.

- *Anatomic snuffbox tenderness:* Palpation of the anatomic snuffbox is the most reliable clinical sign, with a sensitivity exceeding 90% in acute scaphoid fractures.
- *Scaphoid tubercle tenderness:* Volar tenderness over the scaphoid tubercle can aid in the diagnosis, particularly in fractures of the distal third or waist.
- *Axial compression of the thumb and index finger*: Pain elicited with axial loading of the thumb metacarpal is another useful clinical test.

Radiographic Evaluation

- *Standard radiographs:* Initially, four views [posterolateral (PA), lateral, oblique, and dedicated scaphoid view] are taken. However, up to 25% of scaphoid fractures may not be visible on initial radiographs, especially in nondisplaced or incomplete fractures.
- *Computed tomography (CT) scan:* The gold standard for assessing fracture displacement and comminution. CT provides excellent bony detail and is particularly useful for surgical planning and postoperative assessment of union.
- *Magnetic resonance imaging (MRI):* The preferred modality for diagnosing occult fractures or evaluating vascularity, MRI is highly sensitive for detecting bone marrow edema and early signs of AVN.
- *Bone scintigraphy*: While less commonly used today due to the advent of MRI, bone scintigraphy remains a valid option for detecting radiographically occult fractures. It is highly sensitive but less specific.

Management Strategies: Nonsurgical versus Surgical

The treatment of scaphoid fractures is dictated by multiple factors, including fracture location, displacement, vascularity, and patient-specific considerations such as age and activity level. Advances in minimally invasive surgery and fixation techniques have expanded the indications for operative intervention, even in nondisplaced fractures.

Nonsurgical Treatment

Nondisplaced and stable scaphoid fractures, particularly those involving the distal pole, can often be managed conservatively with immobilization.

Casting: Traditionally, a long-arm thumb spica cast was used, but recent studies suggest that short-arm casting is sufficient for most stable waist and distal pole fractures.

Duration: Immobilization for 8–12 weeks is standard, though distal fractures may heal more quickly. Regular radiographic follow-up is crucial to ensure union.

Surgical Management

Surgical intervention is indicated in displaced fractures, unstable patterns, proximal pole fractures, and cases with a high risk of nonunion.

Various surgical modalities include:

- *Percutaneous fixation:* Headless compression screws have revolutionized the management of scaphoid fractures **(Figs. 2A and B)**. Percutaneous fixation allows for minimal soft-tissue disruption, reduced postoperative pain, and faster rehabilitation.
  - The volar or dorsal percutaneous approach can be used depending on the fracture location, with the dorsal approach favored for proximal pole fractures due to better access.
  - *Outcomes:* Studies show union rates exceeding 90% with early intervention and percutaneous screw fixation.
- Open reduction and internal fixation (ORIF) is preferred for fractures with significant displacement, comminution, or delayed presentation. The volar and dorsal approaches are both widely utilized, with the approach chosen based on fracture location and surgeon preference.
  - *Volar approach:* Provides optimal access to the waist and distal pole fractures
  - *Dorsal approach:* Favored for proximal pole fractures due to better visualization and access to this region
  - *Outcomes:* ORIF achieves excellent union rates but requires careful surgical planning to avoid complications such as iatrogenic damage to the dorsal blood supply.
- *Bone grafting:* In cases of nonunion, particularly with AVN, bone grafting becomes essential. Vascularized bone grafts from the distal radius or iliac crest have demonstrated superior outcomes compared to nonvascularized grafts, especially in proximal pole fractures.

Complications and Long-term Outcomes

Despite advances in treatment, complications following scaphoid fractures remain a significant concern.

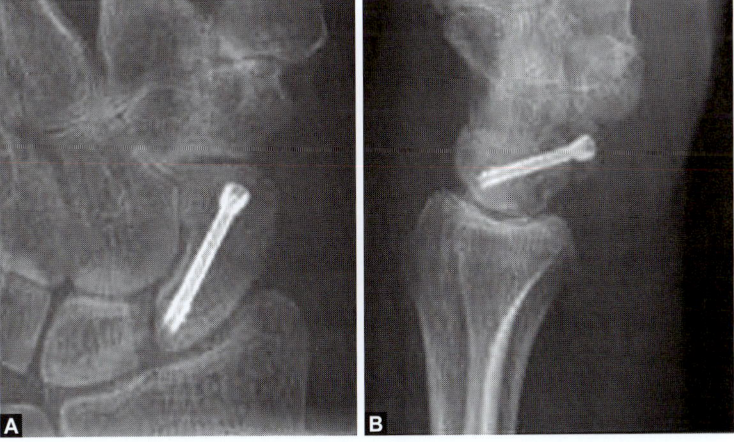

FIGS. 2A AND B: X-rays showing fixation of scaphoid.

- *Nonunion* rates range from 5–15%, with higher rates seen in proximal pole fractures and those with delayed presentation. CT scanning is the gold standard for diagnosing nonunion.
- *AVN* is most commonly seen in proximal pole fractures, with a reported incidence of 15–30%. Early diagnosis via MRI and prompt intervention with vascularized bone grafting can mitigate the risk of collapse.
- *Post-traumatic arthritis:* Chronic nonunion can lead to scaphoid nonunion advanced collapse (SNAC), a progressive form of wrist arthritis that may require salvage procedures such as proximal row carpectomy or wrist fusion.

DISLOCATION OF THE LUNATE

Lunate dislocation is a rare but serious wrist injury that often involves ligamentous instability and potential neurovascular compromise. It can occur with or without associated fractures, notably of the scaphoid, which further complicates diagnosis and treatment.

Anatomy and Mechanism of Injury

The lunate, a crescent-shaped carpal bone, occupies a central role in wrist stability, articulating with the radius, scaphoid, and triquetrum. The injury is typically caused by a high-energy event like FOOSH, which forces the wrist into hyperextension.

Classification of Lunate Dislocation

- *Isolated lunate dislocation:* This involves the lunate being displaced without fracture **(Figs. 3A and B)**. The dislocation is usually anterior, where the lunate rotates and dislocates volarly into the carpal tunnel, potentially compressing the median nerve. At times, the dislocated lunate may displace into the forearm and has to be squeezed distally before reduction.

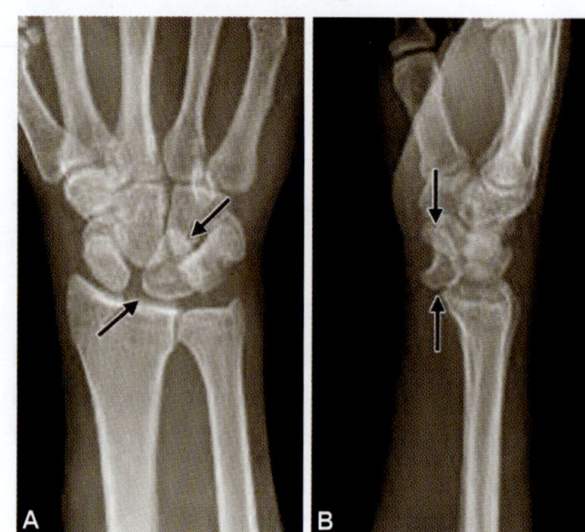

FIGS. 3A AND B: Isolated volar dislocation of the lunate.

- *Lunate dislocation with scaphoid fracture (trans-scaphoid perilunate dislocation):* In this more complex injury, the lunate dislocates and the scaphoid sustains a fracture **(Figs. 4A to D)**. This pattern is classified as a perilunate dislocation, and the injury disrupts the carpal arch, causing greater instability and complicating treatment.

The patient may present with numbness or tingling in the median nerve distribution (due to potential compression in volar dislocations).

Radiographic Evaluation

- *X-rays:* In isolated lunate dislocations, the lateral view may show the lunate in a "spilled teacup" position, rotated and dislocated into the volar space. The PA view may reveal a triangular "piece-of-pie" appearance.
- In cases of *lunate dislocation with scaphoid fracture,* X-rays typically reveal the fractured scaphoid along with displacement of the lunate.
- *CT scans* may be required for more detailed assessment, particularly to evaluate fracture patterns and joint alignment.

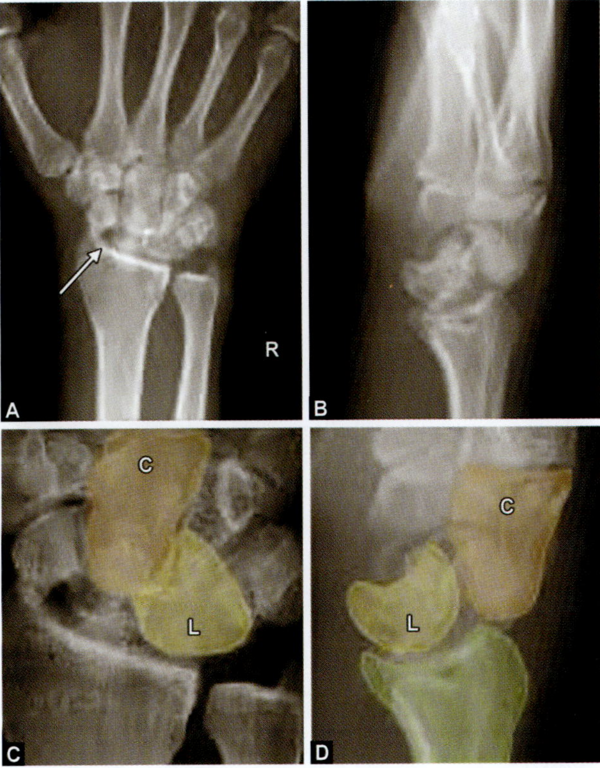

FIGS. 4A TO D: X-rays showing trans-scaphoid perilunate dislocation.

- *MRI* can be useful in assessing ligamentous injuries and any potential compromise of blood flow to the lunate, helping to predict the risk of AVN.

Management

Isolated Lunate Dislocation

- *Emergency reduction:*
  - *Closed reduction* may be attempted in the acute setting (within 24–48 hours). This involves applying longitudinal traction to realign the carpal bones, often under sedation. A successful reduction can provide immediate relief, but due to ligamentous damage, it is often unstable and requires surgical fixation.
  - *Immobilization* is done in a splint or cast (typically in slight wrist flexion) for 4–6 weeks postreduction, with regular monitoring for recurrent dislocation or neurovascular compromise.
- *Surgical treatment:*
  - *ORIF is* often necessary when closed reduction fails or when instability persists after closed reduction. ORIF involves manually realigning the lunate and securing the carpal bones, often with *K-wire fixation.*
  - *Ligament repair or reconstruction* is usually required to restore stability, as ligamentous injury (scapholunate and lunotriquetral) is common in lunate dislocations.
  - In cases of irreducibility or recurrent instability, *partial wrist fusion* may be considered to maintain function while preventing further instability.
- *Rehabilitation:* Postoperative immobilization lasts for 6–8 weeks. This is followed by a tailored *physiotherapy* program

aimed at restoring range of motion, grip strength, and wrist stability. Full recovery may take several months.

Lunate Dislocation with Scaphoid Fracture

- *Initial management:* In these cases, *emergency closed reduction* is less likely to be successful due to the fracture. Immediate stabilization of the scaphoid fracture and realignment of the lunate are priorities.
- *Surgical treatment:*
    - *ORIF*: Both the scaphoid fracture and the lunate dislocation require surgical intervention. The fractured scaphoid is typically fixed with *screws or K-wires*, while the lunate is reduced and stabilized with K-wires **(Fig. 5)**.
    - *Ligament repair* is essential to restore normal wrist kinematics. Given the complexity of trans-scaphoid perilunate injuries, ensuring proper ligament reconstruction is crucial for long-term stability.
- *Postoperative care:* Immobilization remains longer (up to 12 weeks), given the healing requirements of the scaphoid fracture. After the healing period, *physiotherapy* to restore motion and strength follows. In these cases, there is a higher risk of complications, including carpal instability and AVN.

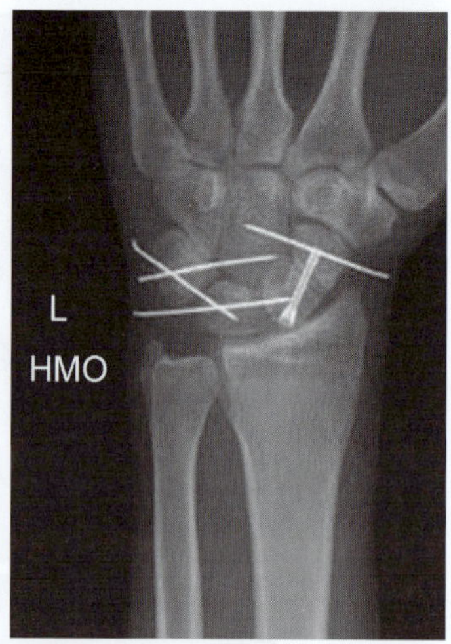

FIG. 5: Open reduction and internal fixation (ORIF) of trans-scaphoid perilunate fracture-dislocation.

Complications

- *AVN:* In lunate dislocations with delayed treatment or complex injuries, AVN may require interventions like *radial shortening osteotomy* or *wrist fusion*.
- *Median nerve compression:* Volar dislocations may compress the median nerve, leading to acute carpal tunnel syndrome, which may require surgical decompression.
- *Chronic instability:* Inadequate treatment of ligamentous injury may lead to long-term instability, resulting in painful wrist movement or degenerative changes like arthritis.
- *Arthritis and stiffness:* Despite appropriate management, lunate dislocations, especially those involving the scaphoid, can lead to degenerative arthritis or chronic wrist stiffness over time.

BIBLIOGRAPHY

1. Cooney WP, Linscheid RL. Scaphoid fractures and their complications. J Hand Surg. 2018;43(5):475-82.
2. Inoue G, Shionoya K. Percutaneous fixation of acute scaphoid fractures. Clin Orthop Relat Res. 2020;483:67-72.
3. Jebson PJ, Adams JE. Vascularized bone grafts in scaphoid non-union. J Hand Surg. 2019;44(7):655-64.
4. Moran SL, Berger RA. Arthroscopic-assisted management of scaphoid fractures. J Wrist Surg. 2019;8(4):322-30.

CHAPTER 6.2

Carpal Bone Fracture and Carpal Instability

Younis Kamal

CARPAL BONE FRACTURES

Fractures of the carpal bones most commonly occur from direct trauma or axial loading of the wrist, often during falls on an outstretched hand (FOOSH).

Anatomy and Biomechanics of Carpus

The carpus is composed of eight bones arranged in two rows: The proximal row (scaphoid, lunate, triquetrum, and pisiform) and the distal row (trapezium, trapezoid, capitate, and hamate). These bones articulate with each other and the adjacent radius and ulna to form a highly intricate structure that facilitates wrist mobility, stability, and load transmission **(Figs. 1A to C)**.

Classification of Carpal Bone Fractures

Carpal bone fractures can be classified based on the specific bone involved, the fracture pattern, and the stability of the injury. The most frequently encountered fractures include:

- *Scaphoid fractures:* These account for 60–70% of carpal fractures.
- *Lunate fractures:* These are rare but significant, as lunate fractures are often associated with perilunate dislocations or Kienböck's disease.
- *Triquetrum fractures:* Typically, these are avulsion fractures from ligamentous attachments or dorsal impaction.
- *Pisiform fractures:* Less common, these are usually seen as a result of direct trauma to the hypothenar eminence.
- *Other carpal bones:* Fractures of the trapezium, capitate, and hamate are rarer and are frequently associated with high-energy trauma or concomitant fractures of other carpal bones.

Diagnostic Imaging

Initial radiographs should include posteroanterior (PA), lateral, and scaphoid views of the wrist. However, up to 30% of scaphoid fractures may be missed on initial X-rays. In these cases, advanced imaging modalities such as computed tomography (CT), magnetic resonance imaging (MRI), or bone scintigraphy can provide a more detailed assessment. CT is particularly useful for evaluating fracture morphology and displacement, whereas MRI is superior for detecting occult fractures and assessing the vascularity of the carpal bones, which is crucial in cases of scaphoid nonunion or avascular necrosis (AVN) risk.

Treatment Strategies

The treatment of carpal bone fractures depends on the specific bone involved, the fracture type, and the degree of displacement. Conservative management with immobilization is appropriate for nondisplaced fractures, while displaced or

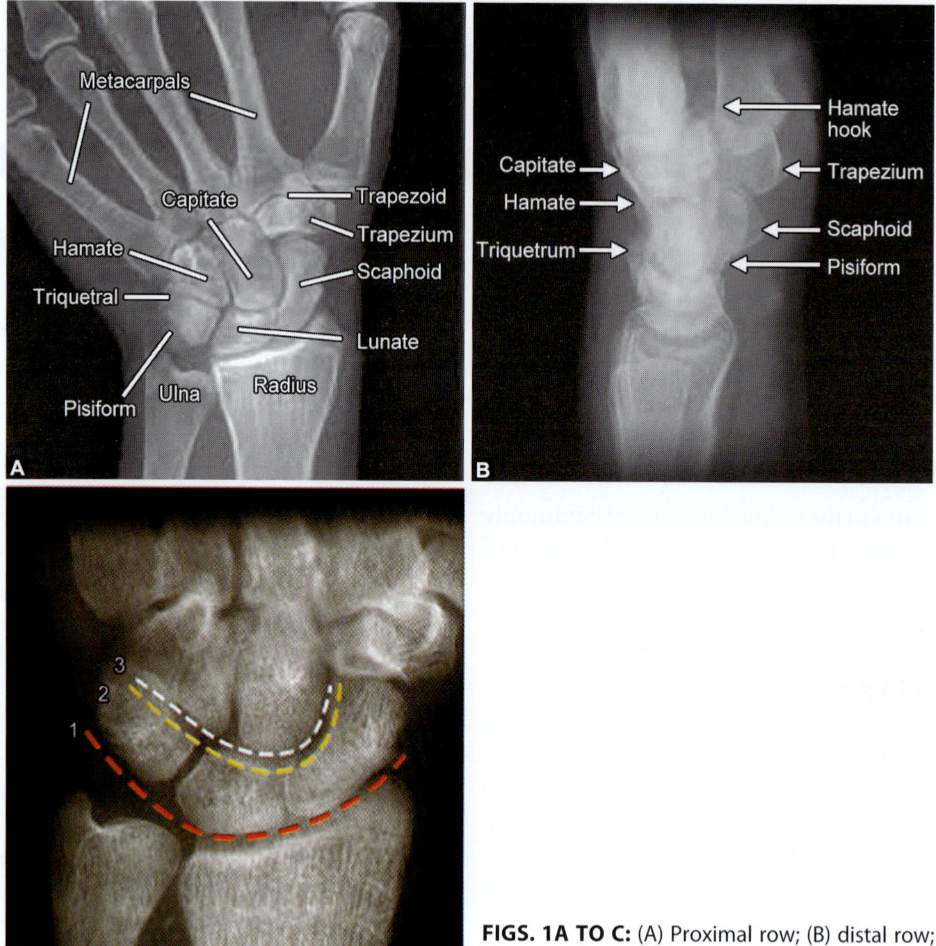

FIGS. 1A TO C: (A) Proximal row; (B) distal row; and (C) gilula lines or three arcs.

unstable fractures often require surgical intervention.

- *Scaphoid fractures*: Detailed management of the scaphoid fracture is already described in the **Chapter 6.1**.
- *Lunate fractures*: Isolated lunate fractures are rare and are often treated conservatively. However, if associated with perilunate dislocations, surgical reduction and stabilization is required.
- *Triquetrum and pisiform fractures*: Triquetrum fractures are usually managed conservatively with splinting for 4–6 weeks. Pisiform fractures, being less common, may also be treated with immobilization, though pisiformectomy can be considered in chronic cases with persistent pain.
- *Fractures of the other carpal bones*: Hamate fractures, especially those involving the hook of the hamate, may necessitate surgical excision in cases of nonunion or ulnar nerve compression. Trapezium fractures can be managed with open reduction and internal fixation (ORIF) if displaced, given their important role in thumb motion and grip strength.

VOLAR AND DORSAL INTERCALATED SEGMENT INSTABILITY

Carpal instability, including both volar intercalated segment instability (VISI) and dorsal intercalated segment instability (DISI), generally occurs due to trauma, typically following a FOOSH. The specific injury mechanism dictates whether scapholunate or lunotriquetral instability occurs. In some cases, these ligamentous injuries may occur gradually due to chronic repetitive stress, particularly in athletes or workers who rely on heavy wrist use, such as gymnasts, weightlifters, or construction workers.

- *DISI* is commonly associated with hyperextension injuries where the scapholunate ligament is torn or attenuated. The scaphoid is unable to maintain its normal relationship with the lunate, leading to dorsiflexion of the lunate and abnormal wrist motion.
- *VISI*, while less common than DISI, usually occurs when there is a disruption to the lunotriquetral ligament. This is often due to a twisting injury or repetitive stress, where the triquetrum and lunate fail to maintain their volar alignment.

Clinical Presentation

- *DISI* is characterized by pain on the dorsal side of the wrist, particularly over the scapholunate interval. Patients often report difficulty with activities that require wrist extension or weight-bearing on the hands.
- *VISI* presents with pain more localized to the ulnar side of the wrist, near the lunotriquetral joint. Ulnar deviation and activities that involve gripping or twisting motions typically exacerbate symptoms.

In both cases, the physical exam may reveal tenderness over the affected ligamentous interval (scapholunate or lunotriquetral), along with a reduced range of motion and instability when performing provocative tests. The Watson test (scaphoid shift test) is often positive for DISI, while the Lunotriquetral Ballottement test may be indicative of VISI.

Radiographic Evaluation

- *Radiographic features* **(Figs. 2A to C)**:
  - In *DISI*, the lateral view typically reveals a dorsal tilt of the lunate, with a *scapholunate angle greater than 60°*. The scaphoid appears flexed, and the carpal alignment may show a widening of the scapholunate interval (Terry-Thomas sign).
  - In *VISI*, the lunate is tilted volarly, resulting in a *scapholunate angle of <30°*. The radiographic features may be subtle in early cases, making diagnosis more challenging.
- *Dynamic radiographs:* These are essential in evaluating carpal instability. Stress views, such as radial and ulnar deviation or clenched fist views, can demonstrate abnormal motion between the carpal

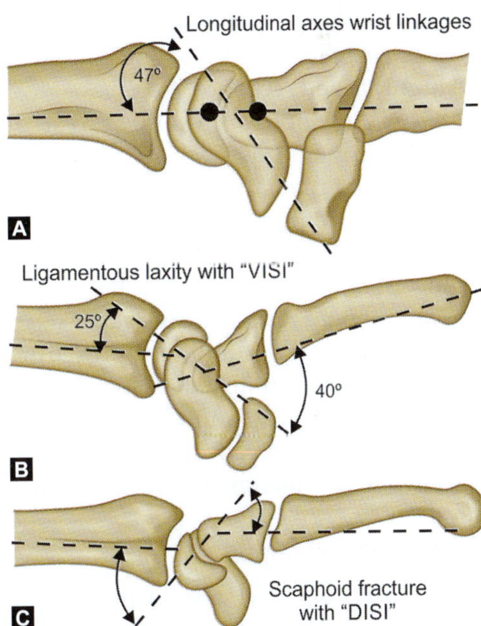

FIGS. 2A TO C: Volar intercalated segment instability (VISI) and dorsal intercalated segment instability (DISI).

bones that may not be visible in static images.

- *Advanced imaging*:
  - *CT scans* provide detailed information about the bony anatomy and alignment, particularly in cases where radiographs are inconclusive.
  - *MRI* is particularly valuable for assessing ligamentous injuries and soft tissue structures. High-resolution MRI can detect partial tears, degenerative changes, and associated pathologies, such as synovitis or ganglion cysts, which may contribute to wrist pain.
  - *Arthroscopy* is particularly helpful for diagnosing and confirming the extent of ligamentous injury. It allows direct visualization of the carpal ligaments and any associated chondral or synovial pathology. Wrist arthroscopy is often utilized when clinical suspicion is high, but imaging findings are equivocal.

CLASSIFICATION

Carpal instability can be classified based on its chronicity and severity:

- *Static instability:* Present at rest on standard radiographs
- *Dynamic instability:* Only evident under specific loading conditions or with stress views

In terms of severity, it can be divided into *predynamic*, *dynamic*, and *static* stages, with predynamic instability representing early ligamentous injury that does not yet manifest on imaging, and static instability being associated with advanced, permanent malalignment visible on plain radiographs.

Treatment Strategies

The management of VISI and DISI depends on the severity of the instability, the presence of symptoms, and the extent of the underlying ligamentous injury. Both conservative and surgical approaches are used, and treatment should be individualized based on patient factors, including age, activity level, and occupational demands.

- *Conservative management*:
  - *Initial treatment* typically involves immobilization in a wrist splint or cast to heal any ligamentous injury and reduce inflammation. Anti-inflammatory medications and activity modifications are recommended to alleviate pain and prevent further damage.
  - However, conservative management is usually insufficient for complete ligament tears, especially in the case of scapholunate or lunotriquetral ligament disruption leading to instability.
- *Surgical management:* Surgical intervention is indicated in cases of persistent instability, failure of conservative treatment, or progressive degenerative changes. The type of surgical procedure depends on the degree of instability and the condition of the ligaments.
  - *Ligament repair or reconstruction:* For acute or incomplete tears, direct repair of the scapholunate or lunotriquetral ligament may be possible. In chronic cases or where ligament repair is not feasible, ligament reconstruction using grafts (e.g., tendon autografts) is performed to restore stability.
  - *Arthroscopic debridement and pinning:* For partial tears or early dynamic instability, arthroscopic debridement of torn ligament fibers combined with temporary pinning of the carpal bones may provide symptom relief and prevent further progression.
  - *Proximal row carpectomy or wrist fusion:* In cases of advanced carpal instability leading to arthritis [e.g.,

scapholunate advanced collapse (SLAC) wrist-scapholunate advanced collapse], salvage procedures such as proximal row carpectomy or partial/total wrist arthrodesis may be necessary to relieve pain and restore function.

Complications of untreated VISI or DISI include:

- Post-traumatic arthritis
- Wrist stiffness
- *Recurrence of instability:* Despite surgical repair or reconstruction, particularly in high-demand individuals or athletes

BIBLIOGRAPHY

1. Adams BD, Steinmann SP. Management of scaphoid fractures. J Orthop Surg. 2019;35(4): 332-9.
2. Garcia-Elias M, Lluch AL. Dorsal intercalated segment instability (DISI) and volar intercalated segment instability (VISI): A comprehensive review. J Hand Surg. 2019;44(6):555-65.
3. Jebson P JL, Adams JE. Vascularized bone grafting for scaphoid nonunion. J Hand Surg. 2018;43(5):475-85.
4. Moran SL, Berger RA. Kienböck's disease: Diagnosis and management. J Wrist Surg. 2020;9(2): 150-6.
5. Watson HK, Ryu J. Carpal instability: Classification and pathomechanics. Clin Orthop Relat Res. 2020;483:69-76.
6. Wolfe SW, Hotchkiss RN, Pederson WC, Kozin SH. Green's Operative Hand Surgery, 7th edition. Philadelphia: Elsevier Health Sciences; 2016.

Injuries of Thumb

Amarjeet Singh

Approximately, 80% of thumb fractures involve the metacarpal base with extra-articular epibasal fractures being the most common variant.

MECHANISM OF INJURY

The primary mechanism involves an axial force applied to the thumb while in a flexed position, e.g., open fist punching.

APPLIED ANATOMY

- The carpometacarpal (CMC) joint of the thumb has a saddle shape, formed by the trapezium and the base of the first metacarpal.
- This joint allows flexion-extension and abduction-adduction motions.
- The CMC joint permits limited axial rotation of thumb.
- Various deforming forces are described in **Figure 1**.

CLASSIFICATION

Green and O'Brien classification **(Fig. 2)**

- *Type I:* Simple intra-articular fracture (Bennett fracture) with a small fragment at the base of the first metacarpal articulating with the trapezium
- *Type II:* Comminuted intra-articular fracture (Rolando fracture) often forming a "Y sign" from the split of the metacarpal base
- *Type III:* Extra-articular, epibasal fracture (pseudo-Bennett fracture)
  - *IIIA:* Transverse fracture
  - *IIIB:* Oblique fracture
- *Type IV:* Epiphyseal fracture

IMAGING

- *X-rays:*
  - *True anteroposterior (AP) (Robert's view):* Taken with the arm fully pronated **(Figs. 3A and B)**

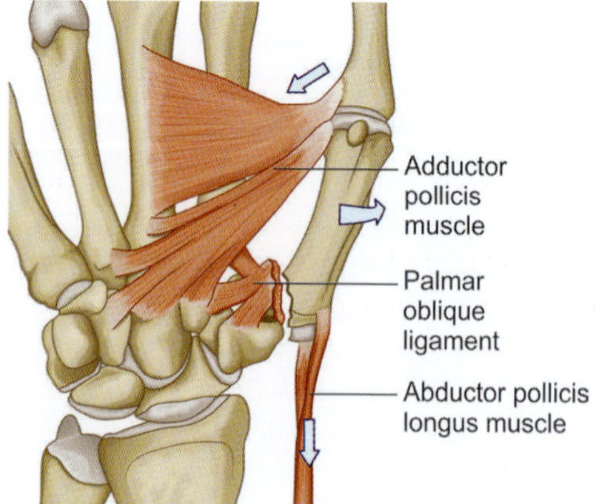

FIG. 1: Forces acting on the fracture fragment.

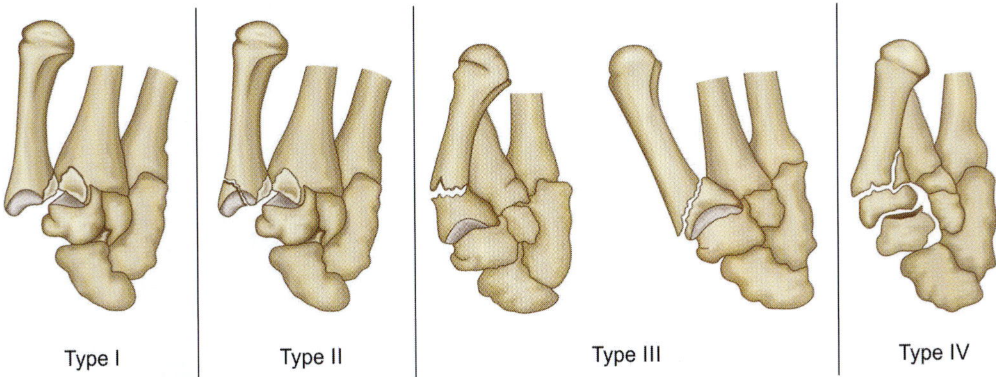

FIG. 2: Green and O'Brien classification.

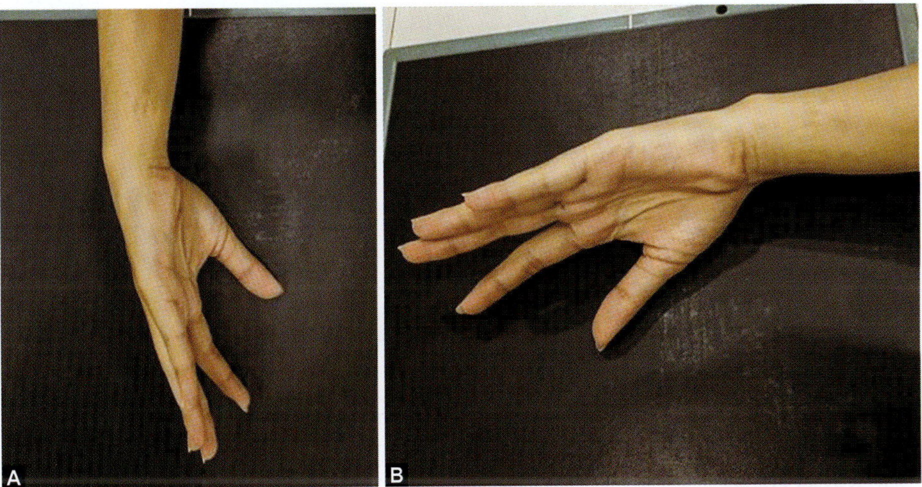

FIGS. 3A AND B: Robert's view of the thumb.

- *True lateral:* Achieved with the hand pronated 30° and a 15° beam tilt.
- *Optional view:* Oblique
- *Additional imaging:*
  - *Traction view:* Helpful for evaluating complex or comminuted fractures
  - A 30° pronated view offers the clearest radiographic assessment
- *CT scan:*
  - Used for complex fractures to better visualize fragment details.

TREATMENT

Nonoperative Treatment

Closed reduction and thumb spica casting:

- *Indications:* Extra-articular fractures with <30° of angulation after reduction and Bennett fractures with <1 mm of displacement.
- *Techniques:* Reduction using traction, palmar abduction, and pronation followed by thumb spica **(Fig. 4)**.

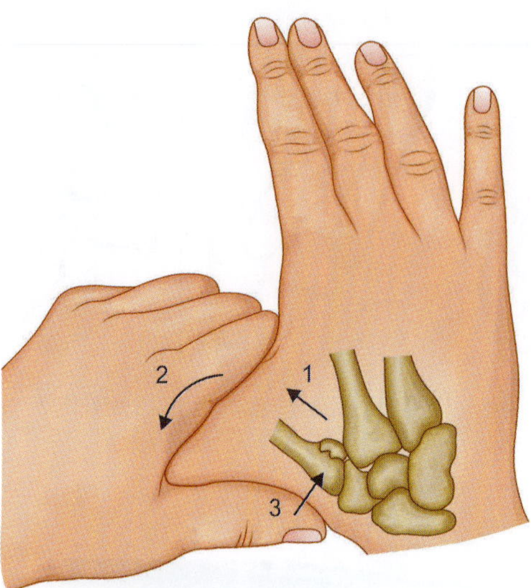

FIG. 4: Technique for closed reduction.

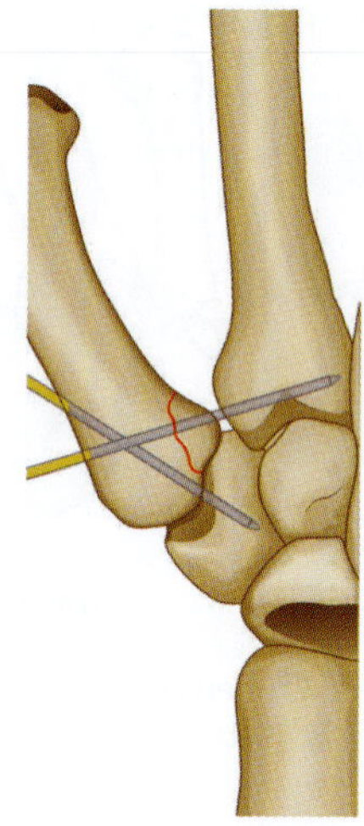
FIG. 5: Iselin technique of transfixing K-wires.

Operative

- *Closed reduction with percutaneous Kirschner wire (K-wire) fixation:*
    - *Indications:* Failure to maintain a reduction under 30° or displacement over 1 mm in Rolando fractures.
    - *Iselin technique:* Transfixing the first metacarpal with the trapezium and the second metacarpal by crossed K-wires **(Fig. 5)**.
- *Open reduction internal fixation (ORIF) indications:* Displacement greater than 1 mm in Bennett or comminuted fractures.
    - *Approach:*
        - Volar (Gedda and Moberg) with careful soft-tissue handling **(Fig. 6)**.
            - The fracture is clamped and stabilized with K-wires or screws.
        - *Dorsal:* Mini plate fixation **(Fig. 7)**
- Distraction and external fixation

Indications: Severely comminuted fractures or significant soft-tissue injury

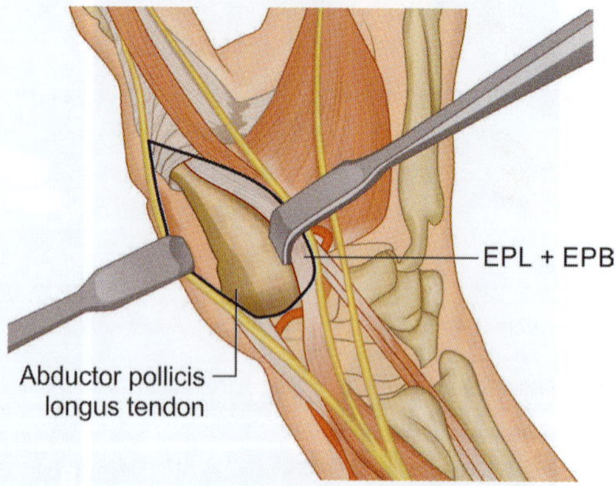

FIG. 6: Dorsal approach to the metacarpal base.
(EPB: extensor pollicis brevis; EPL: extensor pollicis longus)

COMPLICATIONS

- *Post-traumatic arthritis:* Common in highly comminuted intra-articular fractures
- *Malunion:* May cause long-term stiffness or arthritis

PROGNOSIS

Early intervention and proper fracture management generally lead to favorable outcomes, with a high likelihood of regaining

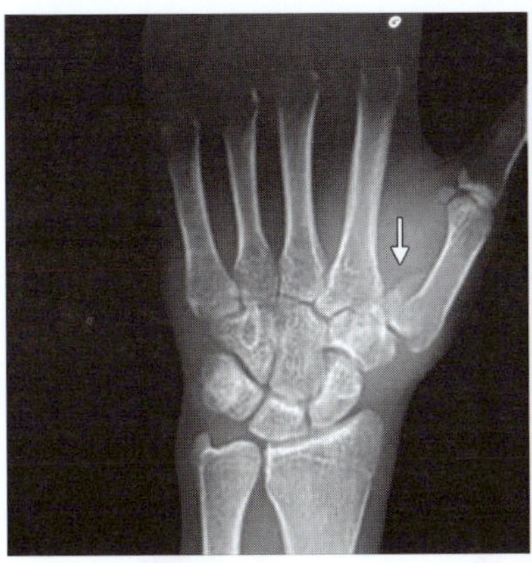

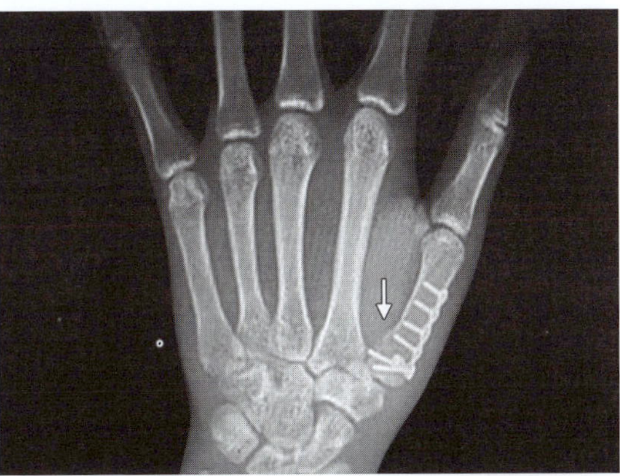

FIG. 7: Mini-plate fixation.

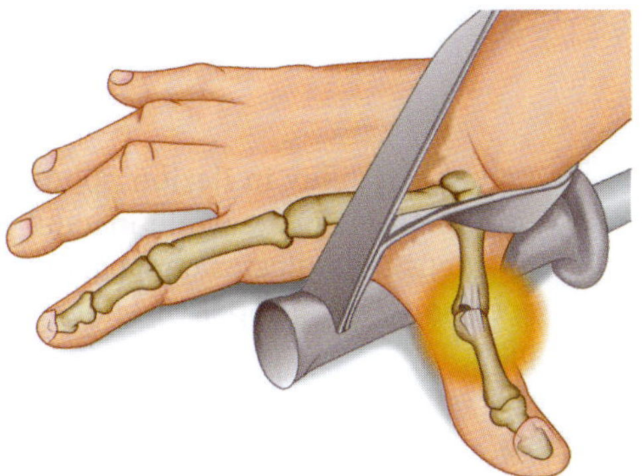

FIG. 8: Mechanism of skier's thumb injury.

function. However, complex fractures like Bennett or Rolando types have a higher risk of long-term complications such as arthritis.

GAMEKEEPER'S THUMB/SKIER'S THUMB: ULNAR COLLATERAL LIGAMENT INJURY OF THE THUMB

- Ulnar collateral ligament (UCL) injuries are more prevalent than radial collateral ligament (RCL) injuries.
- UCL injuries account for >80% of all athletic thumb injuries.
- Men are commonly affected and acute injuries are seen mostly in sports like skiing, baseball, Javelin, football, etc. (both contact and noncontact)
- Known as *"Skier's thumb"* when caused by acute trauma
- Chronic UCL injuries, often due to repetitive stress, are referred to as "Gamekeeper's thumb". Traditionally seen in Gamekeepers [*People who used to maintain and take care of an estate with animals used for hunting. They often had to break the neck of small animals for hunting (rabbits, birds, etc.), which caused repetitive stress on the thumb*].

Etiology

- *Mechanism of injury:* Radial-directed force causes hyperabduction of the thumb's metacarpophalangeal (MCP) joint, such as a skier's thumb being caught by a stationary ski pole and strap **(Fig. 8)**.
- *Pathoanatomy:*
    - *Stener lesion:* The avulsed ligament, with or without bone attachment, is displaced dorsally and superficially to the adductor aponeurosis **(Fig. 9)**.
    - Typically, the ligament's distal end retracts proximally, and healing is not possible without surgery due to the interposition of the adductor aponeurosis.
    - *Stener-like RCL lesions* are rare, but RCL injuries generally result in joint subluxation rather than instability.

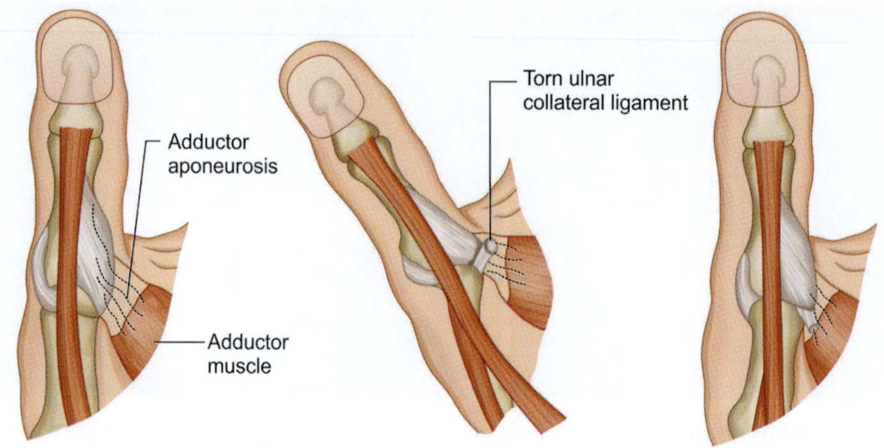

FIG. 9: Stener lesion.

Classification

The UCL/RCL instability grading:

- *Grade 1:* Sprain with no joint instability (incomplete tear)
- *Grade 2:* Asymmetric joint laxity but with an endpoint present (incomplete tear)
- *Grade 3:* Joint instability without an endpoint and joint space opening of 30–35° or 10–15° more than the opposite thumb (complete tear).

Grading/stress testing should preferably be done under local anesthesia.

Clinical Presentation

- UCL tears often result in pain on the ulnar side of the MCP joint, particularly during pinching or gripping, while RCL tears cause pain on the radial side.
- Deformity is rarely visible.
- Tenderness at the site of the ligament injury (distal for UCL and proximal for RCL) and a mass indicating a Stener lesion may be present.
- Radioulnar stress tests should be done in both extension and 30° MCP flexion (preferably under LA).
  - Radial instability in flexion points to proper UCL injury, while instability in extension indicates damage to the accessory UCL, proper UCL, or volar plate.

Imaging

- Standard views include posteroanterior (PA), strict lateral, and oblique. Stress views can be used if a bony avulsion is ruled out.
- *Findings:*
  - UCL injury may show avulsion or condylar fractures or "Sag sign" on lateral views **(Fig. 10)**.
- RCL injuries may exhibit pronation of the proximal phalanx.
- *MRI:* It can be used if clinical findings are inconclusive, offering 100% sensitivity and specificity.
- *Ultrasound:*
  - Operator-dependent accuracy, with sensitivity ranging from 76 to 88% and specificity from 81 to 83%.
  - Hockey stick probe is used.
  - Dynamic testing is extremely helpful.

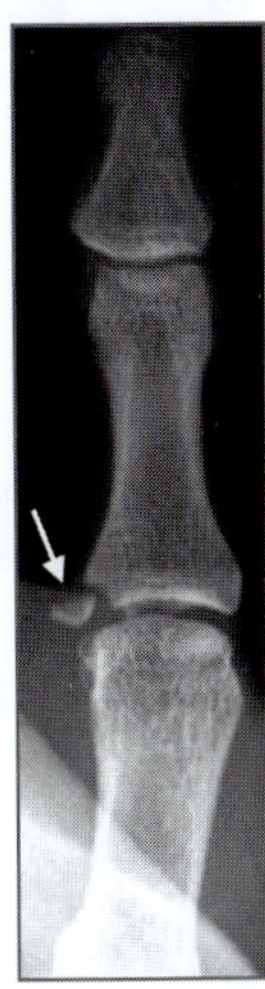

FIG. 10: Sag sign.

Treatment

- *Nonoperative:*
  - Immobilization for 4–6 weeks is recommended for grade 1 and 2 partial UCL and RCL tears, particularly if side-to-side instability is <15°. Excellent outcomes are common, with no residual instability.
  - Immobilization involves splinting (Thumb Spica) for 4–6 weeks, with active and passive motion exercises introduced gradually.
- *Operative:*
  - Surgery is indicated for acute grade 3 injuries, particularly with >15° instability or 30–35° of joint opening, and in cases of Stener lesions. Outcomes are generally excellent for both UCL (over 90%) and RCL repairs (96%).
  - Chronic injuries older than 3–8 weeks may require ligament reconstruction using tendon grafts, with success rates over 90%.
  - *Techniques:*
    - Surgical repair techniques vary, with options such as transosseous sutures, suture tapes, or suture anchors.
    - Tendon reconstruction involves autografts (e.g., palmaris longus) secured with various fixation methods more common in chronic injuries.

Complications

Common complications include stiffness in MCP and interphalangeal (IP) joints and residual instability, particularly in grade 3 injuries treated nonoperatively (15% incidence).

BIBLIOGRAPHY

1. Carlson MG, Warner KK, Meyers KN, Hearns KA, Kok PL. Anatomy of the thumb metacarpophalangeal ulnar and radial collateral ligaments. J Hand Surg Am. 2012;37(10):2021-6.
2. Lark ME, Maroukis BL, Chung KC. The Stener lesion: Historical perspective and evolution of diagnostic criteria. Hand (N Y). 2017;12(3):283-9.
3. Mohseni M, Sina RE, Graham C. Ulnar Collateral Ligament Injury (Gamekeeper's Thumb). In: StatPearls [Internet]. Treasure Island (FL): StatPearls Publishing; 2024. Available from: https://www.ncbi.nlm.nih.gov/books/NBK482383/#
4. Nichols DS, Oberhofer HM, Chim H. Anatomy and biomechanics of the thumb carpometacarpal joint. Hand Clin. 2022;38(2):129-39.

Metacarpals and Phalangeal Fracture

Kamal Ji Pandit

METACARPAL FRACTURES

Metacarpal fractures are among the most common injuries to the hand, accounting for approximately 30–40% of all hand fractures.

Applied Anatomy of the Metacarpals

- *First metacarpal:* Associated with the thumb; shorter and more mobile
- *Second and third metacarpals:* Provide stability to the hand and have limited motion.
- *Fourth and fifth metacarpals:* More mobile, allowing for grip adjustment and increased dexterity

Each metacarpal has a base (proximal end), shaft, neck, and head (distal end). The base articulates with the carpal bones of the wrist, while the head forms the knuckle joint with the proximal phalanx of each finger.

Classification of Metacarpal Fractures

Metacarpal fractures can be classified based on their location, pattern, and whether they are open or closed:

- *Location-based classification:*
    - *Base fractures:* These can involve the carpometacarpal (CMC) joints and may be associated with dislocations.
    - *Shaft fractures:* Fractures of the mid-portion of the metacarpal
    - *Neck fractures:* Commonly occur in the fifth metacarpal (boxer's fracture)
    - *Head fractures:* Involve the distal end of the metacarpal, often intra-articular
- *Angulation-based classification:*
    - Angulation is measured in degrees on lateral X-rays. Generally, the acceptable angulation differs by metacarpal.
    - *Second and third metacarpals:* 10–15°
    - *Fourth metacarpal:* Up to 30°
    - *Fifth metacarpal:* Up to 40°

Clinical Evaluation

The common mechanisms include direct trauma (e.g., punching a hard object and crush injuries) and indirect trauma (e.g., twisting injuries). It is very important to assess clinically for any rotational deformity, apart from assessing for angulation and shortening.

Diagnostic Imaging

- *X-rays:* Standard views include postero-anterior (PA), lateral, and oblique views. X-rays help determine fracture location, displacement, angulation, rotation, and the presence of any intra-articular involvement.
- *CT scans:* These are useful for complex fractures, intra-articular fractures, or when

there is suspected carpal-metacarpal dislocation.

Management

Nonsurgical Management

Nonsurgical management is indicated in nondisplaced or minimally displaced fractures, stable fractures, fractures with no rotational deformity, and fractures involving the second to fourth metacarpals.

- *Techniques:*
  - *Immobilization:* Closed reduction and immobilization are done using a splint or cast. Typically, a gutter splint or short arm cast is used, depending on the metacarpal involved. The metacarpophalangeal (MCP) joint is immobilized in 70–90° of flexion to prevent stiffness and promote healing.
  - *Buddy taping:* This involves taping the injured finger to an adjacent finger to provide support while allowing some movement.
  - *Duration:* Immobilization usually lasts for 3–6 weeks, depending on the fracture's severity and stability.

Surgical Management

Surgical management is indicated in displaced fractures with unacceptable angulation or rotation, comminuted fractures, fractures with multiple fragments, intra-articular fractures, open fractures, and fractures that fail conservative management.

- *Techniques **(Figs. 1A to H)**:*
  - Closed reduction and percutaneous pinning (CRPP)
  - Open reduction and internal fixation (ORIF): It involves a surgical incision to realign the fracture and fixation using plates, screws, or wires. This method is chosen for unstable or severely displaced fractures, especially in young, active patients.
  - *Intramedullary pinning:* Involves inserting Kirschner wires (K-wires) and, rarely, screws within the medullary canal of the bone. It is an option for transverse or short oblique fractures.

BOXER'S FRACTURE

Boxer's fracture, a common injury, often occurs due to a direct impact or punching a hard object. Despite its name, the fracture is not limited to boxers; it is a misnomer, as anyone striking an object with a clenched fist can sustain this type of fracture. A boxer's fracture typically involves a break in the neck or distal shaft of the metacarpal bones, usually the fourth or fifth metacarpal, in the hand.

Most patients are young adults, particularly males aged 15–35, who engage in high-risk behaviors such as sports, fights, or accidental trauma.

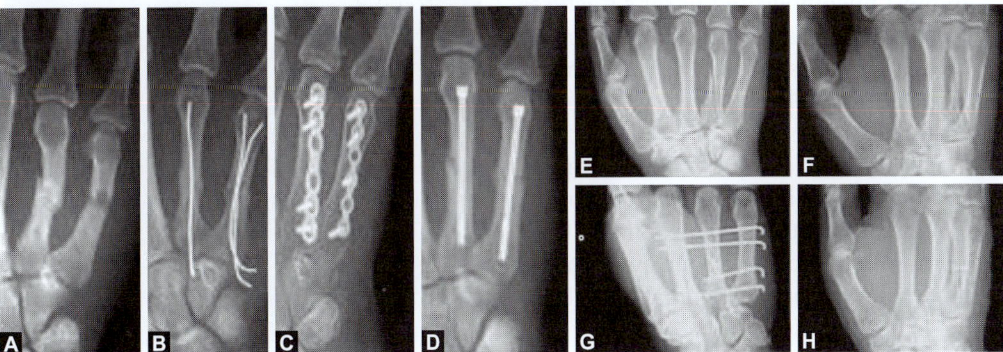

FIGS. 1A TO H: Techniques.

Applied Anatomy

The relatively more mobility of fifth metacarpal bone incresae its susceptibility to fracture, particularly in the metacarpal neck, when subjected to a forceful impact.

Classification

Boxer's fractures can be classified based on the location, pattern, and angulation of the fracture:

- *Location-based classification:*
  - *Head fractures:* Rare but may involve the articular surface
  - *Neck fractures:* Most common type, occurring just below the metacarpal head
  - *Shaft fractures*: Less common; typically require high-energy trauma
  - *Base fractures:* Infrequent and often involve more extensive hand injuries
- *Angulation-based classification*: Generally, the acceptable angulation in fifth Metacarpal is up to 40°.

Diagnostic Evaluation

A characteristic feature is a depression or "loss of knuckle contour" of the injured metacarpal when the fist is clenched.

It is very important to examine and see for any rotational deformity.

Management

- *Nonsurgical management*: It is indicated in most uncomplicated boxer's fractures with minimal angulation that can be managed conservatively. Treatment involves immobilization using a splint or cast.
  - *Ulnar gutter splint:* A common method for immobilizing the fourth and fifth metacarpals, extending from the elbow to the fingertips with the wrist in slight extension and the MCP joints in flexion.
  - *Buddy taping:* For minor fractures or after initial immobilization, buddy-taping the affected finger to the adjacent finger can provide additional support.
- *Surgical treatment*: Surgical intervention is indicated for boxer's fractures with severe angulation (beyond acceptable limits), significant rotation, open fractures, or those involving multiple metacarpals. Various surgical techniques include:
  - *CRPP:* Pins are inserted percutaneously to stabilize the fracture **(Fig. 2)**.
  - *ORIF:* It involves fixation with the plates, screws, or wires. ORIF is typically reserved for comminuted fractures or those with soft-tissue injury **(Fig. 3)**.
  - *External fixation:* It is rarely used, mainly for complex fractures with significant soft-tissue damage.

FRACTURES OF THE BASE OF FIFTH METACARPAL

Fractures of the base of the fifth metacarpal are relatively common injuries, often resulting from direct trauma or forceful twisting motions.

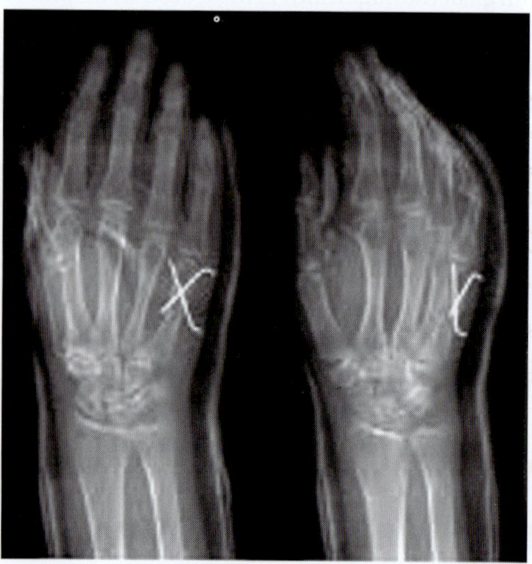

FIG. 2: Closed reduction and percutaneous pinning.

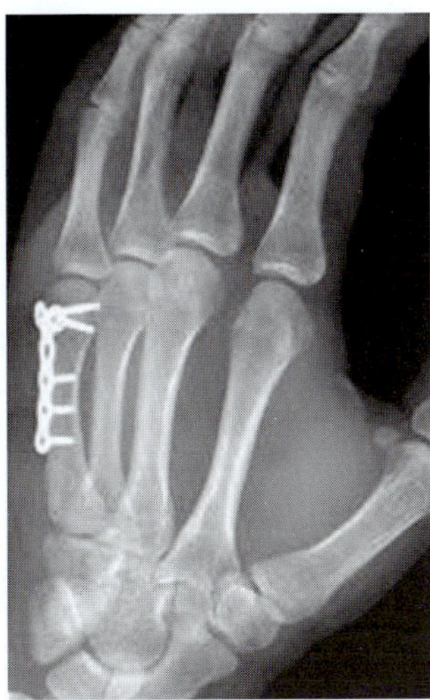

FIG. 3: Open reduction and internal fixation.

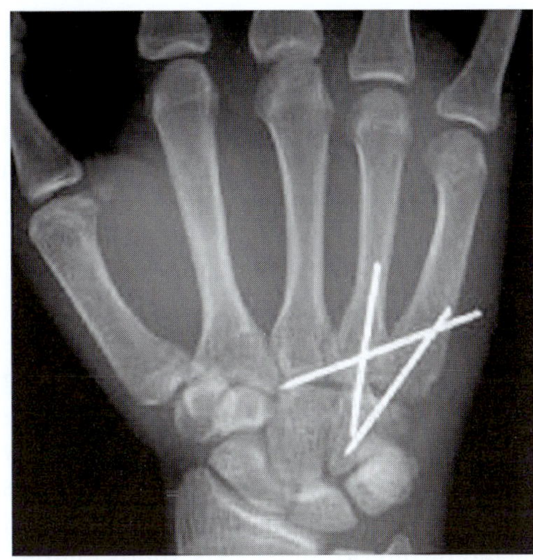

FIG. 4: Fixation of base of fourth and fifth CMP joints.

Applied Anatomy

The base of the fifth metacarpal articulates with the hamate bone and, to a lesser extent, with the fourth metacarpal. This joint is crucial for the function of the hand, providing stability and mobility for gripping, twisting, and a range of other hand movements.

Types of Fractures

Fractures of the base of the fifth metacarpal can be classified into the following based on their location, pattern, and mechanism of injury:

- Intra-articular fractures
- Extra-articular fractures
- Avulsion fractures

Diagnostic Evaluation

A standard set of PA, lateral, and oblique views should be obtained to assess the fracture pattern, displacement, and any involvement of the articular surface.

Management

- Nonoperative management: It is suitable for stable, nondisplaced, or minimally displaced fractures without significant rotational deformity or articular involvement. The mainstay of conservative management includes:
    - *Immobilization:* The use of a splint or cast is the most common method of immobilization. A below-elbow ulnar gutter splint or cast is typically applied to immobilize the wrist, fourth and fifth metacarpals, and the little finger in a functional position. Immobilization is usually maintained for 3–6 weeks, depending on the rate of healing and clinical symptoms.
- *Operative management*: Surgical intervention is indicated for fractures that are displaced, unstable, intra-articular, or associated with significant soft-tissue injury. The primary surgical options include:
    - CRPP **(Fig. 4)**
    - *ORIF:* It is indicated for displaced intra-articular fractures, comminuted fractures, or when closed reduction is unsuccessful. This technique involves the use of plates, screws, or a combination of both to achieve anatomical reduction and stable fixation.

The surgical approach may vary depending on the fracture pattern and surgeon preference.
 - *External fixation:* In cases where there are severe soft-tissue damage or open fractures, external fixation may be employed.

PHALANGEAL FRACTURES OF HAND

Phalangeal fractures of the hand are among the most common skeletal injuries encountered in clinical practice, comprising roughly 10% of all fractures in the body. These fractures can occur due to a variety of mechanisms, including direct trauma, falls, sports injuries, or occupational hazards. Phalangeal fractures can range from simple, nondisplaced fractures to complex, comminuted fractures involving joint surfaces.

Phalangeal fractures can be classified based on their location (proximal, middle, or distal). Intra-articular fractures, which extend into the joint space, present additional challenges due to their potential to disrupt joint congruity and lead to stiffness or osteoarthritis.

Mechanism of Injury

Phalangeal fractures typically result from:
- Direct trauma
- *Indirect trauma*: Twisting or rotational forces may lead to spiral or oblique fractures.
- *Crush injuries:* High-impact trauma or crush injuries may result in comminuted fractures, often involving soft-tissue damage.

Diagnosis

Assess for rotational deformity and angulation.

X-rays: Anteroposterior (AP), *strict lateral* (is a must), and oblique views of the hand and finger are the primary diagnostic tools.

Management

Nonsurgical Management

Nonsurgical management is indicated for stable, nondisplaced, or minimally displaced fractures, especially those with an intact periosteum or minimal rotational deformity. The primary goals are to maintain alignment, prevent stiffness, and promote healing. Methods of nonsurgical management are:
- *Buddy taping/strapping:* It is used for stable, nondisplaced fractures of the proximal or middle phalanx. The injured finger is taped to an adjacent finger to provide support while allowing early mobilization.
- *Splinting:* Common splints include:
  - *Gutter splint:* For stable fractures of the middle or proximal phalanx, holding the finger in a safe, protected position [20–30° of MCP flexion and full proximal interphalangeal (PIP) and distal interphalangeal (DIP) extension]
  - *Aluminum or custom thermoplastic splint:* It is used for distal phalanx fractures or fractures requiring a specific angle of immobilization.
- *Casting:* It is rarely used, but may be considered for noncooperative patients or children to maintain immobilization.

Follow-up and Rehabilitation

- *Regular X-ray monitoring:* Repeat X-rays at 1–2 weeks to ensure proper alignment and detect any secondary displacement.
- *Early mobilization:* Initiate early range-of-motion exercises once there is evidence of fracture stability to prevent joint stiffness and tendon adhesions.

Surgical Management

Indications for surgery:
- *Displaced fractures*: Where closed reduction cannot maintain alignment
- *Unstable fractures:* Comminuted or spiral fractures prone to redisplacement

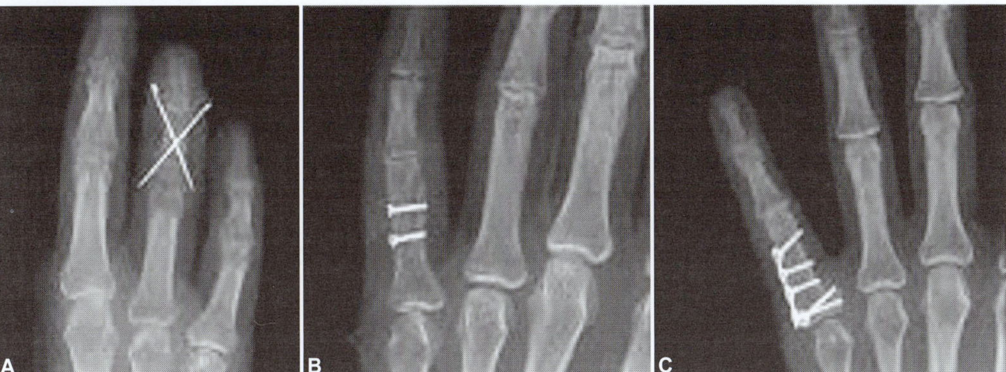

FIGS. 5A TO C: Various different methods of phalangeal fixation.

- *Intra-articular fractures:* To restore joint congruity and prevent arthritis
- *Open fractures:* Require surgical debridement, stabilization, and possible soft-tissue repair
- *Malrotation or angulation:* Where clinical deformity is evident
- *Associated tendon, nerve, or vascular injuries:* Concurrent repair with fracture stabilization

The goal of surgery is to achieve anatomical reduction, stable fixation, and early mobilization to restore hand function.

Techniques

- *CRPP:* It is utilized for simple fractures that can be reduced but require stabilization to maintain alignment. K-wires are inserted percutaneously across the fracture site **(Fig. 5A)**.
- *ORIF:* It is indicated for fractures that cannot be aligned with closed reduction or those requiring precise anatomical restoration. Various fixation methods are used, including:
  - *Plates and screws:* For comminuted or intra-articular fractures **(Fig. 5C)**
  - *Interfragmentary screws:* For oblique or spiral fractures where lag screw fixation can achieve compression **(Fig. 5B)**
- *External fixation:* It is employed in cases of severe soft-tissue damage, comminuted fractures, or when other internal fixation methods are not feasible.

Postoperative Care and Rehabilitation

Immobilization: Typically, for 3–6 weeks, depending on the stability of the fixation and fracture type.

BIBLIOGRAPHY

1. Dell P, Salter RB. Review article: Current concepts in managing fractures of metacarpal and phalangeal bones. J Hand Surg Eur. 2022;47(5):429-36.
2. Kamath JB, Harshvardhan H, Naik DM, Bansal A. Current concepts in managing fractures of metacarpal and phalanges. Indian J Plast Surg. 2011;44(2):203-11.
3. Kopp J, Rhee P. Techniques for metacarpal and phalangeal fracture fixation. J Hand Surg Am. 2022;47(3):295-305.
4. Slade JF III, Schenck RR. Principles of metacarpal and phalangeal fracture management: A new approach to an old problem. J Orthop Sports Phys Ther. 2022;52(6):315-21.
5. Vaudreuil N, Calfee RP. Current outcomes and treatments of complex phalangeal and metacarpal fractures. Hand Clin. 2023;39(4):465-75.

CHAPTER 6.5

Carpometacarpal, Metacarpophalangeal and Interphalangeal Dislocation

Aman Koul

CARPOMETACARPAL DISLOCATION

- Carpometacarpal (CMC) joint dislocations are rare, accounting for 1–1.5% of global hand trauma cases.
- Due to their infrequency, they are often overlooked or misdiagnosed.

Applied Anatomy

- The second to fifth CMC joints are inherently stable due to their joint surfaces and surrounding dorsal, volar, and intra-articular ligaments.
- The trapezoid–metacarpal joint (thumb CMC joint) allows for multiplanar movement and is stabilized by its biconcave–convex shape, ligaments, and capsule.
- The fourth and fifth CMC joints are most commonly dislocated due to their greater mobility compared to other CMC joints.
- Dorsal dislocations are more prevalent due to weaker support on the dorsal side compared to the volar side.

Challenges in Diagnosis

The CMC dislocations **(Figs. 1A and B)** are often misdiagnosed due to:

- Nonspecific symptoms
- *Swelling:* Obscure deformities
- X-ray images can be difficult to interpret due to overlapping structures.

Good anteroposterior (AP), lateral, and oblique X-rays, as well as identifying Gilula's lines and parallel M lines, aid in diagnosis **(Fig. 2)**.

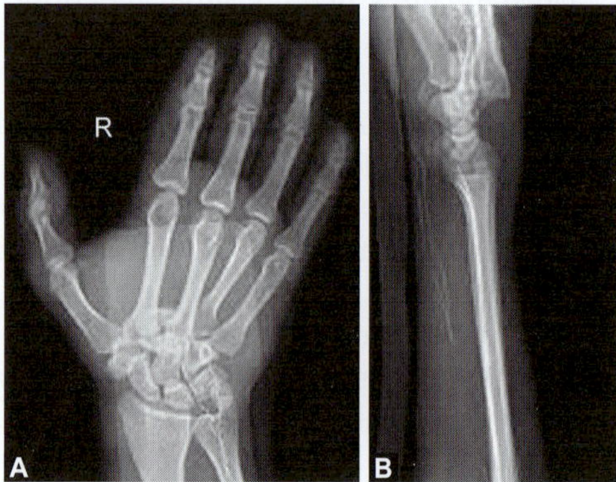

FIGS. 1A AND B: Carpometacarpal (CMC) dislocations.

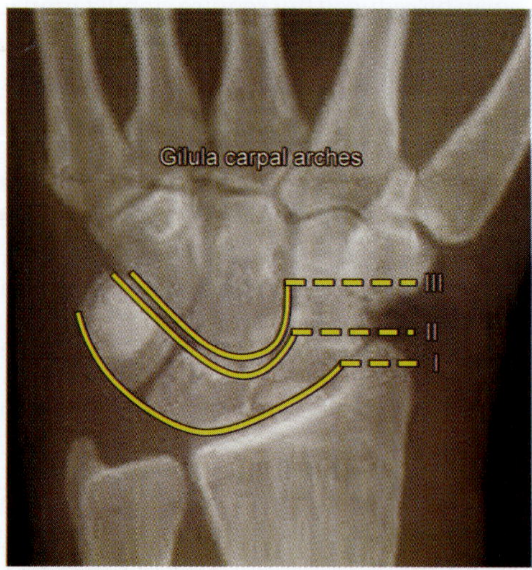

FIG. 2: Gilula carpal arches.

In some cases, computed tomography (CT) scans are used for better visualization and preoperative planning.

Up to 80% of cases involve associated fractures of the metacarpal or carpal bones, complicating diagnosis and treatment.

Clinical signs: Clinical signs are often non-specific (e.g., edema, deformity, and limited motion).

Treatment Approaches

The treatment approach includes the following:

- Management by conservative means is usually unsuccessful despite obtaining a closed reduction.
- Closed reduction and percutaneous pinning (CRPP) is preferred in the majority of cases because it restores joint alignment, limits soft-tissue damage, and is cost-effective for patients.
- Open reduction and internal fixation (ORIF) is reserved for complex or irreducible dislocations.
- Approach via a direct incision on the injured CMC joint on the dorsal surface can also be done.

Surgical timing: Surgery should ideally be performed within 7–10 days after injury, though successful outcomes have been achieved even after 20 days.

METACARPOPHALANGEAL DISLOCATION

- Dorsal dislocations are most common.
- Second digit is most commonly involved followed by thumb.

Mechanism of Injury

Fall on an outstretched hand causes metacarpophalangeal (MCP) joint hyperextension, which leads to avulsion of the volar plate from the metacarpal neck.

Associated conditions: Metacarpal and phalanx fractures

Classification of Metacarpophalangeal Dislocations

- *Anatomic classification:*
    - Volar dislocation
    - Dorsal dislocation
- Based on the complexity, MCP dislocation can be:
    - *Simple (subluxation):* No interposition of the volar plate or sesamoids, and the base of the proximal phalanx remains in contact with the metacarpal head.
    - *Complex (complete dislocation):* Involves interposition of the volar plate or sesamoids, with the metacarpal head becoming trapped by displaced natatory ligaments distally and the superficial transverse metacarpal ligament proximally.

Kaplan's Lesion (Rare)

- Most frequently seen in the index finger.
- The metacarpal head displaces volarly, "buttonholing" into the palm.
- The volar plate becomes lodged between the base of the proximal phalanx and the metacarpal head.

Imaging

Radiographs: AP, lateral, and oblique.

- *Joint space widened:* Interposition of volar plate
- *Entrapped sesamoid in the joint:* Complex dislocation **(Fig. 3)**

Treatment for Metacarpophalangeal Joint Dislocations

Nonoperative Treatment

Closed reduction: Indicated for simple dislocations

- *Dorsal dislocation:*
    - *Reduction technique*: Apply direct pressure to the dorsal aspect of the proximal phalanx while the wrist is flexed to reduce tension on the intrinsic and extrinsic flexors. Avoid

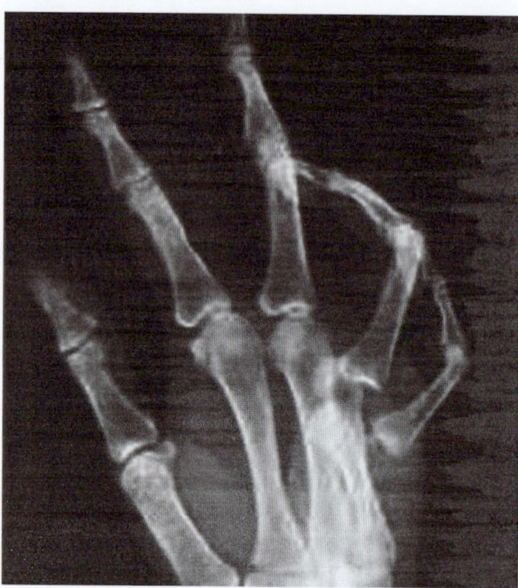

FIG. 3: Entrapped sesamoid in the joint.

using longitudinal traction to prevent pulling the volar plate into the joint, which could make the dislocation irreducible.
    - *Immobilization:* After successful reduction, use a dorsal blocking splint and initiate early range of motion exercises.
- *Volar dislocation:*
    - *Reduction technique:* Direct pressure is applied to the volar aspect of the proximal phalanx with the MCP joint flexed.
    - *Immobilization:* The joint should be immobilized in 30° flexion for 2 weeks, followed by active range of motion exercises in a dorsal blocking splint.

Operative Treatment

Operative treatment is required for complex dislocations or delayed presentations.

Dorsal Approach

- Perform a midline incision, splitting the extensor tendon and joint capsule longitudinally.
- In the thumb, work between the extensor pollicis longus (EPL) and extensor pollicis brevis (EPB) tendons.
- The volar plate may be displaced using a Freer elevator; however, splitting the volar plate might be necessary for complete reduction.

Advantages:
- Lower risk of neurovascular injury
- Better access to treat fractures of the metacarpal head

Volar Approach

An oblique incision is made, taking care to avoid damaging the neurovascular bundle.

The A1 pulley is released to expose the volar plate, which can be manipulated along with surrounding ligaments and tendons using a Freer elevator.

Advantages: This approach provides better access to the volar plate and associated structures.

Disadvantages: Greater risk of neurovascular injury and difficulty in addressing osteochondral fractures.

Complications of Metacarpophalangeal Joint Dislocations

- Joint stiffness
- Post-traumatic arthritis or osteonecrosis
- *Premature physeal closure:* A rare complication that may result from injury in children.

INTERPHALANGEAL DISLOCATION

Interphalangeal dislocations involve the displacement of the finger joints, specifically the proximal interphalangeal (PIP) or distal interphalangeal (DIP) joints. These injuries are frequent in sports and occur when the joint experiences extreme force, leading to misalignment. Immediate and effective management is essential to prevent complications such as chronic instability or arthritis.

Applied Anatomy

The PIP joint is between the first (proximal) and second (middle) phalanges, while the DIP joint is between the second and third (distal) phalanges. Ligaments, tendons, and a joint capsule stabilize these joints. Dislocations are often caused by:

- *Hyperextension:* Forcefully bending the joint beyond its limit
- *Direct impact:* A blow to the fingertip, pushing the joint out of alignment
- *Twisting forces:* Rotational stress on the joint, causing lateral displacement

Types of Dislocations

- *Dorsal dislocation:* It is the most common type, where the distal bone moves backward, usually due to hyperextension.
- *Volar dislocation:* The distal bone moves toward the palm, often resulting from high-impact trauma.
- *Lateral dislocation:* It is caused by sideways displacement, typically from a lateral force.

X-rays (AP, strict lateral, and oblique view) are critical for confirming the type of dislocation and checking for associated fractures. Clinical assessment should include range of motion tests and evaluation for ligament or tendon damage, and neurovascular deficit.

Treatment

- *Closed reduction:* Manual realignment under local anesthesia is usually the first step. Postreduction X-rays verify alignment.
- Following reduction, a splint or buddy taping, generally for 2–3 weeks, stabilizes the joint allowing soft tissues to heal.
- *Surgery:* It is required if there is an associated fracture or if the dislocation is unstable postreduction.

Common Surgical Approaches for Irreducible Interphalangeal Dislocations

- *Dorsal approach:*
  - *Indication:* Primarily used for irreducible dorsal dislocations, especially when the volar plate or other soft-tissue structures are interposed and blocking reduction.
  - *Advantages:* Provides excellent visualization of the joint, making it easier to address interposed structures, such as the volar plate or extensor tendons.
- *Volar approach:*
  - *Indication*: Often selected for irreducible volar dislocations or when there is interposition of the dorsal structures.
  - *Advantages:* It provides direct access to the volar plate, which is often involved in volar dislocations. It is useful for repairing volar plate avulsion fractures and associated ligament injuries.
- *Lateral approach:*
  - *Indication:* It is utilized in cases of lateral dislocations where soft tissue entrapment on one side is suspected.
  - *Advantages:* It provides direct access to lateral soft tissues with minimal disruption to surrounding structures.

Early guided exercises to restore range of motion and strength are useful. Immobilization beyond 3 weeks can lead to stiffness.

Potential Complications

- Joint stiffness
- *Recurrent instability*: If ligamentous structures are compromised
- Post-traumatic arthritis is more common with articular surface damage.

BIBLIOGRAPHY

1. Dunn JC, Koehler LR, Kusnezov NA, Polfer E, Orr JD, Pirela-Cruz MA, et al. Perilunate dislocations in the U.S. military. J Wrist Surg. 2018;7(1):57-65.
2. Garner M, Rudran B, Khan A, Tang Q, Mathew P. Lunate dislocations: Anatomy, diagnosis, and management. Br J Hosp Med (Lond). 2021;82(7): 1-10.
3. Goodman AD, Harris AP, Gil JA, Park J, Raducha J, Got CJ. Evaluation, management, and outcomes of lunate and perilunate dislocations. Orthopedics. 2019;42(1):e1-6.
4. Kazemian GH, Khak M, Ravarian B, Sarzaeem MM, Okhovatpour MA, Amouzadeh Omrani F. Closed K-wire fixation for the treatment of perilunate dislocations and trans-scaphoid perilunate fracture dislocations without ligamentous repair: Short term follow-up. Arch Bone Jt Surg. 2020;8(5):633-40.

Terminal Phalangeal Injuries

Aman Koul, Mozam Hamid Wani

The common mechanisms of injury include crushing the fingertip between objects, getting the finger caught in a door, saw injuries, snowblower accidents, and direct impact from a hammer. Phalanx injuries are frequent hand injuries affecting the distal > middle > proximal segments of the phalanges.

APPLIED ANATOMY

The applied anatomy includes the following:
- *The distal phalanx comprises three main components*: The tuft, the shaft, and the base.
- The tuft, being the most distal, is structurally important for fingertip sensitivity and functional grip but prevalent to injuries.
- Surrounding soft tissues, including the perionychium, are often injured in conjunction with tuft fractures.
- *Perionychium:* Includes the nail, nail bed, and surrounding skin
- *Paronychium:* Refers to the lateral nail folds
- *Hyponychium:* Skin located distal and palmar to the nail
- *Eponychium:* The dorsal nail fold situated just proximal to the nail
- *Lunula:* The white, crescent-shaped part at the base of the nail
- *Matrix:*
    - *Sterile matrix:* Soft tissue located beneath the nail, distal to the lunula, and adhering to the nail
    - *Germinal matrix:* Soft tissue beneath the nail, proximal to the sterile matrix; responsible for most nail growth. The extensor tendon inserts approximately 1.2–1.4 mm proximal to the germinal matrix.

Assessment: The exact mechanism and duration of injury is the key to management. Proper clinical assessment, especially the vascularity and neurological examination, and radiographs [anteroposterior (AP), lateral, oblique views] are essential to rule out distal phalanx fractures.

Various injuries of terminal phalanx include:

SUBUNGUAL HEMATOMA

Treatment options:
- *Drainage:* Indicated when <50% of the nail is involved.
    - *Technique:* Perforation of the nail with a sterile needle or electrocautery
- *Nail removal and repair:* Necessary if >50% of the nail is involved.
    - *Technique:* Nail removal, debridement, and repair of the nail bed

NAIL BED LACERATIONS

Laceration of the nail and nail bed, often accompanied by a subungual hematoma covering > 50% of the nail surface.

Treatment: Most cases require nail removal, debridement, and repair of the nail bed.

AVULSION INJURIES OF THE NAIL AND NAIL BED (WITH OR WITHOUT FRACTURE)

Treatment: Nail removal and nail bed repair

Technique: Remove the nail, repair the nail bed, and fix the fracture as needed. Always provide tetanus prophylaxis and antibiotics.

Nail Removal, Repair, and Matrix Transfer

- *Indications:* Avulsion or crush injuries with significant loss of the nail matrix
- *Technique:* Perform a nail matrix transfer from an adjacent injured finger or the second toe. Provide tetanus prophylaxis, antibiotics, and fracture fixation based on the fracture type.
- *Techniques for nail bed repair:*
    - Extract the nail and soak it in Betadine solution during the repair of the nail bed.
    - Use very fine absorbable sutures (6–0 or smaller) to sew the nail bed.
    - Stabilize the eponychial fold using the original nail, aluminum foil, or nonadherent gauze to ensure proper healing.
- *Complications:*
    - *Hook nail:* This occurs when the nail matrix is advanced to cover the defect without sufficient bony support.
        - *Treatment:* Remove the affected nail and trim the matrix down to the level of the bone to prevent recurrence.
    - *Split nail:* Results from scarring of the nail matrix after a nail bed injury
        - *Treatment:* Excise the scar tissue and reconstruct the nail matrix, which may require a graft for proper healing.

TUFT FRACTURES OF HAND

Tuft fractures refer to distal phalanx fractures involving the fingertip, specifically the terminal segment, which is often accompanied by nail bed injuries.

Treatment:

- Primarily, conservative
- Stable fractures without significant displacement or associated subungual hematomas can be treated with splinting.
- Typically, the injured finger is immobilized in a protective splint for 2–4 weeks, ensuring the distal interphalangeal (DIP) joint remains in slight extension to prevent stiffness.
- Subungual hematomas involving >50% of the nail bed, however, require drainage via trephination or nail removal, followed by nail bed repair if necessary.
- In cases where nail bed lacerations are present, meticulous repair using absorbable sutures is performed to optimize cosmetic and functional outcomes.

MALLET FINGER

Mallet finger is classified as a zone 1 injury according to the Kleinert and Verdant classification of extensor tendon injuries.

Mechanism of injury:

- Typically results from a sudden, forceful blow causing forced flexion of the fingertip while the finger is extended, forcing the DIP joint into flexion.
- A less common cause is a sharp or crushing laceration to the dorsal side of the DIP joint.

Doyle's Classification of Mallet Finger Injuries

According to the Doyle's classification, the mallet finger injuries are classified into the following:

- *Type I:* Closed injury, may include a small dorsal avulsion fracture
- *Type II:* Open injury caused by a laceration
- *Type III:* Open injury with deep soft-tissue damage, including loss of skin and tendon
- *Type IV:* Mallet fracture, further divided into:
    - *A:* Physeal injury of the distal phalanx (common in children)

- *B:* Fracture involving 20–50% of the articular surface (in adults)
- *C:* Fracture involving >50% of the articular surface (in adults)

Imaging

Radiographs: AP and strict lateral views of the finger (without strict lateral view, an oblique view only can easily miss the exact type of injury).

Radiographs may reveal a bony avulsion at the base of the distal phalanx or normal bony anatomy with possible ligamentous injury. Check for distal phalanx subluxation.

Treatment

Nonoperative Treatment

Extension splinting: Maintain the DIP joint in extension for 6–8 weeks, worn 24 hours daily.

- *Indications:* Acute soft-tissue injuries (<12 weeks) or small, minimally displaced bony mallet injuries without joint subluxation; also used for chronic injuries (>12 weeks) if the joint is supple and nonarthritic.
- *Technique*: Keep the proximal interphalangeal (PIP) joint mobile; if the injury caused a swan-neck posture, block PIP extension with a dorsal blocking splint. It is typically followed by 4 weeks of nocturnal splinting (though this is debated). Use volar splints to reduce complications and avoid hyperextension to prevent skin necrosis. Begin progressive flexion exercises at 6 weeks.
- *Outcomes:* Both operative and nonoperative treatments show similar patient satisfaction and extensor lag, with approximately 80% of patients achieving satisfactory outcomes.

Operative Treatment

Indications:

- *Absolute:* Volar subluxation of the distal phalanx
- *Relative:* Involves >50% of the articular surface, an articular gap >2 mm, or open injuries

Techniques:

- *Closed reduction and percutaneous pinning (CRPP):*
  - *Fixation:* Dorsal extension block pinning with the joint pinned in extension. Techniques include Ishiguro and Modified Ishiguro methods.
- *Open reduction and internal fixation (ORIF):*
  - *Approach:* Dorsal midline incision
  - *Fixation:* Simple pin fixation or dorsal blocking pin **(Fig. 1)**
- *Surgical reconstruction of terminal tendon:* Traumatic tendon laceration or chronic injury (>12 weeks) without contracture or segmental tendon loss
  - *Repair options:*
    - Direct repair often with a transarticular pin, including tendon advancement, tenodermodesis, or spiral oblique retinacular ligament reconstruction
    - Lateral band tenodesis, flexor digitorum superficialis (FDS) tenodesis, or Fowler central slip tenotomy; minimal deformities may resolve with the treatment of DIP pathology alone.

Complications

- Extensor lag
- Reduced DIP flexion

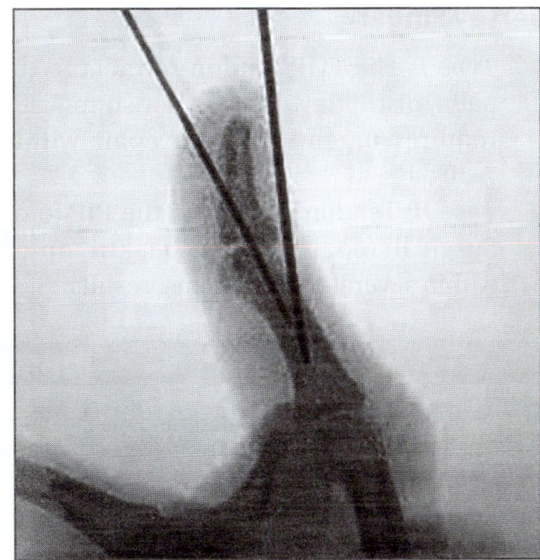

FIG. 1: Fixation of mallet finger.

- Swan-neck deformities
- *Skin issues:* Maceration, ulceration, and nail deformities affect about 70% of non-operatively treated cases, with limited soft-tissue coverage increasing the risk of wound dehiscence and infection.

Treatment of complications:
- *DIP arthrodesis:* For painful, stiff, and arthritic DIP joint
- Swan-neck deformity correction

JERSEY FINGER

- A Jersey finger is a traumatic injury involving the flexor tendon, specifically caused by the avulsion of the flexor digitorum profundus (FDP) from its attachment at the base of the distal phalanx.
- The ring finger is affected in approximately 75% of cases.
- During gripping, the ring finger extends about 5 mm further than the other fingers in around 90% of individuals, making it more vulnerable to higher forces during pull-away movements.
- The injury occurs when the FDP muscle is forcefully contracted while the DIP joint is extended.

Leddy and Packer Classification of Jersey Finger

- *Type I:* The FDP tendon retracts to the palm, disrupting the vascular supply and requires urgent surgical repair within 7–10 days.
- *Type II:* Tendon retracts to the PIP joint. Surgical repair should be attempted within several weeks for best results.
- *Type III:* A large avulsion fracture limits tendon retraction to the DIP joint. Repair should be attempted within several weeks.
- *Type IV:* There is both an avulsion fracture and separation of the tendon from the bone fragment ("double avulsion"). The fracture is treated with ORIF, followed by tendon reattachment as in type I/II.
- *Type V:* This involves tendon rupture with bone avulsion and comminution of the distal phalanx, classified as extra-articular (Va) or intra-articular (Vb).

Imaging: Radiographs may reveal an avulsion fracture fragment.

Operative Treatment

- *Direct tendon repair/tendon reinsertion with dorsal button:* For acute injuries (<3 weeks)
  - Advancing the tendon >1 cm risks DIP flexion contracture or quadrigia.
- *ORIF for fracture fragment:* For types III and IV injuries (type IV is treated similarly to type I/II after fracture fixation)
  - Fixation is done using K-wire, mini frag screw, or pull-out wire. Check for symmetric cascade after fixation.
- *Two-stage flexor tendon grafting:*
  - *Indications:* Chronic injuries (>3 months) with full passive range of movement (ROM) of the DIP joint.
- *DIP arthrodesis:* Used as a salvage procedure for chronic injuries (>3 months) with persistent stiffness

Complications

Advancing the tendon >1 cm increases the risk of DIP flexion contracture or quadrigia.

BIBLIOGRAPHY

1. Guitton TG, Ring D. Diagnosis and management of injuries to the terminal phalanx. J Hand Surg Am. 2020;45(10):939-48.
2. Soejima O, Inagaki K. Distal phalanx fractures and nail bed injuries. Hand Clin. 2020;36(3):287-98.

SECTION

7

Spinal Fractures

CHAPTER 7.1

Cervical Spine Fracture

Nishank Mehta, Prashant Tank

- Traumatic injuries of the cervical spine (fractures and/or dislocations) occur in 1.5–3% of all major trauma patients.
- The overall rate of mortality following cervical spine trauma has been reported to be 2.5%, whereas it is over 10% in patients with spinal cord involvement.
- In obtunded or unconscious patients, cervical spine injuries are often missed—a low Glasgow coma scale (GCS) score, low systolic blood pressure at presentation to the emergency room and severe facial fractures are associated with cervical spine injuries.

ANATOMY AND BIOMECHANICS

- Atlas (C1) has no vertebral body—the two lateral masses are the weight-bearing articulations between the skull and spinal column.
- Stability is provided by the tectorial membrane and alar ligaments. The stability between the anterior tubercle of the atlas and the odontoid process of C2 is provided by the transverse ligament of the atlas.
- Upper cervical spine (occiput to C2) accounts for 50% of total neck movement in the flexion-extension plane.
- Axis (C2) contributes to the atlantoaxial junction (C1-C2)—about 50% of neck rotation occurs at this joint; the stability between anterior tubercle of atlas and the odontoid process of C2 is provided by the transverse ligament of the atlas. Facet joints contribute little to the stability in upper cervical spine.
- The three-column concept can be used to conceptualize the anatomy and mechanics of the subaxial cervical spine
- The vertebral artery enters the foramen transversarium of C6 and ascends through the foramina transversarium to C1. It then emerges from the foramen transversarium and passes between C1 and the occiput, traversing a depression on the superior aspect of the C1 ring.

INITIAL ASSESSMENT

- Patients typically have multiple injuries—so follow Advanced Trauma Life Support (ATLS) protocol.
- Rigid cervical immobilization is a part of airway protection ("A" in the sequence of ABCDE) and an integral component of primary survey and resuscitation.
- *On examination*: Midline neck tenderness in conscious patients, document history of loss of consciousness, look for indirect evidence such as injuries to head, scalp, face
- *Thorough neurological examination*: Sensory and motor testing of all four limbs, cranial nerve examination (often affected in occipitocervical injuries), reflexes (specially, bulbocavernosus

reflex shows recovery from spinal shock), rectal tone, and perianal sensation (sacral sparing)

IMAGING

- *Standard radiographic protocol includes three views*: AP, lateral, and open-mouth view. To visualize C6, C7, and cervicothoracic junction, one may require Swimmer's view or lateral radiograph with shoulders pulled down. The following should be look for in a lateral cervical spine radiograph **(Fig. 1)**—prevertebral soft tissue swelling (increase beyond normal limits for the level), acute change in sagittal alignment (usually kyphosis), loss of continuity in spinal alignment lines (anterior vertebral, posterior vertebral, spinolaminar), loss of vertebral height, and widened or narrowed disk spaces (compare to upper and lower disk spaces).
- Flexion-extension views are controversial—may be considered in awake, symptomatic patient to rule out discoligamentous injury.
- CT scan is the most useful investigation in the setting of acute cervical spine trauma—has superior sensitivity and specificity than plain radiographs. Addition of cervical MRI in patients with normal cervical spine CT and normal neurological examination does not add any additional information that warrants a change in management.

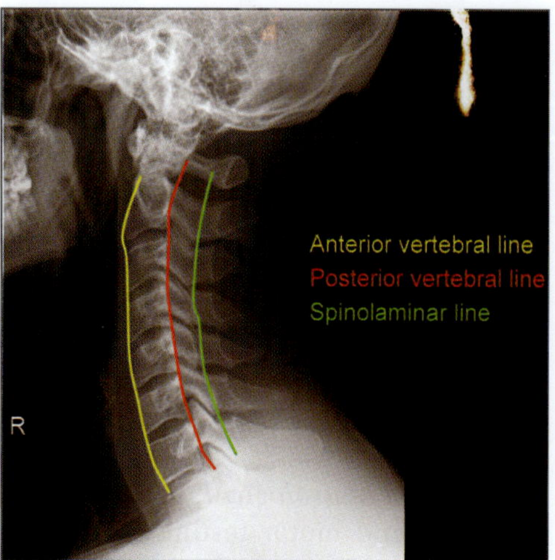

FIG. 1: X-ray cervical spine.

CLEARING THE CERVICAL SPINE

- Integral to the acute management of cervical spine trauma is the concept of "clearing" the cervical spine—this means that a complete evaluation of the cervical spine is done and based on clinical and radiographic findings. Usually this also means that rigid cervical spine immobilization can be discontinued.
- According to NEXUS (National Emergency X-ray Utilization Study Group), clearance of the cervical spine is obtained if following findings are present:
  - No midline cervical pain and tenderness
  - Normal alertness
  - No neurological deficit
  - No evidence of intoxication
  - No painful associated "distracting" injuries
- Another commonly used decision-making tool is the Canadian C-spine rule (CCR) which is illustrated in **Flowchart 1**. The CCR has been found to be more sensitive than NEXUS criteria in detection of cervical spine injuries.

CLASSIFICATION

In 2015, AO Spine published the new AO Spine Subaxial Cervical Spine Injury Classification System. Fractures in C3–C7 are classified into three major morphological types:

1. *Type A*: Compression injury
2. *Type B*: Injury to the anterior or posterior tension band
3. *Type C*: Translational injury

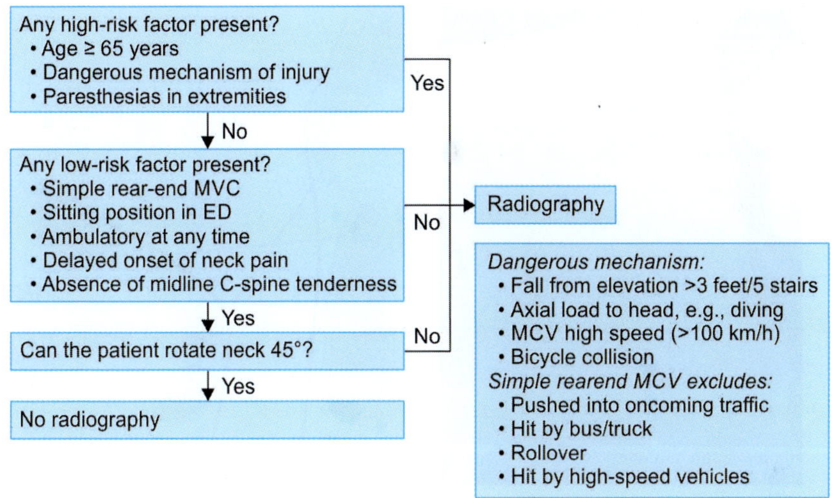

FLOWCHART 1: Canadian C-spine rule.

Furthermore, *the SLIC score* (subaxial injury classification and severity score) can be calculated to guide treatment—SLIC score identifies three major injury characteristics, in addition to morphology of the fracture, it also takes into account the integrity of discoligamentous complex and the neurological status. Each major characteristic is assigned a numerical score depending upon injury severity. Minor injury characteristics include injury level and osseous fractures. The sum of these scores constitutes the injury severity score.

Score greater than 5: Operative therapy consisting of realignment, decompression, and stabilization

INJURIES TO UPPER CERVICAL SPINE (OCCIPUT TO C2)

Occipital Condyle Fractures

- *Presentation*:
  - High cervical pain
  - Motor weakness, possibly lower cranial nerve involvement
  - Transient or persistent loss of consciousness reported in 80% of patients
- *Classification and diagnosis:*
  - *Anderson and Montesano classification system*:
    - Type 1: Axial compression injuries; typically stable; 15% of cases
    - Type 2: Basilar skull fracture; stable injuries; 50% of cases
    - *Type 3*: Avulsion injuries near alar ligament attachment; might be unstable; 35% of cases
  - Best diagnosed in CT scans; plain radiographs likely to miss injury
- *Management*:
  - Surgery is indicated for ligamentous injury and craniocervical instability
  - Most cases managed with rigid external immobilization
  - For patients needing surgery, posterior occipitocervical fusion (occiput to C2 or C3)

Atlanto-occipital Dislocation

It can also occur due to nontraumatic cause like bony dysplasia or ligamentous laxity in certain syndromes (e.g., Down's syndrome).

- *Presentation*:
  - Severe neural deficits, possibly quadriparesis

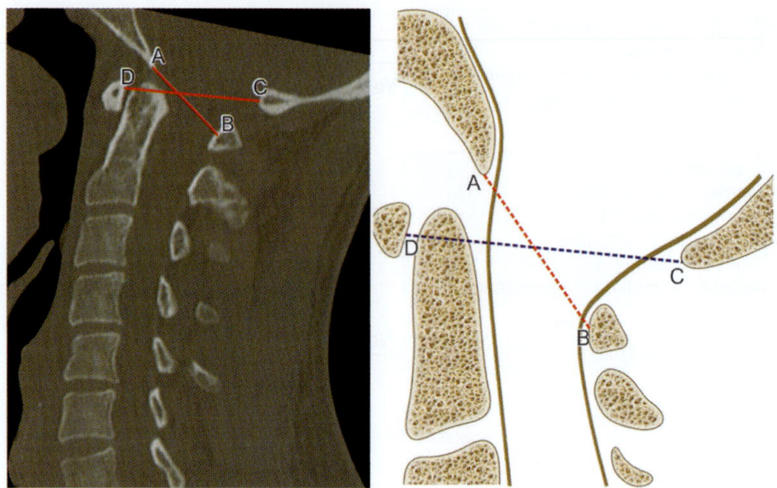

FIG. 2: Power's ratio = AB/CD.

- Cardiorespiratory impairment
- Potentially fatal due to brainstem impingement

- *Imaging*:
  - *Harris' lines*: Suggestive of injury, if basion-dens interval (BDI) > 10 mm, basion-axial interval (BAI) > 12 mm, and atlantodental interval (ADI) > 3 mm
  - *Powers' ratio*: AB/CD **(Fig. 2)** where A-B: distance from basion to posterior arch, C-D: distance from anterior arch to opisthion. Powers' ratio greater than 1 is indicative of anterior subluxation/dislocation, while Powers' ratio < 1 is indicative of posterior dislocation, odontoid fracture.
  - *Wackenheim's line **(Fig. 3)***: Line from the posterior surface of clivus to the upper cervical canal. Line behind odontoid: posterior dissociation, line in front of odontoid: anterior dissociation
  - *MRI*: To look for integrity of the cruciate ligament and the occipitocervical (OC) joint capsule
- *Management*:
  - Stable cases managed with rigid external immobilization

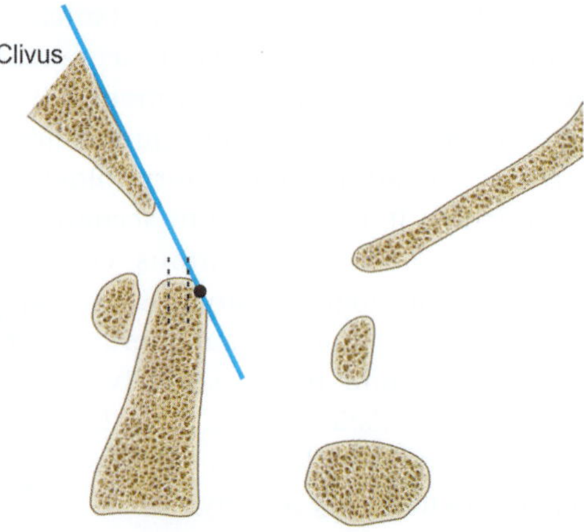

FIG. 3: Wackenheim's line.

  - For patients needing surgery, posterior occipitocervical fusion (occiput to C2 or C3)

Atlas (C1) and Jefferson Fractures

- Occurs due to combination of hyper-extension and axial loading
- Bilateral fractures of anterior and posterior arch—Jefferson's fracture
- *Presentation*:
  - Typically, presents without neural deficits

- If severe, can present with medullary dysfunction:
  - Open-mouth odontoid view—shows unilateral or bilateral overhang of C1 lateral mass over C2 superior articular process (seen only in burst fracture with severe displacement). "Rule of Spence"—C1 overhang should be no more than 6.9–8.1 mm.
  - Lateral view—check anterior atlantodental interval (ADI). Less than 3 mm—normal, 3–5 mm—injury to transverse ligament with intact alar and apical ligaments, greater than 5 mm—injury to transverse, alar ligament, and tectorial membrane
- *CT scan*: Careful study of axial cuts to look for bony avulsion of transverse ligament which suggest instability
- *MRI*: To look for competency of transverse ligament

- *Management*:
  - Depends on status of transverse ligament
  - Stable cases (intact TL) managed with rigid external immobilization
  - Unstable cases (torn TL) require C1-C2 fusion.

Hangman's Fracture (Traumatic Spondylolisthesis of C2 Over C3)

- *Usually occurs in the mechanical sequence*: Hyperextension → compression → rebound flexion
- Bilateral laminae and pedicles of C2 are fractured as a result.
- *Presentation*:
  - Can be asymptomatic if nonangulated and undisplaced
  - Can present with signs and symptoms of vertebral artery injury
    - *Radiographs*: Flexion-extension views to look for subluxation
  - Classified radiologically as per the Levine and Edwards classification, which is a modification of the Effendi classification **(Fig. 4)**:
    - *Type 1*: Nondisplaced fractures with no angulation between C2 and C3 and a fracture dislocation of <3 mm
    - *Type 2*: Fracture with significant angulation (>11°) and displacement (>3.5 mm)
    - *Type 2A*: Fracture with minimum displacement and significant angulation (>11°)
    - *Type 3*: Fractures with severe angulation and displacement associated with unilateral or bilateral C2-3 facet dislocation
- *Management*:
  - *Type 1*: Halo brace for 12 weeks
  - *Type 2*: Reduction by means of cervical traction and halo brace for 12 weeks
  - *Type 2A*: Reduction in extension followed by halo brace; traction to be avoided
  - *Type 3*: Anterior C2–C3 or posterior C1–C3 fusion

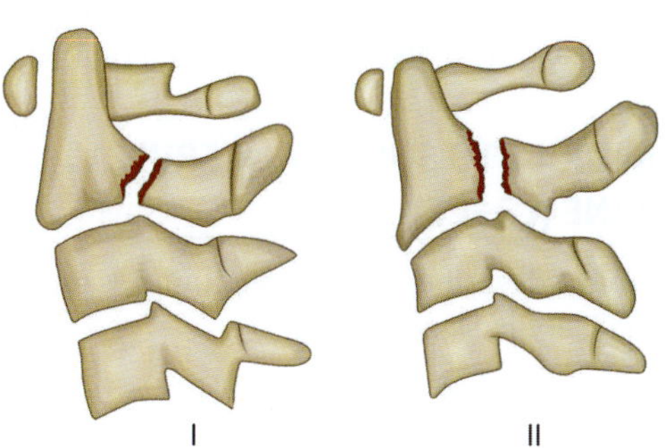

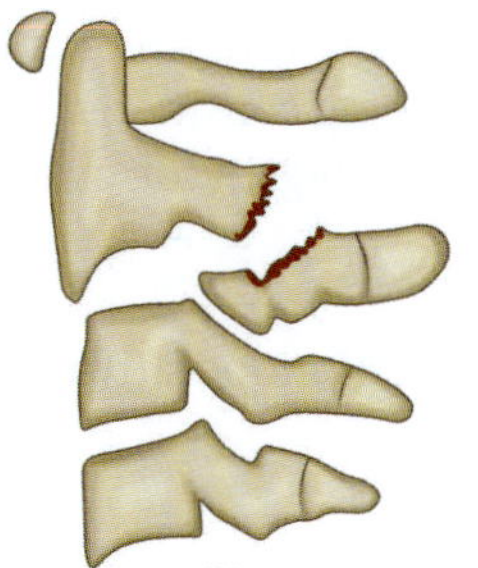

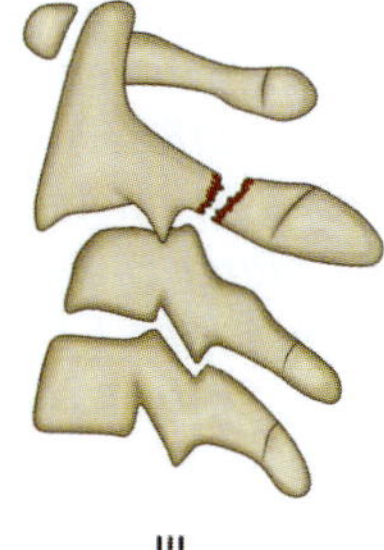

FIG. 4: Levine and Edward classification of Hangman's fracture.

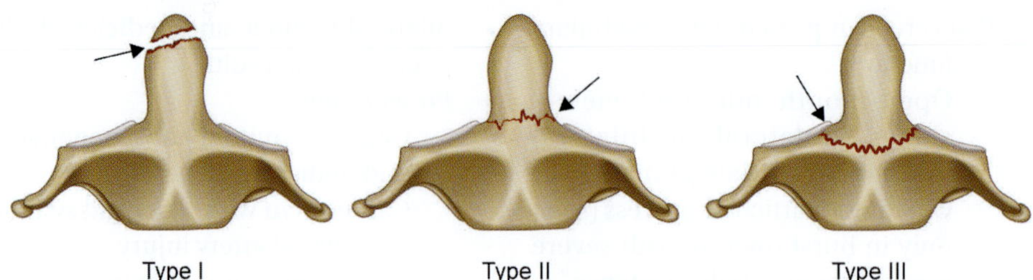

FIG. 5: Anderson and D'Alonzo classification of odontoid fractures.

Odontoid Fractures

- *Background*:
  - Account for 9–18% of all cervical spine fractures—most common cervical spine injuries in elderly
  - Can be caused by both hyperflexion and hyperextension
- *Presentation*:
  - Neck pain and tenderness to palpation
  - Does not usually present with neural deficit—incidence of the same is 5–10%, and can manifest as hemiparesis, cruciate paralysis, or quadriparesis
- *Radiographs*: AP, lateral, open-mouth "odontoid" views
  - *Anderson and D'Alonzo classification **(Fig. 5)***:
    - *Type 1*: Avulsion fracture at the tip of odontoid process
    - *Type 2*: Fracture at the neck of odontoid process **(Fig. 6)**
    - *Type 3*: Fractures that run into the C2 vertebral body
  - Rule out "os odontoideum" (see *Chapter 21.1: Pediatric Spinal Fracture*)
  - *CT scan*: Add angiography to see vertebral artery anatomy if surgical intervention is being considered
  - *MRI*: To assess integrity of cruciate ligament
- *Management*:
  - *Type 1 fractures*: Nonoperative, hard cervical collar

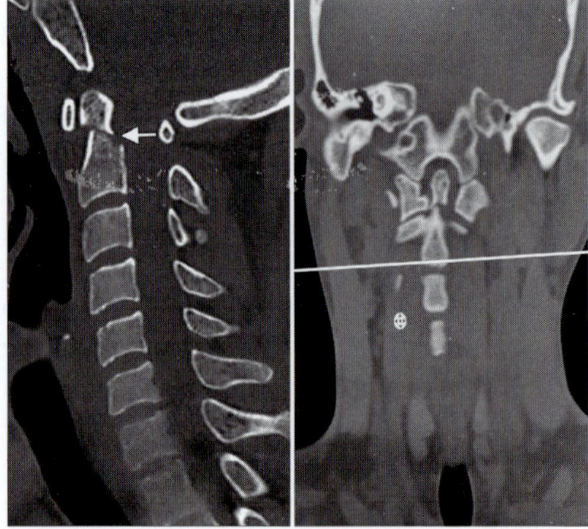

FIG. 6: Type-2 odontoid process fracture.

  - *Type 2 fractures*: Typically unstable injuries; surgical versus nonsurgical based on fracture pattern, patient's age, neural deficit, and comorbidities Treated by anterior odontoid screw fixation or posterior C1–C2 arthrodesis.
  - *Type 3 fractures*: Typically stable, heals well with nonsurgical management (rigid external immobilization with halo) if fracture surface is large; if likely to displace, then needs surgery

INJURIES TO SUBAXIAL CERVICAL SPINE (C3–C7)

Table 1 describes the types of injuries to subaxial cervical spine.

TABLE 1: Types of injuries to subaxial cervical spine.

Type of injury	Etiology	Presentation	Imaging/Evaluation	Management
Flexion–compression injury	Compressive forces, causes fracture of anteroinferior body of vertebra	• Radiculopathy to neurological deficit • Significant retropulsion can cause central cord syndrome	• *Plain X-ray*: Lateral view shows tear drop (fracture of anteroinferior body of vertebra) • *CT scan*: Possible retropulsion of bony fragment into the canal	• *Stable*: Hard cervical collar • *Unstable*: Surgical • ACDF/posterior fusion
Extension–compression injury	Forced extension of neck causing avulsion of anteroinferior part of body of vertebra via ALL disruption	Radiculopathy to neurological deficit	*Plain X-ray*: Lateral view shows tear drop (only corner) and widening of anterior disk space	*Mostly stable*: Brace only
Vertical compression (burst) fracture **(Fig. 7)**	High velocity trauma, vertical compression, both anterior and posterior cortex fractured	Radiculopathy to neurological deficit	• *Plain X-ray*: Lateral view shows loss of height of body • *CT*: Both anterior and posterior cortex fractured	• Stable: Bracing • *Unstable*: Surgical management • ACDF/ACCF/posterior fixation
Bifacet disloca-tion **(Fig. 8)**	Flexion rotation forces	Radiculopathy to neurological deficit	*Plain X-ray:* • Loss of facetal apposition • Interspinous space increased • *CT scan*: Perched/locked facets on sagittal cut • Hamberger/reverse Hamberger sign on axial cut	• Mostly unstable: Surgical management • Reduction (closed/open) followed by ACDF/ACCF ± posterior fixation

Continued

Continued

Type of injury	Etiology	Presentation	Imaging/Evaluation	Management
Unifacetal dislocation	Flexion/distraction with rotation forces	Radiculopathy (70%) to neurological deficit	*Plain X-ray* • Lateral view shows bow tie sign • Increased interspinous space	• *Stable*: Halo bracing for 12 weeks • *Unstable*: Surgical • ACDF/ACCF ± posterior fixation
Clay-Shoveler's fracture	• Direct blow to posterior spine • Most common at C7 spinous process	Radiculopathy to neurological deficit	• *Plain X-ray*: Lateral view: • Fractured spinous process ± displacement of fragment	*Mostly stable*: Bracing
Lateral mass fracture **(Fig. 9)**	Hyperextension, rotation, and compression	Radiculopathy to neurological deficit (66%)	• *Plain X-ray*: Poor sensitivity, disk space narrowing • *CT scan*: Translation of fractured and adjacent vertebra in multiple plains	• *Mostly unstable*: Posterior decompression + fixation • *Stable*: Halo vest

(ACDF: anterior cervical discectomy and fusion; ACCF: anterior cervical corpectomy and fusion)

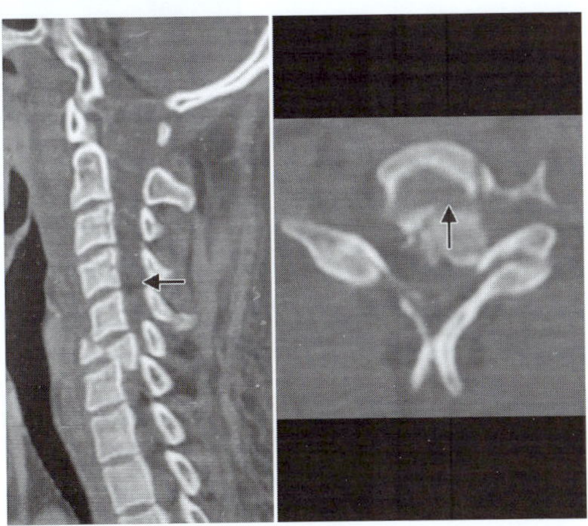

FIG. 7: Burst fracture C6 vertebra (retropulsed fragment marked with arrow).

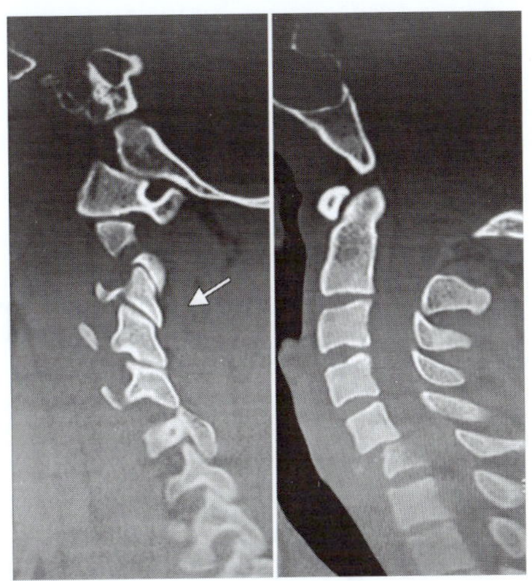

FIG. 8: Facet dislocation (locked facets marked with arrow).

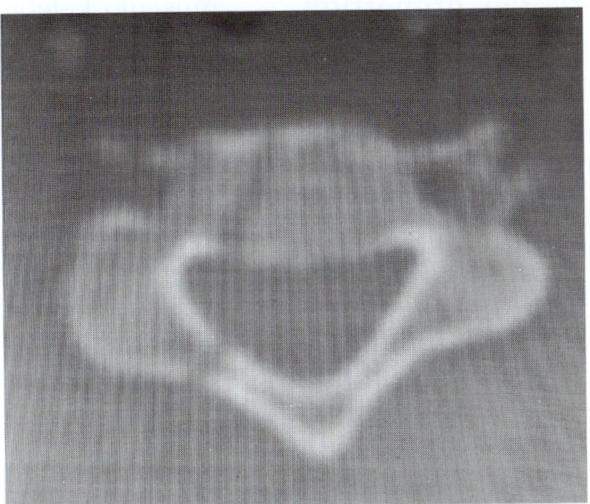

FIG. 9: Lateral mass fracture of cervical vertebra.

BIBLIOGRAPHY

1. Fredø HL, Rizvi SAM, Lied B, Rønning P, Helseth E. The epidemiology of traumatic cervical spine fractures: a prospective population study from Norway. Scand J Trauma Resusc Emerg Med. 2012;20(1):85.
2. Hoffman JR, Mower WR, Wolfson AB, Todd KH, Zucker MI. Validity of a Set of Clinical Criteria to Rule Out Injury to the Cervical Spine in Patients with Blunt Trauma. N Engl J Med. 2000;343(2):94-9.
3. Khanna P, Chau C, Dublin A, Kim K, Wisner D. The value of cervical magnetic resonance imaging in the evaluation of the obtunded or comatose patient with cervical trauma, no other abnormal neurological findings, and a normal cervical computed tomography. J Trauma Acute Care Surg. 2012;72(3):699-702.
4. Stiell IG, Wells GA, Vandemheen KL, Clement CM, Lesiuk H, De Maio VJ, et al. The Canadian C-spine rule for radiography in alert and stable trauma patients. JAMA. 2001;286(15):1841-8.
5. Vaccaro AR, Koerner JD, Radcliff KE, Oner FC, Reinhold M, Schnake KJ, et al. AOSpine subaxial cervical spine injury classification system. Eur Spine J. 2016;25(7):2173-84.

CHAPTER 7.2

Thoracic and Lumbar Spine Fracture

Nishank Mehta, Agnivesh Tikoo, Prashant Tank

- The majority of spinal column fractures are seen in the thoracic and lumbar spine; most commonly these injuries are seen at the thoracolumbar junction (TL junction), with the proportion being quoted as 75–90% in various epidemiological studies.
- Injury to the spinal column can lead to pain in the acute setting, late mechanical instability, loss of function, impaired mobility, and compromise to encased neurological structures leading to incomplete and complete paralysis. The majority of thoracolumbar fractures occur at the thoracolumbar junction (T10–L2) due to the following reasons:
  - It represents a transition area between a mobile spine (lumbar) and a relatively less mobile spine (thoracic, due to the presence of the anchoring rib cage)
  - It represents a transition area between lordotic spine (lumbar) and thoracic spine (kyphotic)
  - The facet joint orientation changes from oblique/more horizontal in the thoracic spine to sagittal orientation in the lumbar spine—making the two parts of the spine resistant to different axis of forces.
- Thoracolumbar spine injuries are also seen in the setting of a multiply injured patient and are often accompanied by injury to visceral structures in the chest, abdomen, and pelvis.
- When the mechanism of injury is a fall from height, it is often accompanied by other musculoskeletal injuries such as bilateral fractures of the calcaneus, injuries of the tibial plafond, ligamentous injuries of the knee, posterior dislocation of the hip, and injuries of the craniovertebral junction.

APPLIED ANATOMY

- Due to disproportionate growth between the spinal cord and vertebral column, the spinal cord ends at L1–L2 in adults as the conus medullaris. As a result of this, there is also a discrepancy between the vertebral level and the corresponding neurological level of the spinal cord located against that particular vertebra.
- In the thoracolumbar spine, each spinal cord segment is located at a level that is higher than the corresponding vertebral level—this difference in most pronounced distally toward the lumbar and sacral segments of the spinal cord.
- Spinal cord levels relative to the vertebral body level **(Table 1)**

CLINICAL EVALUATION

- Complete neurological examination including sensations, muscle weakness, and reflexes

- In particular, one should look for "sacral sparing" (perianal sensations, rectal tone, great toe flexion) since this can differentiate between complete and incomplete spinal cord injury

TABLE 1: Spinal cord levels relative to the vertebral body level.

Spinal cord level	Vertebral body level
Upper cervical level	Same as vertebral level
Lower cervical level	+1
Upper thoracic level	+2
Lower thoracic level	+3
Lumbar	T10–T12
Sacral	T12–L1

RADIOLOGICAL EVALUATION

The features of thoracolumbar injuries seen on plain radiographs are summarized in **Table 2**.

CT scan: Nowadays, this is the investigation of choice to evaluate thoracolumbar injuries. The advantages are better spatial resolution, the ability to clearly depict the pattern of injury, and the extent of spinal canal compromise and investigation for associated visceral injuries (CT Torso). The various features noted in a CT scan and its implications of management are detailed in **Table 3**.

MRI: There is no conclusive evidence to support its routine use. The most common

TABLE 2: Features of thoracolumbar injuries seen on plain radiographs.

Anteroposterior radiographic features	Lateral radiographic features
Loss of vertebral height	Loss of vertebral body height (typically, anterior > posterior)
Fracture of transverse process	Widening of interspinous distance
Loss of alignment of spinous processes	Vertebral body collapse
Translational injury	Retropulsion of posterior wall fragments
Widening of interpedicular distance	Anteroposterior translation
Horizontal splitting of the vertebral body (occasionally)	Facet joint dislocation/subluxation
	Kyphosis
	Spinous process fractures

TABLE 3: Role of CT in thoracolumbar fractures.

Feature identified	Seen in	Comments
Retropulsed posterior wall fragments **(Fig. 1)**	Sagittal, axial cuts	• Depict the extent of spinal canal compromise and need for direct/indirect decompression • Typically seen with burst component
Reversed cortical sign	Axial cuts	Needs direct reduction; rules out possibility of decompressing by ligamentotaxis
Comminution	Coronal, sagittal, axial	Defines possible need for partial corpectomy and anterior column reconstruction
Pedicle fracture **(Fig. 2)**	Sagittal, axial	Precludes screw placement at that level
Lamina fracture	Axial, sagittal	Possibility of nerve roots and dura injury during decompression
Spinous process/posterior element fracture	Axial, sagittal	Injury to PLC; implications on "stability"

(PLC: posterior ligamentous complex)

reason for getting a preoperative MRI is to determine the patient's posterior ligamentous complex (PLC) status and to see the spinal cord status. The sensitivity of preoperative MRI for various PLC components ranges from 78 to 90%, whereas the specificity ranges from 53 to 65%.

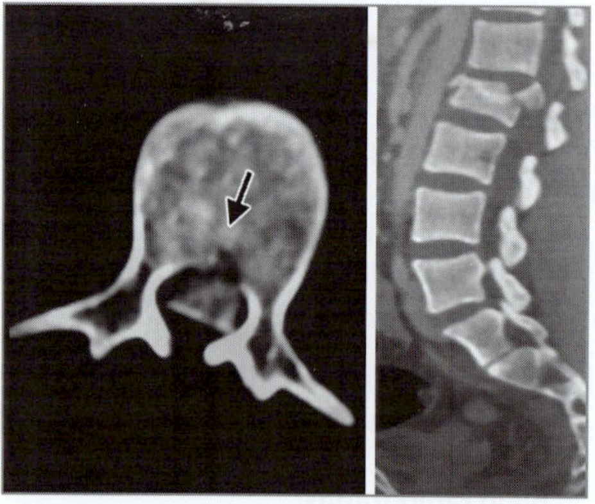

FIG. 1: L2 burst fracture with retropulsed bony fragment into the canal (marked with arrow).

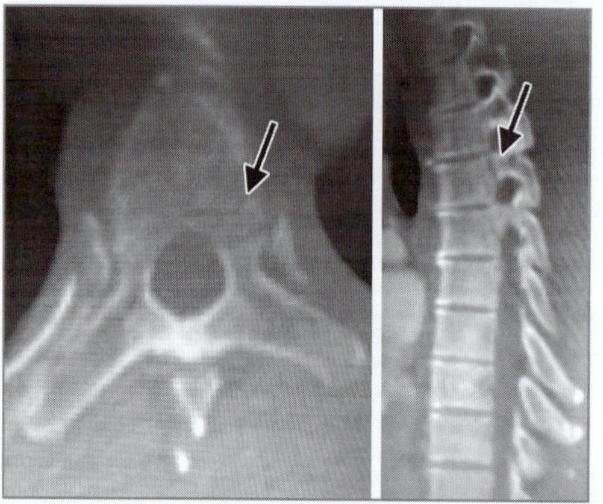

FIG. 2: Left-sided pedicle fracture (marked with arrow).

CONCEPT OF "INSTABILITY"

Much of the decision-making regarding the management of thoracolumbar spine injuries in adults revolves around the concept of recognizing the "instability" of the spinal column. A spinal injury is considered to be unstable if normal physiological loads can cause mechanical pain, progressive deformity, and neurological compromise.

Denis "Three-column" Concept

The most common way of determining the presence of instability is by assessing the injury through the lens of the Denis three-column concept. This is illustrated in **Figure 3** and the implications on instability are highlighted in **Table 4**.

CLASSIFICATION

Thoracolumbar Injury Classification System

This was described by Vaccaro et al. in 2005. This classification system postulates that spinal stability is a function of three independent variables: (1) Morphology of injury (which implies immediate mechanical stability), (2) Status of PLC (which implies long-term mechanical stability), and (3) Neurological status at the time of injury (which portends the ultimate functional

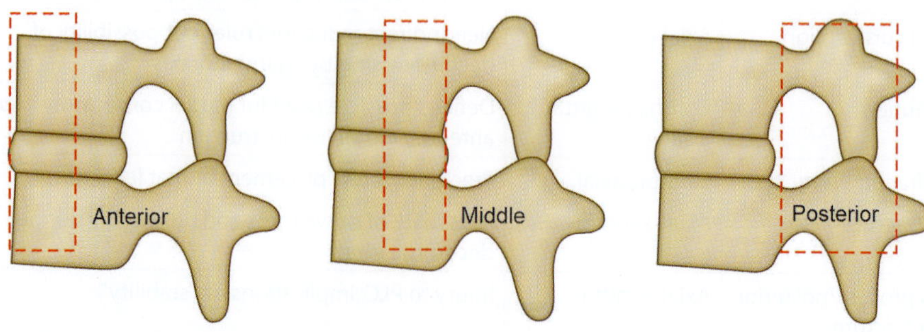

FIG. 3: Denis three-column classification system.

TABLE 4: Determination of stability of a thoracolumbar injury.

Stable injury	
Minimal to moderate compression fracture	May be treated by early ambulation with or without external immobilization
First-degree injury (mechanical instability)	
Severe compression fracture Or Seatbelt-type injury	• Spine buckles around the intact middle column hinge • Spine buckles around the intact anterior column
Second-degree injury (neurological instability)	
Burst fractures	20.3% of burst fractures with intact neurology initially become neurologically compromised during follow-up
Third-degree instability (mechanical + neurological instability)	
Severe burst fracture with neurological compromise and fracture dislocation	Recommended surgical decompression and surgical stabilization in this group

prognosis). The Thoracolumbar Injury Classification System (TLICS) score is used to determine the need for surgery—a TLICS score < 3 suggests that the injury can be managed without surgery, while a score > 4 mandates surgical intervention. The classification has a high validity, sensitivity and specificity—however, there is only moderate agreement on the determination of the status of PLC, which is a major shortcoming on this classification. The scoring system is summarized in **Table 5**.

TABLE 5: Thoracolumbar injury classification and severity score.

1	Morphology (immediate stability)	• Compression • Burst • Translation/ Rotation • Distraction	1 2 3 4
2	Integrity of PLC	• Intact • Suspected • Injured	0 2 3
3	Neurological status	• Intact • Nerve root • Complete cord • Incomplete cord • Cauda equina	0 2 2 3 3
	Need for surgery		For >4

(PLC: posterior ligamentous complex)

AO Classification System

This is the most comprehensive of all classification systems and is based on the direction of injury that helps in determination of stability. The injuries are categorized into three types, and the subdivisions allow for identification of 53 injury patterns.

1. Type A (compression) injuries are either stable or partially compromised but never completely unstable **(Fig. 4)**.
2. Type B (distraction/tensile) injuries have a transverse disruption either anteriorly or posteriorly. B1 and B2 injuries have a transverse disruption posteriorly and are unstable in flexion, but stable in extension/B3 injuries have an anterior tension band disruption and are unstable in extension, but stable in flexion **(Fig. 5)**.
3. Type C (torsional) injuries can be superimposed on Type A or B injuries and represent the most severe of all injury patterns. These injuries are always unstable **(Fig. 6)**

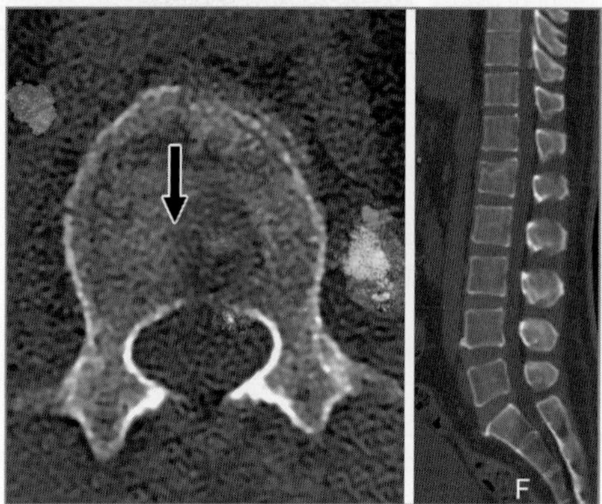

FIG. 4: Anterior wedge compression fracture (intact posterior cortex marked with arrow).

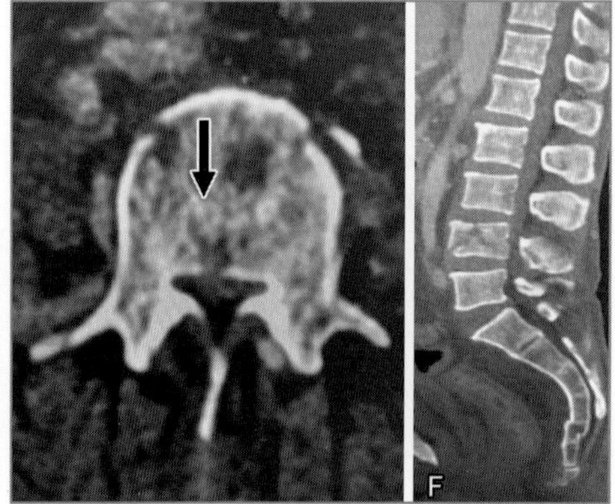

FIG. 5: Burst fracture (fractured posterior cortex marked with arrow).

The complete classification is available on: *(https://surgeryreference.aofoundation.org/spine/trauma/thoracolumbar)*

The classification system is depicted in **Figure 7**.

MANAGEMENT

In general, the decision to operate is based on the implications of the injury on mechanical stability and neurological involvement. The TLICS score provides good guidance for determining the need for surgery.

The goals of surgery are the following:

- To stabilize the spine—provide pain relief and allow for quicker and more efficient rehabilitation

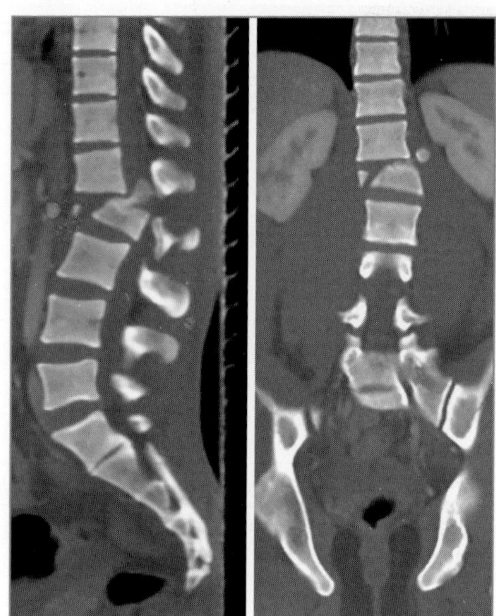

FIG. 6: Translational injury L1–L2.

- To achieve or correct sagittal balance (kyphosis, translation)
- To prevent future kyphosis progression
- To preserve intact neurology (in patients who are neurologically intact at the time of presentation) or to achieve neurological recovery (in patients with neurological deficit at the time of presentation)

For a brief discussion of the current recommendations with regards to surgical timing and the role of steroids, please refer to Chapter 7.3.

Some important considerations with regard to the surgical management of thoracolumbar injuries are listed below:

Surgical approach: The traditional recommendations are as follows–

- Translation injury (AO Type C) and PLC injury—posterior approach
- Incomplete neurological deficit/burst fracture with retropulsion fragments—anterior approach
- Both together—combination of both approaches

However, in recent years, decompression ventral to the cord can be achieved by the posterior approach (transpedicular decom-

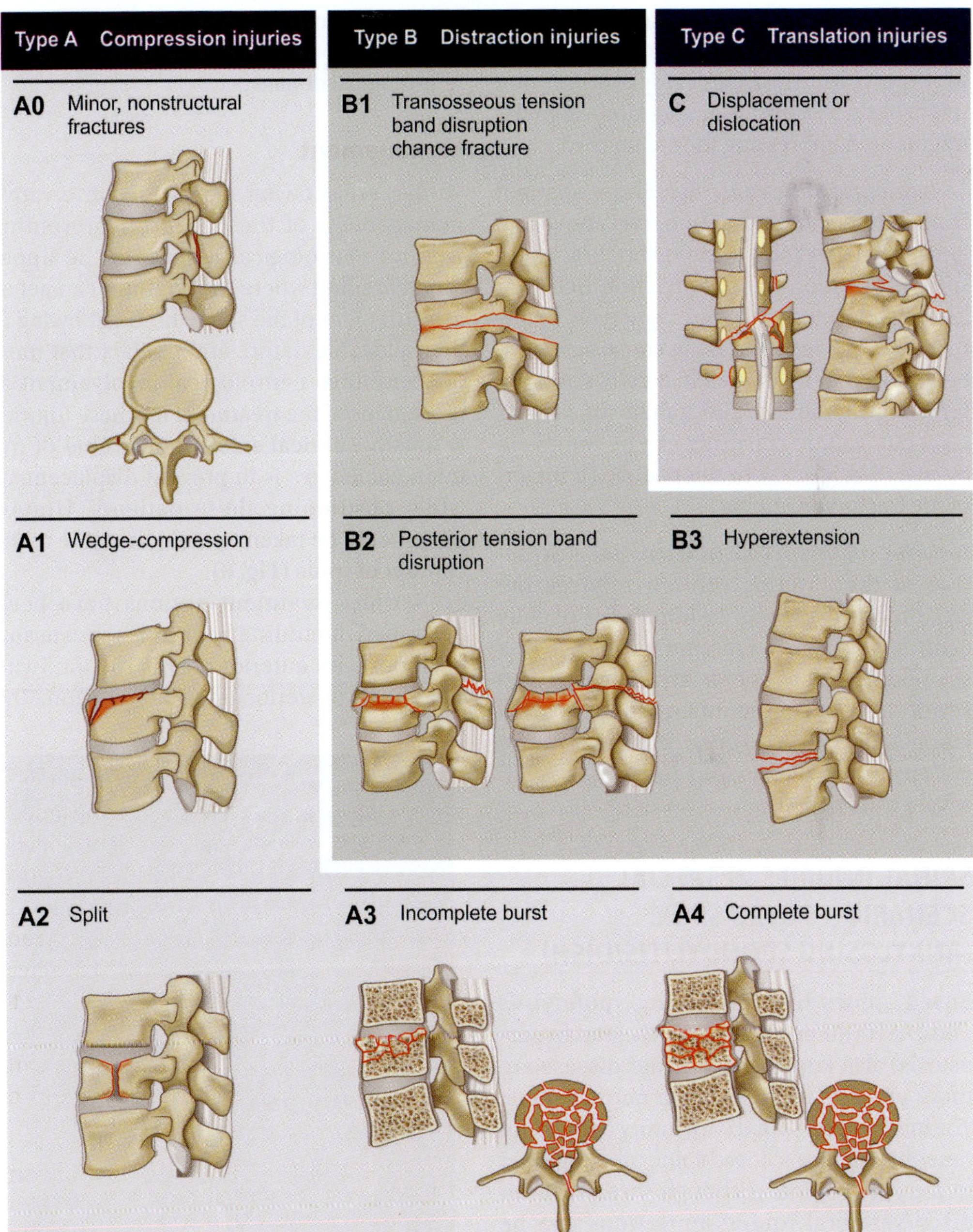

FIG. 7: AO classification system for thoracolumbar fractures.

pression or costotransversectomy approach) and hence, the posterior approach is sufficient to deal with most cases.

Decompression: Decompression of the spinal cord or neural elements is important in patients presenting with neurological compromise. Indirect decompression refers to the falling back of the retropulsion fragments inside the spinal canal due to ligamentotaxis by distraction over pedicle screws in burst fractures. Indirect decompression is also implied when the alignment is restored in Type C injuries. Direct decompression refers to the visualization and removal of the fragments compressing the spinal cord.

Length of fixation/construct: Short-segment fixation refers to fixation one level above and one level below the fractured vertebra. Long-segment fixation refers to fixation that is at least two levels above and two levels below the fractured vertebra. Long constructs have been found to be biomechanically stronger, but clinically similar. The stability of a short-segment fixation construct can be improved by inserting a screw in the pedicle (if intact) of the fractured vertebra.

Anterior column reconstruction: Reconstruction of the anterior column reduces the risk of kyphosis progression and is usually achieved by using a titanium mesh cage or a strut bone graft. It is indicated in cases with severe anterior comminution, where a partial corpectomy has been done, if there is severe collapse or kyphosis and in patients with severe osteoporosis.

SPINAL INJURIES IN SPECIAL SCENARIO—FUSED SPINE (ANKYLOSING SPONDYLITIS/DISH)

Fused spines like ankylosing spondylitis and DISH (diffuse idiopathic skeletal hyperostosis) also known as Forestier disease are more prone to injuries than a normal spine. The incidence of spinal cord injury can be 11.4 times higher in ankylosed spines as compared to a normal spine. Although three-column disco-vertebral Andersson lesions can be traumatic or nontraumatic (inflammatory), the Andersson-like lesions in DISH usually have a traumatic etiology. Conventional radiographs tend to miss these injuries, and it is recommended to do further imaging like a CT scan/MRI based on clinical suspicion for a patient with a fused spine presenting after a fall. These patients are also at higher risk of neurological injuries with >50% developing neurological deficits.

Management

Studies are showing successful conservative management of these injuries presenting without neurological deficits in the upper thoracic spine where the sternum can act as a fourth pillar of the spine, however owing to their unstable nature and the fact that most of them have neurological involvement at presentation, the treatment for these injuries is mostly surgical stabilization. One of the main challenges is to prevent displacement while positioning these patients. Utmost care should be taken to mold the table to the contour of spine **(Fig. 8)**.

Various treatment options have been described including anterior + posterior, posterior with anterior reconstruction (with cage), and posterior-only stabilization. The

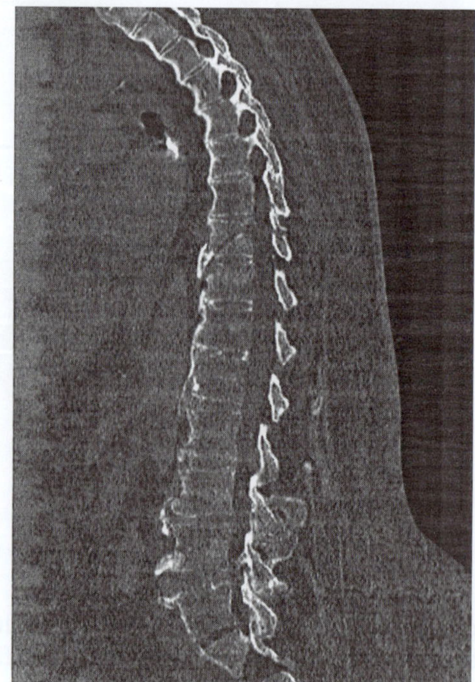

FIG. 8: Spinal injury in AS.

posterior-only stabilization is sufficient in most of the cases as the fusion rates are good. Decompression may be additionally required based on clinical consideration. The fixation should extend long to compensate for long-level arms caused by the fused segments.

BIBLIOGRAPHY

1. Caron T, Bransford R, Nguyen Q, Agel J, Chapman J, Bellabarba C. Spine fractures in patients with ankylosing spinal disorders. Spine (Phila Pa 1976). 2010;35(11):E458-64.
2. Chaudhary SB, Hullinger H, Vives MJ. Management of acute spinal fractures in ankylosing spondylitis. ISRN Rheumatol. 2011;2011:150484.
3. Hu R, Mustard CA, Burns C. Epidemiology of incident spinal fracture in a complete population. Spine. 1996;21(4):492-9.
4. Jacobs WB, Fehlings MG. Ankylosing spondylitis and spinal cord injury: origin, incidence, management, and avoidance. Neurosurg Focus. 2008;24(1):E12.
5. McCormack T, Karaikovic E, Gaines RW. The load sharing classification of spine fractures. Spine. 1994;19(15):1741-4.
6. Oliver M, Inaba K, Tang A, Branco BC, Barmparas G, Schnüriger B, et al. The changing epidemiology of spinal trauma: a 13-year review from a Level I trauma centre. Injury. 2012;43(8):1296-300.
7. Sudhakar PV, Kandwal P, Mch KA, Ifthekar S, Mittal S, Sarkar B. Management of Andersson lesions of spine: A systematic review of the existing literature. J Clin Orthop Trauma. 2022;29:101878.
8. Vaccaro AR, Rihn JA, Saravanja D, Anderson DG, Hilibrand AS, Albert TJ, et al. Injury of the posterior ligamentous complex of the thoracolumbar spine: a prospective evaluation of the diagnostic accuracy of magnetic resonance imaging. Spine. 2009;34(23):E841-7.

Spinal Cord Injury and Spinal Shock

Nishank Mehta, Prashant Tank

- Spinal Cord Injury (SCI) is acute, traumatic lesion of neural elements in the spinal canal (spinal cord and cauda equina) resulting in temporary or permanent neurological deficit.
- Spinal shock is a temporary condition following SCI and can last from days to weeks.
- Spinal shock occurs because of the physiological shutdown of spinal functions secondary to trauma.
- During spinal shock, it is difficult to assess the full extent of injury because of loss of motor and sensory functions and reflexes below the level of injury.

APPLIED ANATOMY

- *Total 33 vertebrae*: 7 cervical, 12 thoracic, 5 lumbar, 5 sacral (fused), and 3–5 coccyx (fused)
- *The spinal cord occupies the spinal canal:*
  - 35% at C1 level (Atlas)
  - 50% at lower cervical spine and thoracolumbar spine
- The remaining volume of the spinal canal is filled with epidural fat, cerebrospinal fluid (CSF), and dura mater.
- *Conus medullaris*: Cone-shaped caudal termination of the spinal cord, lies distal to L1, and contains coccygeal and sacral myelomeres.
- *Cauda equina*: Bundle of spinal nerve roots arising from conus medullaris and supplying lower limbs and bowel bladder functions. They are less likely to get damaged as the canal is roomy in this region. Their compression can result in a surgical emergency—called cauda equina syndrome.

Terminology used to describe SCI **(Table 1)**.

MECHANISM OF SPINAL CORD INJURY

Neural tissue injury can be:

- *Primary*: At the time of trauma (due to tissue disruption because of mechanical forces)
- *Secondary*: Due to biological response resulting from injury

Mechanics

- Structural failure displaces bone/soft tissue components into the spinal canal causing neural compromise.
- Most commonly cord is contused only, rarely transection even in grossly displaced fractures.
- *The extent of damage depends upon:*
  - Rate of force application
  - Degree of compression
  - Duration of compression
  - Preinjury spinal canal diameter

(A narrow spinal canal is associated with more chances of neurological injury and a high likelihood of complete SCI.)

Causes of progressive/secondary neurodeficit following initial injury:
- Cord edema
- Cord hemorrhage
- Inflammatory response
- Progressive myelomalacia because of syrinx formation

ASSESSMENT AND MANAGEMENT

Initial assessment and management include:
- Assessment of detailed neurological function
- Diagnosis of severity of injury
- Assessment of hemodynamic parameters and ruling out of neurogenic shock

Hypovolemic shock versus neurogenic shock:
- Neurogenic shock can complicate hemodynamic resuscitation.
- Loss of sympathetic tone and hence vasoconstrictive effect over peripheral vessels can accentuate hemodynamic effects of blood loss.
- It is imperative to differentiate between neurogenic and hypovolemic shock **(Table 2)** since management is different for both.
- Neurogenic shock requires management with the pharmacologic agent—dopamine to increase vascular tone; on the contrary,

TABLE 1: Spinal cord injuries classification based upon different etiologies.

Type	Causes
Based upon etiology:	
Traumatic	Due to road traffic accidents, fall from height, sports related
Nontraumatic	Due to infections, tumors, etc.
Based upon extent of structural damage to the cord:	
Concussion	Physiological disruption but no anatomical damage
Contusion	Physical disruption leading to swelling and hemorrhage
Laceration	Loss of structural integrity (anatomical damage)
Based upon temporal association:	
Acute	Within few hours of injury
Subacute	Between hours to few days
Chronic	Weeks to months following injury
Functional consequences (prognosis) will depend upon severity of injury:	
Complete	Absence of motor and sensory function in the lowest sacral segment
Incomplete	Partial function preserved

TABLE 2: Comparison of neurogenic and hypovolemic shock.

	Neurogenic shock	Hypovolemic shock
Etiology	Loss of sympathetic outflow	Loss of circulating blood volume
Blood pressure	Hypotension	Hypotension
Heart rate	Bradycardia	Tachycardia
Skin temperature	Warm extremities	Cold extremities
Urine output	Normal	Low

hemorrhagic shock requires replacement for lost blood and blood products.
- Excessive fluid replacement can cause pulmonary edema if the neurogenic shock is not identified and hemodynamic resuscitation is continued solely based on grounds of hypovolemic shock.
- Studies suggest a favorable neurological recovery in patients whose mean arterial pressure (MAP) is maintained >85 mm Hg.

Clinical examination after resolution of spinal shock only clearly reflects the extent of injury, because, during spinal shock, all motor, and sensory functions and reflexes at and below the level of injury are absent and clinical assessment of neurology is not possible.

Physical Examination

The patient must be log-rolled:
- Requires 4 persons—3 for holding the patient position and 1 for assessment

Neurology Assessment

American Spinal Injury Association (ASIA) score **(Fig. 1)**:
- Assessment of strength of 5 specific muscles in each limb
- Pin-prick discrimination at 28 specific points on each side of body

Motor: Sum of total 20 muscles (all 4 limbs) gives maximum score of 100 points for patients without weakness

Sensory: With 28 dermatomes and sensory scoring on a scale of 0 to 2 points, maximum score would be 112 in patients with intact neurology.

Neurological injury level:
The most common caudal segment of the spinal cord with normal motor and sensory function on both sides: Right and left

Complete and incomplete injury **(Table 3)**.

Incomplete spinal cord injury syndromes **(Table 4)**.

Assessment of Recovery from Spinal Shock

- Spinal shock is common in cervical and upper thoracic injuries.
- It almost always resolves within 24-48 hours.
- The bulbocavernosus reflex (S3-S4) is the first to return, followed by the anal wink reflex **(Table 5)**
- Literature shows that deep plantar reflex (DPR) is the first to recover (before bulbocavernosus reflex), and its persistence is poor prognostic sign

Treatment of Spinal Cord Injury

Always follow the basic principles like:
Do no harm:
- Harm to the patient comes from improper immobilization and transfer, missing the spine injury in the emergency room and other associated injuries like:
    - Aortic tear with thoracic fracture dislocation
    - Abdominal injury with lumbar flexion-distraction injury

Role of steroids in spinal cord injury patients: While the trials were influential in shaping treatment guidelines, they have been subjected to significant criticism over past years in view of increased chances of complications like the risk of pneumonia and sepsis and have questionable clinical significance. For these reasons, methylprednisolone is not being used routinely at most of the centers.

Surgical Timing in Acute Spinal Cord Injury Study (STASCIS) trial:
- Compared neurological improvement in early (within 24 hours) versus delayed (after 24 hours) decompressive surgery after a traumatic cervical spine injury
- Decompression within 24 hours following acute SCI can safely be performed and is associated with improved clinical outcomes in terms of neurological improvement, defined as at least a 2 grade AIS improvement at 6 months follow-up.

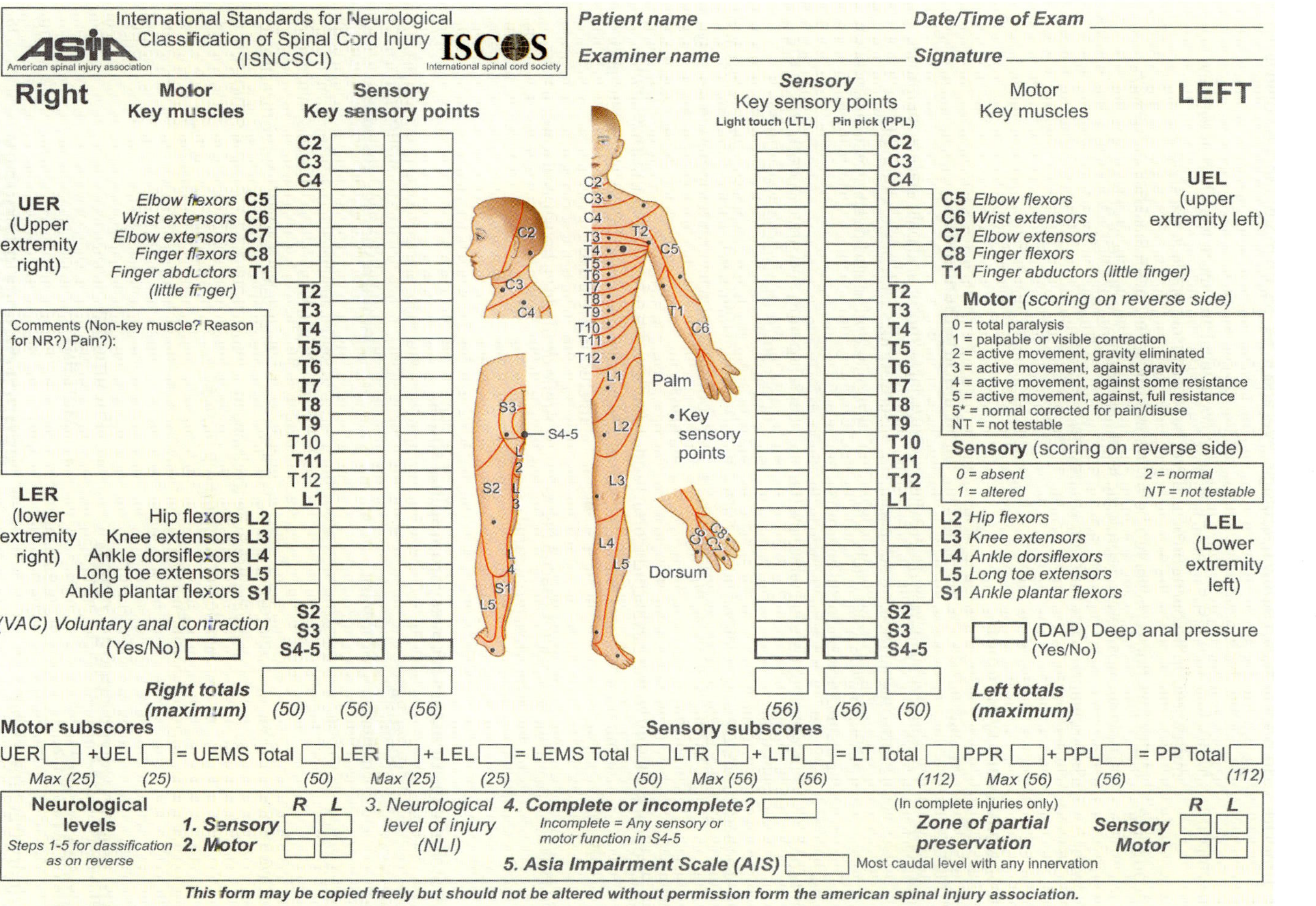

ASIA American spinal injury association
International Standards for Neurological Classification of Spinal Cord Injury (ISNCSCI)
ISCOS International spinal cord society

Patient name ______ Date/Time of Exam ______
Examiner name ______ Signature ______

Right

Motor **Key muscles** | **Sensory** **Key sensory points**

UER (Upper extremity right)
Elbow flexors **C5**
Wrist extensors **C6**
Elbow extensors **C7**
Finger flexors **C8**
Finger abductors (little finger) **T1**

C2, C3, C4, T2, T3, T4, T5, T6, T7, T8, T9, T10, T11, T12, L1, S2, S3, S4-5

Comments (Non-key muscle? Reason for NR?) Pain?):

LER (lower extremity right)
Hip flexors **L2**
Knee extensors **L3**
Ankle dorsiflexors **L4**
Long toe extensors **L5**
Ankle plantar flexors **S1**

(VAC) Voluntary anal contraction (Yes/No)

Right totals (maximum) *(50)* *(56)* *(56)*

Sensory Key sensory points
Light touch (LTL) Pin pick (PPL)

LEFT

Motor Key muscles

UEL (upper extremity left)
C5 *Elbow flexors*
C6 *Wrist extensors*
C7 *Elbow extensors*
C8 *Finger flexors*
T1 *Finger abductors (little finger)*

Motor *(scoring on reverse side)*

0 = total paralysis
1 = palpable or visible contraction
2 = active movement, gravity eliminated
3 = active movement, against gravity
4 = active movement, against some resistance
5 = active movement, against, full resistance
5* = normal corrected for pain/disuse
NT = not testable

Sensory (scoring on reverse side)

0 = absent *2 = normal*
1 = altered *NT = not testable*

LEL (Lower extremity left)
L2 *Hip flexors*
L3 *Knee extensors*
L4 *Ankle dorsiflexors*
L5 *Long toe extensors*
S1 *Ankle plantar flexors*

(DAP) Deep anal pressure (Yes/No)

(56) *(56)* *(50)* ***Left totals (maximum)***

Motor subscores
UER ☐ +UEL ☐ = UEMS Total ☐ LER ☐ + LEL ☐ = LEMS Total ☐
Max (25) *(25)* *(50)* *Max (25)* *(25)* *(50)*

Sensory subscores
LTR ☐ + LTL ☐ = LT Total ☐ PPR ☐ + PPL ☐ = PP Total ☐
Max (56) *(56)* *(112)* *Max (56)* *(56)* *(112)*

Neurological levels
Steps 1-5 for classification as on reverse
R L
1. Sensory
2. Motor

3. Neurological level of injury (NLI)

4. Complete or incomplete?
Incomplete = Any sensory or motor function in S4-5

5. Asia Impairment Scale (AIS)

(In complete injuries only)
Zone of partial preservation
Most caudal level with any innervation
R L
Sensory
Motor

This form may be copied freely but should not be altered without permission form the american spinal injury association.

FIG. 1: American Spinal Injury Association (ASIA) scoring system.

TABLE 3: Impairment scale categories (ASIA score).

A	Complete	No motor or sensory function in the lowest sacral segment (S4–S5)
B	Incomplete	Sensory function below neurologic level and in S4–S5, no motor function below neurologic level
C	Incomplete	Motor function preserved below neurologic level and more than half of the key muscle group below neurologic level have a muscle grade lower than 3
D	Incomplete	Motor function is preserved below neurologic level and at least half of the key muscle groups below neurologic level have a muscle grade of at least 3
E	Normal	Sensory and motor function are normal

TABLE 4: Spinal cord syndromes.

Syndrome	Lesion	Clinical presentation
Anterior cord	Anterior gray matter, descending corticospinal motor tract, and spinothalamic tract injury with preservation of dorsal columns	Variable motor and pain and temperature sensory loss with preservation of proprioception and deep pressure sensation
Central cord	Incomplete cervical white matter injury	Sacral sparing and greater weakness in the upper limbs than in the lower limbs
Brown–Sequard	Injury to one lateral half of cord and preservation of contralateral half	Ipsilateral motor and proprioception loss and contralateral pain and temperature sensory loss
Conus medullaris	Injury to the sacral cord (conus) and lumbar nerve roots within the spinal canal	Areflexic bladder, bowel, and lower limbs. May have preserved bulbocavernosus and micturition reflexes
Cauda equina	Injury to the lumbosacral nerve roots within the spinal canal	Areflexic bladder, bowel, and lower limbs

TABLE 5: Reflexes to assess recovery from spinal shock.

Reflex	Location of lesion	Stimulus	Normal response	Abnormal response
Anal wink reflex	S2–S4	Stroking skin around	Anal sphincter contracts	No contraction of anal sphincter
Bulbocavernosus reflex	S3–S4	Squeezing penis in males, applying pressure to clitoris in females, or tugging the bladder catheter	Anal sphincter contracts	No contraction of anal sphincter

COMPLICATIONS OF SPINAL CORD INJURY PATIENTS

- Urinary tract infection
- Respiratory complications
- Cardiac
- Decubitus ulcer
- Pneumonia
- Mortality

NEUROLOGICAL RECOVERY

- Predominantly determined by patient's age and severity of injury

- Cord hemorrhage is associated with less neurologic recovery.
- The initial motor index score correlates with overall function at the time of discharge from rehabilitation in tetraplegia and complete injuries but not in paraplegia and incomplete injuries.
- Levels that have some motor function at 1 week are likely to recover 3/5th of muscle power at 1-year follow-up.
- Pediatric incomplete injuries have a good prognosis, neurologic deficit improves in 74% and resolves in 59% of children, however complete injury shows improvement in only 10% of patients.

BIBLIOGRAPHY

1. Barbiellini Amidei C, Salmaso L, Bellio S, Saia M. Epidemiology of traumatic spinal cord injury: a large population-based study. Spinal Cord. 2022;60(9):812-9.
2. Burney RE, Maio RF, Maynard F, Karunas R. Incidence, characteristics, and outcome of spinal cord injury at trauma centers in North America. Arch Surg Chic Ill 1960. 1993;128(5):596-9.
3. DeVivo MJ. Causes and costs of spinal cord injury in the United States. Spinal Cord. 1997;35(12):809-13.
4. Kirshblum SC, Burns SP, Biering-Sorensen F, Donovan W, Graves DE, Jha A, et al. International standards for neurological classification of spinal cord injury (Revised 2011). J Spinal Cord Med. 2011;34(6):535-46.
5. Ko HY, Ditunno JF, Graziani V, Little JW. The pattern of reflex recovery during spinal shock. Spinal Cord. 1999;37(6):402-9.
6. Vale FL, Burns J, Jackson AB, Hadley MN. Combined medical and surgical treatment after acute spinal cord injury: results of a prospective pilot study to assess the merits of aggressive medical resuscitation and blood pressure management. J Neurosurg. 1997;87(2):239-46.

Osteoporotic Thoracolumbar Fracture

Agnivesh Tikoo

Thoracolumbar osteoporotic vertebral fractures are becoming more common in older patients. They invariably occur due to trivial trauma, just by bending or due to minor strain on the back. If not managed appropriately, they can have a significant increase in morbidity and mortality.

CLASSIFICATION

AO-DGOU (German Society for Orthopaedics and Trauma) classification:

- *OF1*: No deformation—only edema seen in MRI imaging
- *OF2*: Deformation of one endplate without or with only minor posterior wall involvement (with posterior wall < 1/5 involvement)
- *OF3*: Deformation of one endplate with distinct posterior wall involvement (with posterior wall > 1/5 involved)
- *OF4*: Deformation of both endplates with/without posterior wall involvement (loss of vertebral frame structure, vertebral body collapse, pincer type fracture)
- *OF5*: Injuries with anterior or posterior tension band failure (injuries with signs of distraction, rotation, or translation; hyperextension with anterior tension band failure)

For OF1 and OF2, the recommended course of treatment was nonsurgical whereas for *OF3, OF4, and OF5*, it was surgical **(Fig. 1)**.

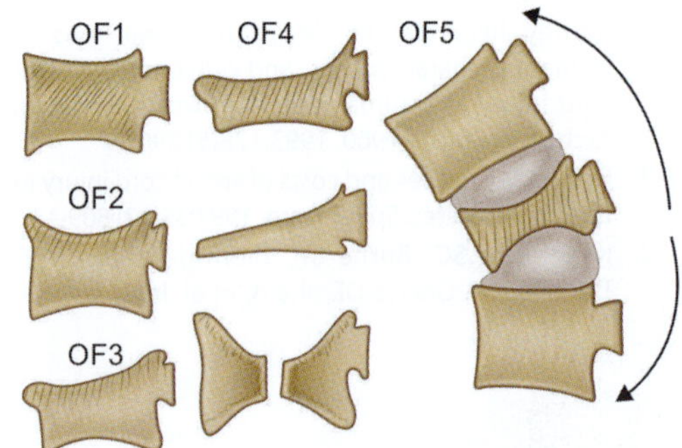

FIG. 1: Osteoporotic fracture (OF) scoring.

Modified osteoporotic fracture (OF) scoring system was also proposed for deciding between surgical and nonsurgical treatment; however, it is yet to be fully validated **(Table 1)**.

Regardless of the classification, the key lies in early detection and instituting medical measures as early as possible **(Figs. 2A and B)**.

TREATMENT FOR OSTEOPOROTIC SPINAL FRACTURES

Mostly it is an osteoporotic fracture which brings the patient to a clinician.

Hematological investigations (CBC, ESR, creatinine, liver function tests, thyroid function, S 25-OH vitamin D, calcium, phosphorus, and PTH among others) and radiological work up are recommended to rule out secondary causes of osteoporosis and pathological fractures.

TABLE 1: Modified score for therapeutic decision-making in OF.*

Parameter	Grade	Points
Morphology (OF 1–5)	1–5	2–10
Severity of osteoporosis	T-Score < –3 or qCT: HU ≤ 90	1
Deformity progression	Yes, No	1, –1
Pain (under analgesia)**	VAS ≥ 5, < 5	1, –1
Neurological symptoms (N2–N4)	Yes	2
Mobilization (under analgesia)	No, Yes	1, –1
Health status	ASA > 3, ***mFI > 2, Anticoagulation	Each –1, Maximum –2

*The severity score system has not been validated yet and should be used as a reference only.

**According to step II WHO pain ladder.

*** 5-item modified frailty index (mFI) = COPD, or recent pneumonia; Congestive heart failure; Functional status (not independent); Hypertension requiring medication; Diabetes mellitus.

Note: 0 points if a parameter is unknown or not determinable; 0–5 points = Conservative therapy; 6 points = Conservative therapy or surgery; >6 points = Surgery.

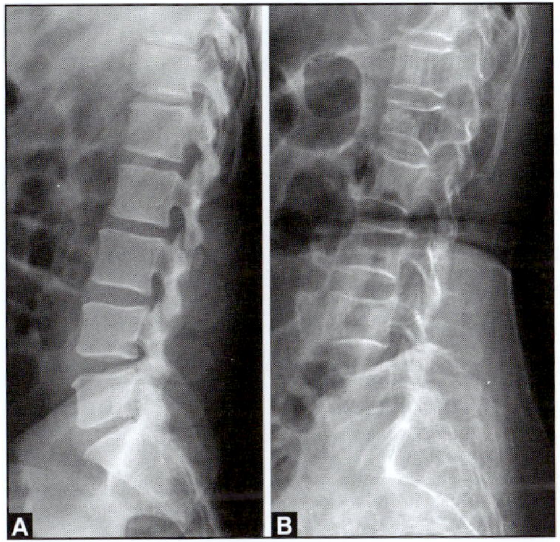

FIGS. 2A AND B: Lumbar spine lateral X-rays showing (A) normal bone density and (B) osteoporotic bones with multiple compression fractures.

Nonoperative Treatment

Most of osteoporotic spinal fractures heal with nonoperative management though with varying degrees of collapse. Timely instituted conservative management can prevent worsening pain, instability, and development of neurological deficit.

Rest

Initial few days of bed rest is helpful in alleviating pain. During this time, patient may be allowed bed chair mobilization as and when pain allows. As per pain tolerance, the activities may be increased with time. Various authors have recommended rests ranging from 3 days to a few weeks. Bed rest has also been shown to be beneficial in preventing surgery in patients with poor prognostic MRI findings. Author recommends that 5–7 days bed rest should be preferably given and as per pain tolerance, gradual mobilization should be slowly encouraged. It is essential that all preventive precautions for deep vein thrombosis (DVT), prevention hypostatic pulmonary complications, and pressure sores be taken into consideration while prescribing bed rest.

Bracing

Bracing is optional based on patient tolerability as there is no compelling evidence that bracing is essential. Some authors have shown the benefits of bracing, whereas others have contradicted it with no added advantage. Some have suggested that semirigid bracing could offer the same advantage as rigid bracing. Various braces that can be used include ASH brace, Jewett's brace, and Taylor's brace. Taylor's brace may appear more comfortable but has a kyphogenic effect on the spine. Many patients do not tolerate bracing, it requires assistance to put on and remove them, and they feel that it hinders mobilization more than it can help. The author recommends bracing wherever the patient can tolerate it. Usually after a few days of use, patients start tolerating braces.

Analgesics

Nonsteroidal anti-inflammatory drugs (NSAIDs) (if no contraindication) are better than opioids. Opioids, though renal safe, tend to make elderly patients drowsy (thereby further increasing the propensity for falls) and can cause severe constipation. It is advisable to use a combination of medications in low doses to achieve desired pain relief and to reduce side effects.

Calcitonin Nasal Spray

Calcitonin has an analgesic effect on pain due to vertebral fractures. Calcitonin is usually used as a nasal spray with doses ranging from 200 to 400 IU once a day for 2–4 weeks. Also, it acts as an antiresorptive and prevents acute bone loss due to recumbency. It is not meant to be used as an antiosteoporotic agent.

Antiosteoporotic Medications

Appropriate antiosteoporotic therapy, preferably with an anabolic drug unless contraindicated, should be started early.

Intervention/Operative Treatment

Indications

- Unstable fractures
- Neurological deficit
- Failure to respond to conservative treatment for 3–6 weeks

Various treatment modalities are proposed based on the type of osteoporotic fracture and the type of reconstruction required.

Standalone Cement Augmentation Procedures (Vertebroplasty and Kyphoplasty)

Vertebroplasty and kyphoplasty are different techniques in which a polymethylmethacrylate (PMMA) cement is injected under fluoroscopy control in the vertebral body. A subacute vertebral fracture with a cleft (Kümmell's sign) which appears as a fluid-filled cleft on the MRI where the posterior wall of the vertebral body is intact (stable but painful) is an ideal case for vertebroplasty. *Kyphoplasty* involves inflating a balloon with a pressure gauge mechanism inserted from the transpedicular route within the fractured vertebral body **(Fig. 3)**. The balloon is used to elevate the endplate or the collapsed fracture fragments of the vertebral body thereby creating a cavity which is filled with cement later. However, the benefits and advantages of kyphoplasty are still debatable. Neurological involvement, endplate breaches, or posterior cortex breaches are contraindications for standalone cement augmented procedures (**Figs. 4A to E**; vertebral compression fracture—treated with vertebroplasty).

Vertebral fractures with gross instability, with or without neurology, requires a more aggressive approach. It is important to address the anterior void which is formed because of a fractured vertebra. As the bone stock is poor, the screw purchase is likely to loosen. However, strategies to mitigate screw pullouts/implant failures have been proposed.

Vertebral Cement Augmentation with Cement Augmented Pedicle Screw Fixation

Cement augmentation can be combined with screw fixation in the adjacent vertebra to protect the cement from dislodging in osteoporotic fracture where there is high risk of cement dislodgement or retropulsion of fracture fragment. The fixation with pedicle screws (which may be cement augmented) helps to protect the "vertebroplastied" vertebra from collapsing. The procedure can be done percutaneously especially if its only requiring a single-level fixation above and below.

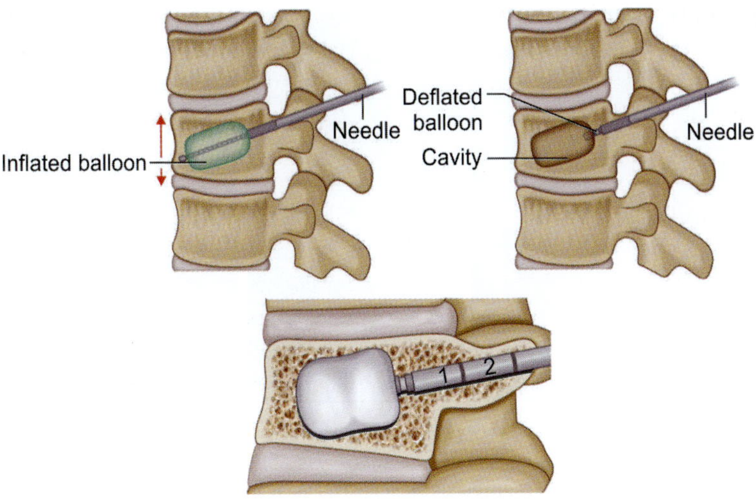

FIG. 3: Kyphoplasty.

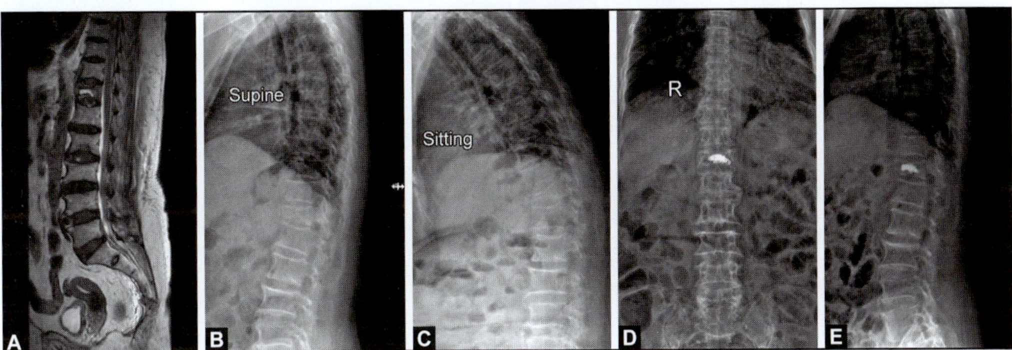

FIGS. 4A TO E: A 74-year-old female with history of fall with (A) T2w sagittal MRI showing Kummell's sign, (B) lying down and (C) sitting X-rays showing significant compression. Postprocedure AP and lateral view (D and E) showing vertebroplasty cement in the cleft/fractured vertebra.

Cement Augmentation with Multiple-level Fixation

A case of neurological deficit with significant vertebral instability, where there is auto decompression on recumbent position, can be treated with cement augmentation and multiple-level screw fixation. Decompression may be required if there is persistent neural compression or significant retropulsion of the posterior vertebral body **(Figs. 5A to E)**.

Anterior Intravertebral Reconstruction

Anterior intravertebral reconstruction can be done using an interbody cage inserted from the transpedicular route **(Figs. 6A to D)**.

Vertebral Shortening Procedure

Transpedicular decompression and shortening procedure to collapse the adjoining vertebral margins of Kümmell's sign preferably after filling in the bone graft can prevent an anterior void as the two com-

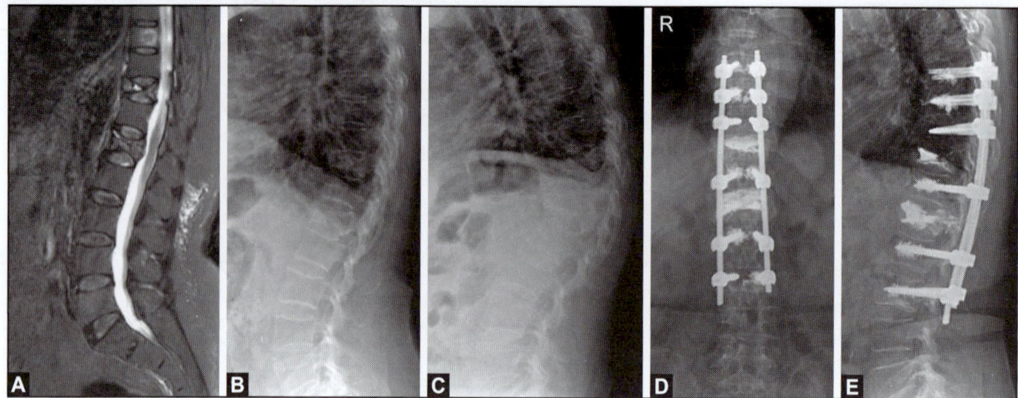

FIGS. 5A TO E: A 69-year-old female—preoperative MRI (A) and lateral lying down (B) and sitting (C) X-rays showing unstable D12 and D10 vertebral fractures. Patient was ASIA C at presentation. AP and lateral (D and E) postoperative X-rays of cement augmented pedicle screws with 2 level vertebroplasty.

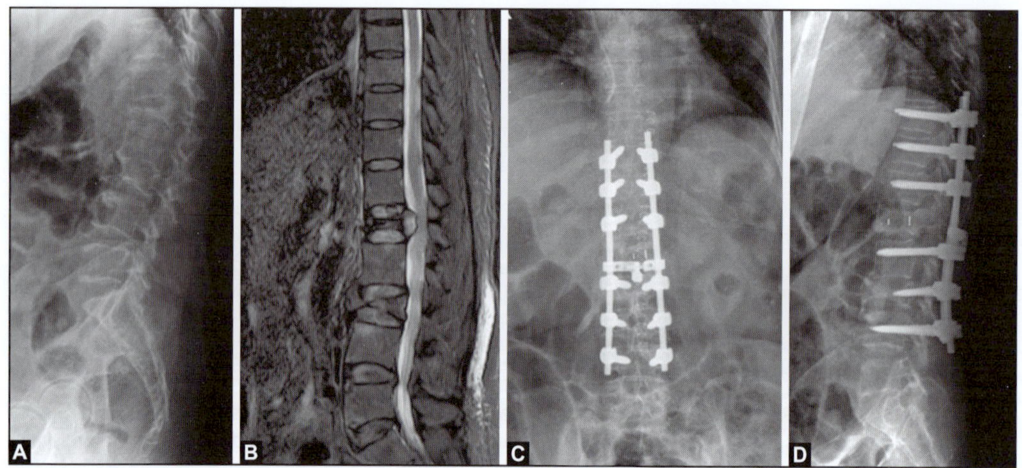

FIGS. 6A TO D: A 73-year-old female—with history of fall and ASIA C at presentation—preoperative X-ray (A) and sagittal STIR MRI sequence (B) showing L1 vertebral fracture with retropulsion and cord compression/ edema. Postoperative AP and lateral (C and D) X-rays of anterior cage reconstruction with pedicle screw fixation.

(AP: anteroposterior; STIR: short TI inversion recovery)

pressed endplates of the same vertebra help in anterior load sharing reducing stress on posterior fixation.

Anterior Intervertebral Reconstruction

If one endplate of the fractured vertebra is so destroyed that it cannot function as a load-bearing surface, then reconstruction has to be done between viable bone margins.

Hartshill/Sublaminar Wires

Laminae are part of the vertebrae, which get affected very late in osteoporosis. Sublaminar wiring can act as a primary modality of treatment in severe osteoporosis, or as a salvage if the pedicle screw fixation fails. Because laminae encase two cortical layers of bone they are much more resistant to pull out, than the pedicle screw which essentially

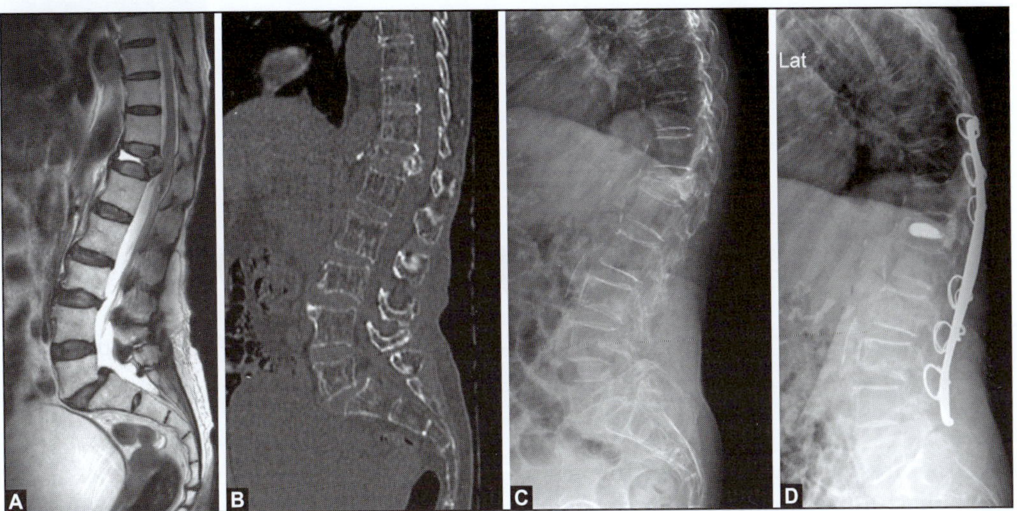

FIGS. 7A TO D: An 82-year-old female—with history of fall and ASIA C at presentation with urinary retention—preoperative (A) sagittal T2W MRI sequence and sagittal CT reconstruction (B) and lateral X-ray (C) showing D12 vertebral fracture with retropulsion and cord compression/edema. Postoperative lateral (D) X-ray showing Hartshill–sublaminar wiring spanning D9–L3.

has a cancellation purchase. There are other modifications as sublaminar tapes which have been shown to have better pullout strength than sublaminar wires **(Figs. 7A to D)**.

No surgery for an osteoporotic spinal fracture will be successful unless osteoporosis is treated. It is very essential to initiate an appropriate antiosteoporotic therapy as early as possible. Osteoporosis is a medical disease and fracture is just a small aspect of the presentation of that medical disease. If we just treat the effect, and not the cause, we are doomed to fail.

BIBLIOGRAPHY

1. Phillips FM. Minimally invasive treatments of osteoporotic vertebral compression fractures. Spine (Phila Pa 1976). 2003;28(15 Suppl):S45-53.
2. Morse LR, Battaglino RA, Stolzmann KL, Hallett LD, Waddimba A, Gagnon D, et al. Osteoporotic fractures and hospitalization risk in chronic spinal cord injury. Osteoporos Int. 2009;20(3):385-92.
3. Sudo H, Ito M, Kaneda K, Abumi K, Kotani Y, Nagahama K, et al. Anterior decompression and strut graft vs. posterior decompression and pedicle screw fixation with vertebroplasty for osteoporotic thoracolumbar vertebral collapse. Spine J. 2013;13:1726-32.
4. Tsoupras A, Tessitore E, Biver E, Dominguez DE. Multidisciplinary and Coordinated Management of Osteoporotic Vertebral Compression Fractures: Current State of the Art. J Clin Med. 2024;13(4): 930.

Management of Ribs Fracture

Meganath V Pawar, Tejpal Singh

Rib fractures, frequently resulting from blunt chest trauma, carry significant morbidity, especially in older adults. Effective management is critical to reducing the risk of complications like pneumonia, respiratory failure, and chronic pain.

CLINICAL ASSESSMENT AND RISK STRATIFICATION

Rib fractures can range from minor injuries to complex cases involving multiple fractures and flail chest. Accurate assessment and risk stratification are key to guiding treatment. Imaging with chest X-rays or CT scans is essential for identifying associated injuries, such as pneumothorax or hemothorax, that may require immediate intervention.

The *pain inspiration cough (PIC)* score **(Table 1)** is increasingly used for assessing injury severity. It evaluates pain intensity, inspiratory effort, and cough strength to aid in clinical decision-making. High PIC scores suggest a need for closer monitoring and possible ICU admission, especially in patients over 65 years old, who are more prone to complications.

PAIN MANAGEMENT

Pain control is central to managing rib fractures as it directly impacts respiratory function. Unmanaged pain can lead to hypoventilation, atelectasis, and pneumonia.

Multimodal Analgesia

The recommended approach is *multimodal analgesia*, combining nonsteroidal anti-inflammatory drugs (NSAIDs), acetaminophen, and opioids when necessary. Non-opioid analgesics reduce the need for opioids, which can depress respiration. While opioids remain essential for severe pain, careful dosing is vital, particularly in elderly patients.

TABLE 1: PIC Score.

Pain (Patients-reported, 0–10 scale)	Inspiration (Inspiratory spirometer; goal and alert levels set by respiratory therapist)	Cough (Assessed by bedside nurse)
3 — Controlled (Pain intensity scale 0–4)	4 — Above goal volume	3 — Strong
2 — Moderate (Pain intensity scale 5–7)	3 — Goal to alert volume	2 — Weak
	2 — Below alert volume	
1 — Sever (Pain intensity scale 8–10)	1 — Unable to perform incentive spirometry	1 — Absent

Multimodal strategies, which may include gabapentinoids and muscle relaxants, help reduce reliance on opioids.

Regional Anesthesia

For severe or refractory pain, regional anesthesia techniques such as *epidural analgesia, paravertebral blocks,* and *erector spinae plane (ESP) blocks* are effective. ESP blocks, e.g., can be safer than epidural anesthesia in patients with contraindications to epidurals. Regional analgesia can reduce ICU stays and ventilator dependence, demonstrating significant benefits in terms of recovery and overall outcomes.

RESPIRATORY SUPPORT AND MONITORING

Given that rib fractures can significantly impair respiratory function, especially in high-risk patients, respiratory support is a priority.

Incentive Spirometry and Noninvasive Ventilation

Incentive spirometry (IS) is universally recommended to encourage deep breathing and prevent atelectasis. Noninvasive positive pressure ventilation (NIPPV) is useful for patients with severe fractures, particularly those with compromised respiratory function, as it supports breathing and may prevent the need for intubation. Early initiation of NIPPV can lower the risk of pneumonia and other complications.

Intensive Care Unit Monitoring

Patients with multiple fractures or significant comorbidities, particularly those over 65, should be considered for ICU admission. Regular assessment of respiratory function, using tools like the PIC score, can help guide the need for escalation of care, ensuring early intervention for those at risk of respiratory failure.

SPECIAL CONSIDERATIONS FOR ELDERLY PATIENTS

Older adults face increased risks of complications from rib fractures. Their management often requires ICU monitoring and tailored analgesia strategies that minimize the use of opioids. Regional anesthesia, such as ESP blocks, is particularly beneficial for elderly patients as it provides effective pain control without the respiratory risks associated with systemic opioids. In this population, proactive respiratory support and careful monitoring are essential to prevent complications.

Surgical Stabilization

Surgical management, generally involving open reduction and internal fixation (ORIF), is reserved for cases where nonoperative measures are insufficient.

Flail chest or fractures that impair respiratory function are clear indications for surgery. Surgical intervention, typically performed within 72 hours, can reduce pain, improve pulmonary function, and decrease the need for prolonged mechanical ventilation. Early ORIF has been associated with reduced ICU and hospital stays, as well as lower rates of long-term complications.

Other relative indications for surgical fixation of rib fractures include:

- *Severely displaced fractures*: These can lead to prolonged pain and poor healing.
- Respiratory compromise from multiple rib fractures
- *Nonunion or delayed healing*: When fractures fail to heal over time, leading to chronic pain and functional issues
- *Intractable pain despite analgesia*: Techniques for rib fracture fixation and choice of implants

Various techniques and implants are selected based on fracture characteristics, fracture location, and patient-specific factors. **The primary techniques and types of implants used include:**

- *Low-profile titanium plates* are preferred due to their flexibility, strength, and

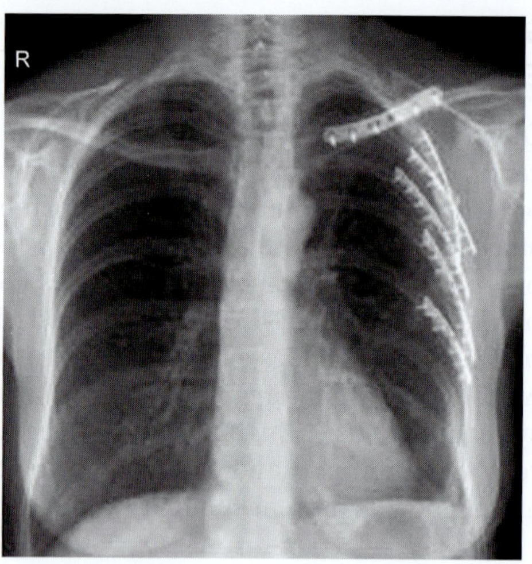

FIG. 1: X-rays showing internal fixation of multiple ribs with plating.

reduced risk of irritation. Some systems, like *locked plates,* offer additional stability, particularly useful in osteoporotic bone or complex fractures **(Fig. 1)**.

- Intramedullary splints or *flexible titanium nails*
- Suture or wire cerclage

FUTURE DIRECTIONS IN RIB FRACTURE MANAGEMENT

Emerging trends in rib fracture management include *enhanced recovery protocols (ERPs),* which emphasize early mobilization and optimized pain control. Novel analgesic approaches, such as ketamine infusions for opioid-tolerant patients, are also being explored.

BIBLIOGRAPHY

1. Kasotakis G, Hasenboehler EA, Streib EW, Patel N, Patel MB, Alarcon L, et al. Operative fixation of rib fractures after blunt trauma: A practice management guideline from the Eastern Association for the Surgery of Trauma. J Trauma Acute Care Surg. 2017;82(3):618-26.
2. Franssen AJPM, Daemen JHT, Luyten JA, Meesters B, Pijnenburg AM, Reisinger KW, et al. Treatment of traumatic rib fractures: an overview of current evidence and future perspectives. J Thorac Dis. 2024;16(8).
3. Hemati K, Gray AT, Agrawal A. (2024). A Comprehensive Review of the Non-operative Management of Traumatic Rib Fractures. [online] Available from https://link.springer.com/article/10.1007/s40140-024-00645-w [Last accessed November, 2024].
4. Mukherjee K, Schubl SD, Tominaga G, Cantrell S, Kim B, Haines KL, et al. Non-surgical management and analgesia strategies for older adults with multiple rib fractures: A systematic review, meta-analysis, and joint practice management guideline from the Eastern Association for the Surgery of Trauma and the Chest Wall Injury Society. J Trauma Acute Care Surg. 2023;94(3):398-407

SECTION

8

Pelvic Fracture

Pelvic Fracture

Imran Ahmed Hajam, Zubair Ahmad Lone, Mohammad Farooq Butt

Pelvic fractures are critical injuries with potentially life-threatening consequences. The mortality rate associated with pelvic fractures ranges from 5 to 20%, depending on the severity, stability, and associated injuries. Prompt diagnosis and timely appropriate intervention are essential for optimizing outcomes.

SURGICAL ANATOMY

The pelvic ring comprises the sacrum and two innominate bones joined anteriorly at the symphysis and posteriorly at the paired sacroiliac joints. The innominate bone is formed at maturity by the fusion of three ossification centers—the ilium, the ischium, and the pubis through the triradiate cartilage at the dome of the acetabulum. Ligamentous structures confer inherent stability of the pelvis, such as sacroiliac ligament which is very strong ligament and is divided into posterior and anterior, sacrotuberous ligament and sacrospinous ligament.

The integrity of the pelvis depends on both the anterior and posterior arches; damage to both structures indicates instability, which has critical implications for treatment.

MECHANISM OF INJURY

High-energy trauma, such as motor vehicle accidents and falls from heights, can cause significant damage to the pelvic ring and associated vascular and visceral structures, while low-energy trauma (common in the elderly) can lead to fragility fractures, particularly in osteoporotic patients. Pelvis behaves like a "polo mint". It is impossible to break a polo mint in one place. The same principle applies to the normal bony pelvic ring. If there is an anterior ring injury, always look for the associated posterior fracture or joint disruption. Pediatric pelvic ring fractures with open triradiate cartilage, the iliac wing is weaker than the elastic pelvic ligaments, resulting in bone failure before pelvic ring disruption usually involve the pubic rami and iliac wings and rarely require surgical treatment.

Avulsion type or straddle type injury results from sudden muscular contractions in young athletes.

CLINICAL PRESENTATION

Check for limb length discrepancy, swelling, and bruise over the groin and lower abdomen. Palpation of the posterior aspect of the pelvis may reveal a large hematoma, a defect representing the fracture, or a dislocation of the sacroiliac joint. Palpation of the symphysis may also reveal a defect.

The anterior-posterior and lateral compression test for pelvic instability should be performed once only (ideally to be done by the seniormost member of the orthopedic emergency team) and involves rotating the pelvis internally and externally. Digital rectal in all and vaginal examination in women should be done in all patients with pelvic injury. Neurological examination is important in pelvic fracture especially sacral fracture with injury to lumbosacral plexus.

RADIOLOGY

Standard anteroposterior (AP) view of the pelvis and special views for pelvic injury are inlet and outlet views.

The inlet view shows rotational deformity or anteroposterior displacement of the hemipelvis and is taken as a 40° caudal inlet. Outlet view shows vertical displacement of the hemipelvis, sacral fractures, and widening or fracture of the anterior pelvis taken at a 40° cephalad outlet.

Judet views are used in suspected acetabulum fractures. CT, an essential part of the evaluation of any significant pelvic injury as allows evaluation of the posterior portion of the pelvic ring that may be poorly seen on standard radiographs.

Stress views such as the push-pull test are used under radiographic control, to check the vertical instability.

CLASSIFICATION OF PELVIC FRACTURES

Pelvic fractures are classified based on stability and the mechanism of injury, which helps guide treatment and predict complications. The most commonly used classifications include:

- *Young and Burgess classification*:
  - This classification is based on the direction of the force vector applied during trauma *(mechanism of injury)*
  - This classification predicts the severity of injury and guide surgeon how to correct the deformity.
  - *Anteroposterior compression (APC)*: Common in frontal collisions; can result in widening of the symphysis pubis and disruption of sacroiliac joints.
  - *Lateral compression (LC)*: Common in side impacts, causing internal rotation of the hemipelvis, potentially leading to fractures of the iliac wing or pubic rami.
  - *Vertical shear (VS)*: Resulting from falls, with vertical displacement, causing significant instability.
  - *Combined mechanisms*: Often seen in severe trauma with complex fracture patterns.
- *Tile classification*: This classification is based on stability of the pelvic ring and guides surgeon whether fixation is needed or not **(Fig. 1)**.
  - *Type A:* Stable fractures—
    - *A1*: Avulsion fractures (often involving the iliac crest or ischial tuberosity) or fractures of the pelvic wings. These do not disrupt the integrity of the pelvic ring.
    - *A2*: Isolated fractures of the pubic rami. The pelvic ring remains intact, as only one side is affected.
    - *A3*: Transverse sacral fractures that do not affect the stability of the pelvic ring.
  - *Type B:* Partially stable (rotationally unstable) fractures—
    - *B1 (open book)*: Anterior-posterior compression fracture, where the pelvis opens like a book. There is disruption of the symphysis pubis and/or the sacroiliac ligaments. The pelvis is stable vertically but not rotationally.
    - *B2 (lateral compression)*: Unilateral compression injuries. The pelvic ring is impacted on one side, with the other side usually remaining intact.
    - *B3 (bilateral compression)*: Bilateral compression injuries with partial rotational instability. The pelvis remains stable in the vertical plane.

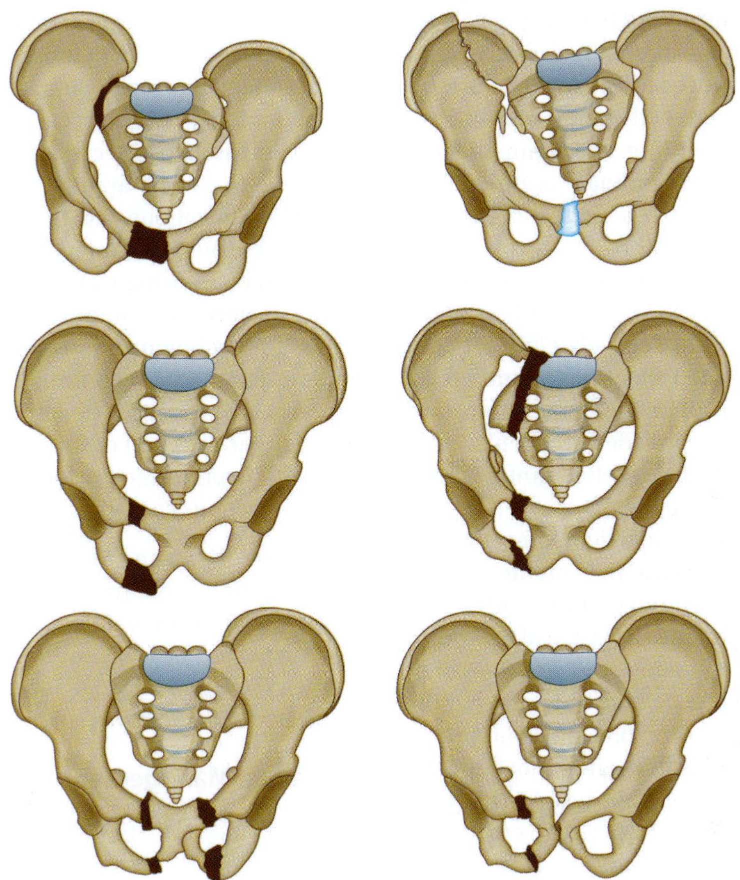

FIG. 1: Types of fractures.

- *Type C:* Unstable (both rotationally and vertically) fractures—
  - *C1*: Unilateral disruption of the sacroiliac complex with vertical and rotational instability on one side only.
  - *C2*: Unilateral injury with contralateral sacral involvement, resulting in both sides of the pelvis being vertically and rotationally unstable.
  - *C3*: Bilateral injuries with complete disruption of the sacroiliac complex on both sides. These fractures are vertically and rotationally unstable.

Another classification for pelvic fracture is the AO/OTA classification. This classification labels pelvic fracture as 61 and comprises 61A1, A2, A3 for stable pelvic injury, 61B1, 61B2, 61B3 under partially stable injury, and 61C1, C2, C3 for unstable injury.

MANAGEMENT OF PELVIC FRACTURES

The management of pelvic fractures can be divided into initial stabilization and definitive management.

Initial Management and Hemodynamic Stabilization

Employing the Advanced Trauma Life Support (ATLS) principles, immediate resuscitation with fluids and blood products is critical. Pelvic fractures often require additional measures for hemorrhage control. Bleeding from the injured pelvis occurs from displaced fracture surfaces, veins, arteries, and soft tissues, with veins and fracture surfaces representing the main bleeding sources. A multidisciplinary approach with orthopedic surgeons, general surgeons, and anesthesiologists is critical to optimizing outcomes. On recognition of an unstable pelvic ring injury, apply a pelvic binder around the pelvis. The pelvic binder could be a simple folded sheet or a commercially available one, both documented to provide sufficient stability provided proper placement over the trochanters. Pelvic binder is fast, cheap, and easily applicable.

After circumferential tightening, the sheet is clamped to decrease the volume, increase stability, and encourage tamponade. It will result in less motion in all tested planes during bed transfer, log rolling, and elevation of the head of the patient's bed. This can stabilize the pelvic ring, reduce bleeding, and provide temporary stabilization. It is most effective for AP compression injuries. As the pelvic volume increases by 10–20% by 5 cm opening up of the pelvic ring, closing up and stabilizing the pelvic ring represent a first-line measure to halt low-pressure hemorrhage, by limiting space and facilitating early tamponade. Pelvic binders can provide false reassurance by reducing a pelvic fracture, therefore, the clinical assessment remains critical and X-rays should be taken without the binder to ensure no displacement of fracture. The *FAST* (Focused Assessment with Sonography for Trauma) examination is a rapid bedside tool used to detect hemoperitoneum in hemodynamically unstable patients, helping guide initial management.

Early use of blood products, particularly in balanced transfusion ratios, has been shown to improve outcomes.

External fixator: Anterior external fixator or frame and C clamp are used for the stabilization of unstable pelvic fractures but they are time-consuming compared to pelvic binder. Supraacetabular pin placement is preferred when applying anterior frames and can be applied without fluoroscopic guidance in the emergency room. Supraacetabular pin configuration also creates good compression force compared to iliac crest frames.

C clamp can be applied to an unstable pelvis. Modifications of C clamp are applied over the greater trochanter called as T clamp and thereby exerting its compressive forces to the posterior pelvic ring through the hip joints. This technique is fast and easy to apply without fluoroscopic control, and the frame can also in most cases be left in place until final fracture fixation of the posterior pelvic ring can be performed, without an elevated risk of infectious complication.

Angioembolization: It is indicated for ongoing hemodynamic instability after initial stabilization and in cases where there is a suspected arterial source of bleeding. Studies show that early angioembolization is associated with improved survival rates.

Definitive Management

- *Nonoperative treatment*: Fractures amenable to nonoperative treatment include avulsion fractures, LC-I and APC-I fractures, and gapping of pubic symphysis <2.5 cm. Rehabilitation measures are protecting weight-bearing typically with a walker or crutches initially. If the displacement of the posterior ring >1 cm is noted, weight-bearing should be stopped. Operative treatment should be considered for gross displacement.
- *Operative treatment*:
    - *Absolute indication*: Open pelvic fractures or those in which there is an associated visceral perforation requiring operative intervention, open-book fractures, or vertically unstable fractures with associated patient hemodynamic instability
    - *Relative indications*: Symphyseal diastasis >2.5 cm, leg-length discrepancy >1.5 cm, rotational deformity, sacral displacement >1 cm, and intractable pain

The principle of operative fixation is to convert an unstable pelvic ring to a stable one.

Various operative techniques:

- External fixation is a resuscitative fixation and can only be used for the definitive fixation of anterior pelvis injuries, it cannot be used as the definitive fixation of posteriorly unstable injuries.
- *Percutaneous fixation*: Often used in minimally invasive procedures for posterior pelvic fractures, particularly in hemodynamically stable patients. It offers a quicker recovery with a reduced risk of infection.

Open reduction and internal fixation (ORIF): ORIF is the mainstay for displaced fractures, providing anatomical alignment and stability. This significantly increases the forces resisted by the pelvic ring compared with external fixation.

- *For iliac wing fractures*: Open reduction and stable internal fixation are performed using lag screws and neutralization plates **(Fig. 2)**.
- For diastasis of the pubic symphysis, plate fixation is used if no open injury or cystostomy tube is present.
- For sacral fractures, transiliac bar fixation may be inadequate or may cause compressive neurologic injury in these cases, plate fixation or sacroiliac screw fixation may be indicated **(Fig. 3)**.

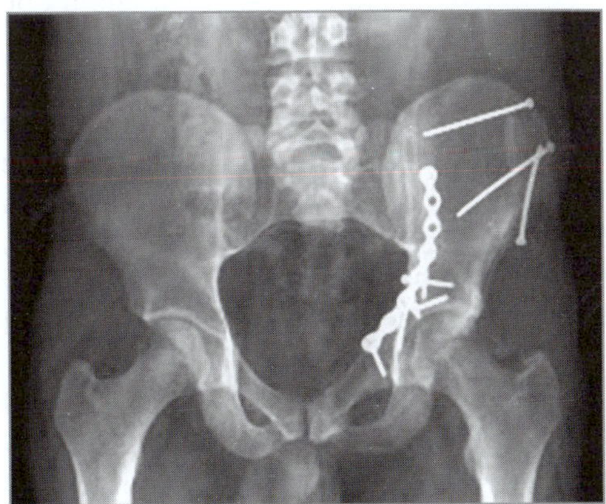

FIG. 2: Iliac wing fractures.

- For unilateral sacroiliac dislocation, direct fixation with cancellous screws or anterior sacroiliac plate fixation is used. Bilateral posterior unstable disruptions involve fixation of the displaced portion of the pelvis to the sacral body and may be accomplished by posterior screw fixation **(Fig. 4)**.

COMPLICATIONS

Complications from pelvic fractures can be immediate or delayed.

Immediate Complications

- Hemorrhagic shock
- *Urinary tract injury*: This injury can be worsened by injudicious attempts at catheterization

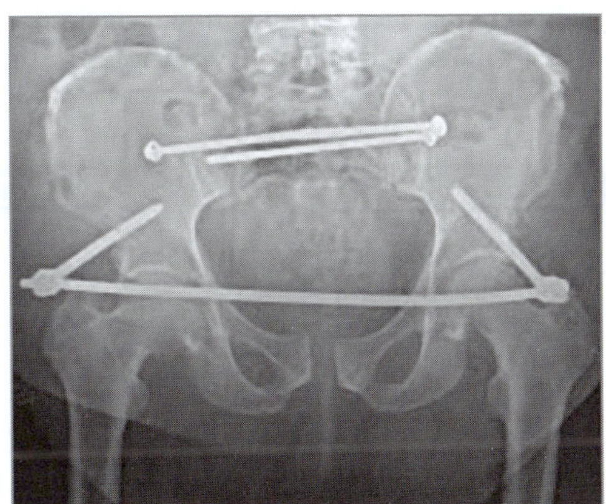

FIG. 3: Transiliac bar fixation.

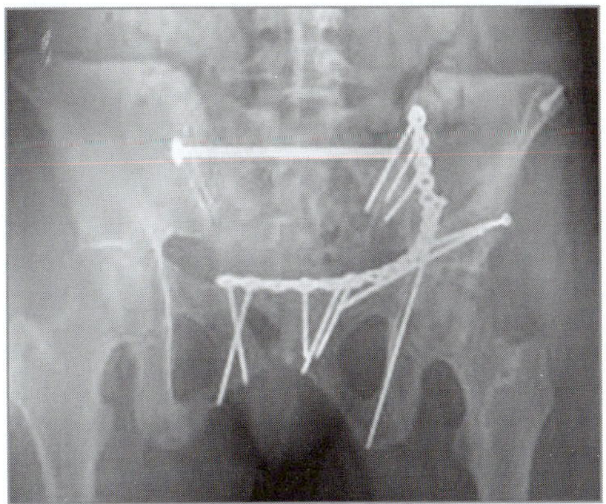

FIG. 4: Unilateral sacroiliac dislocation.

- Nerve injury
- Pelvic fracture may develop systemic inflammatory response syndrome (SIRS) and acute respiratory distress syndrome (ARDS).
- Deep venous thrombosis and pulmonary embolism

Late Complication

Including malunion, chronic pain, and sexual or urinary dysfunction, infection, including erectile dysfunction, mechanical pelvic pain, and psychological disturbance

POSTOPERATIVE CARE AND REHABILITATION

Comprehensive postoperative protocol:
- In general, early mobilization is desired.
- Prophylaxis against thromboembolic phenomena

Weight-bearing status may be advanced as follows:
- Full weight bearing on the uninvolved lower extremity/sacral side occurs within several days.
- Partial weight bearing on the involved side is recommended for at least 6 weeks. Recently, weight bearing as tolerated has been supported in low-energy LC-I fractures.
- Full weight bearing on the affected side without crutches is indicated by 12 week.

SPECIAL CONSIDERATIONS IN GERIATRIC PATIENTS

Geriatric patients present unique challenges due to comorbidities and reduced bone quality. Fragility fractures require careful management to prevent complications such as malunion and to facilitate mobilization as early as possible.

BIBLIOGRAPHY

1. American College of Surgeons. ATLS Guidelines. Chicago: ACS; 2023.
2. Tile M. Acute pelvic fractures: I. Causation and classification. J Am Acad Orthop Surg. 1996;4(3): 143-51.
3. Giannoudis PV, Grotz MR, Tzioupis C, Dinopoulos H, Wells GE, Bouamra O, et al. Prevalence of pelvic fractures, associated injuries, and mortality: The United Kingdom perspective. J Trauma. 2007;63(4):875-83.
4. Rommens PM, Hofmann A. Comprehensive classification of fragility fractures of the pelvic ring: Recommendations for surgical treatment. Injury. 2013;44(12):1733-44.
5. Manson TT, Nascone JW, Sciadini MF, O'Toole RV. Percutaneous fixation of the posterior pelvic ring: Techniques and outcomes. J Orthop Trauma. 2010;24(5):285-90.
6. Höch A, Schneider I, Pieroh P, Josten C, Böhme J. Management of pelvic ring injuries: Differences between specialists and nonspecialists. Injury. 2019;50(12):2233-8.

Sacrum and Coccyx Fracture

Barkat Anwar Shah, Zubair Ahmad Lone, Mohammad Farooq Butt

FRACTURE OF THE SACRUM

Sacral fractures are relatively rare injuries that pose significant challenges due to their complex anatomy, functional importance, and association with other pelvic injuries.

Applied Anatomy

The sacrum is a triangular bone at the base of the spine, forming the posterior portion of the pelvis. It consists of five fused vertebrae (S1-S5), which articulate with the lumbar spine superiorly and the coccyx inferiorly. Laterally, it articulates with the ilium at the sacroiliac (SI) joints, which are important weight-bearing joints.

The sacrum serves as a conduit for several vital neural structures. The sacral plexus, comprising nerve roots from L4 to S4, lies within the sacral canal and exits through the sacral foramina. Injuries to the sacrum can, therefore, lead to neurological deficits, particularly if they involve the S1 and S2 levels, which contribute to the sciatic nerve **(Fig. 1)**.

Classification of Sacral Fractures

Sacral fractures are classified based on their location, morphology, and the extent of displacement. The Denis classification remains widely used for its simplicity and clinical relevance. However, the recent

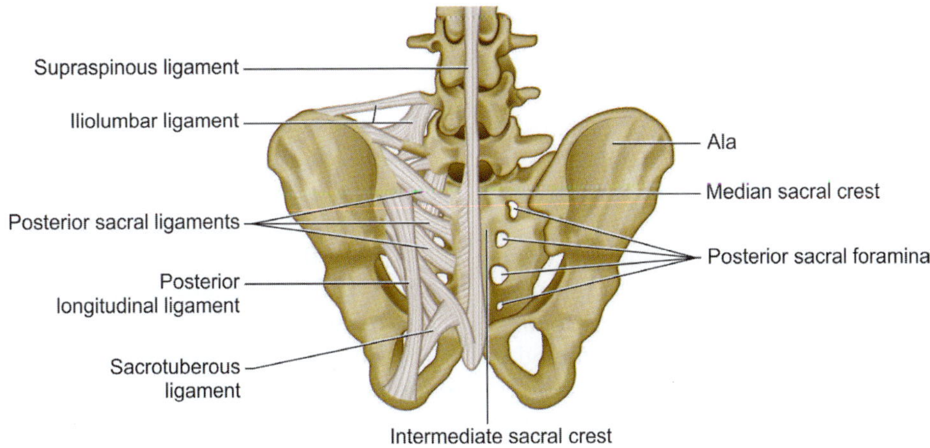

FIG. 1: Applied anatomy.

advancements in imaging have led to a more refined classification, the AO/OTA system, which is now often used to guide treatment decisions.

- *Denis classification*:
  - *Zone I*: Fractures lateral to the foramina, usually involving the alae
  - *Zone II*: Fractures through the foramina, with potential neurological impairment
  - *Zone III*: Fractures involving the sacral canal, often with high risk of neurological injury
- *AO/OTA classification*:
  - *Type A*: Stable fractures with minimal displacement
  - *Type B*: Unstable fractures, often associated with pelvic ring injuries
  - *Type C*: Vertically unstable fractures with disruption of the posterior pelvic ring

Taxonomy of classification system of sacral fractures is shown in **Figure 2**.

Clinical Presentation

Patients with sacral fractures often present with lower back pain, sacral tenderness, and, in some cases, neurological deficits such as radiculopathy or cauda equina syndrome. A high index of suspicion is necessary, particularly in polytrauma cases where sacral fractures may be overlooked.

- Plain radiographs can identify gross fractures but are often inadequate for detailed assessment.
- CT is the gold standard for diagnosing sacral fractures, offering detailed visualization of the fracture pattern and displacement.
- MRI is useful for evaluating soft tissue injuries, including nerve root impingement, hematoma, or ligamentous injury.
- *Dual-energy CT (DECT)*: This emerging modality allows for the assessment of bone bruises and early microfractures, which may not be visible on conventional CT.

Management of Sacral Fractures

Nonoperative Treatment

Nonoperative treatment is generally reserved for stable fractures without neurological deficits or severe displacement. It involves:

- *Bed rest and analgesia*: Patients may require initial bed rest to reduce pain and inflammation, along with appropriate analgesia.
- *Bracing*: Lumbosacral orthoses can help immobilize the area, promoting healing in stable fractures.
- *Weight-bearing restrictions*: Partial weight-bearing is typically advised, progressing to full weight-bearing as tolerated over 6–12 weeks.

Operative Treatment

Surgical intervention is often indicated for unstable fractures, displaced fractures, or fractures associated with neurological deficits. Advancements in surgical techniques have made minimally invasive options more feasible, reducing recovery time and improving outcomes.

- *Percutaneous sacroiliac screw fixation*:
  - *Indications*: Stable fractures with minimal displacement but high risk of further instability.
  - *Technique*: Screws are inserted under fluoroscopic or CT guidance through the ilium and into the sacrum. Navigation systems have improved accuracy and reduced radiation exposure.
- *Trans-sacral screw fixation*:
  - *Indications*: Vertically unstable fractures, particularly those involving Zone III
  - *Technique*: Screws are placed transversely across the sacrum, from one ilium to the other **(Fig. 3)**.
- *Spinopelvic fixation*:
  - *Indications*: Unstable fractures involving the sacral canal and sacroiliac joints

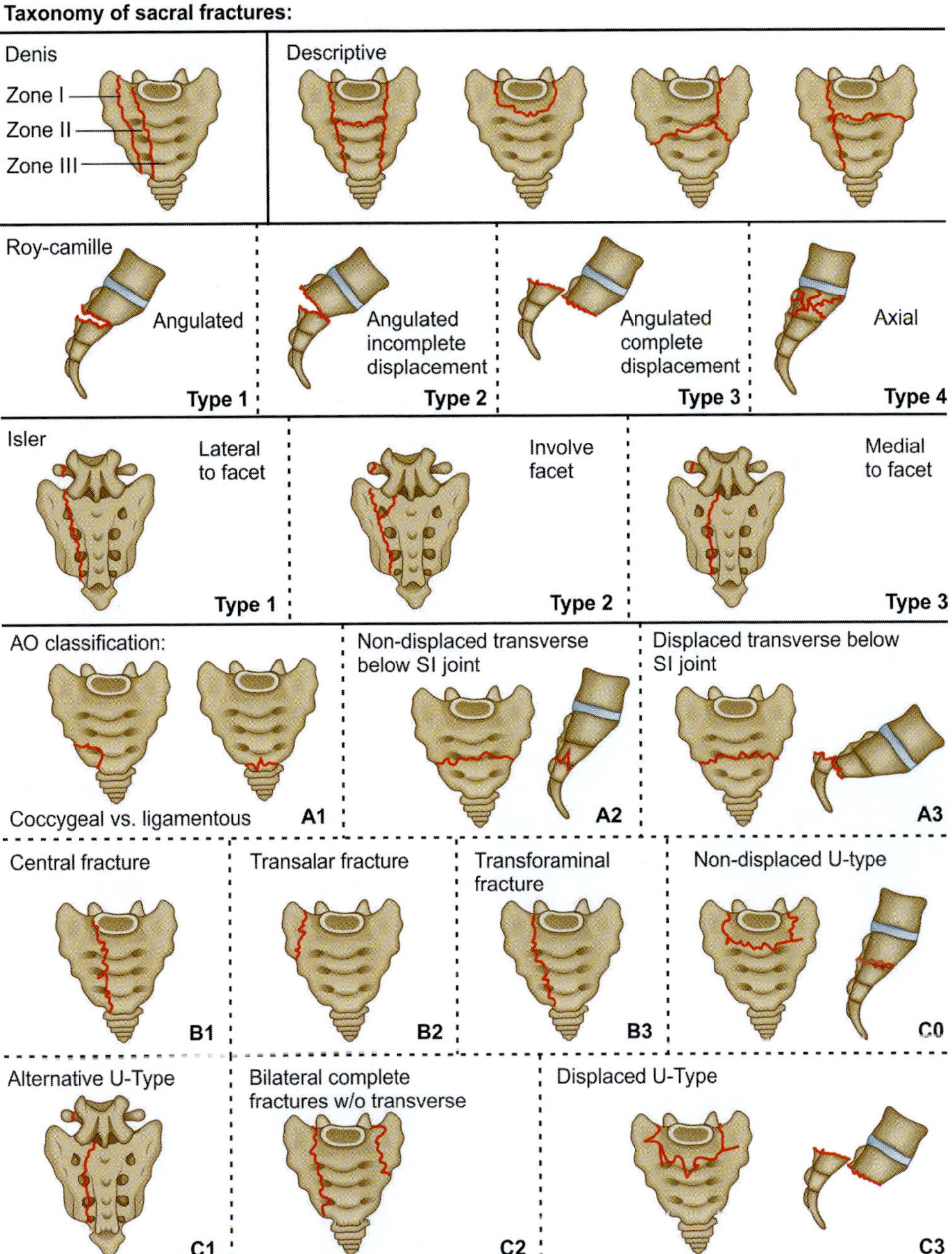

FIG. 2: Classification system of sacral fractures.
Source: Taken and adapted from Barber LA, Katsuura Y, Qureshi S. Sacral Fractures: A Review. HSS J. 2023;19(2):234-46.

    - *Technique*: Utilizes pedicle screws in the lumbar spine connected to iliac screws **(Fig. 4)**.
- *Minimally invasive techniques*:
    - *Balloon kyphoplasty and cement augmentation*: Emerging options for patients with osteoporotic fractures or those unsuitable for traditional surgery. These techniques involve inserting a balloon into the sacrum to restore height and filling the space with bone cement.

- *Advances in navigation and robotics*: Computer-assisted navigation and robotic guidance enhance the precision of screw placement, reducing complications related to misalignment or neural damage.
- *Neurological considerations*:
  - Neurological deficits may require decompression, particularly in Zone III fractures. Decompression can be achieved via a posterior approach, which allows for direct visualization and protection of the neural elements.

FRACTURE OF THE COCCYX

Coccyx fractures, although less common than other spinal injuries, can cause significant pain and discomfort due to the coccyx's role in supporting weight-bearing activities, particularly in seated positions.

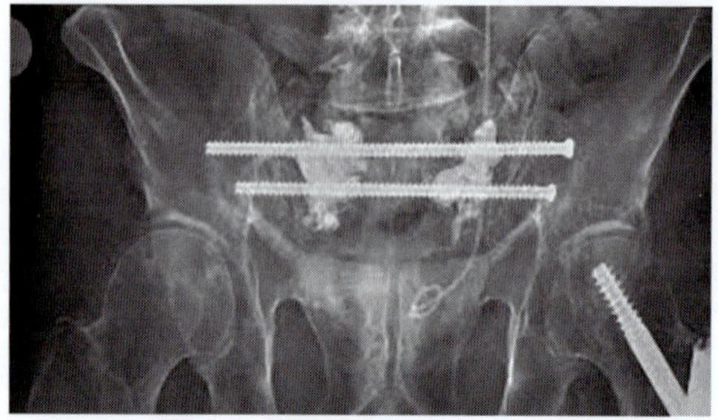

FIG. 3: Trans-sacral screw fixation.

Anatomy of the Coccyx

The coccyx, or tailbone, is the terminal portion of the vertebral column, comprising three to five small, fused vertebrae. It articulates superiorly with the sacrum at the sacrococcygeal joint. The coccyx serves as an attachment site for several muscles, tendons, and ligaments, including the gluteus maximus, levator ani, and sacrococcygeal ligaments, which play a role in maintaining pelvic floor integrity and supporting seated posture.

The coccyx is highly susceptible to injury from direct trauma, such as falls or repetitive strain, particularly in sports or activities involving prolonged sitting. Although typically nondisplaced, coccygeal fractures can lead to chronic pain, termed coccydynia, which can significantly impact a patient's quality of life.

Classification of Coccyx Fractures

Coccyx fractures are classified based on the location, type of displacement, and the presence of angulation. Although there is no universal classification system, the types below help guide treatment approaches:

- *Types of fractures*:
  - *Transverse fractures*: Often occur at the sacrococcygeal junction due to direct impact or fall

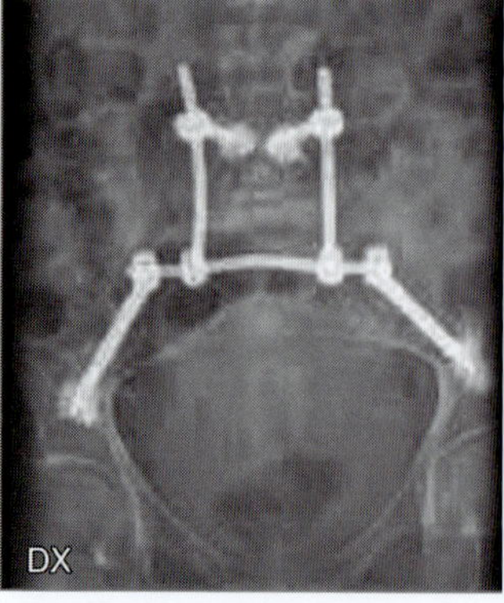

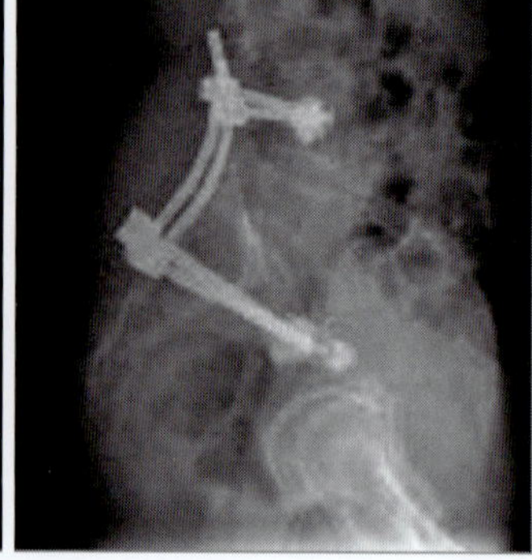

FIG. 4: Spinopelvic fixation.

  - *Comminuted fractures*: Less common, usually seen with high-impact trauma, resulting in multiple fragments
  - *Avulsion fractures*: Occur when a ligament or tendon pulls off a portion of the coccyx, frequently seen in younger patients or athletes
- *Displacement*:
  - *Nondisplaced*: Fracture fragments remain aligned.
  - *Displaced*: Fracture fragments shift, leading to angulation, which can contribute to chronic pain or coccygeal instability.
- *Chronic versus acute*:
  - *Acute fractures*: Result from recent trauma and typically present with sharp, localized pain
  - *Chronic fractures*: Result from repetitive stress or untreated acute fractures, often presenting with chronic pain

It is essential to differentiate between coccydynia from trauma versus other potential causes, such as sacroiliac joint dysfunction or referred pain from the lumbar spine.

- *Radiography*: Lateral radiographs of the coccyx are the initial imaging modality, although their utility is limited due to the small size of the coccyx and the potential for overlapping structures.
- CT scans offer better visualization, particularly for complex fractures or those involving displacement or angulation.
- *Magnetic resonance imaging (MRI)*: Useful for evaluating soft tissue injuries, including ligamentous damage, hematoma, or coccygeal instability, particularly in chronic coccydynia.
- *Dynamic radiography*: This involves comparing coccygeal angles in sitting versus standing positions, aiding in the assessment of coccygeal mobility and instability.

Management of Coccyx Fractures

Nonoperative Treatment

Most coccyx fractures can be managed conservatively. Nonoperative treatment is the first line of management, focusing on pain control and minimizing coccygeal stress.

- *Rest and activity modification*: Patients are advised to avoid activities that exacerbate pain, such as prolonged sitting or cycling, for 4–6 weeks.
- *Analgesia*: Nonsteroidal anti-inflammatory drugs (NSAIDs) and acetaminophen are commonly prescribed for pain relief. Local anesthetic injections may be considered for persistent pain.
- *Cushions and seating modifications*: Use of specialized coccygeal cushions or doughnut-shaped cushions to alleviate pressure on the tailbone during sitting. Adjustable seats or reclining chairs may also aid in reducing discomfort.
- *Physical therapy*: Pelvic floor therapy, postural training, and gentle stretching exercises can help improve coccygeal alignment and reduce muscular tension around the coccyx.

Operative Treatment

Surgical intervention is considered for cases where conservative treatment has failed, or when there is significant displacement, instability, or persistent pain beyond 6 months.

- *Coccygectomy*:
  - *Indications*: Persistent coccydynia unresponsive to conservative treatment, displaced fractures with angulation, and cases with severe coccygeal instability
  - *Procedure*: Removal of part or all of the coccyx through a posterior approach. Care is taken to preserve surrounding soft tissues and neural structures.

- *Minimally invasive interventions*:
    - *Steroid injections*: Corticosteroid injections into the sacrococcygeal joint can reduce inflammation and pain in cases where surgery is not immediately feasible.
    - *Radiofrequency ablation*: An emerging modality for patients with chronic pain unresponsive to injections, targeting the sensory nerve fibers that innervate the coccyx.
- *Neuromodulation techniques*:
    - *Transcutaneous electrical nerve stimulation (TENS)*: TENS therapy may provide temporary relief for chronic coccydynia by modulating pain signals. It is generally used as an adjunct to other therapies rather than a standalone treatment.
    - *Spinal cord stimulation (SCS)*: In rare cases, SCS may be considered for refractory pain that has not responded to other modalities.

Emerging Modalities and Techniques

- Ultrasound-guided injections
- Stem cell and platelet-rich plasma (PRP) therapy
- Biomechanical cushions and seating devices

BIBLIOGRAPHY

1. Denis F, Davis S, Comfort T. Sacral fractures: an important problem. Retrospective analysis of 236 cases. Clin Orthop Relat Res. 1988;227:67-81.
2. Keating JF, Werier J, Blachut P, Broekhuyse H, Meek RN, O'Brien PJ. Early fixation of the vertically unstable pelvis: the role of iliosacral screw fixation of the posterior lesion. J Orthop Trauma. 1999;13(2):107-13.
3. Rommens PM, Wagner D, Hofmann A. Minimal invasive surgical treatment of fragility fractures of the pelvis. Chirurgia (Bucur). 2017;112(5):524-37.
4. Lee Y, Lambrechts M, Narayanan R, Bransford R, Benneker L, Schnake K, et al. The Surgical Algorithm for the Management of Sacral Fractures and Associated Conditions: An Evidence-Based Approach. J Am Acad Orthop Surg. 2017;25(9):610-22.

Acetabular Fracture

Yassir Mehmood, Bhaarath KS

Acetabular fractures have been generally associated with high-velocity injury mostly in the younger age group. This trend has lately been changing from young adults to elderly and children.

APPLIED ANATOMY

It is a partial ball and socket joint which has an inverted horseshoe-shaped articular surface and deficient inferior margins. Acetabulum development includes both endochondral growth and intramembranous growth. It is formed from triradiate cartilage, ilium (superiorly), ischium (inferior and lateral), and pubis (medially) which articulates with the femoral head. It is composed of the anterior wall, anterior column, posterior wall, and posterior column. The columns are connected to the sacral bone with a sciatic buttress.

- *Anterior column*: It is composed of the anterior wall and extends from the sacroiliac joint up to the ipsilateral pubic symphysis **(Figs. 1A and B)**.
- *Posterior column*: It includes the posterior wall and extends from the sciatic notch up to the ischial tuberosity **(Figs. 1A and B)**.

The main weight-bearing portion of the acetabulum is the dome which supports the acetabulum. The posterior wall extends laterally and is larger as compared to the anterior wall.

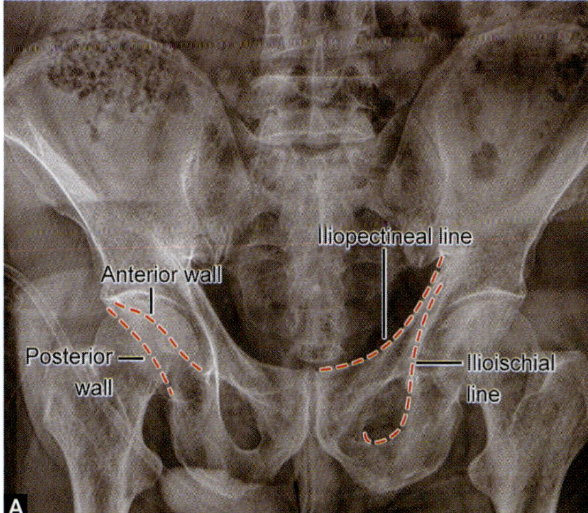

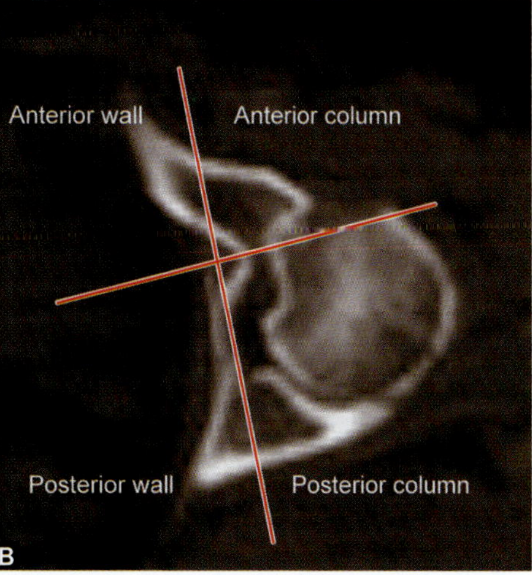

FIGS. 1A AND B: Landmarks corresponding to the columns and walls (on X-ray and CT scan).

CLINICAL PRESENTATION

Fracture-dislocation of the femoral head, combined with a femoral neck fracture, necessitates a thorough assessment to rule out associated neurological injuries. There is an incidence of 9% of sciatic nerve injuries which are post-traumatic and 5% of injuries are iatrogenic. The neurological injury associated with fracture acetabulum is most commonly found in posterior wall fractures. Compromised soft tissue cover may further add to the grievousness of the injury. Due to these injuries, patients may present with hemodynamic shock for which urgent diagnostic modalities and management options must be explored on initial presentation.

RADIOLOGICAL EVALUATION

To evaluate these injuries, anteroposterior (AP) and Judet views are taken.

Judet views:
- *Iliac oblique view*: This is a 45° external rotation view in which the X-ray beam is targeted perpendicular to the iliac wing. This view helps diagnose anterior wall fractures and posterior column fractures **(Fig. 2)**.
- *Obturator view*: This is a 45° oblique view in which the X-ray beam is perpendicular to the obturator foramen. This view is helpful in diagnosing anterior column fracture and posterior wall fractures **(Fig. 2)**.

CT scan: A CT (2D/3D) scan is further needed for a better understanding of fracture patterns and planning of surgery **(Fig. 3)**.

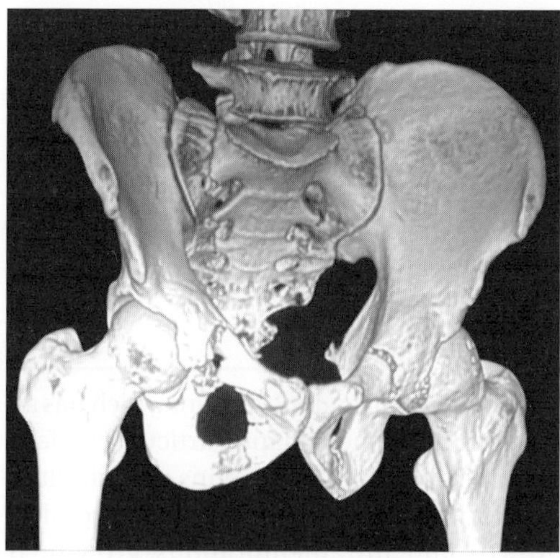

FIG. 3: A 3D scan for better understanding acetabular fracture.

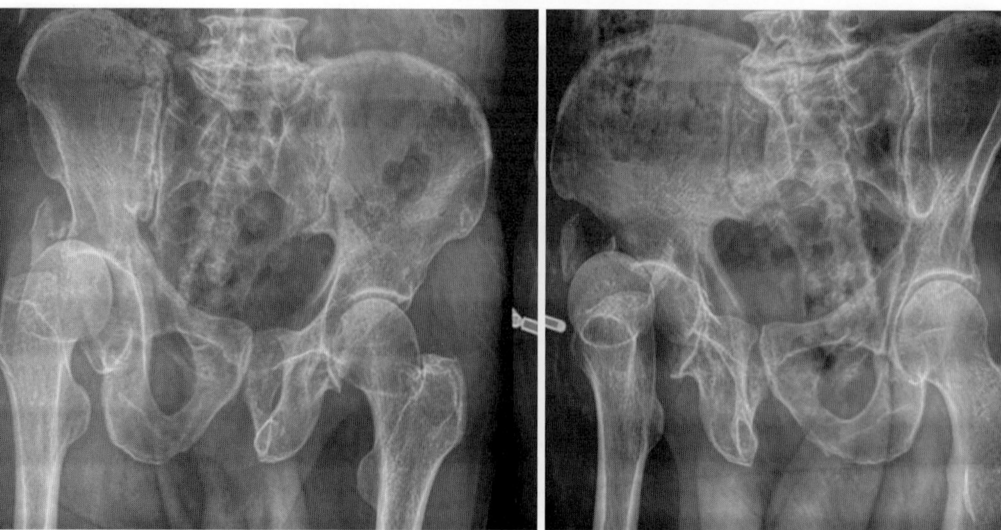

FIG. 2: Judet views of the acetabulum.

It also provides information regarding any incarcerated fragment, marginal impaction, sacroiliac joint disruption, and other occult fractures which are difficult to diagnose on plain radiographs.

CLASSIFICATION

Judet and Letournel's Classification

This classification groups the fractures into 10 subtypes with 5 being elementary type and 5 being associated acetabular fractures. This is most common classification to describe the acetabular fractures **(Fig. 4)**.

Elementary fractures:
- Anterior wall fractures **(Fig. 5)**
- Posterior wall fractures **(Fig. 6)**
- Anterior column fractures
- Posterior column fractures
- Transverse fractures **(Fig. 7)**

Associated fractures:
- T type **(Fig. 8)**
- Posterior column and posterior wall
- Transverse and posterior wall
- Anterior column posterior hemi transverse
- Associated both column

TIPS TO IDENTIFY FRACTURE PATTERN

If there is no involvement of column, it can be categorized as a wall fracture.
- Anterior wall fracture (fracture line only passing through anterior wall)
- Posterior wall fracture (fracture line only passing through the posterior wall)

If there is involvement of only one column then it can be categorized as:
- Posterior column fracture (broken ilioischial line)
- Anterior column fracture (broken iliopectineal line)
- Posterior column and posterior wall (broken ilioischial line as well as broken posterior wall)

If there is involvement of two columns, then it can be categorized as:
- *Transverse (iliac wing not involved)*:
  - Transverse
  - T type
  - Transverse and posterior wall
- *If there is involvement of the iliac wing*:
  - Associated both column fractures
  - Anterior column posterior hemi transverse

TREATMENT

Initial Management

Most of the patients suffering from fracture acetabulum are generally hemodynamically unstable. Initially, ATLS protocol is followed and the patient is evaluated with urgent medical intervention. Associated hip dislocation is reduced initially and traction is applied to minimize the acetabular cartilage damage. This is followed by the post-reduction CT scan.

Definitive Management

- *Conservative treatment*:
  - Elderly patients who are not fit for surgery.
  - *Matta's roof arc angle*: This rule is applied when the posterior wall is intact and the hip joint is stable. When the angle is >45° in all views (medial, anterior, and posterior), the patient is managed conservatively **(Fig. 9)**.
  - Associated both-column fractures can be managed conservatively when there is a secondary congruence and in elderly patients with low functional demands and underlying comorbidities. Femoral head reduction into acetabulum can be achieved by applying skin/skeletal traction.
- *Operative intervention (ORIF) indications*:
  - >2 mm displaced fractures
  - Roof arc angle of <45° in Judet views

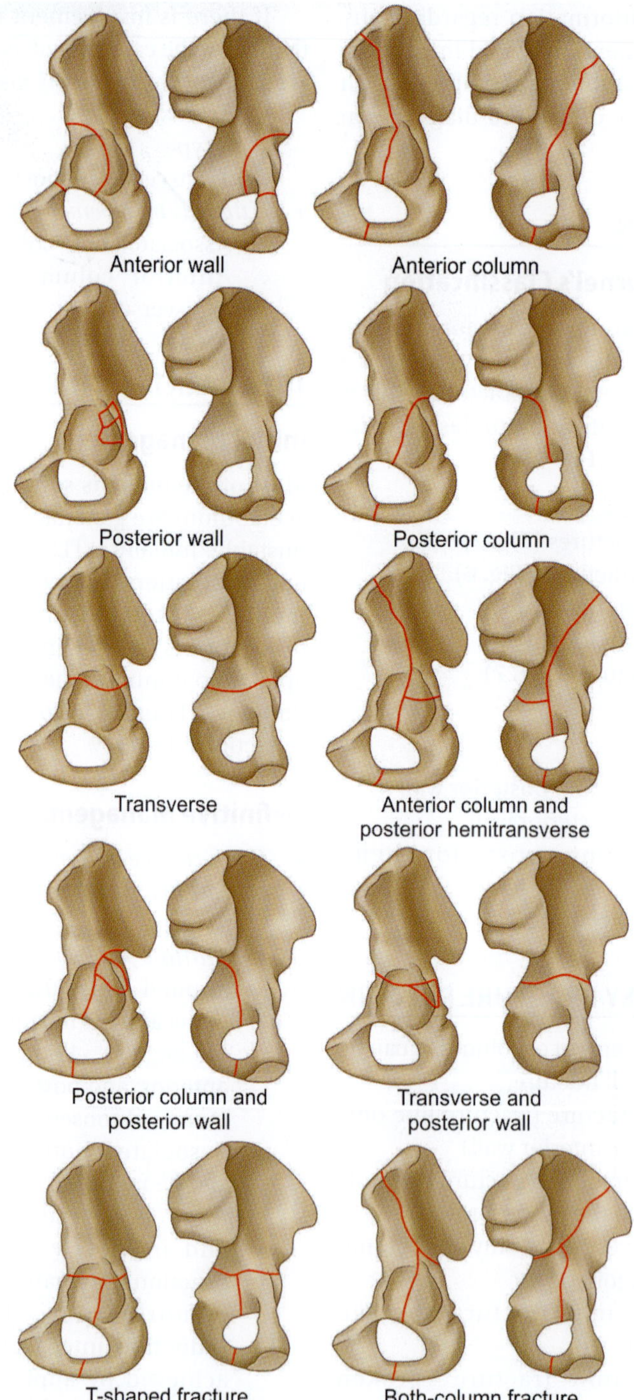

FIG. 4: Letournel's classification (fracture acetabulum)

Source: Adapted from Moed BR. Acetabular fractures: Kocher–Langenbeck approach. In: Wiss DA (Ed). Master Techniques in Orthopaedic Surgery: Fractures, 3rd edition. Philadelphia, PA: Lippincott Williams & Wilkins; 2012. pp. 817-68.

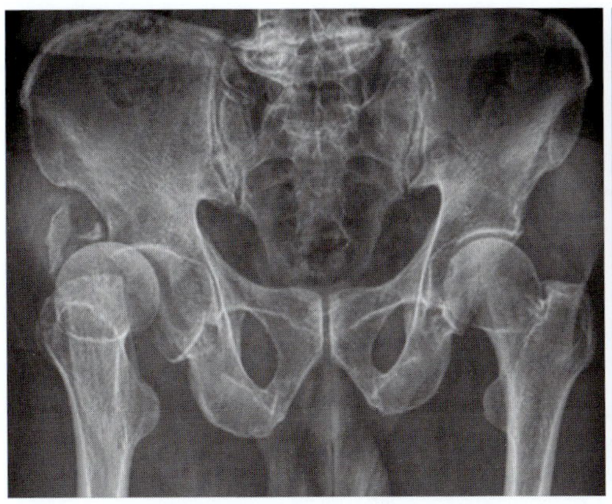

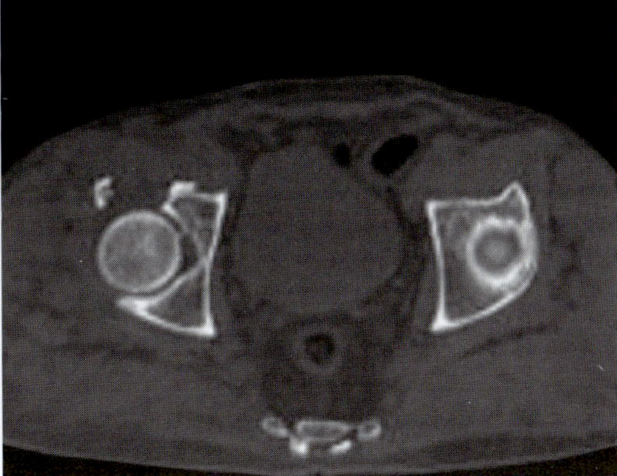

FIG. 5: CT scan and X-ray of anterior wall fracture dislocation.

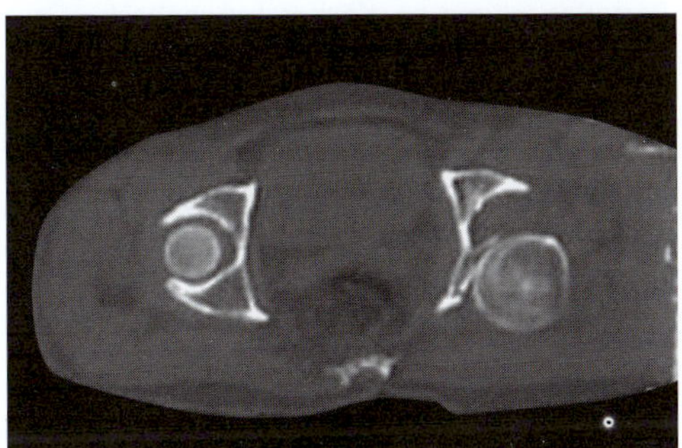

FIG. 6: A CT scan showing post wall fracture dislocation.

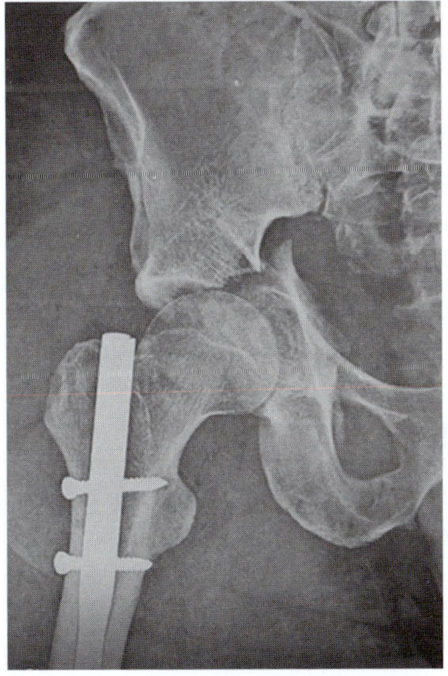

FIG. 7: A transverse acetabular fracture.

- >40% involvement of posterior wall fragment
- Unstable posterior wall fractures of (<40% fragment size)
- Presence of incarcerated fragments after closed reduction of hip joint dislocation
- Younger patients with higher functional demands

Surgical Approaches

Patients suffering from fracture acetabulum need to be medically fit for surgery as these patients generally have associated injuries **(Fig. 10)**. All the fracture patterns with associated irreducible hip dislocations, vascular injury, or worsening neurological deficit need urgent surgical care. ORIF should not be delayed as there are increased chances of early callus formation and soft tissue contractures leading to difficult reduction intraoperatively. According to a study, it was found that reduction was challenging in delayed ORIF (15 days after elementary fractures and 5 days after associated fractures post-injury). The most favorable time to operate such fractures is as soon as the patient is fit for anesthesia preferably within 7 to 10 days of injury.

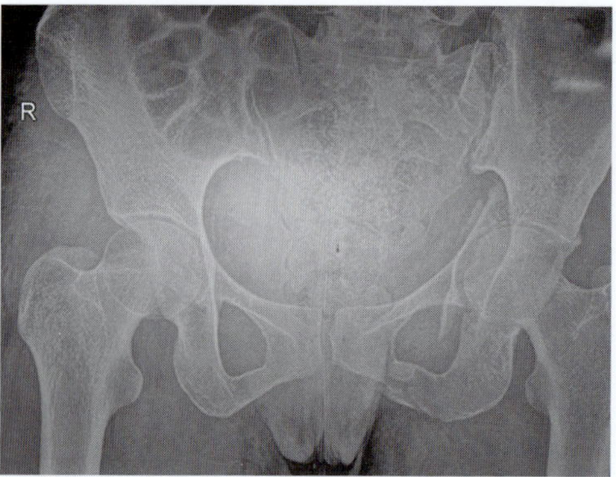

FIG. 8: X-ray showing comminuted T type fracture.

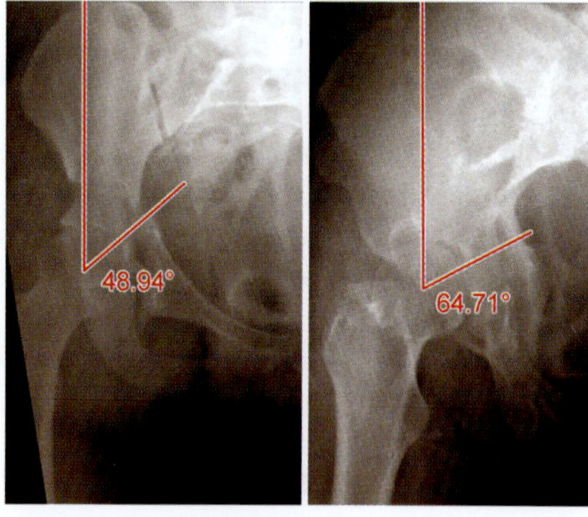

FIG. 9: Roof arc measurements.

Source: Adapted from Azar FM, Beaty JH. Matta roof arc measurement. In: Campbell's Operative Orthopaedics, 14th edition, Volume 3. Amsterdam: Elsevier; 2020. p. 2967.

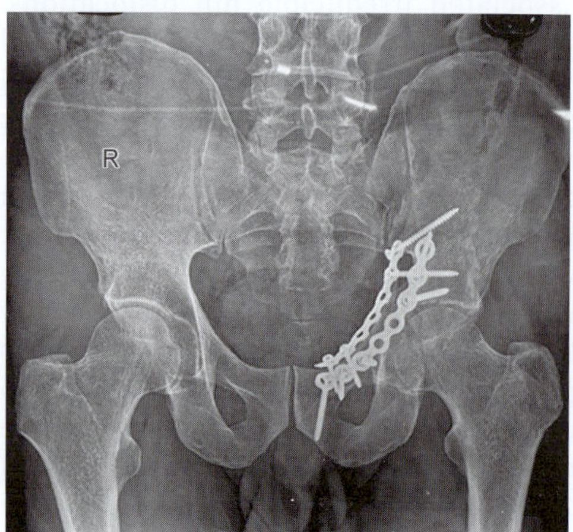

FIG. 10: X-ray showing an operated case of acetabular fracture.

TABLE 1: Preferred approaches for the specific fracture pattern.

Fracture pattern	Preferred approach
Anterior column/ anterior wall fractures	• Ilioinguinal approach • Lateral window with an ASIS osteotomy
Posterior column fractures	• Kocher–Langenbeck approach • More chances of sciatic nerve injury
Transverse fractures	• Kocher–Langenbeck • Ilioinguinal approach • Combined approach
Posterior column with posterior wall fractures	• Kocher–Langenbeck • Combined approach
T-shaped fractures	• Kocher–Langenbeck • Anterior approach • Combined approach
Anterior column posterior hemitransverse	• Anterior intrapelvic approach (AIP) • Ilioinguinal approach
Associated both column fractures	• Anterior intrapelvic approach (AIP) • Ilioinguinal approach • Staged posterior approach

Approaches:
- *Anterior approaches*:
  - Ilioinguinal
  - Stoppa
  - Iliofemoral
- *Posterior approach*:
  - Kocher–Langenbeck **(Table 1)**

COMPLICATIONS

The common complications are described in **Table 2**.

TABLE 2: Postoperative complications of acetabular fractures.

Early	• Surgical site infection • Iatrogenic sciatic nerve injury • Heterotopic ossification • Deep vein thrombosis
Late	• Post-traumatic arthritis • Osteonecrosis

REHABILITATION PROTOCOL

- Physiotherapy with passive movements at hip joint is started immediately.
- Assisted ambulation with a walker and minimal/partial weight bearing till (8–12 weeks) can be started depending upon the type of fixation and osteoporosis.
- Full weight-bearing after 12 weeks.

BIBLIOGRAPHY

1. Arbash M, Alzobi OZ, Salameh M, Alkhayarin M, Ahmed G. Incidence, risk factors, and prognosis of sciatic nerve injury in acetabular fractures: a retrospective cross-sectional study. Int Orthop. 2024;48(3):849-56.
2. Azar FM, Beaty JH. Campbell's Operative Orthopaedics, 14th edition, Volume 3. Philadelphia: Elsevier; 2020. p. 2972.
3. Madhu R, Kotnis R, Al-Mousawi A, Barlow N, Deo S, Worlock P, et al. Outcome of surgery for reconstruction of fractures of the acetabulum. The time dependent effect of delay. J Bone Joint Surg Br. 2006;88(9):1197-203.
4. Parvaresh KC, Pennock AT, Bomar JD, Wenger DR, Upasani VV. Analysis of acetabular ossification from the triradiate cartilage and secondary centers. J Pediatr Orthop. 2018;38(3):e145-50.

SECTION

9

Hip and Proximal Femur

Hip Dislocation

Shubhranshu Choudhary

Since the native hip joint is inherently stable and requires much power to dislocate, hip dislocation in native joints frequently results from stressful experiences. 95% of patients who present with a hip dislocation also had an accompanying injury needing treatment. A prosthetic joint has less inherent stability than a native joint, hip dislocations resulting from nonnative or prosthetic hips are more common and can happen even after trivial trauma.

EPIDEMIOLOGY

- The incidence of these injuries is two times higher in women than in males.
- Posterior hip dislocations are far more common than anterior hip dislocations, accounting for 90% of cases.
- Other associated injuries include acetabular fracture, hip/femur fracture, sciatic nerve damage, bone bruise (33%), ipsilateral knee meniscal tears (30%), knee effusion (37%), and labral tear (30%) rate.
- Nonorthopedic injuries are documented to be prevalent in 67% of patients with hip dislocations. These injuries include 24% closed head injuries, 21% craniofacial fractures, 21% thoracic injuries, and 15% abdominal injuries.
- 10–20% of posterior dislocations involve sciatic nerve damage.
- Furthermore, it has been noted that abrupt deceleration forces are linked to posterior hip dislocation, in 8% of cases can have thoracic aortic damage.

ANATOMY

- The hip articulation consists of a ball and socket structure, with the femoral head and acetabulum being congruent to provide stability and bony and ligamentous constraints.
- At any hip motion location, the bony acetabulum covers 40% of the femoral head. The labrum deepens the acetabulum and improves the stability of the joint.
- To limit excessive hip extension, the iliofemoral, pubofemoral, and ischio-femoral ligaments—much stronger ligamentous condensations—supplement the thick longitudinal fibers that comprise the hip joint capsule in a spiral pattern **(Figs. 1A and B)**.
- At the greater sciatic notch, the sciatic nerve leaves the pelvis. There is some variation in how the nerve exists with the piriformis muscle and the short external rotators of the hip. The sciatic nerve often leaves the pelvis deep in the piriformis muscle belly.
- The two anatomic variations of the hip that have been described as predisposing a person to hip dislocation are decreased femoral anteversion and femoroacetabular impingement.

Clinical Significance of Vascular Anatomy

The two most severe and prevalent consequences of hip dislocations are post-

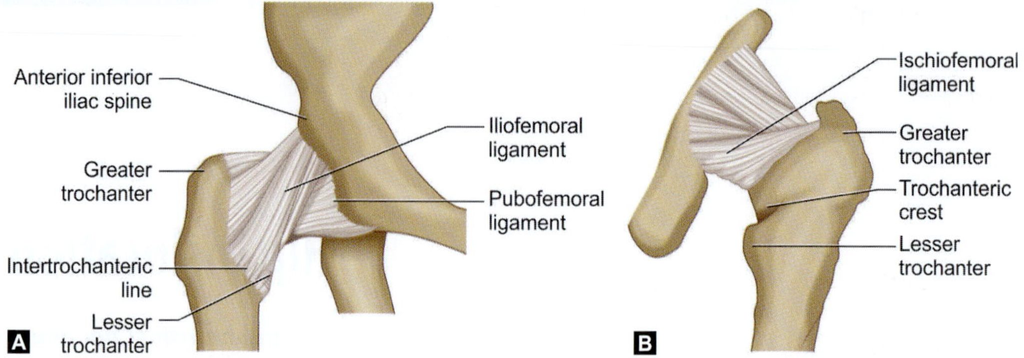

FIGS. 1A AND B: The hip capsule and its thickenings (ligaments) as visualized from anteriorly (A) and posteriorly (B).

Source: Adapted from Bucholz RW, Heckman JD, Court-Brown C, Tornetta P, Koval KJ. Rockwood and Greens Fractures in Adults, 6th edition. Philadelphia: Lippincott Williams & Wilkins; 2006.

traumatic degenerative hip and avascular necrosis of the femoral head. Understanding the reasons behind it requires a thorough understanding of vascular anatomy **(Fig. 2)**. There are three sources of femoral head circulation:

1. The medial and lateral femoral circumflex arteries, which are branches of the profunda femoral artery, provide most of the circulatory supply to the femoral head.
2. At the base of the femoral neck, an extracapsular vascular ring forms, with ascending cervical branches piercing the hip joint at the level of the capsular insertion. These branches climb along the femoral neck and penetrate the bone just inferior to the cartilage of the femoral head.
3. The artery of the ligamentum teres, a branch of the obturator artery, may contribute blood supply to the epiphyseal region of the femoral head. These branches climb along the femoral neck and penetrate the bone just inferior to the cartilage of the femoral head.

Delays in diagnosis and treatment, along with damage to these vessels during dislocation or reduction, can lead to avascular necrosis of the femoral head and, eventually, degenerative arthritis. An incidence of osteoarthrosis of 75% is found in long-term follow-up.

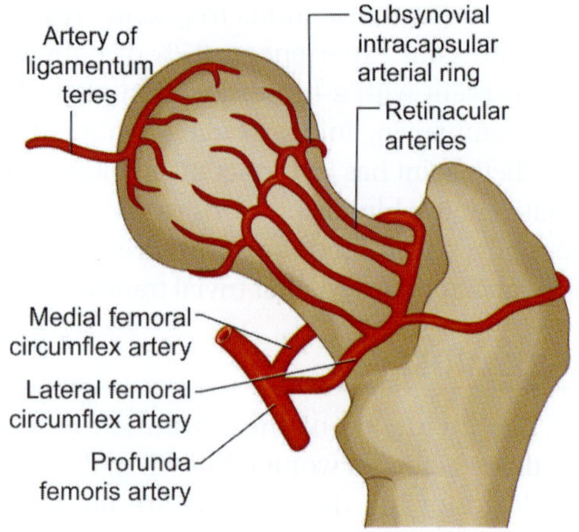

FIG. 2: Blood supply of proximal femur.

MECHANISM OF INJURY

- An object is struck by the anterior portion of the flexed knee (dashboard events).
- With the ipsilateral knee extended, starting at the soles of the feet.
- From the greater trochanter.
- The posterior pelvis is a rare possible source.

The dislocation can be classified as follows: (1) Anterior, (2) Posterior, (3) Central, and (4) any of the dislocations, as mentioned earlier, combined with an acetabulum or femoral head fracture.

Posterior dislocation: Due to high-energy trauma, posterior dislocations with or without fractures are becoming more frequent.

TABLE 1: Direction of hip versus injury pattern.

Flexion, adduction, internal rotation	Pure posterior dislocation
Partial flexion, less adduction, internal rotation	Posterior fracture dislocation
Abduction, extension, ER	Anterior pubic dislocation
Abduction, flexion, ER	Anterior obturator dislocation

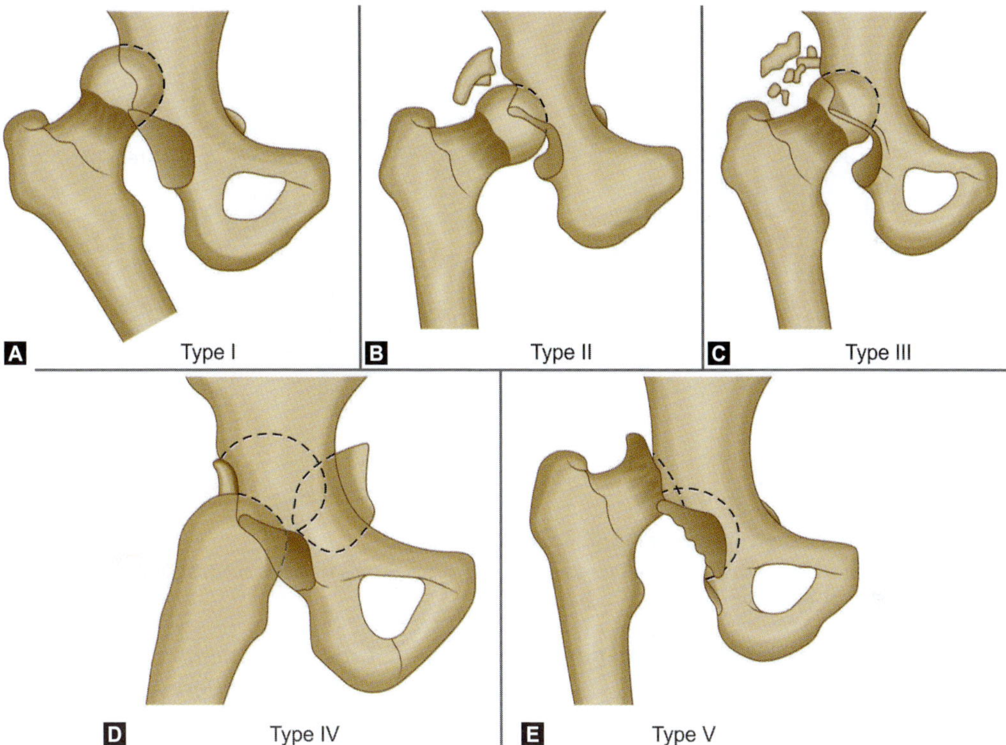

FIGS. 3A TO E: Posterior dislocations of the hip: Type I—with or without minor fracture, type II—with a large single fracture of the posterior acetabular rim, type III—with comminution of the rim of the acetabulum with or without a major fragment, type IV—with a fracture of the acetabular floor, and type V—with a fracture of the femoral head.
Source: Adapted from DeLee JC. Fractures in Adults. In: Rockwood CA Jr, Green DP, editors. Rockwood and Green's Fractures in Adults. 4th ed. Philadelphia: Lippincott Williams & Wilkins; 1996.

The term "dashboard injury" refers to the mechanism of injury, often the longitudinal force imparted to the flexed knee with the hip at varied degrees of flexion. An example is the dashboard striking the knee in a car accident.

Anterior dislocation: Due to the forces of an RTA, when the knee strikes the dashboard with the thigh abducted; a violent fall from the height, forceful blow to the back of the patient in a squatted position.

Central dislocation: It may result from a fall on the sides or a direct blow, as in the case of RTA, on the greater trochanter. It is always linked to acetabulum fractures, which makes treating it very challenging **(Table 1)**.

CLASSIFICATION

Posterior dislocation: It is classified as per Thompson and Epstein classification as described in **Table 2** and **Figure 3**.

Anterior dislocation: It is classified using Epstein classification which is described in **Figure 4** and **Table 3**.

TABLE 2: Thompson and Epstein classification of posterior dislocation.

Type I	Dislocation with or without minor fracture
Type II	Dislocation with single large fracture of the posterior rim of the acetabulum
Type III	Dislocation with comminuted fracture of the rim, with or without a large major fragment
Type IV	Dislocation with fracture of the acetabular floor
Type V	Dislocation with fracture of the femoral head

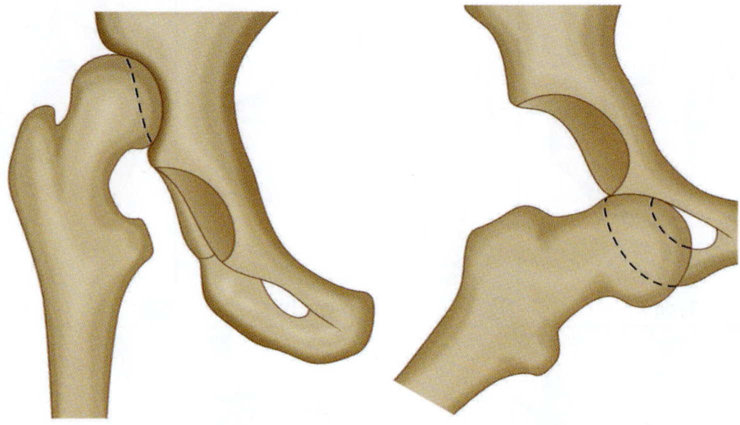

FIG. 4: Epstein classification of anterior hip dislocations.

Source: Adapted from Rockwood CA Jr, Green DP, editors. Rockwood and Green's Fractures in Adults. 3rd ed. Philadelphia: Lippincott-Raven; 1991. pp. 1576–79.

TABLE 3: Epstein classification of anterior hip dislocation.

Type I	Superior dislocations, including pubic and subspinous
IA	No associated fractures
IB	Associated fracture or impaction of the femoral head
IC	Associated fracture of the acetabulum
Type II	Inferior dislocations, including obturator, and perineal
IIA	No associated fractures
IIB	Associated fracture or impaction of the femoral head
IIC	Associated fracture of the acetabulum

Central dislocation: It is classified by Judet's classification system which is described in **Table 4**.

- *Radiographs*:
  - *Recommended views*:
    - Anteroposterior (AP)
    - *Cross-table lateral*:
      - Used to differentiate between anterior versus posterior dislocation
      - Scrutinize the femoral neck to rule out fracture before attempting closed reduction
    - Obtain AP, inlet/outlet, and Judet views after reduction

The important points which should be noted in the initial X-rays are:

- Are the femoral heads symmetric in size?
- Is the joint space symmetric throughout?
- Is the head large (anterior dislocation) or small (posterior dislocation) **(Fig. 5C)**?
- Is the Shenton line maintained or broken?
- Is the greater trochanter prominent (posterior) **(Fig. 5B)** or inconspicuous

TABLE 4: Judet's types.

Type I	Undisplaced fractures (either single-line or stellate types)
Type II	Inner wall fractures
IIA	Femoral head concentrically reduced beneath the dome on initial X-rays
IIB	Femoral head not reduced under the acetabular dome but centrally dislocated
Type III	Superior dome fractures
IIIA	Gross outline of the acetabular dome intact and congruous with the femoral head
IIIB	Gross outline of the acetabular dome not intact and not congruous with the femoral head
Type IV	Bursting fractures (all elements of the acetabulum are involved)
IVA	Fractures in which congruity remains between the femoral head and acetabular dome
IVB	Fractures in which there is incongruity between the femoral head and acetabular dome

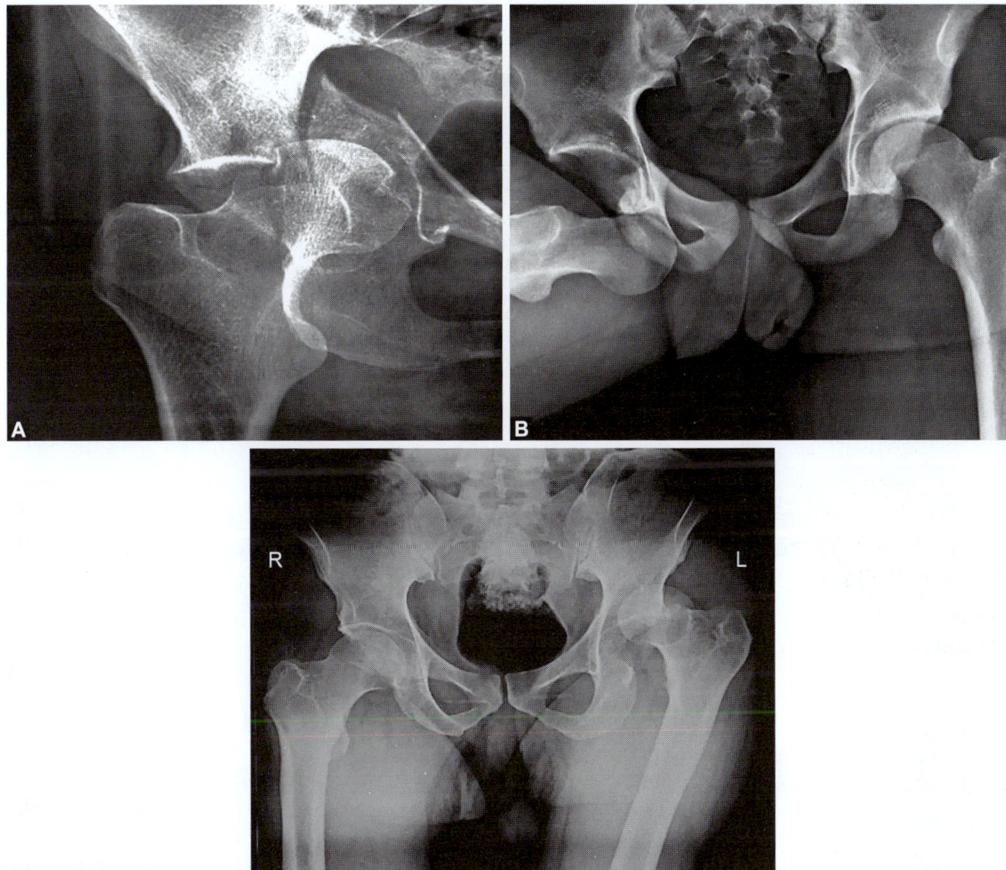

FIGS. 5A TO C: Radiographs showing central (A), anterior (B), and posterior (C) dislocation, respectively.

(anterior) **(Fig. 5A)** reverse with the lesser trochanter **(Figs. 6A and B)**?
- ◦ Is the femoral neck normal?

- *MRI*:
  - ◦ Controversial and routine use is not currently supported.
  - ◦ Useful to evaluate labrum, cartilage, and femoral head vascularity

TREATMENT

The dislocation should be reduced as early as possible under general anesthesia.

Contraindications to close reduction are:

- Ipsilateral displaced or nondisplaced femoral neck fracture

Methods of Reduction

Allis Method

For posterior dislocation, place the patient in the supine position and, stand next to the bed. The knee of the ipsilateral leg is grasped by the surgeon, who then flexes it to 90° using traction in line with the femur while an assistant stabilizes the pelvis against the bed **(Fig. 7)**. Allis's initial description states that there is not any rotation. To enable the femoral head to enter the acetabulum, the doctor gradually extends the hip and externally rotates the leg while the hip reduces.

For anterior dislocation, the surgeon grasps the ipsilateral leg at the knee and applies

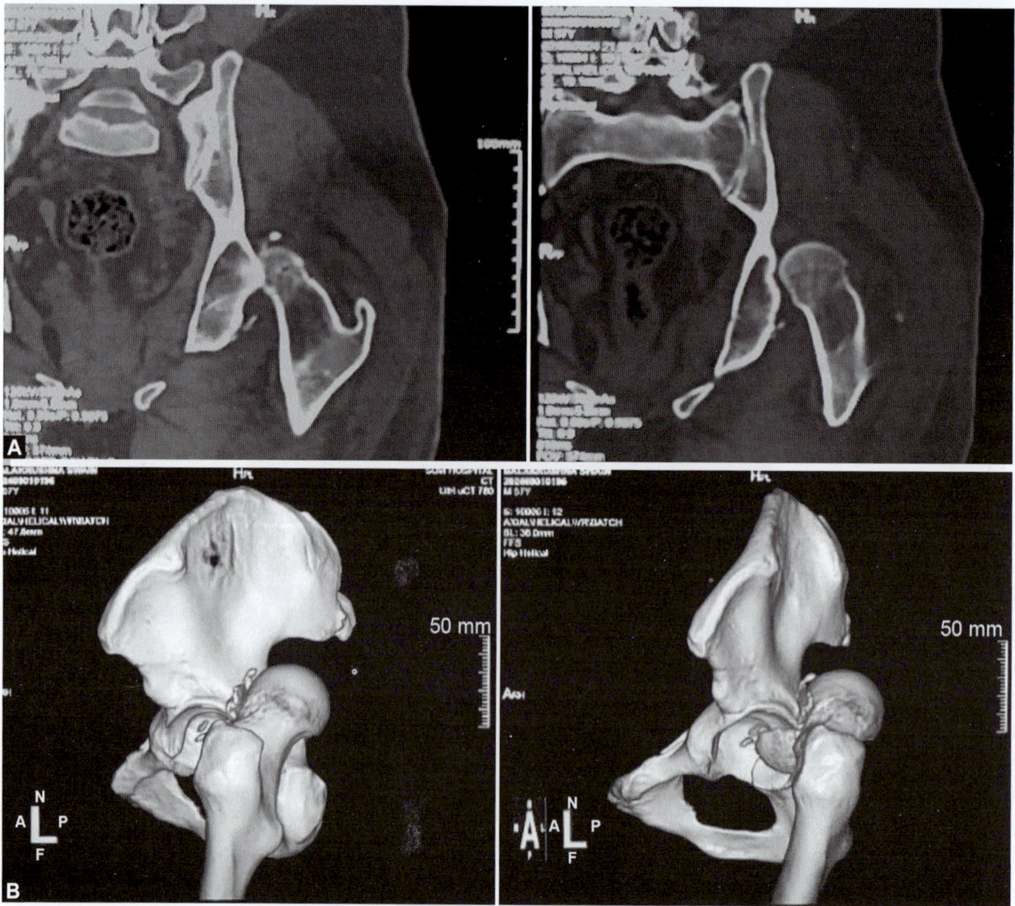

FIGS. 6A AND B: CT showing posterior dislocation of the hip.

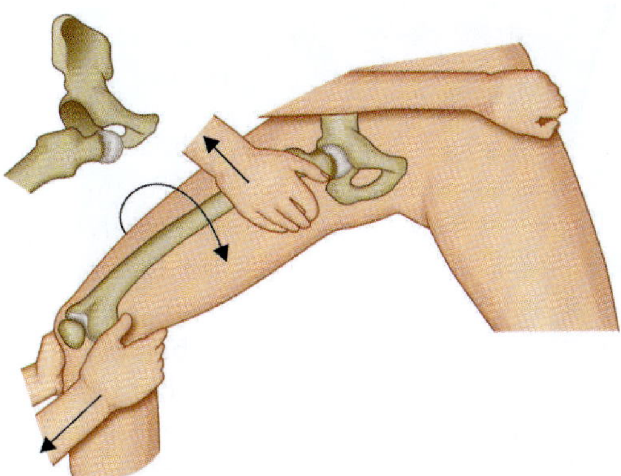

FIG. 7: Allis reduction maneuver for anterior dislocation.

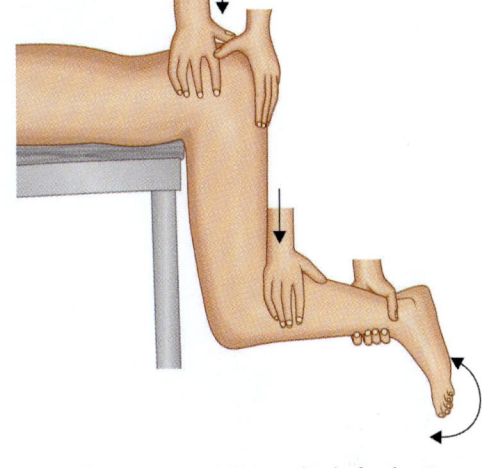

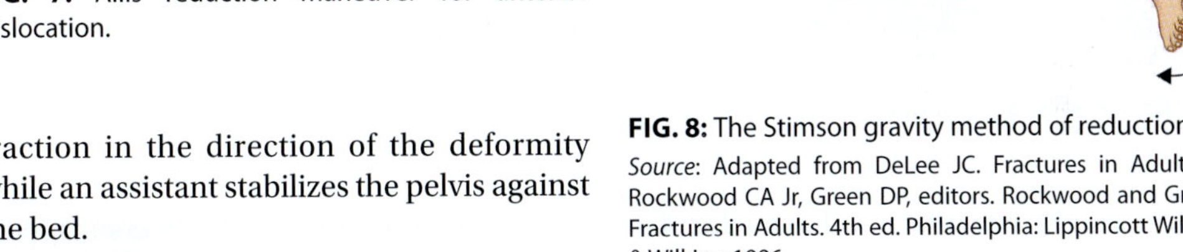

FIG. 8: The Stimson gravity method of reduction.

Source: Adapted from DeLee JC. Fractures in Adults. In: Rockwood CA Jr, Green DP, editors. Rockwood and Green's Fractures in Adults. 4th ed. Philadelphia: Lippincott Williams & Wilkins; 1996.

traction in the direction of the deformity while an assistant stabilizes the pelvis against the bed.

Bigelow and Reverse Bigelow Maneuver

The Bigelow maneuver involves the surgeon placing longitudinal traction on the patient's limb while they are in a supine position. After that, the thigh is internally rotated and adducted to at least 90° of flexion. The hip is then extended, rotated externally, and abducted to lever the femoral head into the acetabulum.

In the reverse Bigelow maneuver, used for anterior dislocations, traction is again applied in the line of the deformity. The hip is then adducted, sharply internally rotated, and extended.

Stimson's Gravity Method

The patient is placed prone on the stretcher with the affected leg hanging off the side of the stretcher. This brings the extremity into a position of hip flexion and knee flexion of 90° each. In this position, the assistant immobilizes the pelvis, and the surgeon applies an anteriorly directed force on the proximal calf. Gentle rotation of the limb may assist in reduction **(Figs. 8 and 9)**.

Postreduction Management

- Following closed reduction, radiographs should be obtained to confirm the adequacy of the reduction.
- The hip should be examined for stability while the patient is still sedated or under anesthesia. If there is an obvious large displaced acetabular fracture, the stability examination need not be performed.
- Stability is checked by flexing the hip to 90° in a neutral position. A posteriorly directed force is then applied. If any sensation of subluxation is detected, the patient will require additional diagnostic studies and possibly surgical exploration or traction.
- Postoperative CT scan is essential to:
    - To assess whether the reduction is concentric or not
    - Detect any osteochondral fragments in the joint
    - Evaluate any fractures of the acetabulum or head of the femur
- Light skin or skeletal traction (5–8 lbs), for 1–2 weeks is recommended

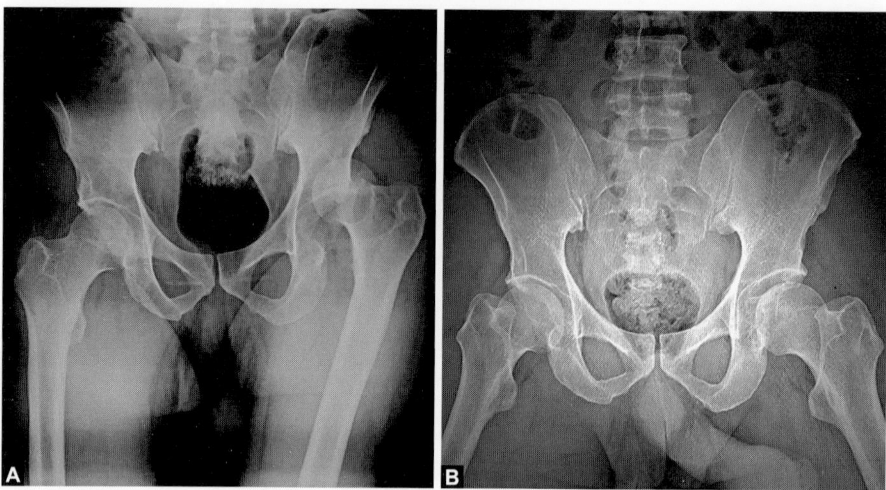

FIGS. 9A AND B: Posterior hip dislocation: (A) Prereduction radiograph, (B) Postreduction radiograph.

- No weight bearing is allowed for 4–8 weeks, then gradually full weight bearing is allowed at 12 weeks.

Operative:
- Open reduction and removal of incarcerated fragments
- *Indications*:
    - Irreducible dislocation
    - Radiographic evidence of incarcerated fragment
    - Delayed presentation
    - Nonconcentric reduction
    - Should be performed on an urgent basis

Open reduction and internal fixation (ORIF):
- *Indications*:
    - Associated fractures of the acetabulum, femoral head, and femoral neck
    - Examining the sciatic nerve, extracting posteriorly impacted fragments, treating significant posterior labral disturbances or instability, and fixing posterior acetabular fractures can all be accomplished using a typical posterior approach (Kocher-Langenbeck).
    - The anterior (Smith-Peterson) technique is advised when dealing with isolated femoral head fractures. Complete vascular disruption is a risk when attempting a posterior dislocation via an anterior route. Injury to the lateral circumflex artery or its branches should be prevented by avoiding the removal of the capsule from the femoral neck and trochanters (i.e., taking down the capsule from the acetabular side).
    - When treating the majority of anterior dislocations and coupled femoral head and neck fractures, anterolateral treatment (Watson-Jones technique) is helpful.
    - It is possible to expose both the anterior and posterior regions through a single incision using a direct lateral (Hardinge) approach.
    - It is not advisable to undertake closed reduction of the hip in the event of an ipsilateral displaced or nondisplaced femoral neck fracture. A lateral technique should be used to stabilize the hip fracture temporarily. A final fixation

of the femoral neck is subsequently carried out after a mild reduction.

COMPLICATIONS

- *Early complications*:
  - Sciatic nerve palsy
  - Superior gluteal artery injury
  - Thrombophlebitis
  - Aseptic necrosis
  - Recurrent central dislocations
- *Delayed complications*:
  - Post-traumatic osteoarthritis is an escapable complication in central dislocation.
  - Myositis ossificans
  - Avascular necrosis of the femoral head
  - A stiff and disabling hip

BIBLIOGRAPHY

1. Dawson-Amoah K, Raszewski J, Duplantier N, Waddell BS. Dislocation of the Hip: A Review of Types, Causes, and Treatment. Ochsner J. 2018;18(3):242-52.
2. Nicholson JA, Scott CEH, Annan J, Ahmed I, Keating JF. Native hip dislocation at acetabular fracture predicts poor long-term outcomes. Injury. 2018;49(10):1841-7.
3. Schmidt GL, Sciulli R, Altman GT. Knee injury in patients experiencing a high-energy traumatic ipsilateral hip dislocation. J Bone Joint Surg Am. 2005;87(6):1200-4.
4. Suraci AJ. Distribution and severity of injuries associated with hip dislocations secondary to motor vehicle accidents. J Trauma. 1986;26(5):458-60.

Femoral Head Fracture

Shubhranshu Choudhary

Femoral head fracture occurs mostly in young people, making up about two-thirds of the patient population, and associated injuries are very common, occurring in up to 75% of cases.

EPIDEMIOLOGY

- Nearly all have a history of hip dislocations.
- 10% of posterior hip dislocations are complicated by these fractures.
- Between 25 and 75% of anterior hip dislocations are linked to indentation fractures.

APPLIED ANATOMY

70% of the femoral head articular surface is involved in load transfer; damage to this surface may result in nontraumatic arthritis.

Clinical assessment:

- Lower limb deformity with associated hip dislocation
- The ipsilateral knee ligamentous stability, needs to be evaluated, as it can be an associated injury
- *Neurovascular status*: There could be indications of sciatic nerve damage.

RADIOGRAPHIC EVALUATION

- *Radiographs*:
  - *Recommended views*:
    - Anteroposterior (AP) pelvis, hip series:
      - Both pre-reduction and post-reduction
    - Judet views:
      - Associated acetabular fracture
    - Inlet and outlet views to see associated pelvic ring injury
- *CT scan*:
  - *Indications*:
    - Post-reduction to evaluate for loose bodies and the presence/size of fracture fragments
  - *Findings*:
    - Femoral head fracture (size, location, comminution)
    - Plane of femoral head fracture
    - Intra-articular fragments
    - Posterior pelvic ring injury
    - Impaction
    - Acetabular fracture

CLASSIFICATIONS

Type V posterior fracture dislocation occurs in 6–7% of posterior dislocations.

- *Pipkin classification*: Pipkin classified this type of fracture into four types **(Figs. 1 to 4) (Table 1)**.
- *Other classification*:
  - Brumback et al. classification

TREATMENT

Pipkin type I: The femoral head fracture is inferior to the fovea. These fractures occur in the nonweight-bearing surface.

- Closed treatment is advised if the hip is stable and the reduction is sufficient (<1 mm step-off).
- If the reduction is insufficient, open reduction and internal fixation using small subarticular screws via an anterior approach are advised.
- If small fragments do not compromise stability, they may be removed.

Pipkin type II: The femoral head fracture is superior to the fovea. These fractures involve the weight-bearing surface.

- The guidelines for the nonoperative management of type II fractures are the same as those for type I fractures, except that anatomic reduction, as seen on CT and follow-up radiographs, is the only one that can be accepted for nonoperative care.
- Open reduction and internal fixation are typically the preferred treatments through an anterior approach.

Pipkin type III: A femoral head fracture occurs with an associated fracture of the femoral neck.

- The degree of dislocation of the femoral neck fracture affects the prognosis, which is poor.
- In younger patients, internal fixation of the femoral head is carried out after emergency open reduction and internal fixation of the femoral neck. Anterolateral (Watson–Jones) approaches can be used for this.
- Prosthetic replacement is recommended for elderly patients with displaced femoral neck fractures.

Pipkin type IV: A femoral head fracture occurs with an associated acetabulum fracture.

- The acetabular fracture should guide the surgical approach, and the femoral head fracture, even if nondisplaced, should be internally stabilized to allow for early hip joint motion.

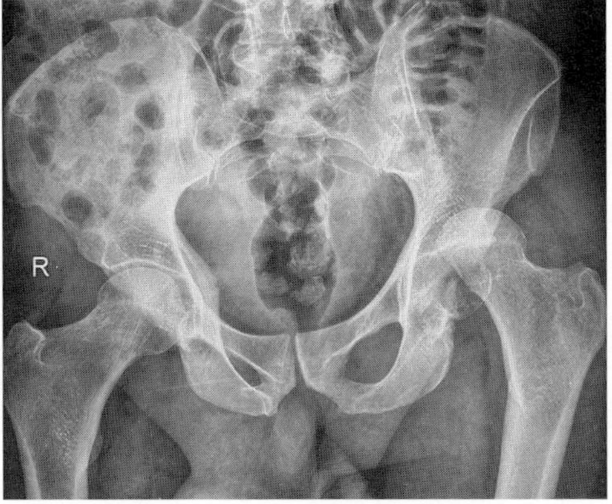

FIG. 1: Radiograph showing femoral head fracture.

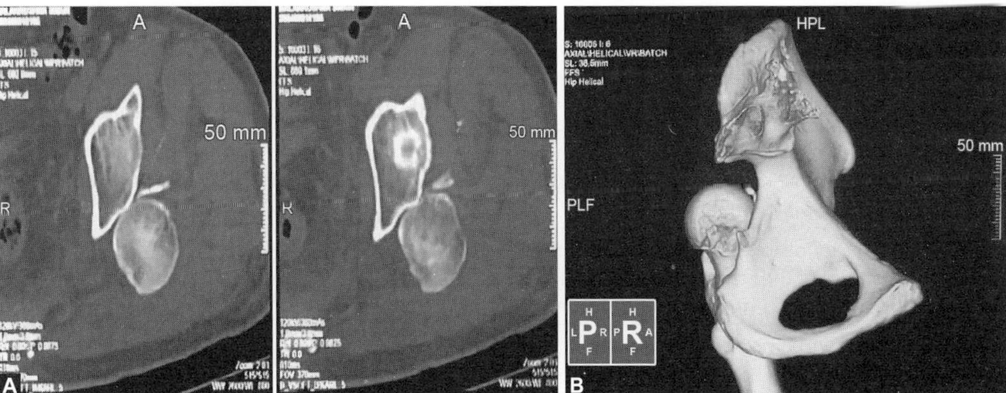

FIGS. 2A AND B: CT scan showing femoral head fracture.

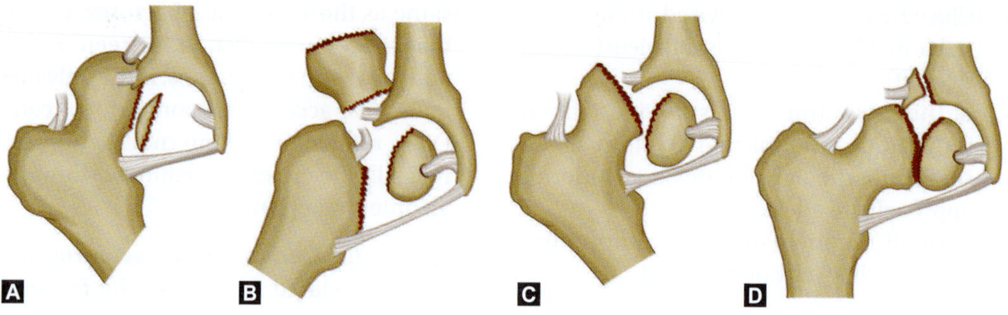

FIGS. 3A TO D: Pipkin classification.

Source: Adapted from DeLee JC. Fractures in adults. In: Rockwood CA, Green DP, editors. *Rockwood and Green's fractures in adults*. Philadelphia: Lippincott Williams and Wilkins; 1996.

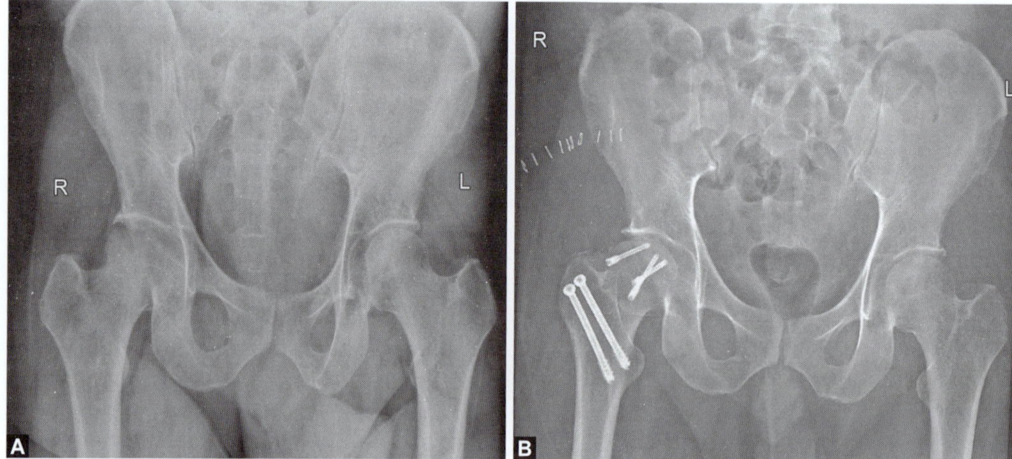

FIGS. 4A AND B: Pipkin type II fracture: (A) Preoperative radiograph of Pipkin type II fracture; (B) ORIF done for Pipkin type II fracture.

(ORIF: open reduction and internal fixation)

TABLE 1: Pipkin's classification of fracture head.

Type I	Posterior dislocation of the hip with fracture of the femoral head caudad to the fovea centralis
Type II	Posterior dislocation of the hip with fracture of the femoral head cephalad to the fovea centralis
Type III	Type I and type II with associated fracture of the femoral neck
Type IV	Type I, II, or III with associated fracture of the acetabulum

- This fracture must be treated concurrently with the concomitant acetabular fracture.

Femoral Head Fractures Associated with Anterior Dislocations

- Managing these fractures is challenging.
- Although indentation fractures, usually found on the superior aspect of the femoral head, do not need special care, the fractures' position, and size impact prognosis.

Depending on the size and position of the fragment, open reduction and either excision or internal fixation are necessary for displaced transchondral fractures that produce a nonconcentric reduction.

Surgical Approaches

- *Anterior approach (Smith-Petersen)*: Provides direct access to the anterior aspect of the hip and is often used for type I fractures or when approaching an anterior acetabular fracture.
- *Posterior approach (Kocher-Langenbeck)*: Commonly used for posteriorly displaced and type II fractures involving the weight-bearing portion of the femoral head. This approach allows good visualization for acetabular involvement as well.
- *Surgical dislocation technique*: This technique, developed by Ganz, is often used in complex cases as it allows complete visualization of the femoral head and acetabulum while minimizing the risk of avascular necrosis (AVN).

Additional Considerations

- *Timing*: Prompt surgical treatment is often critical to prevent complications like AVN and post-traumatic arthritis.
- *Postoperative care*: Weight-bearing restrictions, physical therapy, and close follow-up are essential for optimal recovery.

COMPLICATIONS

- *Osteonecrosis*: 10% of patients with anterior dislocations develop osteonecrosis. Risk factors include a time delay in reduction and repeated reduction attempts.
- *Post-traumatic osteoarthritis*: Risk factors include transchondral fracture, indentation fracture greater than 2 mm in depth, and osteonecrosis.
- *Heterotopic ossification*:
    - The overall incidence is 30–40%.
    - The anterior approach has increased heterotopic ossification compared with the posterior approach.

BIBLIOGRAPHY

1. Alonso JE, Volgas DA, Giordano V, Stannard JP. A review of the treatment of hip dislocations associated with acetabular fractures. Clin Orthop Rel Res. 2000;377:32-43.
2. Giordano V, Costa PRL, Esteves JD, Félix S Junior J, Franklin CE, Amaral NP. Luxações traumáticas do quadril em pacientes esqueleticamente maduros. Rev Bras Ortop. 2003;38(8):462-72.
3. Özcan M, Çopuro!glu C, Sarido!gan K. Fractures of the femoral head: what are the reasons for poor outcome? Turk J Trauma Emerg Surg. 2011;17(1):51-6.
4. Sen RK, Tripathy SK, Goyal T, Aggarwal S, Kashyap S, Purudappa PP, et al. Complications and Functional Outcome of Femoral Head Fracture-Dislocation In Delayed and Neglected Cases. Indian J Orthop. 2021;55(3):595-605.
5. Stannard JP, Harris HW, Volgas DA, Alonso JE. Functional outcome of patients with femoral head fractures associated with hip dislocations. Clin Orthop Relat Res. 2000;377:44-56.

Femoral Neck Fracture

Apoorva Kabra, Samarth Mittal

Femoral neck fractures (FNFs) have a bimodal age distribution being prevalent in the elderly population (osteoporosis and low-energy falls) and following high-energy trauma like road traffic accident (RTA) in young adults.

- In the young, patients' complications (avascular necrosis and nonunion) following a neck femur fracture can have significant morbidity.
- In the elderly, the patients need to return to mobility as early as possible, to avoid the morbidity (especially cardiopulmonary complications) and mortality.

APPLIED ANATOMY

- Intra-articular (within the joint capsule) nature differentiates its management significantly compared to the adjacent trochanteric region.
- The femoral neck has a relatively poor blood supply compared to other bones. The primary blood supply comes from the medial and lateral circumflex femoral arteries, which provide blood through the retinacular vessels.
- *Chief arterial supply*: Medial circumflex femoral artery. Ascending cervical arteries are at risk, especially in displaced fractures.
- This blood supply is easily compromised during a fracture, especially when the fracture is displaced. The lack of collateral circulation means that if these vessels are disrupted, the bone's ability to receive necessary nutrients and oxygen is severely impaired, increasing the risk of avascular necrosis and nonunion.

Complexity of the Femoral Neck Fracture

- The femoral neck is located within the hip joint capsule, which creates an environment with higher intra-articular pressure. This pressure can impede blood flow and slow the healing process.
- Additionally, the synovial fluid within the joint capsule can interfere with fracture healing by washing away the early bone healing matrix, such as hematomas, that forms at the fracture site. This matrix is crucial for the initial stages of bone healing.
- The periosteum is a two-layered membrane covering the bones' outer surface, with the cambium layer as the inner layer. This layer contains osteoprogenitor cells (precursors to osteoblasts) that are essential for bone growth, repair, and remodeling. This layer is absent in the femoral neck region.
- *Biomechanics*: The major concern in neck of femur fractures is with regards to the mechanical forces at the fracture site. Shear forces are predominant in vertical fractures and these are almost perpendicular to the (compression) forces needed at the fracture site for promoting union **(Figs. 1A and B)**.

COMMON CLASSIFICATION SYSTEMS

Classification systems for neck of femur fractures are crucial in guiding treatment and predicting outcomes. Here, we delve into four widely recognized classifications: (1) anatomical, (2) Garden, (3) Pauwels, and (4) the AO/OTA classification.

Anatomical Classification

- Anatomical classification categorizes neck of femur fractures based on the location of the fracture along the femoral neck like **(Figs. 2A to C)**:
  1. *Subcapital fractures* occur just below the head of the femur.
  2. *Transcervical fractures* are located along the mid portion of the femoral neck.

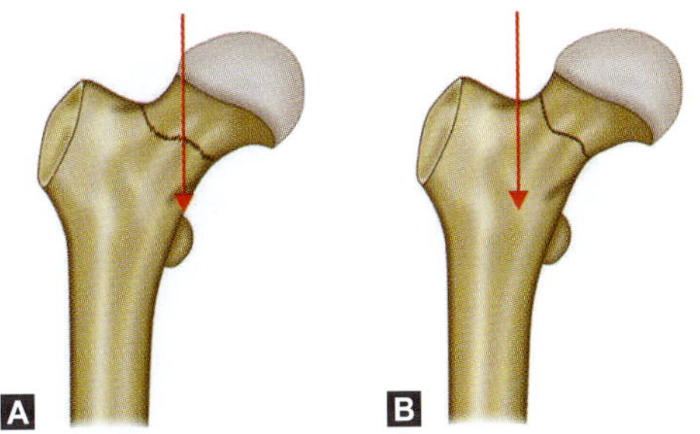

FIGS. 1A AND B: Forces acting at the fracture site. In Figure A, the body weight provides a significant amount of compression force across the fracture site (red arrow). In Figure B, the vertical fracture line has almost no significant compression force across it, in turn creating a shearing force at the fracture site.

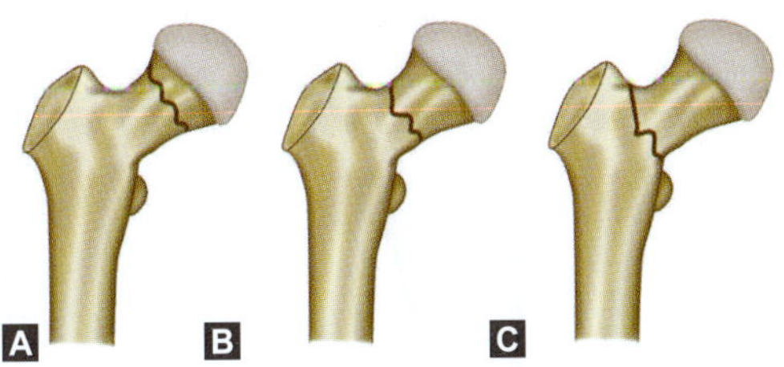

FIGS. 2A TO C: Schematic diagram of anatomical classification of femoral neck fracture—(A) subcapital fracture, (B) transcervical fracture, and (C) basicervical fracture.

  3. *Basicervical fractures* involve the base of the neck near the intersection with the trochanters.
- *Drawback*: This does not consider fracture displacement.

Garden Classification

- The Garden classification system is primarily focused on the displacement of the fracture, which is directly correlated with the disruption of the blood supply to the femoral head and subsequent risk for avascular necrosis **(Figs. 3A to D)**. It consists of four grades:
  - *Type I—incomplete or valgus impacted fractures*: These are typically undisplaced, with the bone valgus impacted into itself.
  - *Type II—complete but undisplaced*: The fracture goes through the entire neck but does not move out of its normal anatomical position.
  - *Type III—complete with partial displacement*: The bone ends partially shift out of alignment, jeopardizing the stability and blood supply.
  - *Type IV—complete and fully displaced*: There is no contact between the fractured ends, leading to a high risk of complications including nonunion and avascular necrosis.
- *Drawback*: Does not consider fracture location on the neck.

Pauwels Classification

- The Pauwels classification system categorizes FNFs based on the angle of the fracture line to the horizontal **(Fig. 4)**. This angle is crucial as it influences the mechanical stress on the fracture site during healing. The classification includes:
  - *Type I*: Fractures with an angle up to 30°, these are generally stable and have a good prognosis as the shear forces are minimal.

- *Type II*: Fractures with an angle between 30° and 50°, these fractures experience more shear forces which may impair healing.
- *Type III*: Fractures with an angle >50°, these are highly unstable and prone to nonunion and avascular necrosis due to the high degree of shear forces.
- *Drawback*: Has a large amount of inter- and intraobserver variability.

AO/OTA Classification

- This system categorizes fractures based on the anatomic location of the fracture and the extent of the fracture through the bone. It is useful for determining the stability of the fracture and potential complications.

Overall, the key aspect to note about neck femur fractures is that subcapital fracture and fracture with high pauwels angle has got

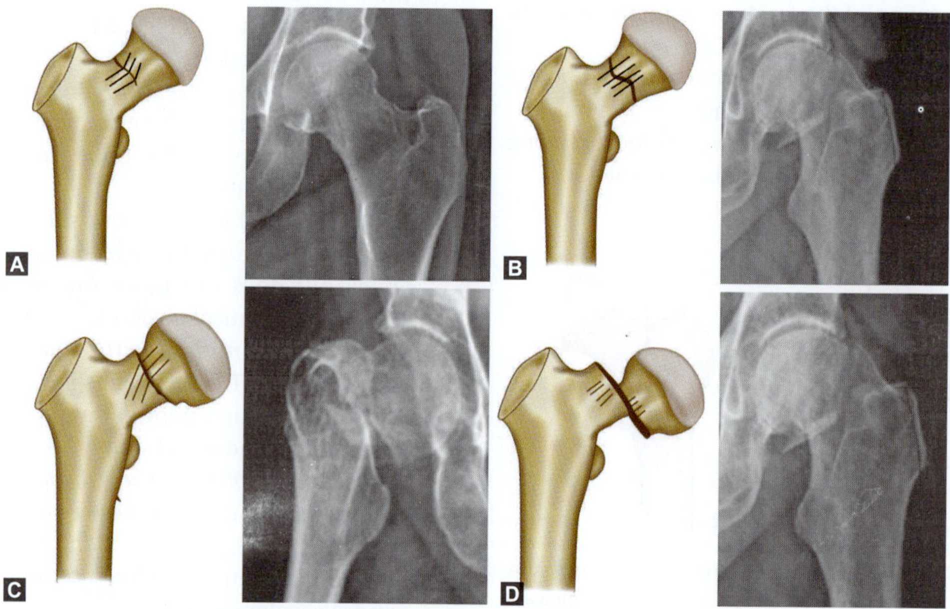

FIGS. 3A TO D: Garden's classification.

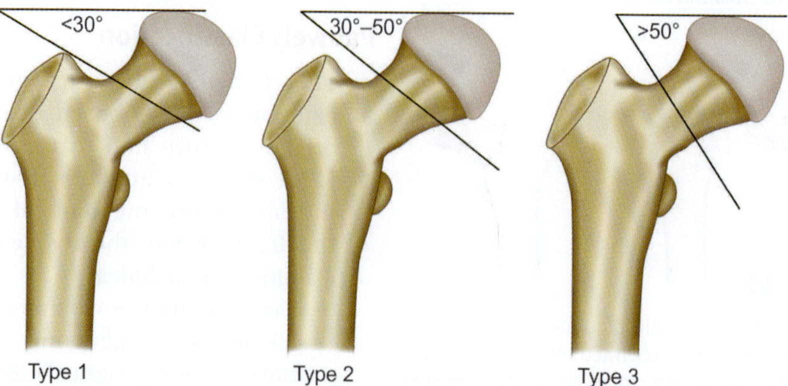

FIG. 4: Schematic diagram of Pauwels classification.

poor prognosis even after good reduction and fixation due to greater disruption of blood vessels at the time of initial injury.

Typically, the injured leg may appear shortened and externally rotated due to muscle forces pulling on the fracture fragments.

- *X-rays*:
  - *Standard views*: Anteroposterior (AP) pelvis and cross-table lateral of the hip are essential. Often the fracture may be missed if the AP view is not done with the leg in 15° internal rotation. A good understanding of the X-rays is a must to identify adequate reduction of the fracture **(Fig. 5)**.
- *Computed tomography (CT)*:
  - A CT scan is particularly useful in cases where the fracture details are not clearly visible on X-rays. It also provides a detailed view of the fracture configuration, including comminution and Pauwels angle of the fracture. This is helpful in surgical planning, especially for complex fractures (comminution).
- *Magnetic resonance imaging (MRI)*: While not routinely used, MRI may be indicated in cases where there is a suspicion of occult fractures/stress fractures where X-rays and CT scans are inconclusive.

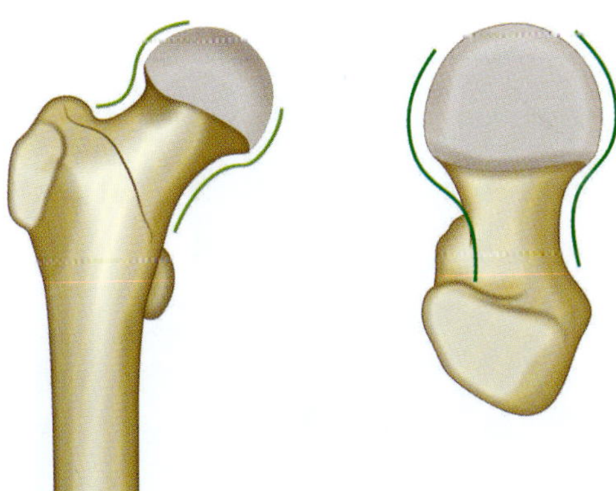

FIG. 5: Schematic diagram of Lowells "S" in anteroposterior and lateral suggestive of anatomical reduction.

MANAGEMENT

- The management of intracapsular FNFs is guided by the fracture's characteristics—whether it is displaced or nondisplaced—and patient-specific factors such as age, mobility, and overall health.
- The goal of management differs based on the patients age group. In younger individuals, open reduction and internal fixation must be attempted with a goal of preservation of the femoral head.
- Whereas, in the elderly population, the goal of treatment is early mobilization and weight bearing which can be achieved by replacement surgeries.
- *Management options*: Reduction (closed/open) followed by internal fixation:
  - *Closed reduction maneuvers* **(Fig. 6)**:
    - *Whitman's method*:
      - *Procedure:* This method involves initial traction, followed by internal rotation and abduction.
      - This method can be used in the extension of the fracture table.
    - *Leadbetter's method*:
      - *Procedure:* Traction is combined with a series of hip movements including flexion, internal rotation, full flexion, abduction, and external rotation.
      - This method is noted as the most successful one.
  - *Open reduction*:
    - In cases when closed reduction is not deemed satisfactory, open reduction must be undertaken.
    - The key aspect in neck femur fracture management in the young is accurate reduction. No compromise must be made with the reduction.
    - The hip can be approached by any of the defined approaches, however,

anterior (Smith-Peterson) or the lateral approaches are usually preferred.
- Visualization of the neck is best via the anterior approach, however, placement of a dynamic hip screws (DHS)/femoral neck system (FNS) or screws may not be possible via this approach and another incision will be needed for the same.
- In patients where open reduction is done, a small plate over the medial aspect of the neck can be placed in the buttress mode. This has been shown to have improved outcomes when compared with DHS/CCS alone.

○ *Internal fixation devices* ***(Figs. 7A to D)***:
- No clear consensus on the best device for fixation.
- However, fixed angle constructs (DHS/FNS) have been shown to have better outcomes when compared with CCS.
- A derotation screw placed along with an DHS provides the strongest construct with a downside of increased surgical time and blood loss.
- This, however, has been mitigated with the development of the FNS. FNS has an in-built antirotation screw and is usually available in

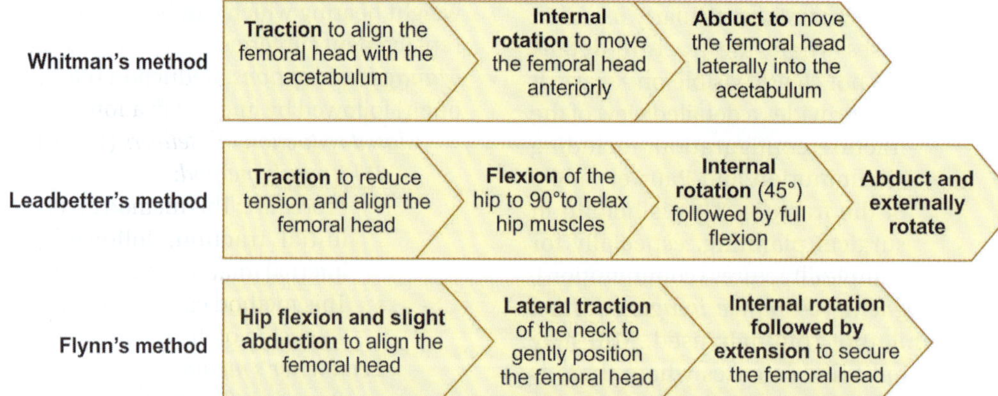

FIG. 6: Closed reduction maneuvers for fracture neck femur.

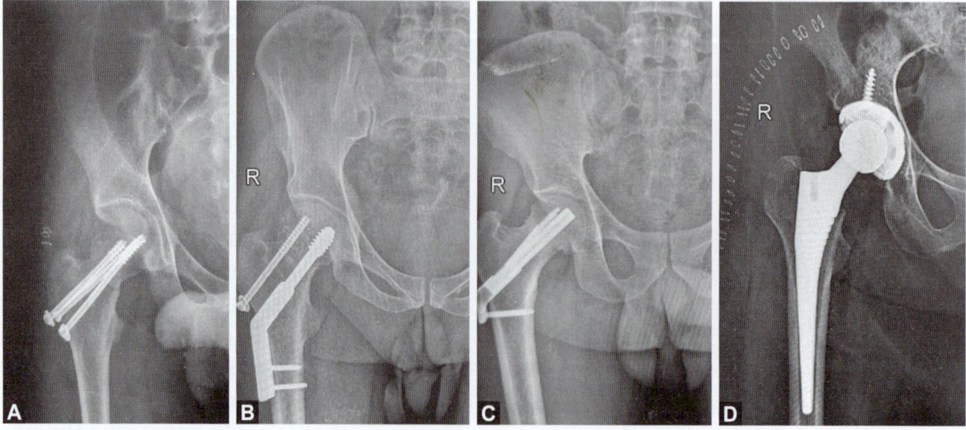

FIGS. 7A TO D: Various fixation options for fracture of neck of femur.

a one/two screw plate size. It has a central barrel which provides fixation in the femoral head across the fracture.
- However, further studies are warranted to determine if FNS is as stable as DHS as a construct for displaced neck femur fractures, especially in middle-aged patients.

The best configuration for screw placement in a FNF depends on factors like the fracture pattern, patient anatomy, and surgeon preference. However, a few widely accepted principles guide screw placement for optimal stability and outcomes:

- *Inverted triangle or triangular configuration*:
  - This configuration typically involves three screws placed in an inverted triangle, which is one of the most commonly used and studied arrangements.
  - *Screw placement*:
    - *Superior screw:* Placed close to the superior cortex, offering stability against varus collapse
    - *Inferior screw:* Positioned near the calcar, which is the thick cortical bone near the medial aspect of the femoral neck, providing rotational stability and support against compression forces.
    - *Posterior screw:* Positioned posteriorly to add further rotational stability
  - The screws should be parallel to each other and avoid penetrating the joint surface. The tips should ideally converge toward the subchondral bone just below the femoral head.
- *Diamond configuration (quadrilateral)*:
  - This method involves placing four screws, providing additional rotational stability, particularly for comminuted fractures.
  - *Screw placement*:
    - Screws are placed in two rows, with one pair superior and one pair inferior, arranged in a quadrilateral pattern.
    - Ensures even more stability, but is technically more challenging to achieve.
- *Medial calcar support*:
  - The inferior screw should be positioned close to the medial calcar (cortical bone), as it is a key area for structural support.
  - This can help prevent varus collapse, which is a common complication in FNFs.
- *Avoidance of the central part of the neck*: Avoid placing screws in the central portion of the neck, as this area is relatively weak. Instead, screws should be placed to optimize cortical support.
- *Angle of screw placement*:
  - The screws should generally be placed at 130–135° relative to the femoral shaft axis.
  - Cannulated screws are often preferred for their ease of placement and the ability to achieve accurate positioning through guidewires.

Arthroplasty: Arthroplasty is the choice of surgery for osteoporotic patients **(Fig. 7D)**. The choice between hemiarthroplasty and total hip arthroplasty is based on numerous factors (patient age, cognitive status, life expectancy, etc.). These factors will be discussed in the subsequent section.

*Algorithm for planning management **(Flowchart 1)***: The algorithm divides treatment options into two primary categories based on the displacement of the fracture:

1. *Nondisplaced fractures (all age groups)*:
   - Fixation is typically recommended to prevent displacement and promote healing.

- Surgical options include cannulated screws, DHS or the FNS, or screws depending on the exact nature and location of the fracture.

2. *Displaced fractures*:
   - *Younger patients (physiological age < 60 years)*:
     - *No osteoporosis risk*: Reduction and internal fixation to restore the anatomy and function of the hip, as their bones generally have better healing potential.
   - *Middle-aged patients (physiological age 40–60 years)*:
     - *With osteoporosis risk/chronic alcohol use*: Total hip arthroplasty may be considered, especially if they are active and have good bone quality to support the prosthesis.
   - *Older patients (physiological age ≥ 60 years)*:
     - *Independently mobile*: For those who are active and have no major cognitive impairments or medical comorbidities, a total hip replacement is typically recommended.
     - *Limited mobility or cognitive impairment*: Hemiarthroplasty may be preferred as it involves less extensive surgery and is generally sufficient for patients with limited mobility expectations.
     - *Institutional care or severe comorbidities*: May be considered for unipolar hemiarthroplasty, focusing on pain relief and minimal mobility restoration to improve quality of life.

Considerations in Management

- *Surgical timing*: The goal of hip fracture management dictates that they be fixed within the first 6–24 hours in most cases. In rare instances, relaxation up to 48 hours can be made due to patient/equipment/logistical constraints.
- *Postoperative mobilization and weight bearing*: In patients who have undergone internal fixation in young patients—6 weeks of nonweight-bearing mobilization must be followed by a further 6 weeks of partial weight bearing. Patients are usually expected to mobilize without support by

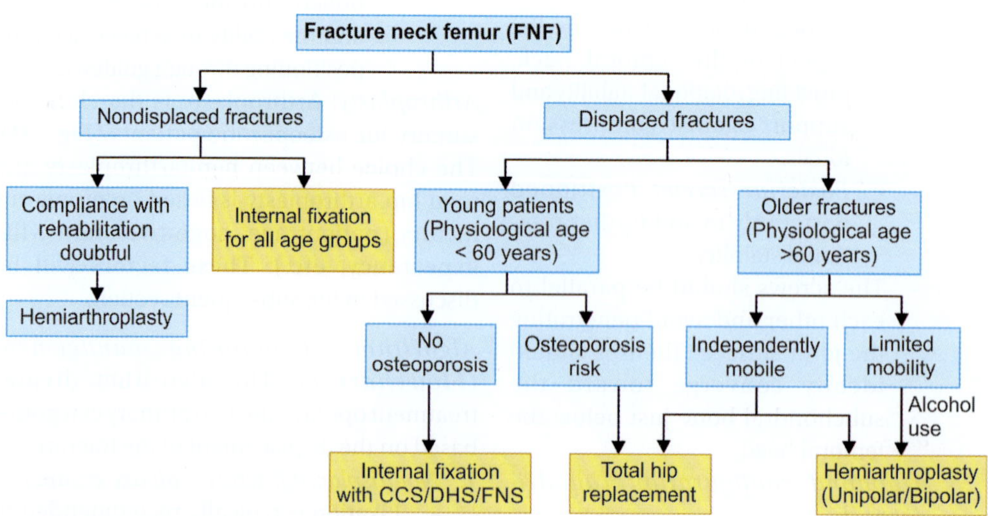

FLOWCHART 1: Algorithm for neck femur management.
(DHS: dynamic hip screws; FNS: femoral neck system)

3 months and return to preinjury activity levels by 6–12 months. Whereas in old patients, full weight bearing from the next day of surgery should be the target.

COMPLICATIONS AND THEIR MANAGEMENT

The major complications include nonunion and avascular necrosis in addition to wound-related and implant-related complications (dislocations in case of THA).

- *Nonunion*:
  - Nonunion is a significant complication following FNFs.
  - *Risk factors*: Malreduction, inadequate stabilization, poor blood supply, and initial displacement of the fracture.
  - *Management*:
    - Revision surgery may be necessary, which could involve an osteotomy (valgus osteotomy) and internal fixation with a more robust construct along with bone grafting to promote healing.
- *Avascular necrosis (AVN)*:
  - *Risk factors*: Displacement of the fracture and damage to vascular supply during injury or surgery.
  - *Management*:
    - *Surgical options*: Depending on the extent of necrosis, treatment might involve bisphosphonates and restriction of weight bearing in early stages, core decompression to reduce pressure and stimulate blood flow prior to head collapse/crescent sign development, or joint replacement if the damage is extensive.

  Elderly patients require a holistic approach to manage the complications associated with neck of femur fractures effectively, focusing not only on the surgical or immediate clinical needs but also on long-term functional and psychological outcomes.
- *Hip dislocation*:
  - *Description*: Postoperative dislocation of the hip is a notable risk, especially after total hip replacement following a FNF. This is more common when compared with nontraumatic indications.
  - *Risk factors*: Advanced age, muscle weakness, poor soft tissue tension, fracture-related capsular injury, improper implant position, and noncompliance with postoperative precautions.
  - *Management*:
    - Initial management of a dislocated hip may involve closed reduction under anesthesia, followed by immobilization.
    - *Revision surgery*: If dislocations recur, surgical intervention to correct the position of the implants or replace the prosthesis may be necessary.
- *General complications in the elderly*: In addition to specific surgical complications, elderly patients are at an increased risk for systemic complications due to immobilization and prolonged recovery periods:
  - *Deep vein thrombosis (DVT) and pulmonary embolism (PE)*: Prophylactic measures include anticoagulation therapy, mechanical compression devices, and early mobilization.
  - *Pneumonia and urinary tract infections (UTIs)*: Due to decreased mobility and general vulnerability, maintaining good respiratory and personal hygiene, along with adequate hydration, is crucial.
  - *Muscle atrophy and loss of independence*: Early physiotherapy and occupational therapy are vital to maintaining muscle tone and supporting independent living as much as possible.

CONCLUSION

- Neck of femur fractures are associated with a high rate of complications, affecting approximately one-fourth of patients.
- A significant contributor to these adverse outcomes, including nonunion and avascular necrosis, is often linked to inadequate fracture reduction.
- Achieving anatomical reduction is critical; therefore, the orthopedic community emphasizes striving for 100% accuracy in reduction alignment.
- When perfect reduction is in doubt, surgical protocols recommend an open reduction to directly visualize and correctly align the fracture fragments.
- In the pursuit of enhancing clinical outcomes, novel treatment devices have been introduced, such as the FNS, which has shown promising initial results in providing stable fixation with minimal invasiveness.
- Although early data is encouraging, longer-term and more comprehensive studies are necessary to fully establish the efficacy and safety of such devices.
- Additionally, the application of a medial support plate in cases where open reduction is performed has been noted to improve outcomes.
- This technique offers additional stability, particularly in unstable or comminuted fractures, by providing medial cortical support, which is crucial in load-bearing areas of the hip.

BIBLIOGRAPHY

1. Borges FK, Bhandari M, Guerra-Farfan E, Patel A, Sigamani A, Umer M, et al. Accelerated surgery versus standard care in hip fracture (HIP ATTACK): an international, randomised, controlled trial. Lancet. 2020;395(10225):698-708.
2. Collinge CA, Harris P, Sagi HC, Rodriguez-Buitrago A, Beltran MJ, Mitchell PM, et al. Comparative Analysis of Supplemental Medial Buttress Plate Fixation for High-Energy Displaced Femoral Neck Fractures in Young Adults. J Orthop Trauma. 2023;37(5):207-13.
3. Gausden EB, Cross WW, Mabry TM, Pagnano MW, Berry DJ, Abdel MP. Total Hip Arthroplasty for Femoral Neck Fracture: What Are the Contemporary Reasons for Failure? J Arthroplasty. 2021;36(7):S272-6.
4. Hoskins W, Rainbird S, Peng Y, Graves SE, Bingham R. Hip Hemiarthroplasty for Fractured Neck of Femur Revised to Total Hip Arthroplasty: Outcomes Are Influenced by Patient Age Not Articulation Options. J Arthroplasty. 2021;36(8):2927-35.
5. Johnell O, Kanis JA. An estimate of the worldwide prevalence and disability associated with osteoporotic fractures. Osteoporos Int. 2006;17(12):1726-33.
6. Kazley J, Bagchi K. (2023). Femoral Neck Fractures. [online] Available from https://www.ncbi.nlm.nih.gov/books/NBK537347/. [Last accessed November, 2024]
7. Kazley JM, Banerjee S, Abousayed MM, Rosenbaum AJ. Classifications in Brief: Garden Classification of Femoral Neck Fractures. Clin Orthop Relat Res. 2018;476(2):441.
8. Liu P, Zhang Y, Sun B, Chen H, Dai J, Yan L. Risk factors for femoral neck fracture in elderly population. Zhong Nan Da Xue Xue Bao Yi Xue Ban. 2021;46(3):272-7.
9. Major LJ, North JB. Predictors of mortality in patients with femoral neck fracture. J Orthop Surg (Hong Kong). 2016;24(2):150-2.
10. Max Hoshino C, O'Toole RV. Fixed angle devices versus multiple cancellous screws: what does the evidence tell us? Injury. 2015;46(3):474-7.
11. Nand S. Revisiting Pauwels' classification of femoral neck fractures. World J Orthop. 2021;12(11):811.
12. National Institute for Health and Care Excellence (NICE). (2023). Hip fracture: management. [online] Available from https://www.ncbi.nlm.nih.gov/books/NBK553768/. [Last accessed November, 2024]
13. O'Connor MI, Switzer JA. AAOS Clinical Practice Guideline Summary: Management of Hip Fractures in Older Adults. J Am Acad Orthop Surg. 2022;30(20):E1291-6.
14. Osterhoff G, Morgan EF, Shefelbine SJ, Karim L, McNamara LM, Augat P. Bone mechanical properties and changes with osteoporosis. Injury. 2016;47(Suppl 2):S11.
15. Papakostidis C, Panagiotopoulos A, Piccioli A, Giannoudis PV. Timing of internal fixation of femoral neck fractures. A systematic review and meta-analysis of the final outcome. Injury. 2015;46(3):459-66.

16. Schweitzer D, Melero P, Zylberberg A, Salabarrieta J, Urrutia J. Factors associated with avascular necrosis of the femoral head and nonunion in patients younger than 65 years with displaced femoral neck fractures treated with reduction and internal fixation. Eur J Orthop Surg Traumatol. 2013;23(1):61-5.
17. Slobogean GP, Sprague SA, Scott T, Bhandari M. Complications following young femoral neck fractures. Injury. 2015;46(3):484-91.
18. Stoffel K, Michelitsch C, Arora R, Babst R, Candrian C, Eickhoff A, et al. Clinical performance of the Femoral Neck System within 1 year in 125 patients with acute femoral neck fractures, a prospective observational case series. Arch Orthop Trauma Surg. 2023;143(7):4155-64.
19. Stoffel K, Zderic I, Gras F, Sommer C, Eberli U, Mueller D, et al. Biomechanical Evaluation of the Femoral Neck System in Unstable Pauwels III Femoral Neck Fractures: A Comparison with the Dynamic Hip Screw and Cannulated Screws. J Orthop Trauma. 2017;31(3):131-7.

Intertrochanteric Femur Fracture and Fracture Greater Trochanter

Arpan Upadhayay, Samarth Mittal, Sakib Arfee

Intertrochanteric (IT) fractures are extracapsular proximal femur fractures occurring between greater and lesser trochanter, which may or may not extend into the subtrochanteric region.

EPIDEMIOLOGY

About 50% of all hip fractures are IT fractures. They are more common in the elderly age group and occur more than twice as frequently in females than males.

MECHANISM OF INJURY

Most fractures in the elderly result from a fall from standing height, typically with direct impact on the trochanteric region, and often occur in the early hours of the day.

Conversely, IT fractures in younger individuals are generally caused by high-velocity trauma, such as road traffic accidents.

ANATOMY

Multiple muscle groups insert into the IT region, and their pull leads to deformities in these fractures. The abductors displace the greater trochanter (GT) laterally and proximally, while the iliopsoas pull the lesser trochanter medially and proximally. The hip flexors, extensors, and adductors tend to pull the distal fragment proximally.

CLASSIFICATION

There are many classifications described for these fractures. We will discuss the two most used classification systems.

Boyd and Griffin

Boyd and Griffin were the first to describe a classification of IT fractures based on treatment recommendations. They divided these fractures into four types **(Fig. 1)**:

1. *Stable fractures*: These were simple two-part fractures.
2. *Unstable fractures* which had posteromedial comminution.
3. *Subtrochanteric extension*: In these fractures, the lateral shaft extension of the fracture ended at or just below the lesser trochanter. These fractures are also known as reverse oblique fractures.
4. *Subtrochanteric fractures with IT extension*: The fractures were in at least two planes.

Orthopaedic Trauma Association Classification of Intertrochanteric Fractures

The Orthopaedic Trauma Association (OTA) classification divided fractures into three groups, namely A1, A2, A3. The A1 fractures are stable fractures, while the A2 and A3 are classified as unstable fractures. Fractures with lateral wall thickness of <20.5 mm were classified as A2 fractures, while reverse oblique fractures were classified as A3 fractures.

Source: For further details please refer to Fracture and Dislocation Classification Compendium at: https://ota.org/research/fracture-and-dislocation-compendium

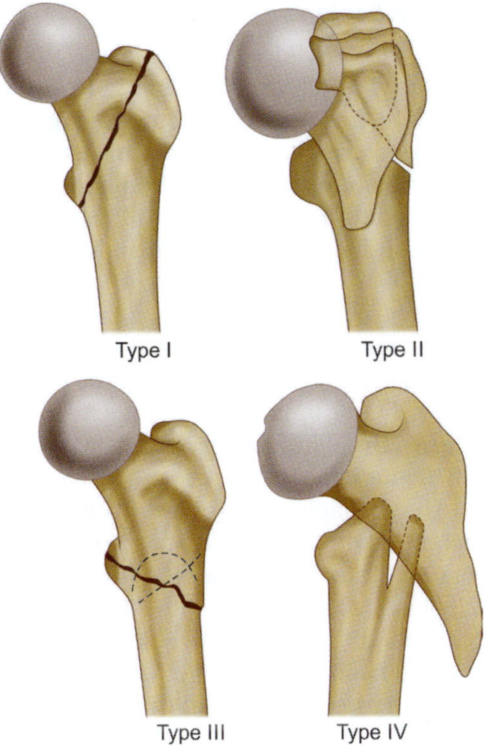

FIG. 1: Boyd and Griffin Classification.

Unstable fracture patterns are those with a lateral wall thickness of <20.5 mm, comminuted posteromedial cortex, subtrochanteric extension, or reverse oblique fractures.

CLINICAL EVALUATION

Patients typically present as nonambulatory with a shortened, externally rotated limb. They experience pain and swelling in the ipsilateral hip and are unable to raise the limb from the affected hip. Initially, the Advanced Trauma Life Support (ATLS) protocol must be followed. A thorough history should be taken, including the mode of injury, associated comorbidities, current medications, preambulatory status, and potential dehydration. Basic laboratory studies, including a complete blood count, comprehensive metabolic panel, and coagulation studies, should be obtained to identify any abnormalities that need to be addressed before proceeding with surgical stabilization. A secondary survey should be performed on all patients to check for any other fractures.

RADIOGRAPHIC EVALUATION

An anteroposterior (AP) view of the pelvis and an AP and lateral view of the involved proximal femur are enough to diagnose most IT fractures **(Figs. 2A and B)**. An X-ray

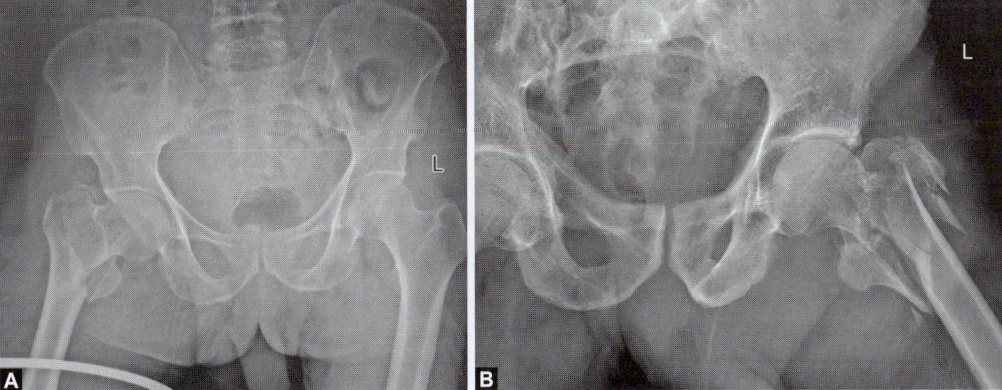

FIGS. 2A AND B: Pelvis with both hips radiograph showing intertrochanteric fracture of right hip.

in traction and internal rotation is the most useful view to decide about the treatment plan. A CT scan (though rarely) can be done to delineate the different fracture lines, and fragments, and help in better planning and fixation of these fractures **(Figs. 3A to C)**.

Magnetic resonance imaging (MRI) is usually reserved for occult fractures which are not obvious on radiographs and CT scans.

TREATMENT

These patients are usually old aged with multiple comorbidities. Most of them need prior optimization. The primary goal of treating an IT fracture is to restore early mobility, reducing the risk of medical complications, and helping the patient return to their preoperative functional status. The management should start promptly with multidisciplinary involvement.

Nonoperative

Nonsurgical intervention is rarely indicated only in grossly unfit, nonambulatory patients or those with a very high risk of perioperative mortality, as outcomes.

Operative

These fractures should be operated as early as possible once the patient is stabilized, preferably within the first 48–72 hours. Early surgery and ambulation play a crucial role in achieving better outcomes. Stable internal fixation enables early mobilization in these patients, which significantly improves their quality of life and enhances long-term survivability.

Fixation Implants

Sliding hip screw [dynamic hip screw (DHS)]:

These implants are commonly used in stable trochanteric fractures **(Fig. 4)**. However, screw cut-out, varus collapse, and fixation failure are frequent complications. Most fixation failures result from poor reduction and improper implant position.

To avoid these issues, the lag screw should be positioned 10–25 mm from the tip of the femoral head, measured by the tip-apex distance (TAD). It should also be placed center-center in both AP and lateral views **(Fig. 5)**. Distal fixation can be achieved with two or four screws.

Any breach in the lateral wall or incompetent lateral wall (<2.1 cm) is a contraindication for using DHS. If any breach happens intraoperatively then DHS should be used with trochanteric stabilization plate (TSP) to maintain the lateral wall otherwise medialization of the distal fragment will occur.

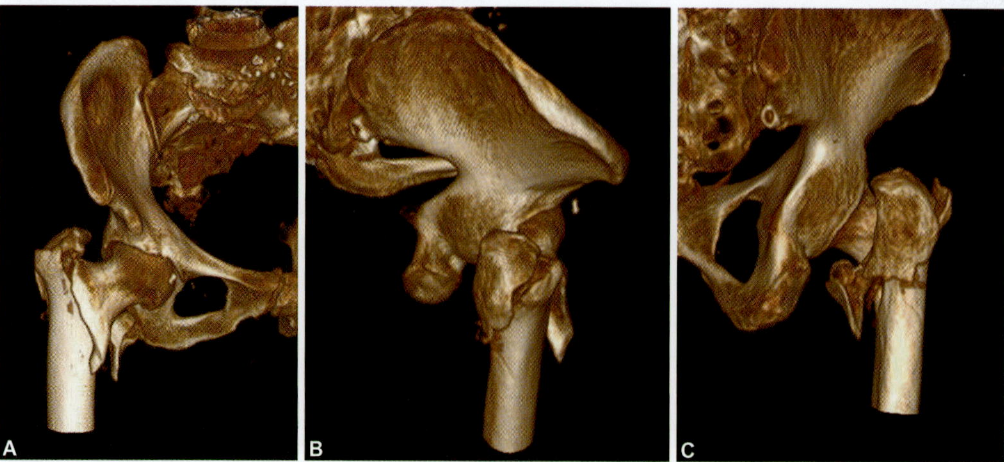

FIGS. 3A TO C: A CT scan demonstrating different fracture lines and fragments in an intertrochanteric fracture.

Cephalomedullary nail: These are the implants of choice for trochanteric fractures although for stable fractures, sliding hip screws (SHS) are equally good. Cephalomedullary nails combine an intramedullary nail with SHS design, addressing the limitations of SHS. Acting as an intramedullary strut, they experience a lower bending moment compared to SHS, reducing the risk of varus collapse and fixation failure. Since they are intramedullary, the thickness of the lateral wall becomes irrelevant, making them suitable for unstable fractures **(Figs. 6A and B)**. Additionally, the procedure can be performed in a closed manner, resulting in shorter surgery times, less blood loss, and reduced tissue damage.

When selecting the nail length, there is no clear consensus among surgeons. Recent literature indicates that standard-sized nails can be used effectively in both stable and unstable fractures with similar outcomes. Despite the advantages of intramedullary implants, proper reduction and fixation are still critical for successful outcomes. Even

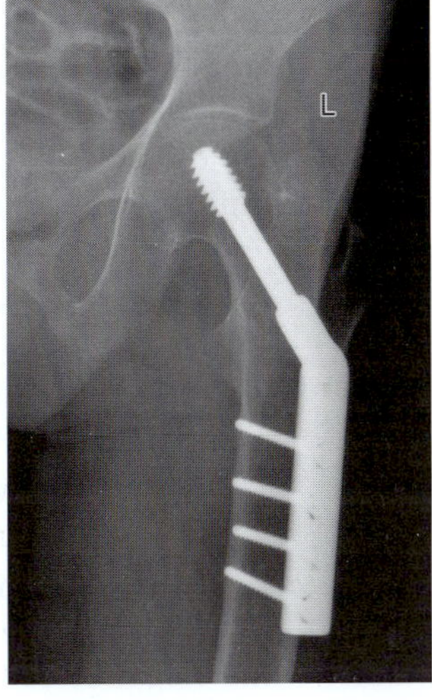

FIG. 4: Dynamic hip screw fixation.

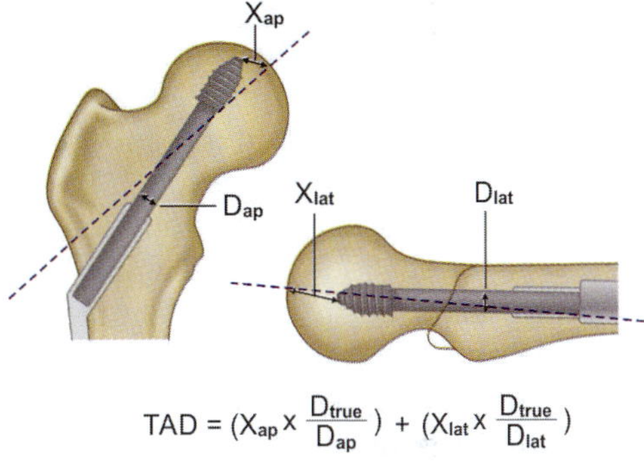

$$TAD = (X_{ap} \times \frac{D_{true}}{D_{ap}}) + (X_{lat} \times \frac{D_{true}}{D_{lat}})$$

FIG. 5: Tip–apex distance calculation (X_{ap} and X_{lat}—a distance of the tip of the screw from the tip of the head, D_{true}—true diameter of the screw, D_{ap} and D_{lat}—measured diameter of screw).

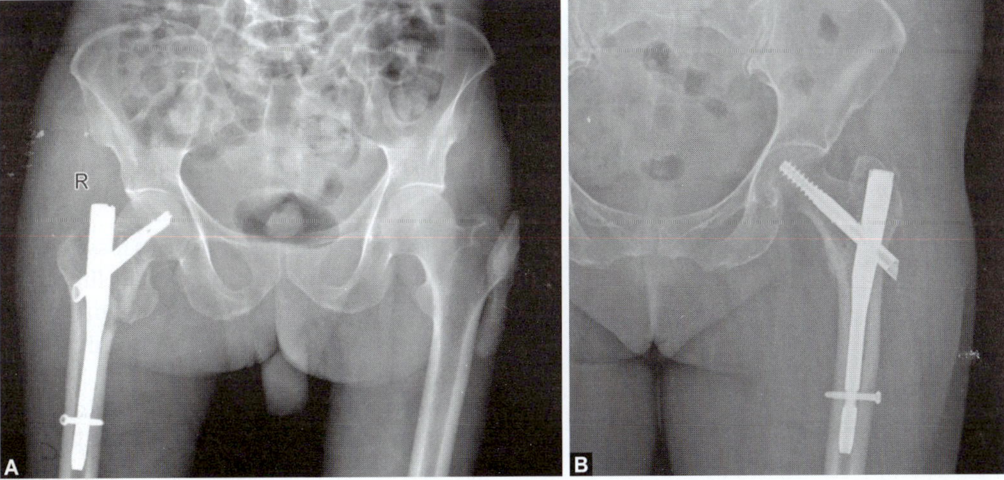

FIGS. 6A AND B: Cephalomedullary nail fixation of an intertrochanteric fracture with a helical blade and lag screw devices.

with an intramedullary implant, a poorly reduced or fixed fracture will likely fail.

Controversies and consensus about cephalomedullary nailing: Short or long nails?

- Both short and long proximal femoral nails (PFNs) are effective in treating proximal femoral fractures, the choice of implant should be tailored to the patient's specific clinical scenario, considering factors such as fracture type, bone quality, and the surgeon's experience.

Various designs of nails:

- *Single-screw versus double-screw designs*:
  - While the double-screw design may provide an advantage in faster fracture healing, especially in comminuted and unstable fractures but is associated with a slightly longer and more complex surgical procedure. A single screw is good enough for stable fracture and has got faster surgical time.
- *Helical blade versus screws*: The helical blade and lag screw designs perform similarly in terms of mechanical stability, pain, and functional outcomes. Therefore, the choice of implant may depend on specific clinical factors, surgeon experience, and patient characteristics.
- *Proximal femoral nail antirotation (PFNA) versus InterTAN*: The studies suggest that while both methods are effective, the choice may depend on surgeon preference and specific patient characteristics.

Distal locking: Static versus dynamic distal locking in PFN:

- *Static locking*:
  - Provides rigid fixation, which is beneficial in unstable fractures or cases where rotational stability is crucial.
  - Prevents axial shortening and rotation, which can be particularly important in osteoporotic bones or highly comminuted fractures.
  - Some studies suggest that static locking may be associated with a slightly higher risk of implant-related complications, such as screw breakage or stress shielding, but these risks are generally outweighed by the need for stability in complex fractures.
- *Dynamic locking*:
  - Meta-analyses and clinical trials have shown that dynamic locking may lead to faster healing times and reduced rates of implant failure in selected patients, particularly those with stable fracture patterns.
  - Some studies suggest that a single distal locking screw can be adequate for stable fractures and may result in similar healing rates compared to two screws, with a lower risk of implant-related complications and faster recovery times.
- *Single versus two distal locking*: Meta-analyses and clinical studies indicate that two distal locking screws provide better stability for complex and unstable fractures, reducing the risk of fixation failure and nonunion.

Type of fracture reduction: Positive and neutral reductions are considered good or acceptable, while negative reductions are classified as poor in the AP view **(Figs. 7A to C)**. In the lateral view, only neutral reduction is considered acceptable, while all other reductions are classified as poor. In both positive and neutral reduction in AP view, there is adequate anteromedial cortical support enabling limited sliding and cortical support providing a favorable environment for fracture healing.

Entry point: GT versus piriformis fossa—

- Almost all recent studies and literature converge on the GT as the preferred entry point due to its anatomical and biomechanical advantages.

The positioning of the screw or blade and TAD follows the same guidelines as for SHS devices.

In osteoporotic bones: Studies have found that cement augmentation *significantly*

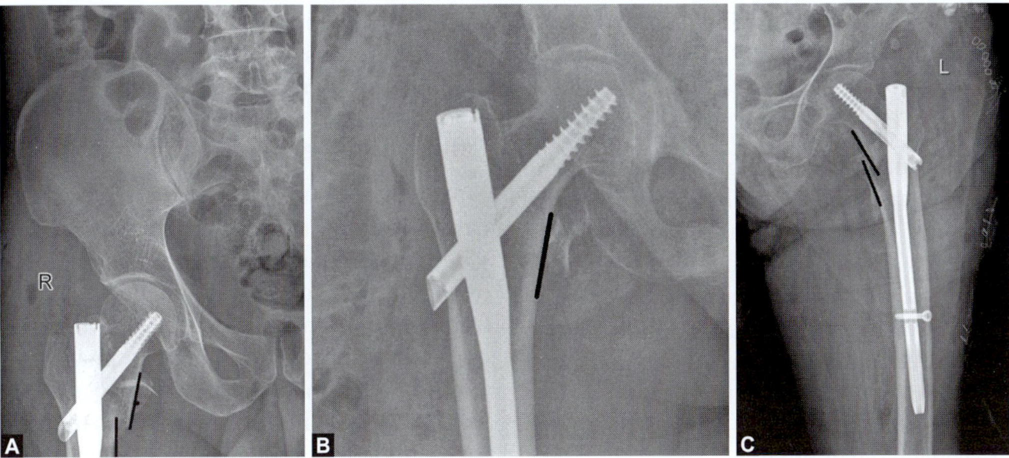

FIGS. 7A TO C: Positive, neutral, and negative reduction of intertrochanteric fractures.

improved the mechanical stability of the fixation, reducing the rate of implant failure and improving early functional outcomes compared to standard PFN without augmentation.

Diameter of nail: Given a choice of larger and optimal diameter nails will have a better outcome.

Reamed or unreamed nails: Reamed is preferred over undreamed.

Dynamic hip screw:
For stable fractures: Not necessarily 4-hole plate—

- *2- or 3-hole plate* is sufficient with advantages of less surgical time, less blood loss, and less morbidity.

Dynamic hip screw versus nail: *In stable fracture*, compared with DHS fixation, PFN fixation had a similar operation time, blood loss and transfusion, weight-bearing protocol, hospital stay, and wound complication (mortality and reoperation).

In unstable fracture, nailing is preferred.

Prosthetic Replacement

This is reserved for failed internal fixation or in patients with a pre-existing arthritic hip.

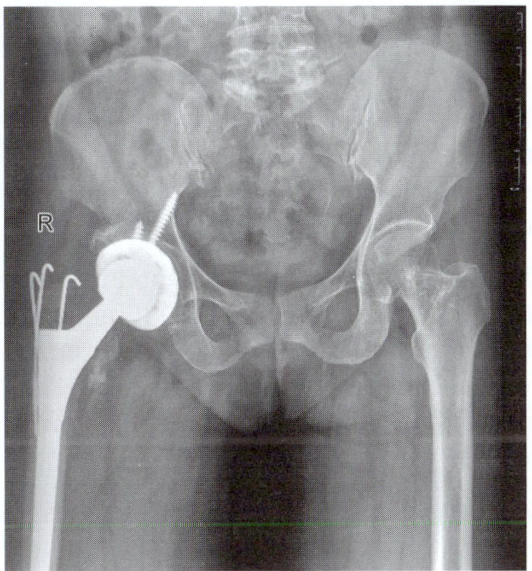

FIG. 8: Total hip replacement with a diaphyseal fitting stem in a case of intertrochanteric fracture with pre-existing arthritis of the right hip.

These patients may need a diaphyseal fitting stem owing to the deformity in the proximal femur **(Fig. 8)**.

COMPLICATIONS

Mortality

Intertrochanteric fractures are linked to a high mortality rate. Despite prompt treatment, nearly 20% of patients do not survive beyond 1 year after the injury.

Fixation Failure

Cut-out and varus collapse of the screw or blade from the femoral head are the most common causes of fixation failure in IT fractures. While some degree of collapse occurs in all cases, uncontrolled collapse leads to failure. This can be prevented through proper reduction and fixation techniques. A neutral or positive reduction, center-center screw positioning, and a TAD of 10–25 mm are considered optimal.

If failure occurs, revision surgery with cement augmentation, wider diameter screw (InterTAN nailing), or prosthetic replacement may be necessary. Anterior blowout fractures from using long nails with a different radius of curvature can happen during or after surgery. Preoperative planning, including assessing the femoral bow, is crucial to avoid this, and shorter nails or those with a greater radius of curvature (ROC) should be considered.

Nonunion: It is quite uncommon for these fractures to go into nonunion. If sequential radiographs reveal nonunion, then resurgery with a wider screw diameter nail (InterTAN nail), osteotomy with bone grafting, or a hip replacement can be performed.

Z-effect: It is generally seen in two screw types of nails. The proximal screw migrates into the joint while the distal screw backs out.

Osteonecrosis of the femoral head: This is rare following an IT fracture.

FRACTURE GREATER TROCHANTER OF FEMUR

Greater trochanter serves as an important lever arm for these attached muscles, which are responsible for stabilizing the hip joint, controlling leg movement, and performing functions such as walking, running, and climbing stairs. GT provides attachment to several key muscles of hip, including the gluteus medius and gluteus minimus in addition to external rotators of hip.

Causes and Mechanism of Injury

Fractures of the GT are relatively rare but can occur due to various mechanisms. In elderly, particularly those with osteoporosis, low energy fall can be sufficient to cause a fracture. In young patients, GT fractures are commonly due to high-energy trauma.

Greater trochanter fracture can occur as a part of a more complex pattern of hip injuries, including femoral neck or IT fractures. The mechanism often involves a direct impact to the hip or a sudden twisting motion that exceeds the bone's capacity to withstand stress especially in osteoporotic bones.

Diagnosis

A plain X-ray is first investigation, to see for visible fractures. For a detailed assessment, particularly if the X-ray is inconclusive, a computed tomography (CT) scan is advised and magnetic resonance imaging (MRI) is advised to see for any associated soft tissue injuries especially abductors of hip. These modalities offer high-resolution images that can reveal subtle fractures and assess the involvement of associated fracture.

Classification (Fig. 9)

- *Type A*: Fracture with transverse direction above the inferior border of the GT
- *Type B*: Fracture with oblique direction above the inferior border of the GT
- *Type C*: Fracture with transverse direction below the inferior border of the GT
- *Type D*: Fracture with oblique direction below the inferior border of the GT

Treatment Strategies

Management of a GT fracture depends on several factors, including the fracture's displacement, the patient's age, activity level, and overall health status.

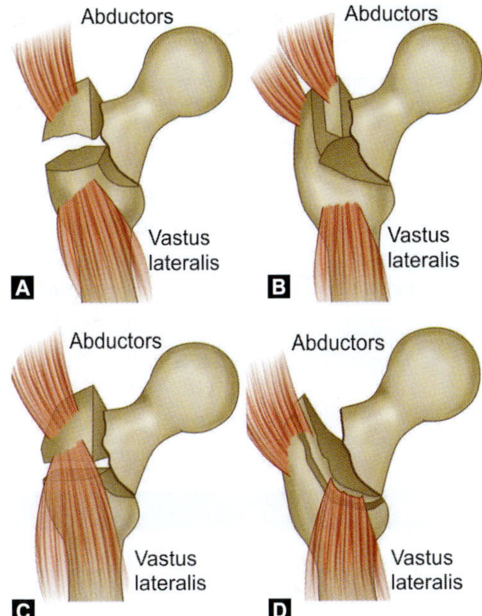

FIGS. 9A TO D: Classification of greater trochanter fractures.

Conservative management: For undisplaced or minimally displaced fractures, conservative treatment is advised. The patient is usually advised to rest and restrict weight-bearing activities within comfort to allow for natural healing.

Surgical intervention: In cases where the fracture is displaced or associated with significant functional impairment, surgical intervention is often necessary. The main aim of surgery is to reduce the fracture and fix it in place. Common surgical techniques include:

- *Internal fixation*: This involves the use of screws, trochanteric plates, or K wires (TBW) to stabilize the fracture. The choice of fixation method depends on the fracture's specifics and the surgeon's expertise **(Figs. 10A to C and Flowchart 1)**.

Patients are encouraged to increase their weight-bearing activities as tolerated.

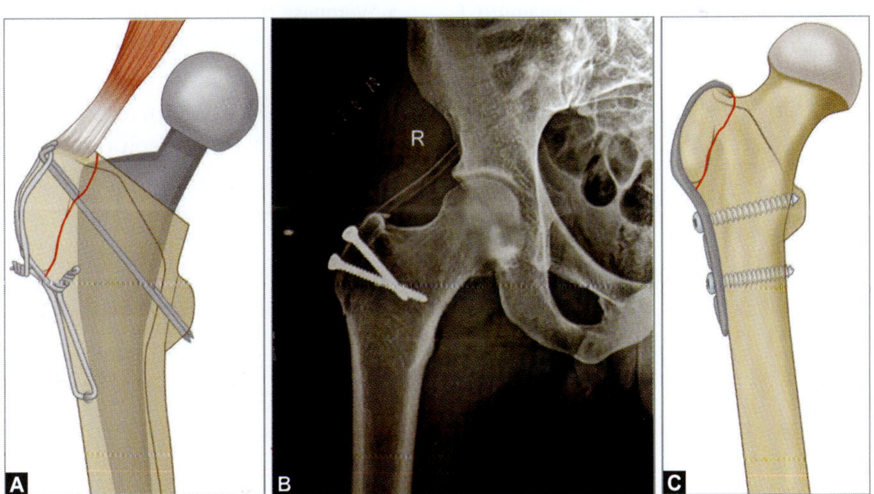

FIGS. 10A TO C: Fixation options for greater trochanter fractures.

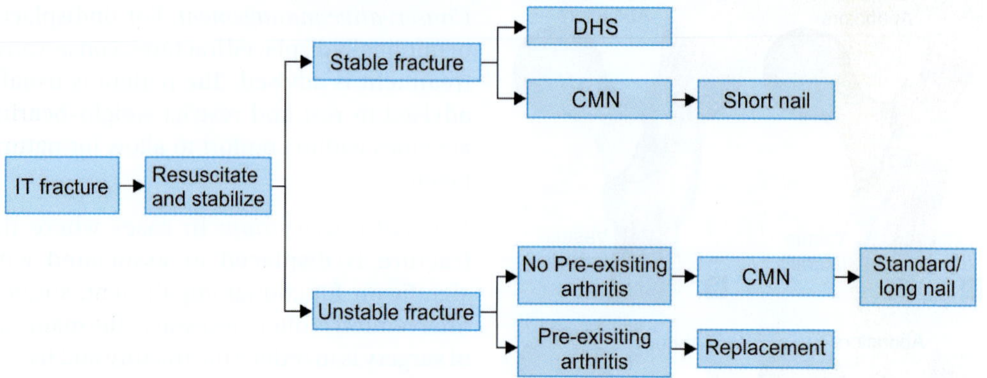

FLOWCHART 1: Operative management of IT fracture in elderly patient.
(CMN: cephalomedullary nailing; DHS: dynamic hip screw; IT: intertrochanteric)

BIBLIOGRAPHY

1. Baumgaertner MR, Curtin SL, Lindskog DM, Keggi JM. The value of the tip-apex distance in predicting failure of fixation of peritrochanteric fractures of the hip. J Bone Joint Surg Am. 1995;77(7):1058-64.
2. Chang SM, Hou ZY, Hu SJ, Du SC. Intertrochanteric Femur Fracture Treatment in Asia: What We Know and What the World Can Learn. Orthop Clin North Am. 2020;51(2):189-205.
3. Iwata T, Nozawa S, Dohjima T, Yamamoto T, Ishimaru D, Tsugita M, et al. The value of T1-weighted coronal MRI scans in diagnosing occult fracture of the hip. J Bone Joint Surg Br. 2012;94(7):969-73.
4. Rockwood CA, Bucholz RW, Green DP, Court-Brown CM, Heckman JD, Tornetta P. Rockwood and Green's Fractures in Adults. Philadelphia: Wolters Kluwer Health/Lippincott Williams & Wilkins; 2010.
5. Veronese N, Maggi S. Epidemiology and social costs of hip fracture. Injury. 2018;49(8):1458-60.

SECTION

10

Femur

Subtrochanteric Fracture

Sakib Arfee

Subtrochanteric fractures of the femur are a specific type of hip fracture involving approximately 5 cm area just below the lesser trochanter and above the femoral diaphysis. This area is important as it acts as a bridge between the femoral head and neck with the shaft of the femur, which bears the load of the body during activities such as walking and running.

Subtrochanteric fractures are complex injuries requiring careful evaluation, planning, and management.

MECHANISM

Subtrochanteric fractures often occur in younger patients due to high-energy trauma or significant stress, especially in individuals with compromised bone quality. In old age patients, especially those with osteoporosis, these fractures can result from relatively low-energy falls **(Figs. 1A to C)**.

Computed tomography: It is indicated for detailed visualization. CT provides high-resolution cuts of the bone and can help identify complex fracture patterns or associated injuries.

CLASSIFICATION

Seinsheimer (Fig. 2)

- *Type 1*: <2 mm displacement
- *Type 2*: Two part fracture—
  - *2A*: Transverse
  - *2B*: Spiral with lesser trochanter proximal to fracture lines
  - *2C*: Spiral with lesser trochanter distal to fracture line

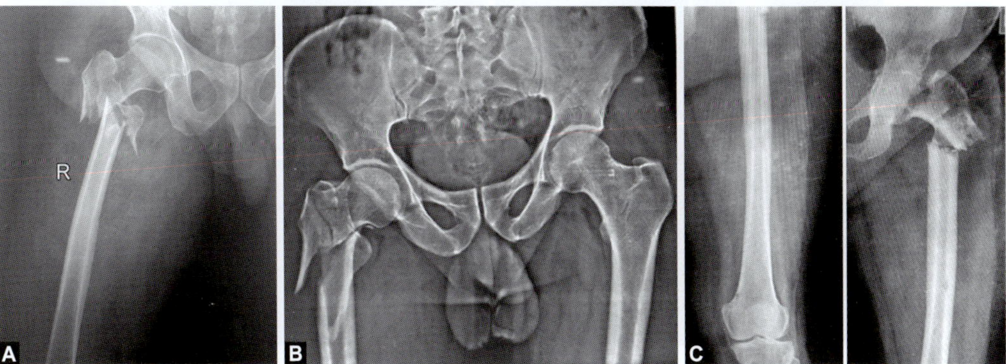

FIGS. 1A TO C: Fractures can result from relatively low-energy falls.

- *Type 3*: Three part—
  - *3A*: Lesser trochanter butterfly
  - *3B*: Lateral butterfly
- *Type 4*: Four part
- *Type 5*: Greater trochanteric extension

TREATMENT

Nonoperative Management

This is rarely used for subtrochanteric fractures due to the high risk of malunion and nonunion.

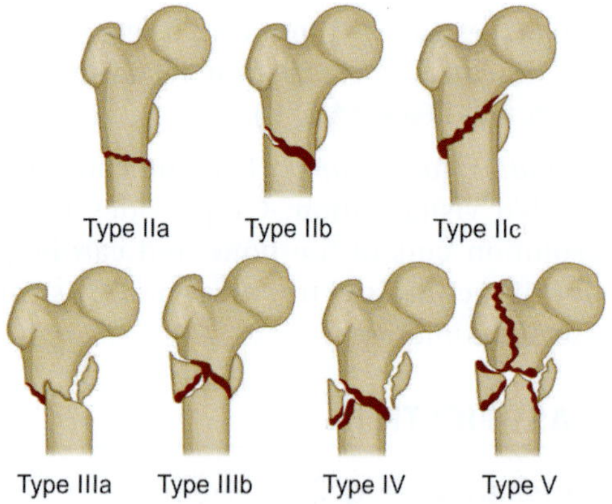

FIG. 2: Types of Seinsheimer.

Operative Management

This is preferred mode of treatment for subtrochanteric fractures due to the complexity of these fractures and the need for precise alignment and stabilization. Surgical options include:

- *Internal fixation*: This common approach to fixing subtrochanteric fractures includes the use of various fixation devices:
  - *Cephalo-intramedullary nails*: The proximal femoral nail (long PFNA2) is the most commonly used implant these days to fix subtrochanteric fractures **(Figs. 3A and B)**. This method is often preferred for its ability to provide strong internal support and minimize soft tissue disruption and blood loss. Enders nail can also be used in a few circumstances.
  - *Plate and screw fixation*: Dynamic condylar screw (DCS) system and proximal femoral plate or occasionally condylar blade plate as shown in **Figures 4A to C** can be used to stabilize the subtrochanteric fracture. This method is less commonly used

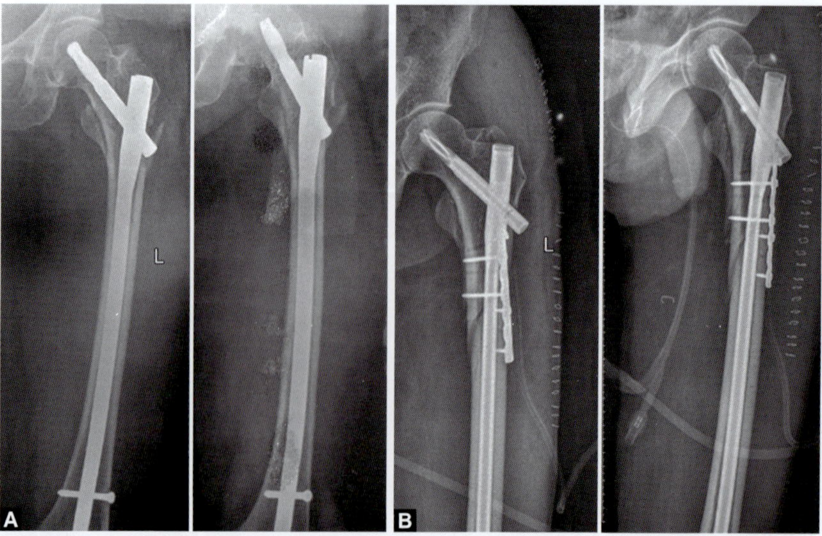

FIGS. 3A AND B: Cephalo-intramedullary nails.

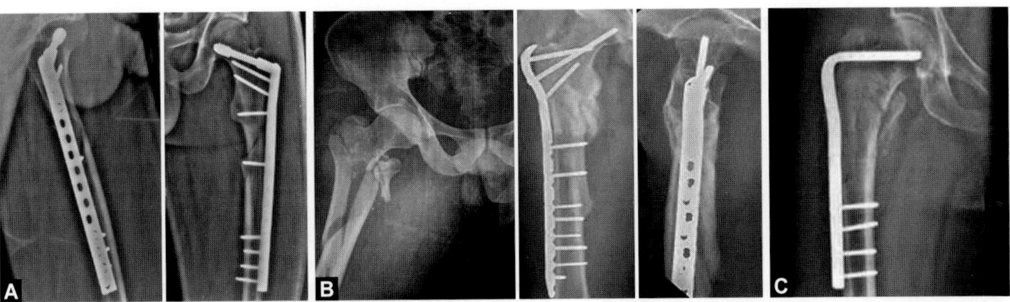

FIGS. 4A TO C: Plate and screw fixation.

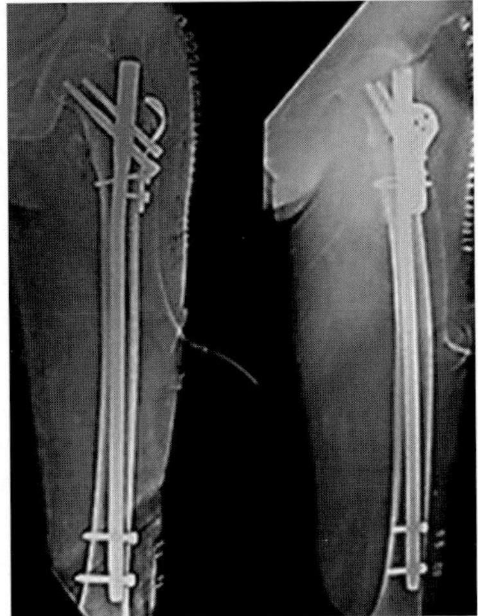

FIG. 5: Lateral wall augmentation, along with nail.

but can be effective for certain fracture patterns.

- *Hip replacement*: Subtrochanteric fracture when associated with severe joint degeneration or if the fracture is complex where fixation is not going to serve the purpose or in cases of failed osteosynthesis (not amenable to refixation), a partial or total hip replacement may be considered. This approach addresses both the fracture and any underlying joint pathology, potentially offering a more comprehensive solution for hip function.
- *Lateral wall augmentation, along with nail*:

It can be done using a plate (buttress plate or auxiliary plate) or cerclage wire alone or cerclage wire with lag screw as in **Figure 5**.

There is *growing evidence supporting the use of lateral wall augmentation* in improving the outcomes of PFN for treating unstable intertrochanteric fractures. It has been found that this technique helps to provide additional lateral support, thereby improving stability and reducing the risk of complications such as cut-out of the implant or fracture displacement. This method is particularly useful in cases with a deficient lateral wall due to fracture comminution or intraoperative damage.

COMPLICATIONS OF SUBTROCHANTERIC FRACTURES

These complications may arise due to the nature of the fracture, treatment methods, or during recovery.

- *Delayed union or nonunion*: Due to limited blood supply in the subtrochanteric region, healing can be slower.
- *Malunion*: Which can result in limb length discrepancy, abnormal gait, or persistent pain
- *Infection*: Open fractures or surgical treatments, especially involving internal fixation, can introduce bacteria, leading to infections that may require antibiotic therapy or further surgical intervention.
- *Hardware complications*: Issues related to internal fixation devices, such as screws, plates, or intramedullary nails, can occur. This might include breakage, loosening, or migration of hardware, which could necessitate a revision surgery.

Prevention and Management

To minimize these complications, it is essential to:

- Ensure proper preoperative planning and implant selection
- Ensure proper surgical technique and fixation
- Monitor the patient closely during recovery
- Regular follow-up imaging and assessments to ensure proper healing and alignment

BIBLIOGRAPHY

1. Bedi A, Toan Le T. Subtrochanteric femur fractures. Orthop Clin North Am. 2004;35(4):473-83.
2. Panteli M, Mauffrey C, Giannoudis PV. Subtrochanteric fractures: Issues and challenges. Injury. 2017;48(10):2023-6.
3. Roberts CS, Nawab A, Wang M, Voor MJ, Seligson D. Second generation intramedullary nailing of subtrochanteric femur fractures: a biomechanical study of fracture site motion. J Orthop Trauma. 2003;17(8):57-64.

CHAPTER 10.2

Fracture Shaft of Femur

Tejpal Singh, John Mohd

A fractured femur shaft is one of the most common injuries due to major violent trauma. It has a bimodal distribution.

- Incidences of femoral shaft fracture are more common in males—15–24 years of age and females—75 years of age or older.
- The most common cause in young men is after high-energy trauma and in elderly women after a low-energy fall.

Elderly patients have a low index of suspicion for pathological fractures.

ASSOCIATED INJURIES

These occur in 5–15% of cases like:

- The ipsilateral neck of the femur fractures (2–6%)
- Bilateral femur fractures
- Ipsilateral tibia shaft fractures
- Ipsilateral acetabular fractures
- Chest injuries
- Cerebral and subdural hemorrhage

BIOMECHANICS OF FRACTURE

Here, the musculature around the shaft femur acts as a deforming force which leads of a series of events leading to shaft femur fracture.

- *Proximal part*:
  - *Abducted*: Gluteus medius and gluteus minimus
  - *Flexed*: Iliopsoas flexes fragment as its insertion is on lesser trochanter
- *Distal part*:
  - *Varus*: Due to pull of adductors
  - *Extension*: Due to pull of gastrocnemius muscle

CLASSIFICATION

- Descriptive classification
- Winquist and Hansen's classification
- AO/OTA classification

- *Descriptive classification*:
  - Open versus closed injury
  - *Based on location*: Proximal, middle, or distal one-third isthmal, infraisthmal, or supracondylar
- *AO/OTA classification*: Refer to **Figure 1** and **Table 1**.
- *Other classification*:
  - *Winquist and Hansen classification*: Based on fracture comminution

CLINICAL EVALUATION

Extremely important to rule out neurovascular injury.

Investigatory Evaluation

- *X-rays **(Fig. 2)***:
  - Anteroposterior (AP) and lateral views of the entire femur including knee and hip
  - AP view of pelvis with bilateral hip to rule out neck of femur fracture
- *CT scan*:
  - To rule out undisplaced incomplete ipsilateral fracture neck of femur

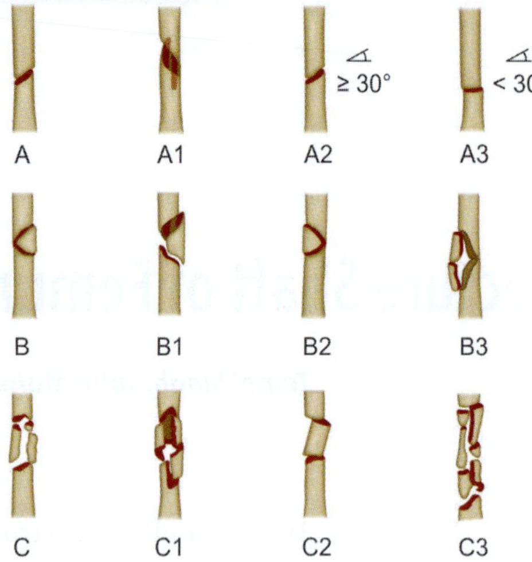

FIG. 1: AO/OTA classification.

TABLE 1: AO/OTA classification of femur.

32A	Simple	A1—spiral A2—oblique, angle >30° A3—transverse, angle <30°
32B	Wedge	B1—spiral wedge B2—bending wedge B3—fragmented wedge
32C	Complex	C1—spiral C2—segmental C3—irregular

INITIAL MANAGEMENT

- As soon as the patient is received in the emergency room, Advanced Trauma Life Support (ATLS) protocol is followed.
- A blood transfusion is done. Blood loss in the fractured shaft of the femur is approximately 1,000–1,500 mL.
- The patient is put on oxygen support.
- Immobilization of the affected limb is done by application of a splint or Thomas splint (used for transportation of patient as well).
- Appropriate multimodal analgesia which may include nerve block as well.

TREATMENT STRATEGIES

Nonoperative Management

Nonoperative management is rare and typically reserved only for a patient who is completely unfit for surgery.

Operative Management

Operative intervention is the gold standard. The choice of surgical technique depends on the fracture pattern, location, and patient factors.

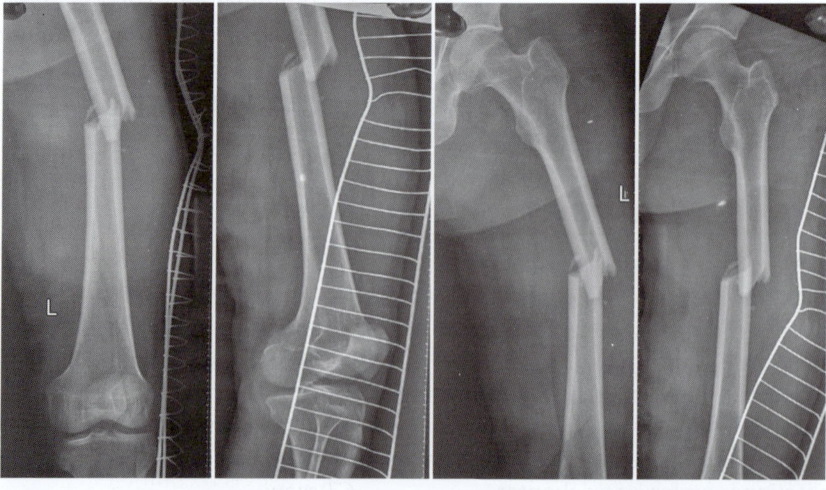

FIG. 2: Radiographs anteroposterior (AP) and lateral views with shaft of femur fracture with one joint above and below.

Intramedullary Nailing (Figs. 2 to 4)

It is commonly used as an antegrade technique.

- This technique is preferred for most femoral shaft fractures due to its minimally invasive nature and effectiveness in promoting healing.
- *Contraindication*:
    - A narrow canal that will not accommodate a nail
    - Open growth plates
    - Previous malunion that prevents nail placement
    - History of intramedullary infection
    - Polytraumatized patients with associated thoracic injury (relative contraindication)
- *Advantages*:
    - Provides stable fixation
    - Preserves soft tissue
    - Allows for early mobilization being the load-sharing device

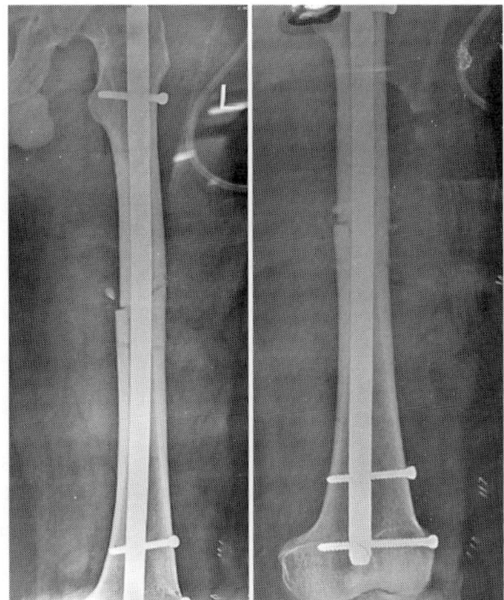

FIG. 3: Immediate postoperative X-rays.

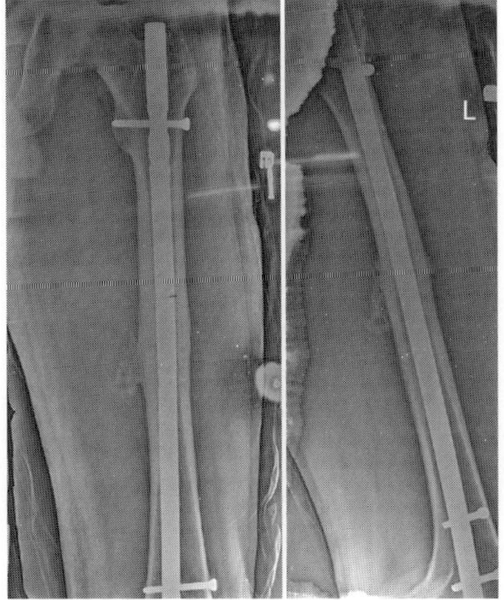

FIG. 4: Radiographs at union.

Relative indications for retrograde nails:

- Multiply injured patients or polytrauma
- Bilateral femur fractures
- Morbid obesity
- Distal metaphyseal fractures
- Pregnancy
- Associated vascular injury
- Associated spine fracture
- Ipsilateral femoral neck fracture
- Ipsilateral acetabular fracture
- Ipsilateral patella fracture
- Ipsilateral tibia fracture
- Ipsilateral through knee amputation

Relative contraindications for retrograde nails:

- Subtrochanteric fracture
- Limited knee motion (if starting point inaccessible)
- Patellar baja

Plating (Figs. 5 to 7)

4.5-mm broad dynamic compression plate (DCP) is used, with at least 4 screws and 8 cortices on either side of the fracture.

Indications:

- The extremely narrow medullary canal where IM nailing is impossible or difficult
- Fractures that occur adjacent to or through a previous malunion
- Fractures that have associated proximal or distal extension into the pertrochanteric or condylar regions (relative indication)
- In patients with an associated vascular injury, the exposure for vascular repair frequently involves a wide exposure

of the medial femur. If rapid femoral stabilization is desired, a plate can be applied quickly through the medial open exposure.
- Used for specific cases such as complex fractures

Advantages: Allows for direct visualization and fixation of the fracture.

External Fixation

- *Technique*: Involves placing pins or screws through the skin into the bone, connected to an external frame
- *Indications*: Often used in cases with significant soft tissue injury, infections, or when internal fixation is not feasible. Used as a damage control orthopedic measure
- *Advantages*: Minimally invasive and can stabilize the fracture while addressing soft tissue injuries

Postoperative Care

Rehabilitation

Effective rehabilitation is crucial for restoring function and promoting recovery:
- *Early mobilization*: It is initiated based on fracture stability and surgical intervention, aiming to prevent complications and enhance recovery. It focuses on range of motion, strengthening exercises, and gait training to restore function and mobility.
- *Physical therapy*: It focuses on range of motion, strengthening exercises, and gait training to restore function and mobility.

Complications

- Heterotopic ossification
- Pudendal nerve injury—while using fracture table with traction
- Femoral artery or nerve injury

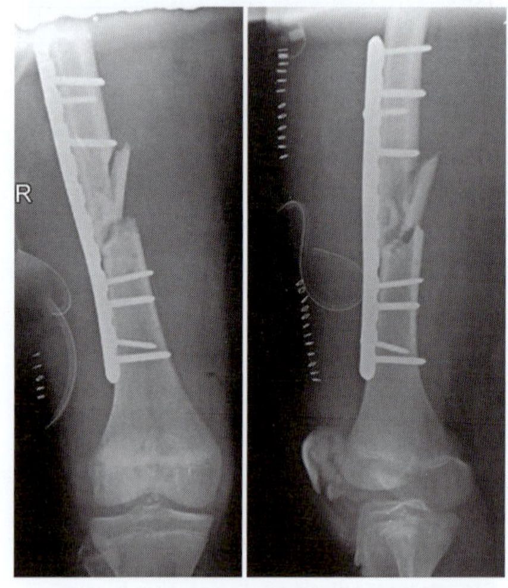

FIG. 6: Postoperative X-rays with plating.

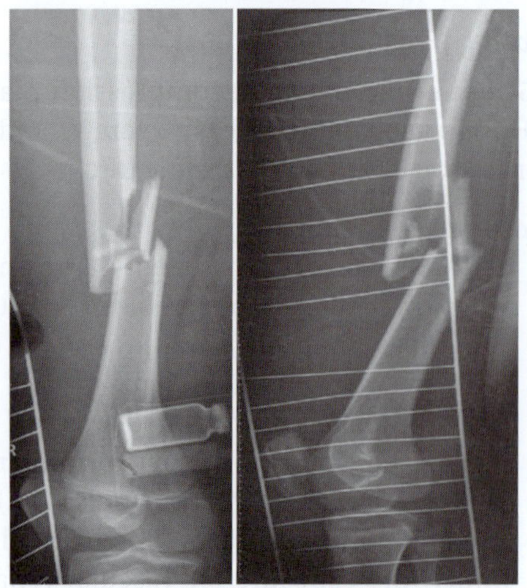

FIG. 5: Preoperative X-rays.

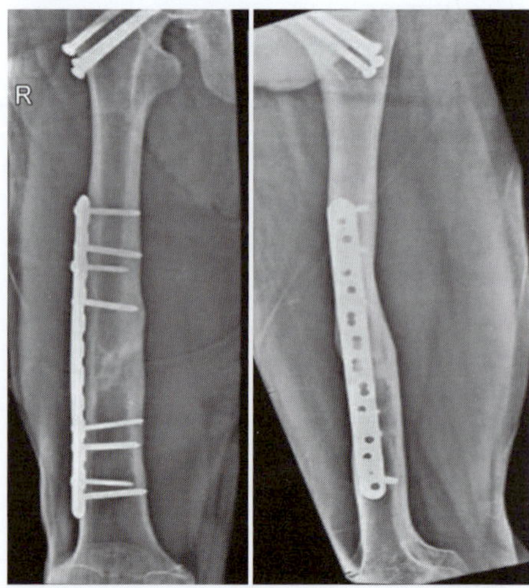

FIG. 7: X-rays at union.

- Malunion, angular malalignment, and rotational malalignment
- Delayed union
- Nonunion
- Infection
- Quadriceps and hip abductors weakness
- Knee stiffness, knee pain, and hip pain

JUNCTIONAL FRACTURES OF THE FEMORAL SHAFT

Junctional fractures of the femoral shaft, specifically those occurring near the proximal or distal ends of the bone, present unique challenges in orthopedic surgery. These fractures, located between the diaphysis and metaphysis, are complex due to their anatomical location, abnormal stress, and the need to balance stability, vascular supply, and functional recovery.

Challenges in Management

- *High risk of malalignment*: Malalignment is a common issue due to the biomechanical forces at play in these regions. Precision in fracture reduction and fixation is essential to avoid long-term complications like malunion, which can lead to pain, functional impairment, and the need for revision surgery.
- *Healing and union rates*: These have been associated with delayed union or nonunion. Recent studies emphasize the importance of achieving absolute stability, particularly in fractures with poor healing potential and using biological adjuncts like bone grafts when necessary.

Current Treatment Approaches

- *Intramedullary nailing (IMN)*: IMN remains the standard of care for many femoral shaft fractures, including junctional types. For fractures closer to the diaphysis, IMN provides stability with relatively low complication rates. However, its application in junctional fractures—especially near the subtrochanteric or supracondylar regions—requires precise technique to ensure optimal alignment and avoid malunion. The use of longer nails and specialized locking techniques (multiple locking screws in smaller fragments), use of cephalomedullary nail in proximal fracture, has shown improved outcomes in maintaining stability.
- *Plate fixation*: In cases where IMN is not feasible or in fractures extending into the metaphysis, plate fixation may be preferred. Plates, including locking compression plates (LCPs), offer the benefit of rigid fixation and can be anatomically contoured to accommodate junctional regions. Dual plating and bridging techniques have been beneficial in complex fractures, especially those involving comminution or extensive soft tissue injury.
- *Minimally invasive techniques*: Minimally invasive plate osteosynthesis (MIPO) has gained popularity for junctional femoral fractures, as it reduces soft tissue disruption and preserves periosteal blood supply. Studies have shown that MIPO techniques may reduce healing time and improve functional outcomes, particularly in distal femoral junctional fractures.
- *Hybrid fixation*: For some junctional fractures, combining IMN and plate fixation can provide superior stability. This approach, often referred to as "plate-over-nail," is particularly beneficial in fractures with extensive comminution or where additional support is required to achieve adequate fixation. Hybrid fixation helps address the limitations of each individual method by providing increased rotational stability.

Management of ipsilateral femoral neck and shaft fracture

IPSILATERAL SHAFT AND PROXIMAL FEMUR FRACTURE

Ipsilateral proximal femur and shaft fractures are rare which makes it very challenging to manage, and they usually occur due to high-velocity trauma in young adults having incidence around 1–9% among all femoral shaft fractures. This scenario is usually seen in polytrauma cases.

Surgical fixation is the standard treatment. Important considerations:

- The fracture morphology of the proximal femur (neck femur intra- or extracapsular/peritrochanteric) may need more imaging like noncontrast computed tomography (NCCT) to study the fracture morphology for implant selection.
- The sequence of tackling and fixing these fractures is an unresolved and equally important subject of contention.
- Most of the maneuvers applied in the reduction of fracture proximal femur use the shaft femur as a lever arm but in the absence of a functional lever arm, these maneuvers become obsolete.
- Ideal fixation strategy—individualized or common approach
- Implant choice—single versus separate
- Usually a polytrauma case with associated multisystem derangement and factors like operative time, blood loss, and anesthesia modes and risks come into play.
- *Missed injury*: A missed fracture neck femur in concomitant injury may surprise a surgeon during fluoroscopy intraoperatively. Many times, the associated proximal femur fracture like fracture neck femur is occult, and is diagnosed late on secondary survey or on operation table during traction and radiography, adding to its complexity.
- *Iatrogenic fracture of neck femur during shaft femur nailing*: Some centers have all the armamentarium of implants autoclaved and ready to use and these cases might not pose a big challenge in such set-up and the standard algorithm can be followed. In those cases, management will depend on degree of displacement and the nail system in situ. If the fracture is not displaced or minimally displaced and the nail system in situ possesses a reconstruction option, then the proximal interlocking bolts can be removed and fracture neck femur is fixed using two cephalomedullary screws. This may need caudal or cranial readjustment of the nail to bring the proximal holes in alignment for screwing of neck fracture, meanwhile holding the fracture provisionally with guide pins. If the nailing system does not have a reconstruction option then a surgeon has to utilize the available ready to use implant for best possible outcome. One such approach to tackle it is "Miss-A-Nail Technique" for Neck of Femur Screw Fixation, where available screws (CCS or noncannulated) can be used to fix the iatrogenic fracture using the bone stock spanning on anterior/posterior aspect of the in situ nail.

Diagnosis

Besides high clinical suspicion and assessment, a planned and focused radiology is of paramount importance.

Advise pelvic CT to study the proximal femur/neck femur as it is painful and nearly impossible to get a true lateral and internal rotation view of the proximal femur/hip in presence of ipsilateral shaft femur fracture.

Some authors like Tornetta et al. have recommended the use of a thin-cut CT scan of pelvis with reconstructed images of sagittal, coronal, and axial sequences.

MANAGEMENT

Broadly the line of management will depend upon the fracture pattern as depicted in clinical algorithm **(Flowchart 1)**.

All these methods of management have been described in literature with their own set of conditions for each scenario. Being a

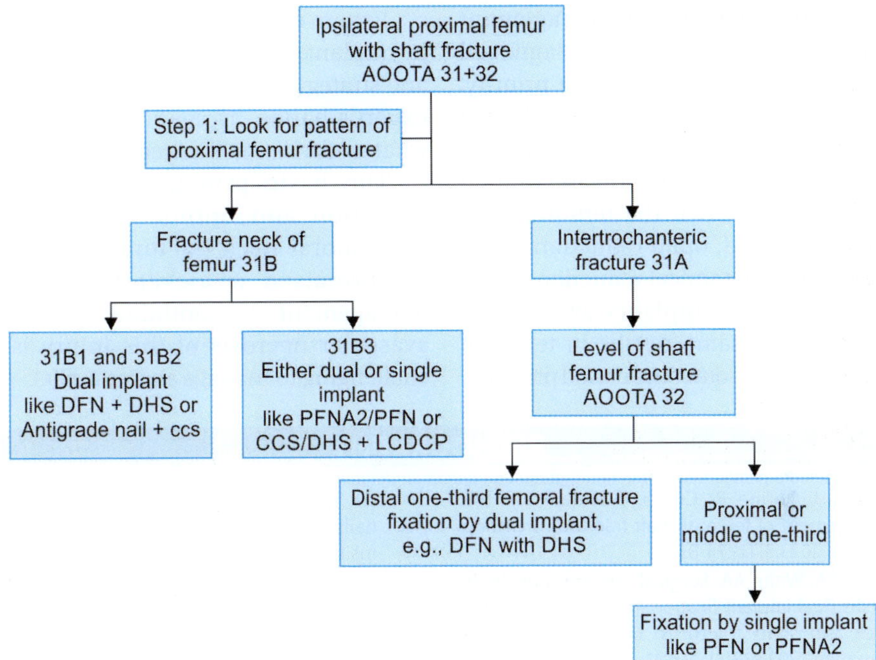

FLOWCHART 1: Clinical algorithm for management of the fracture.

(DFN: distal femoral nail; DHS: dynamic hip screw; CCS: cannulated cancellous screws; PFN: proximal femoral nail; PFNA2: proximal femoral nail antirotation; LCDCP: limited contact dynamic compression plate)

Source: Copyright © 2024, Rai et al. Clinical algorithm based on fracture pattern of ipsilateral proximal and shaft of femur fractures.

rare injury with limited studies, it lacks a level 1 evidence to support or refute a particular management protocol. Still, some general guidelines have been proposed in many studies to guide in planning for each pattern of fracture.

A brief overview of different modalities:

- *Cephalomedullary nails*:
  - *Demerits*: Technically more demanding and challenging to use in displaced femoral neck fractures leading to higher rates of malreduction, fixation failure, nonunion, and avascular necrosis
  - *Merits*: Ideal for a well reduced/undisplaced femoral neck fractures, more quick, short operative time, minimally invasive, less blood loss, single implant
- *Individualized approach*:
  - Distal femoral nail (DFN) for shaft fracture and cannulated cancellous screws (CCS)/dynamic hip screw (DHS) for femoral neck fracture has been found to be more promising in displaced neck fractures in terms of union rates as reported by Ostrum et al.
  - The closed nailing of shaft fracture with DFN primarily will restore the broken lever arm of the shaft to aid in subsequent closed femoral neck reduction.
  - Plating of the femoral shaft is mainly done in distal femur fractures and has the disadvantage of more invasive, higher blood loss, higher nonunion rates, delayed weight bearing, and more invasive implant removal.

As the central focus in management is the neck femur and if it is diagnosed before surgery, its treatment is the priority, followed by the femoral shaft. Usually, the neck fracture is minimally displaced or undisplaced and close reduction and fixation will suffice. However, if the femoral neck fracture is displaced, open reduction might be necessary for anatomical reduction.

Dual and single implants are equally effective and give same results in terms of union and functional outcome if used properly.

Pattern of fracture will be a deciding factor in implant selection. Finally, best implant and strategy is what gives best results in each expert's hands, as every surgeon executes what works best in his/her hands.

The basic principle for anatomical reduction and optimal stabilization of the femoral neck fracture should not be compromised whatever be the line of management, as nonunion, malunion, or avascular necrosis of this injury is more challenging to manage successfully.

BIBLIOGRAPHY

1. Griffen J, Torine R, Cox J. Advances in the management of femoral shaft fractures. J Orthop Trauma. 2023;37(2):75-83.
2. Harris DA, White AA. Surgical outcomes of single versus dual implant fixation in ipsilateral femoral neck and shaft fractures. Eur J Orthop Surg Traumatol. 2023;33(5):723-31.
3. Jones CB, Walker JB. Diagnosis and management of ipsilateral femoral neck and shaft fractures. J Am Acad Orthop Surg. 2018;26(21):e448-54.
4. Liu Y, Cui G, Li Z. Comparison of reconstruction nails versus dual implants in the treatment of ipsilateral femoral neck and shaft fractures in adults: A meta-analysis and systematic review. BMC Musculoskelet Disord. 2023;24:105.
5. Wolinsky PR, Johnson KD. Ipsilateral femoral neck and shaft fractures. Clin Orthop Relat Res. 1995;(318):81-90.

CHAPTER 10.3

Distal Femur Fracture and Hoffa's Fracture

Dibyendu Biswas, Samarth Mittal

- Distal femur fractures have become increasingly prevalent, now representing up to 6% of all femoral fractures.
- These fractures often are unstable and comminuted, which has historically rendered their treatment challenging.
- These fractures exhibit a bimodal age distribution. In the younger population, they are predominantly caused by motor vehicle accidents and falls from height. In contrast, the elderly population experiences a second peak in incidence due to minor falls.
- There is a 1:2 ratio of men to women.
- Because of the proximity of these fractures to the knee joint, regaining full knee range of motion and function may be difficult.
- Compound fractures account for 5–10% of all distal femur fractures.

ANATOMY

- The shaft of the femur is cylindrical, but at the lower end, it broadens into two curved condyles.
- Distal femur includes both supracondylar and condylar regions **(Fig. 1)**.
- Supracondylar region comprises area between femoral condyles and junction of shaft with metaphysis.
- With end on view, distal femur is trapezoidal with posterior part of condyle being wider than anterior, creating 25° inclination angle on medial surface and 15° on lateral surface **(Figs. 2A to C)**.
- In coronal plane, medial condyle extends more distally and is more convex than the lateral condyle.
- Anteriorly, the articular surfaces of the two condyles come together to form trochlear groove and posteriorly they are separated by intercondylar notch which gives attachment to cruciate ligaments.
- Medial surface contains medial epicondyle which gives origin to medial collateral ligament and proximally to it is adductor tubercle which gives attachment to adductor magnus tendon.
- Normally, knee joint is oriented parallel to ankle joint and ground level.
- The anatomic axis of femoral shaft relative to knee amounts to 6–7° of valgus.

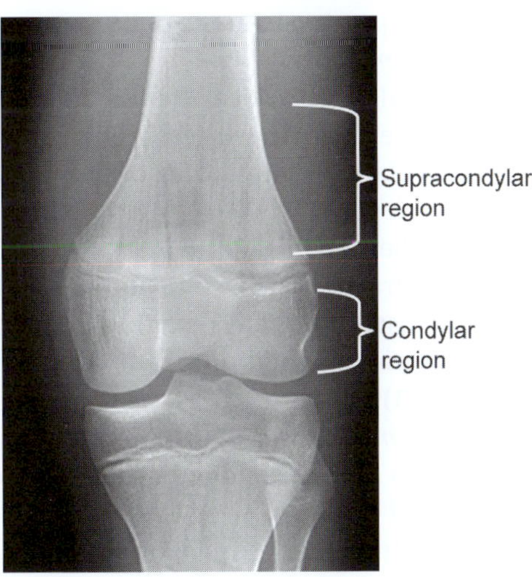

FIG. 1: Radiograph detailing the supracondylar and condylar regions of distal femur.

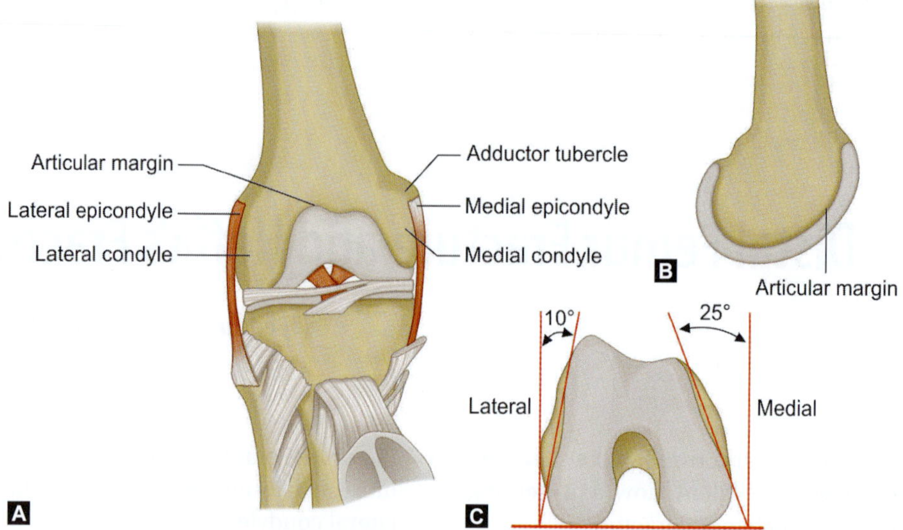

FIGS. 2A TO C: Anatomy of distal femur: (A) Anterior view, (B) Lateral view, (C) Axial view.

Source: Adapted from Court-Brown C, Heckman J, McQueen M, McKee M, Ricci W, Tornetta P III. Rockwood and Green's Fractures in Adults, 8th edition. Philadelphia: Wolters Kluwer; 2014.

BIOMECHANICS AROUND DISTAL FEMUR

- *Quadriceps femoris*:
  - Lies anteriorly and supplies power to extensor apparatus. Tendon envelops patella and terminates via patellar tendon into the tibial tuberosity.
  - Supplied by femoral nerve
  - Results in shortening post fracture due to proximal muscle pull
- *Gastrocnemius*:
  - Medial and lateral heads of this muscle form the inferomedial and inferolateral boundaries of popliteal fossa respectively.
  - Supplied by tibial nerve
  - Post fracture, this muscle extends the distal fragment resulting in apex posterior angulation of the fracture **(Fig. 3)**.
- *Adductor magnus*:
  - Inserts onto the adductor tubercle on medial condyle
  - Supplied by dual innervation. Adductor part is supplied by posterior division of obturator nerve and hamstring part by tibial nerve.
  - Post fracture, this muscle leads to varus deformity of distal fragment.
- *Hamstrings*:
  - Comprises biceps femoris, semitendinosus, semimembranosus, and hamstring part of adductor magnus
  - Supplied by tibial part of sciatic nerve
  - Post fracture causes shortening

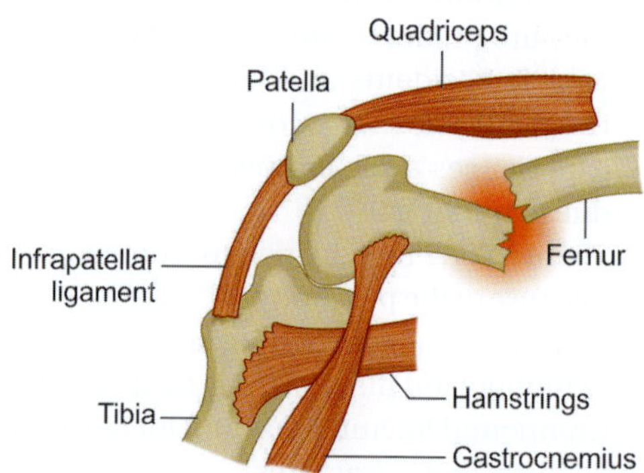

FIG. 3: Biomechanical deforming forces around distal femur.

- *Femoral artery*:
  - Runs anteromedially through mid-thigh between extensor and adductor compartments underneath the sartorius muscle
  - These vessels pierce the adductor magnus 10 cm above the knee joint to enter into posterior compartment.
  - In posterior compartment, it joins sciatic nerve in popliteal fossa.

MECHANISM OF INJURY

- In younger population, these fractures are a result of high-energy trauma such as road traffic accidents or fall from height.
- In elderly population, trivial trauma like slip and fall can result in distal femur fracture.

CLASSIFICATION

- The *AO/OTA classification system* categorizes distal femoral fractures into three distinct groups—A, B, and C with increasing gradient of complexity and severity **(Fig. 4)**.
- Distal femur fracture's prefix is 33, indicating the femur (3) and the distal portion of the femur (3).
- *33A*: Extra-articular—
  - *33A1*: Avulsion
  - *33A2*: Simple
  - *33A3*: Wedge or multifragmentary—
    - *33A3.1*: Intact wedge
    - *33A3.2*: Fragmentary wedge
- *33B*: Partial articular, the fracture involves one part of the articular surface, yet the rest of the joint is still attached to the metaphysis and diaphysis.
  - *33B1*: Lateral sagittal—
    - *33B1.1*: Through the notch
    - *33B1.2*: Through load-bearing lateral condyle
    - *33B1.3*: Sagittal fragmentary
  - *33B2*: Medial sagittal—
    - *33B2.1*: Through the notch
    - *33B2.2*: Through load-bearing medial condyle
    - *33B2.3*: Sagittal fragmentary

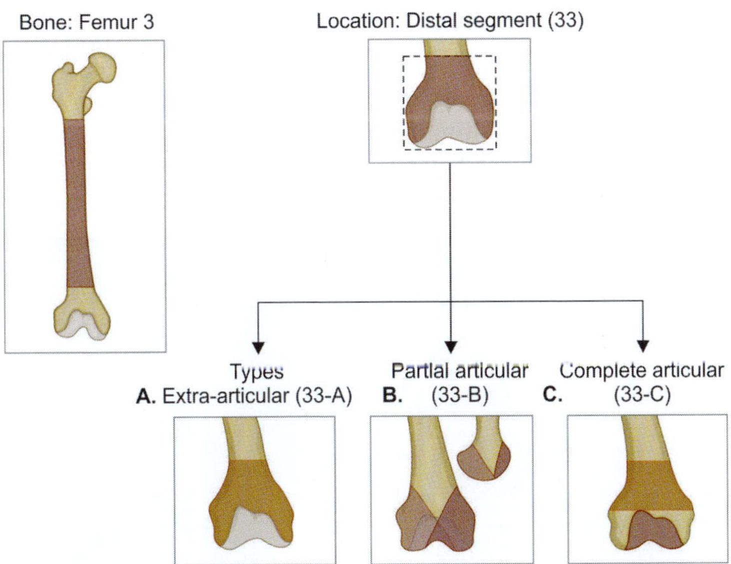

FIG. 4: OTA classification distal femur.

Source: Adapted from Meinberg EG, Agel J, Roberts CS, Karam MD, Kellam JF. AO/OTA fracture and dislocation classification compendium 2018. J Orthop Trauma. 2018;32 Suppl 1:S1-S170.

- *33B3*: Frontal/coronal—
  - *33B3.1*: Anterior and lateral flake fracture
  - *33B3.2*: Unicondylar posterior
  - *33B3.3*: Bicondylar posterior
- *33C*: Complete articular, the fracture is distributing the joint surface and separated from the diaphysis—
  - *33C1*: Simple articular—
    - *33C1.1*: Above transcondylar axis
    - *33C1.3*: Through or below transcondylar axis
  - *33C2*: Simple articular with a fragmentary metaphyseal component—
    - *33C2.1*: Intact metaphyseal wedge
    - *33C2.1*: Fragmentary metaphyseal wedge
  - *33C3*: Multifragmentary articular—
    - *33C3.1*: Simple metaphyseal
    - *33C3.2*: Wedge metaphyseal
    - *33C3.3*: Metaphysio-diaphyseal multifragmentary
- *Descriptive classification* is based on location of fracture:
  - Supracondylar fractures
  - Intercondylar fractures
  - Condylar fractures
- *Hoffa's fracture*: The Hoffa fracture of the distal femur is a rare injury described as a coronal fracture of the femur involving one or both of the condyles **(Figs. 5A to C)**.

In AO classification, these fractures represent 33B3 group.

CLINICAL EVALUATION

- Presenting features in emergency are those of pain, swelling, bluish skin discoloration, deformity in lower thigh and around knee along with inability to bear weight.
- Assessment of neurovascular status is essential, as the popliteal artery is susceptible to injury in this region due to its tethering proximally at the adductor hiatus and distally at the soleus arch.
- Signs of vascular injury include absent or diminished pulse, tense unusual swelling due to expanding hematoma, diminished ankle-brachial index, bruit, injury to anatomically related nerves.
- Concomitant ligamentous injuries, while infrequent, should be thoroughly assessed and identified.
- In massive open wounds, clinical evaluation along with radiographs helps in assessing bone loss.

RADIOGRAPHIC EVALUATION

- *X-rays*: Anteroposterior and lateral views are first line of investigation. Special traction radiographs help in determining

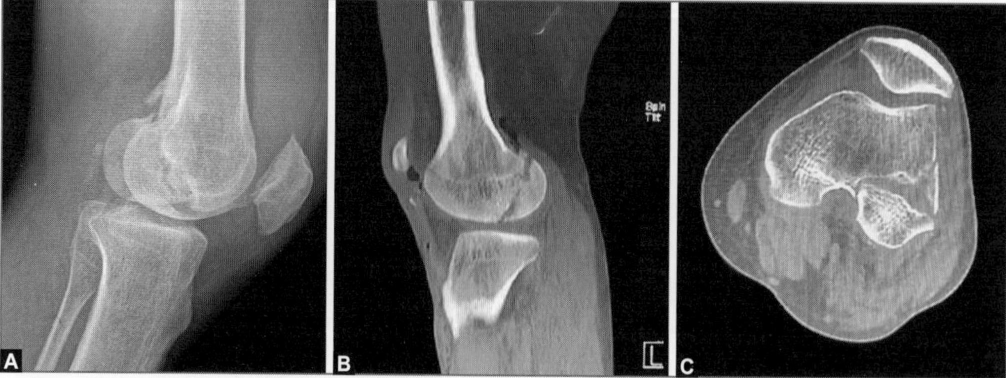

FIGS. 5A TO C: (A) Lateral radiograph showing Hoffa's fracture of distal femoral condyle. (B) Sagittal CT cut. (C) Axial CT cut demonstrating coronal plane fracture.

fracture pattern, joint involvement, and facilitate preoperative planning. Double density sign on AP radiograph is suggestive of a Hoffa's fragment **(Fig. 6)**.

- *Computed tomography (CT)*: Complex intra-articular fractures require CT scan with 3D-reconstructions images to further classify and help in better surgical planning.
- *Magnetic resonance imaging (MRI)*: Very limited role, whenever there is a suspected ligamentous injury associated.
- *Arteriography*: To identify any vascular disruption, especially when associated with knee dislocation.

MANAGEMENT

- *Nonoperative management*:
  - Very limited role as operative treatment is treatment of choice.
  - *Indications*:
    - Nonambulatory patient with significant comorbidities
    - Undisplaced or incomplete fractures
  - In stable, undisplaced fractures, treatment initially includes long leg casts followed by mobilization in hinge ROM knee brace with partial weight bearing.

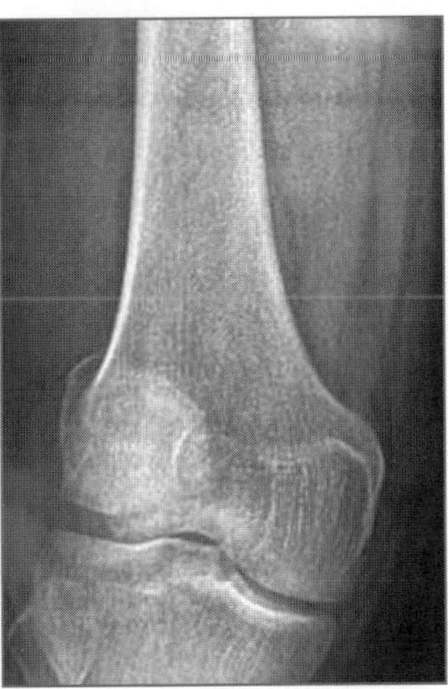

FIG. 6: Double density sign seen in Hoffa's fracture.

  - In displaced fractures, initially skeletal traction is given to restore length and alignment followed by 6–12 weeks of casting with strict nonweight bearing.
  - Limitations of nonoperative management include residual deformity, knee stiffness, prolonged hospitalization or bed rest, and future gait abnormalities due to residual varus.
- *Operative management*:
  - Treatment of choice for most distal femur fractures
  - Emergency surgical intervention is indicated; however, in cases where there is a delay in surgery, it is recommended to apply temporary immobilization using a long knee slab or tibial skeletal traction.
  - *Supracondylar fractures*: Aim of surgery is restoration of length, coronal, sagittal and rotational alignments. Methods of fixation are:
    - *Retrograde femur nailing*: Load sharing device with improved distal fixation with maintained biology **(Figs. 7A and B)**. Disadvantages include violation of knee joint and inability to use in skeletally immature population due to risk of physeal growth arrest.
    - *Locking plates*: Biological minimally invasive plate osteosynthesis (MIPO) **(Figs. 8A and B)** is preferred over conventional open reduction. Can be used in skeletally immature patients as physeal sparing plating.
    - *Antegrade femur nail*: Can be used in case of large supracondylar distal fragment where there is unavailability of retrograde nail. Very limited use due to limited distal locking options.
    - *Dynamic condylar screw (DCS) and 95° condylar blade plate*: Less frequently used these days due to technical demanding nature of

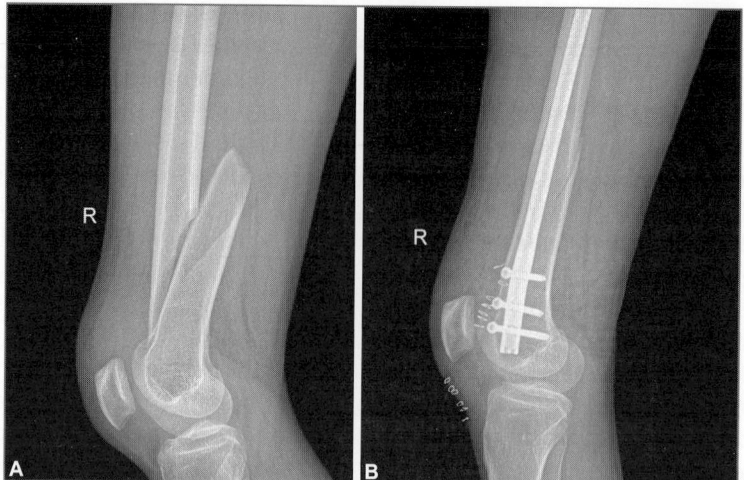

FIGS. 7A AND B: Supracondylar femur fracture managed by retrograde nailing.

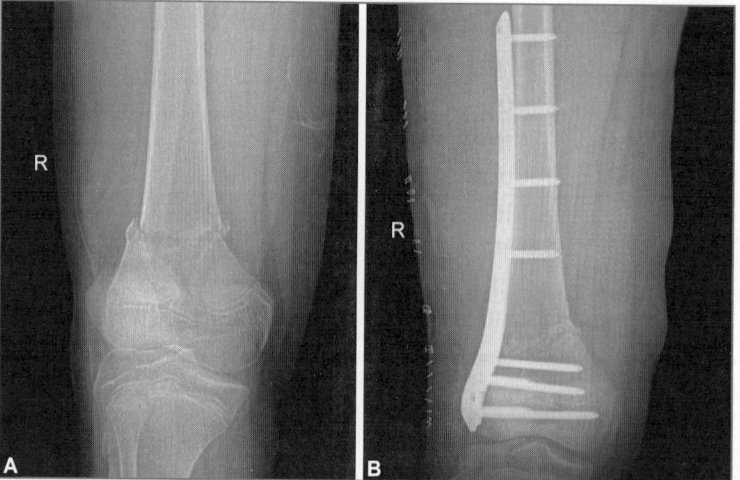

FIGS. 8A AND B: Supracondylar femur fracture managed by MIPO plating.
(MIPO: minimally invasive plate osteosynthesis)

surgery. Mostly used nowadays for treatment of malunions and nonunions.

- *Intercondylar fractures*: Aim of surgery is complete anatomical reduction of articular surface to prevent early arthritis along with restoration of length and alignment. Methods of fixation are:
  - *Open reduction and internal fixation (ORIF) with locked plating*: Treatment of choice for most intra-articular intercondylar fractures. Can be single lateral plate or dual plate based on fracture morphology **(Figs. 9A and B)**.
  - *Retrograde femur nailing*: Increased usage in C1 and C2 fractures after anatomical reduction due to advantage of early weight bearing being a load sharing device.

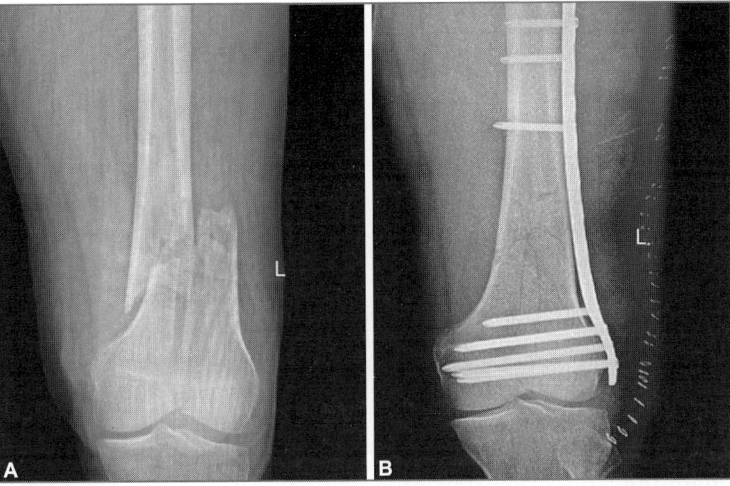

FIGS. 9A AND B: Intercondylar femur fracture managed by locking plate.

- *Combination of nail and locked plate*: There is a growing trend toward the use of this method, as it integrates the advantages of both intramedullary nails and external plates.

- *Hoffa's fractures*: Aim of surgery is anatomical reduction of articular surface to prevent early arthritis and preserve range of motion postsurgery. Methods of fixation are:
  - *Screws*: Anterior to posterior or posterior to anterior screws used alone are most common mode of fixation for such fractures **(Fig. 10)**. Interfragmentary compression can be achieved using cannulated cancellous screws or headless compression screws.
  - *Plating*: Supplementary buttress plating or locked plating is often required in addition to screws when there is associated comminution.
- *Compound fractures*: Up to grade 3a open fractures can be managed on closed lines. Beyond this, compound fractures are managed by thorough debridement, wound wash, and external fixator application followed by definitive fixation at a later date.

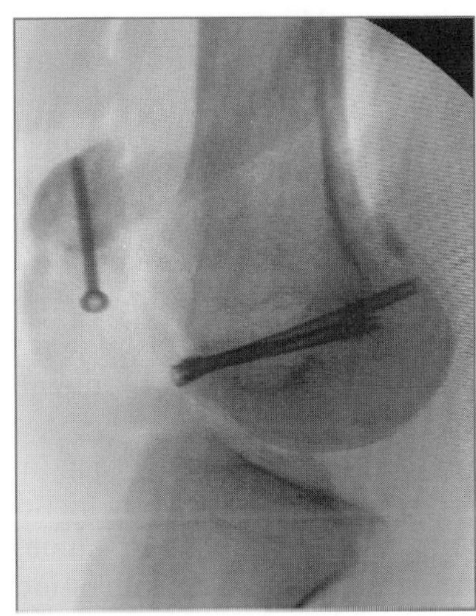

FIG. 10: Hoffa's fracture managed by anterior to posterior screws.

POSTOPERATIVE REHABILITATION

- Postoperatively, early range of motion is started on day 1 to prevent knee stiffness.
- Patients are kept nonweight-bearing postsurgery, and weight bearing is encouraged typically 6–8 weeks after surgery once there is radiographic evidence of callus formation.
- Supportive physiotherapy is form of quadriceps strengthening exercises, knee ROM exercises are continued throughout the process of recovery.

COMPLICATIONS

- *Knee stiffness*: Most common complication post injury. Causes include quadriceps scarring, articular discontinuity, and lack of rehabilitative efforts by the patient. This complication can be mitigated by initiating early range of motion exercises, ensuring accurate anatomical reduction, and performing meticulous dissection during the intraoperative period.
- *Failure of fixation*: Causal factors include nonunion, osteoporosis, inadequate surgical fixation and early weight bearing by patient. Can be prevented by proper surgical planning and execution and using supplementary fixation tools to add stability to the construct.
- *Malunion*: More commonly seen in patients managed nonoperatively. Malalignment can lead to gait disturbances as residual varus being the most common deformity. This can be countered with osteotomy at a later date.
- *Nonunion*: Uncommon due to rich vascular supply in metaphyseal region. When encountered, can be addressed using bone grafting and supplementary fixation.
- *Infection*: More commonly seen in open fractures. Best prevented by meticulous debridement and copious irrigation at the time of first surgery. Treatment includes serial debridement and lavage, antibiotic cement application and sometimes warrants implant removal.
- *Post-traumatic arthritis*: Casual fractures include inability to maintain articular congruity at the time of surgery or impaction cartilage injuries at the time of trauma. Can be managed at a later date with total knee arthroplasty.
- *Vascular injury*: Can occur at the time of injury or during surgery. Management necessitates prompt vascular exploration and repair, followed by prophylactic fasciotomy, executed in close collaboration with the vascular surgery team.

OUTCOMES AND EVIDENCE-BASED GUIDELINES

- Recent studies have proposed that segmental bone loss, open fractures, chronic anemia, and increasing body mass index are significant risk factors in the occurrence of distal femoral nonunion.
- Implant failure is a concern post fracture fixation in many patients. A recent study by Hou et al. concluded that elderly age, fracture type (A3 and periprosthetic fracture after TKA), poor reduction quality, and the ratio of the length of the plate/fracture area above the condylar were the possible risk factors of the revision in distal femoral fractures treated with lateral locking plate.
- A recent trend is toward fixation using nail and plate combination. According to Garala et al., using nail plate combination gives surgeons confidence for early weight bearing and therefore decreases immobility related morbidity, and is of particular value in older patients with poor quality distal femur metaphyseal bone and subsequent metaphyseal comminution.

CONCLUSION

- Distal femur fractures are prevalent lower limb injuries that generally necessitate prompt fixation to facilitate early rehabilitation and enable weight bearing.
- Open fractures present a risk of infection, which can potentially involve the knee joint and exacerbate the condition. Therefore, immediate intervention with lavage, debridement, temporary stabilization, and intravenous antibiotics is crucial.
- Vascular assessment in all patients with distal femur fractures is of paramount importance due to the potentially catastrophic implications of vascular compromise.

- Adherence to stringent acceptability criteria regarding articular congruity, length, and alignment during surgical intervention is crucial for achieving optimal functional outcomes.
- Early rehabilitation, including knee range of motion exercises commencing on postoperative day 1, is crucial for optimal recovery.
- Given the wide range of available implants, the choice of implant is determined by the patient's profile and the surgeon's expertise.

BIBLIOGRAPHY

1. Cone R, Roszman A, Conway Y, Cichos K, McGwin G, Spitler CA. Risk Factors for Nonunion of Distal Femur Fractures. J Orthop Trauma. 2023;37(4):175-80.
2. Garala K, Ramoutar D, Li J, Syed F, Arastu M, Ward J, et al. Distal femoral fractures: A comparison between single lateral plate fixation and a combined femoral nail and plate fixation. Injury. 2022;53(2):634-9.
3. Hou G, Zhou F, Tian Y, Ji H, Zhang Z, Guo Y, et al. Analysis of risk factors for revision in distal femoral fractures treated with lateral locking plate: a retrospective study in Chinese patients. J Orthop Surg Res. 2020;15(1):318.

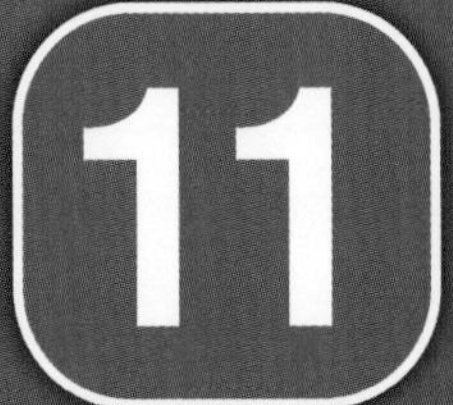

SECTION 11

Knee

CHAPTER 11.1

Patella Fracture

Tejpal Singh

Patella is the largest sesamoid bone in our body.

It is an emergency condition as the patella plays a vital role in extensor mechanism and knee biomechanics, hence fracture of the patella leads to the impairment of its functions. If not managed timely, it may lead to substantial functional disability and its treatment varies from conservative to surgical.

INCIDENCE

- 1% of all the skeletal injuries in the human body.
- 6–9% are open fractures.

APPLIED ANATOMY

Superiorly quadriceps tendon is attached at superior pole of patella and the strong tensile force of contraction of quadriceps tendon is transmitted to ligamentum patellae which extends from inferior pole of patella to tibial tuberosity, thus helps in extension of knee joint. Fascia gets condensed into medial retinacula and lateral retinacula and gets attached at medial and lateral margins of patella. Total of seven facets are there at posterior surface of patella, among them lateral facets being the largest and inferior surface is covered by articular cartilage which is approximately 1 cm thick.

MECHANISM OF INJURY

- *Indirect mechanism (most common)*: This happens secondary to extensor mechanism function of patella which produces such a strong powerful contraction force with knee in a semiflexed position which results in transverse type of fracture pattern with greater degree of retinacular rupture.
- *Direct mechanism*: Due to the anatomical location, i.e., anterior subcutaneous location, direct traumatic impact due to motor vehicle dashboard injury (high energy), trauma due to fall from height with direct impact to anterior knee (low energy). These types of traumatic impact to patella usually produce simple, incomplete, stellate or comminuted type of fracture patterns. Active knee extension function of knee may be intact.
- *Combined direct and indirect mechanism*: This type of injury involves combination of both indirect and direct traumatic impact to the knee joint which is seen in fall from height, leading to transverse fracture of patella.

Associated injuries with patellar fractures:

- Ipsilateral distal femur
- Ipsilateral proximal tibia fracture

CLASSIFICATION

Descriptive:

- Open versus closed
- Displaced versus undisplaced
- *Fracture configuration/pattern* **(Fig. 1)**:
  - Undisplaced
  - Stellate (undisplaced multifragmented)

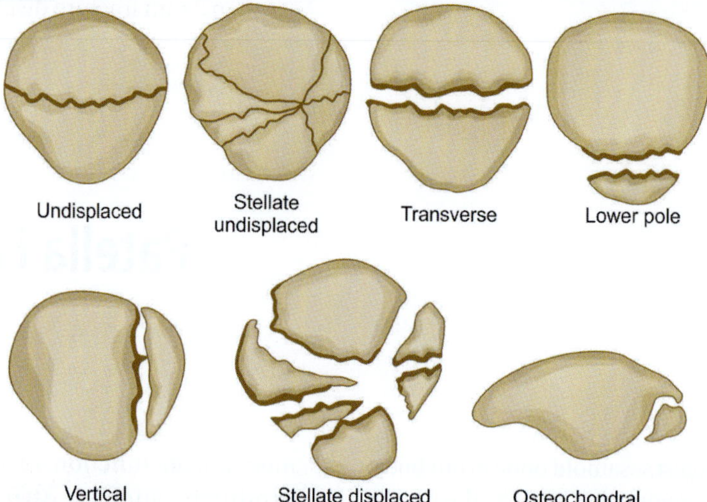

FIG. 1: Classification on the basis of fracture pattern.

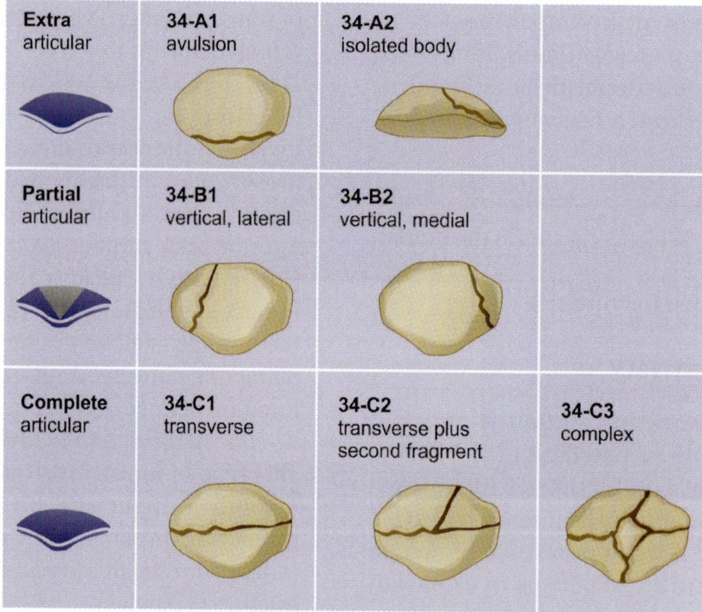

FIG. 2: AO/OTA classification.

- Transverse
- Stellate (displaced multifragmented)
- Vertical
- Polar osteochondral
- Lower or upper pole

AO/OTA classification of patellar fractures ***(Fig. 2)***:

- *34-A*: Extra-articular
- *34-B*: Partial articular
- *34-C*: Complete articular

CLINICAL EVALUATION

- Active knee extension or straight leg raise should be done, if the patient is unable to perform the straight leg, this signifies disruption of the extensor mechanism and disruption of the retinaculum. Sometimes, patient is unable to perform straight leg raise due to a painful knee, then we can aspirate hemarthrosis and

locally inject lignocaine and again check for straight leg raise.
- To rule out involvement of concomitant knee joint, a saline load test should be done.

INVESTIGATIONS

- *Radiographs*: View advised or recommended—
  - Anteroposterior view **(Fig. 3)**
  - Lateral view **(Fig. 4)**
  - *Axial/sunrise/merchant view* ***(Fig. 5)***: Vertical fractures are well viewed with this view (if pain permits).
- *Computed tomography*: Indications are as follows—
  - Suspected fracture of distal pole
  - Stress fracture of patella
  - Malunion
  - Nonunion
  - Also, it is needed to differentiate between the bipartite patella and fracture.

TREATMENT

Conservative/Nonoperative

Indications:
- Intact extensor mechanism
- Undisplaced patella fracture
- Less than 2 mm articular incongruity
- Less than 3 mm fracture displacement
- Severe medical condition
- Severe osteopenia

These patients are managed with extensor splinting/bracing or with a long leg cylindrical cast for a period of 4–6 weeks. Then serial of radiographs will be done for evaluating fracture healing.

Surgical/Operative

Indications:
- Loss of extensor mechanism, i.e., loss of active extension

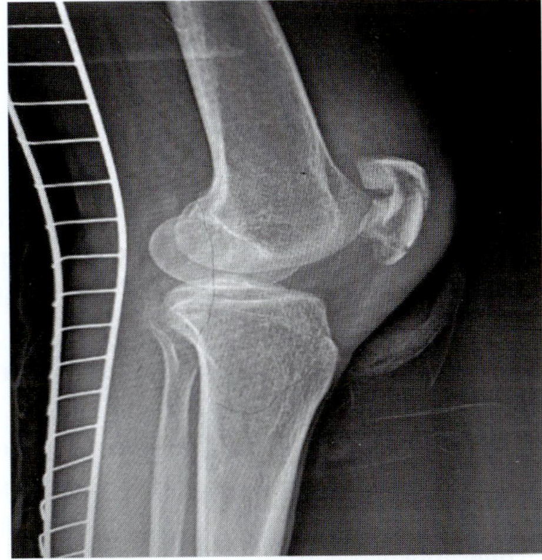

FIG. 4: Lateral view showing fracture of patella.

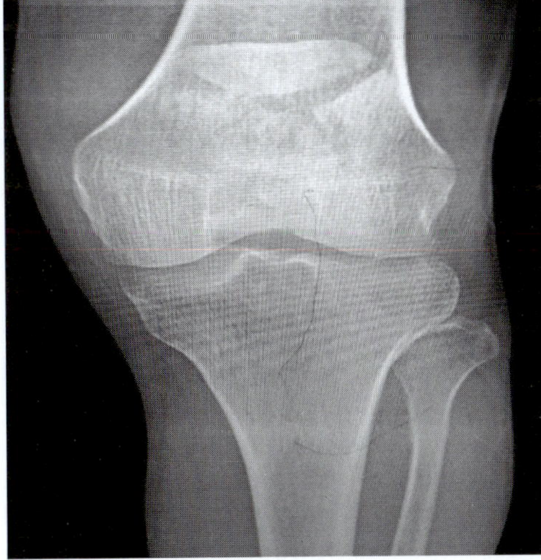

FIG. 3: Anteroposterior (AP) view showing fracture of patella.

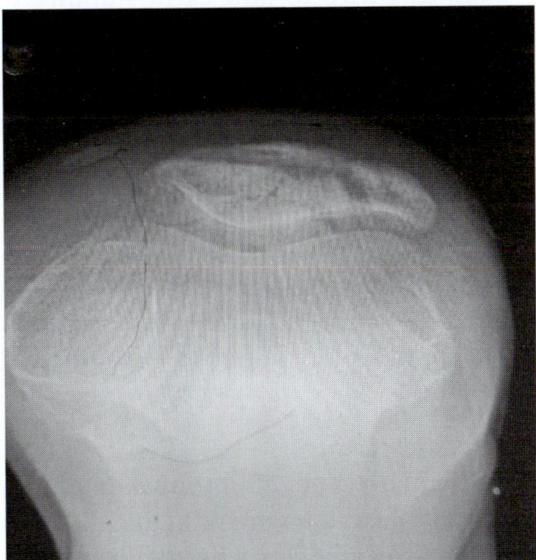

FIG. 5: Merchant view showing fracture of patella.

- Displaced patella fracture with retinacular disruption
- More than 2 mm articular incongruity
- More than 3 mm fracture displacement
- Open fracture
- Loose bodies

Target of operative intervention: To achieve the intact extensor mechanism of the knee joint and congruity of patellofemoral articulation.

Various surgical options are:
- *Open reduction with tension band wiring* ***(Figs. 6 and 7)***: Most common procedure
- Interfragmentary screws
- Locking plate system
- Cerclage wiring
- Partial patellectomy
- Complete patellectomy

Indicated in the transverse pattern of fracture:
- Here two parallel Kirschner wires were used and stainless wires in a figure-of-eight were combined which use distraction forces and covert compression forces to achieve compression at fracture sites.
- Postoperatively, early passive range of motion exercises were initiated to prevent knee stiffness and weight bearing as bearable was started.
- Sometimes, cerclage is done using stainless wire to add extra stability to construct.

Cannulated screws with tension band ***(Fig. 8)***:
- Indicated in patients having large fragments
- Provide superior stability
- Follows the same principle as in TBW

Locked plating systems ***(Fig. 9)***: Indicated in comminuted pattern fractures, especially in osteoporotic bone, anatomically contoured locked plates offer superior fixation and alignment.

Partial patellectomy:
- Indicated when comminution of the distal pole or a fragment of the patella is extensive and cannot be stabilized with internal fixation.

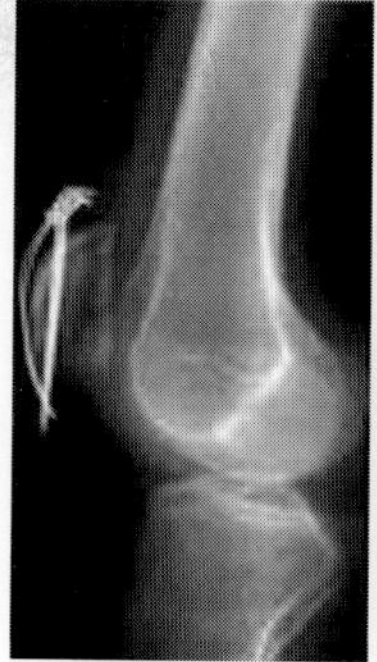
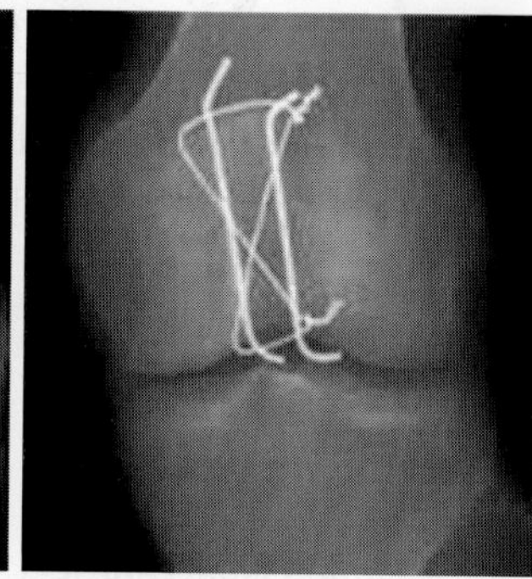

FIG. 6: Tension band wiring using figure-of-eight.

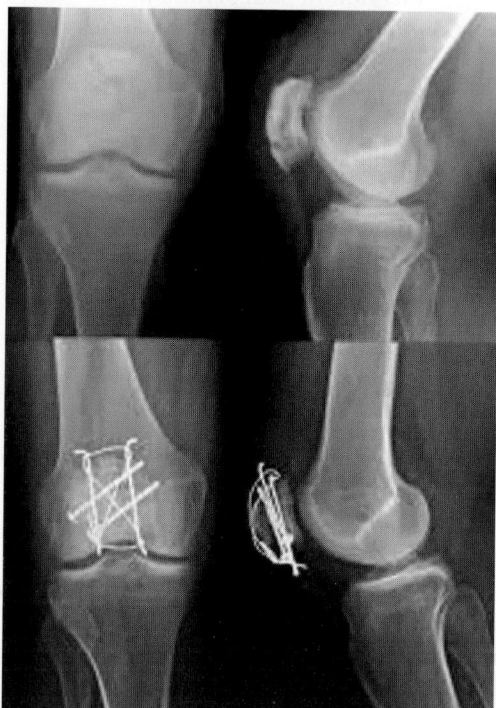

FIG. 7: Anteroposterior (AP) and lateral views showing fracture of patella (preoperative and postoperative).

- Fragments that are avascularized or free with limited soft tissue attachments and likely to become loose bodies within the knee joint should be removed.
- The patellar tendon may be reattached with nonabsorbable sutures placed longitudinally through drill holes or via suture anchors along the long axis.

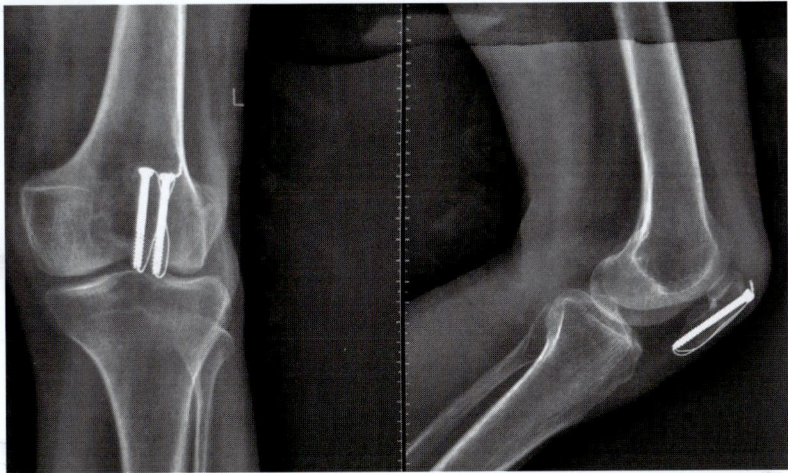

FIG. 8: Postoperative X-ray showing cannulated cancellous screws being used for fixation.

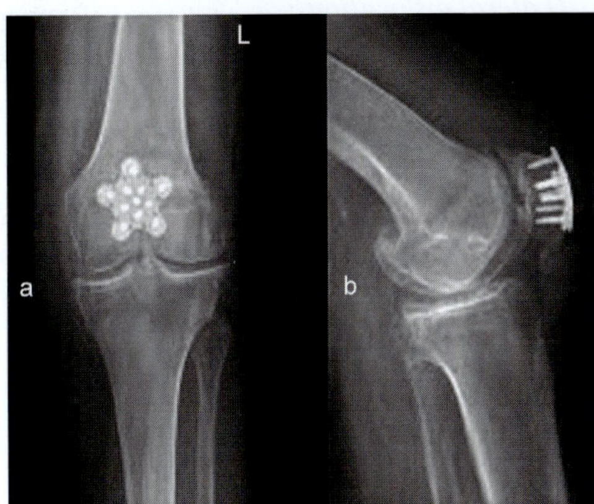

FIG. 9: Locking plating system.

Total patellectomy:

- Indicated in those fracture patterns that are severely comminuted fractures which cannot be fixed by internal fixation or suture repair, infection of the patella, an internal fixation which has failed and tumors of the patella.
- Here almost half of the peak torque of quadriceps is reduced.
- Here all the fragments of the patella are removed, then the redundant extensor mechanism tissue is sutured using a nonabsorbable suture, and then extensor mechanism tension at 90° of flexion is checked.

COMPLICATIONS

- Postoperative infection
- Fixation failure
- Refracture
- Nonunion
- Osteonecrosis (proximal fragment)
- Post-traumatic osteoarthritis
- Loss of knee motion
- Painful retained hardware
- Loss of extensor strength and extensor lag
- Patellar instability

BIBLIOGRAPHY

1. Bucholz RW, Court-Brown CM, Heckman JD, Tornetta P. Rockwood and Green's Fractures in Adults. 9th edition. Philadelphia, PA: Lippincott Williams & Wilkins; 2020. (Chapter on patellar fractures)
2. Egol KA, Koval KJ, Zuckerman JD. Trauma and Orthopaedic Surgery: Principles of Management and Practice. 2nd edition. Springer; 2017. (Patellar fracture management)
3. Koval KJ, Zuckerman JD. Handbook of Fractures. 6th edition. Philadelphia, PA: Wolters Kluwer Health; 2021. (Section on patella fractures)

Acute Patella Dislocation

Manish Singh

The patellofemoral (also called as anterior knee) joint stability depends on osteoarticular conformation and static and dynamic stabilization structures. Any change in anatomy, such as extensor apparatus alignment defect, patellofemoral dysplasia, or trauma, can induce patellar instability. There are two patellar facets—medial and lateral, these are symmetric and congruent with the femoral trochlea. Trochlear morphology remains relatively constant but, with growth, the thick trochlear cartilage thins in the middle, creating an illusion of a trochlear "hollow".

BIOMECHANICS

The medial patellofemoral ligament (MPFL) provides 50–80% of the stability. Outward/lateral patellar dislocation renders it incompetent, causing recurrence of dislocation.

The patellomeniscal or patellotibial ligaments and the superficial medial retinaculum are less contributors to patellar stability.

The vastus medialis oblique (VMO) muscle is very important, acting as a dynamic stabilizer, and works in synergy to the MPFL.

With the knee in complete extension, the patella lies above the trochlear sulcus. It enters the trochlea when the knee is in 10–30° flexion.

TYPES OF DISLOCATION

Patellar dislocation can be classified into:

- *Lateral dislocation*
- *Medial dislocation,* which is exclusively iatrogenic
- *Intra-articular dislocation* is very rare.
- *Acute or chronic*
- *Recurrent dislocation and habitual dislocation* will not be included in this section.

TRAUMATIC MECHANISM AND PREDISPOSING FACTORS

The typical mechanism underlying patellar dislocation is a movement of the knee in flexion and valgus without direct contact, accounting for >90% of traumatic patellar dislocations.

Almost all patients with traumatic patellar dislocation will present with hemarthrosis, MPFL lesion, and medial patellar wing fracture.

Osteochondral fracture occurs in 20–25% of traumatic patellar dislocations.

Recurrence risk is increased sixfold in case of history of ipsilateral or contralateral patellar dislocation.

Predisposing Factors

- Trochlear dysplasia
- Patella alta

- Elevated TT-TG distance
- Patellar tilt (normal 10° and 20°)
- Increased Q angle
- Elevated femoral anteversion
- Vastus medialis hypoplasia
- Genu recurvatum
- Patellar hypoplasia

PRESENTATION

- *Inability to move*: Difficulty or inability to straighten or move the knee
- *Bruising*: Discoloration around the knee
- X-rays to confirm the diagnosis **(Fig. 1)**

CT assesses bony risk factors like:
- Patellofemoral malalignment
- Osteochondral defects
- Patellar tilt and lateral subluxation
- Elevated TT-TG distance
- Trochlear dysplasia

It is also useful to screen for lower-limb rotational abnormality.

MRI: MRI is more specific in precisely diagnosing soft tissue structures and thus helping/guiding in treatment and decision-making. It also assesses the patellofemoral joint cartilage surfaces.

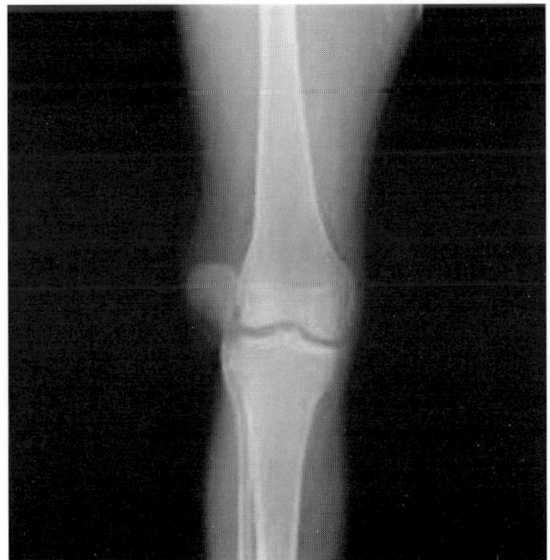

FIG. 1: X-rays showing lateral dislocation of patella.

MRI may reveal:
- Hemarthrosis
- Bone edema of the medial patellar facet and lateral femoral condyle
- Osteochondral lesions of the medial patellar facet and the anterolateral part of the lateral femoral condyle
- Deformity of the inferomedial patella, due to impaction, which is a specific sign of lateral patellar dislocation

TREATMENT

- *Immediate care*:
  - *Reduction*: Most of the times, it reduces spontaneously; only rarely need arises to manually reposition the patella into its proper place.
  - *Imaging*: X-rays or MRI may be required to assess the extent of the injury and check for any associated damage.
  - *Bracing*: A knee brace or splint may be used to stabilize the knee during healing.
  - *Rest to the part*: Avoid putting weight on the affected leg.
  - *Ice packs*: Apply ice to reduce swelling.
  - *Elevation*: Keep the leg elevated to minimize swelling.
  - Use an elastic bandage to reduce swelling.
- *Rehabilitation*:
  - *Physical therapy*: Exercises to strengthen the muscles around the knee and improve flexibility
  - *Range-of-motion exercises*: To regain normal movement in the knee
- *Surgery*: In the case of acute patellar dislocation, immediate surgery is only indicated in the event of a large loose body during which primary MPLF ligament repair can be undertaken.

Prevention:
- *Strengthening exercises*: Focus on strengthening the quadriceps and hamstrings to support the knee.

BIBLIOGRAPHY

1. Fithian DC, Paxton EW, Stone ML, Silva P, Davis DK, Elias DA, et al. Epidemiology and natural history of acute patellar dislocation. Am J Sports Med. 2004;32(5):1114-21.
2. Harilainen A, Myllynen P, Antila H, Seitsalo S. The significance of arthroscopy and examination under anaesthesia in the diagnosis of fresh injury haemarthrosis of the knee joint. Injury. 1988;19(1):21-4.
3. Sillanpaa P, Mattila VM, Iivonen T, Visuri T, Pihlajamäki H. Incidence and risk factors of acute traumatic primary patellar dislocation. Med Sci Sports Exerc. 2008;40(4):606-11.
4. Stefancin JJ, Parker RD. First-time traumatic patellar dislocation: a systematic review. Clin Orthop Relat Res. 2007;455:93-101.

CHAPTER 11.3

Knee Dislocation

Tejpal Singh

Knee dislocation (KD) is an orthopedic medical emergency which if not dealt with seriously may lead to limb loss due to the involvement of vascular injury. Traumatic KD is an uncommon injury which occurs mostly due to the high-energy mechanism of injury. However, KD due to low-energy injury is seen in morbidly obese patients. Multiligament injury is associated with true KD. Hence, vigilant clinical assessment and further management of KD patients are crucial for optimizing outcomes and minimizing long-term disability.

INCIDENCE

- Majority of the KDs were usually not reported due to spontaneous reduction (20–50%) and are misdiagnosed.
- 5% of cases are bilateral.
  - *Popliteal artery*: Injury to the popliteal vessel occurs due to tethering at the level of the popliteal fossa.
    - Proximal—fibrous tunnel at the adductor hiatus
    - Distal—fibrous tunnel at the soleus muscle
- Anterior dislocation of the tibia occurs due to hyperextension with or without varus/valgus.
- Posterior dislocation occurs due to flexion with posterior force (dashboard injury).

ASSOCIATED INJURIES

- Associated with fracture of the femur, proximal tibia, tibial eminence, tibial tubercle, fibular head or neck, and capsular avulsions
- Damage to menisci and cartilage
- Nerve injury—peroneal nerve

CLASSIFICATION

- Kennedy classification—classified on the basis of the direction of the tibia
- Schenck classification—classified on the basis of multiligamentous injury of KD

Kennedy classification **(*Fig. 1*)**:

- *Anterior type*:
  - The most common type
  - 30–40%
  - Posterior cruciate ligament (PCL) tear is commonly associated with injury.
  - Highest incidence of peroneal nerve injury
  - Popliteal vessel occurs here due to traction.
- *Posterior type*:
  - Second most common
  - 30–40%
  - Dashboard injury
  - Highest incidence of popliteal artery injury
- *Lateral type*:
  - 13%
  - Occurs due to varus or valgus force

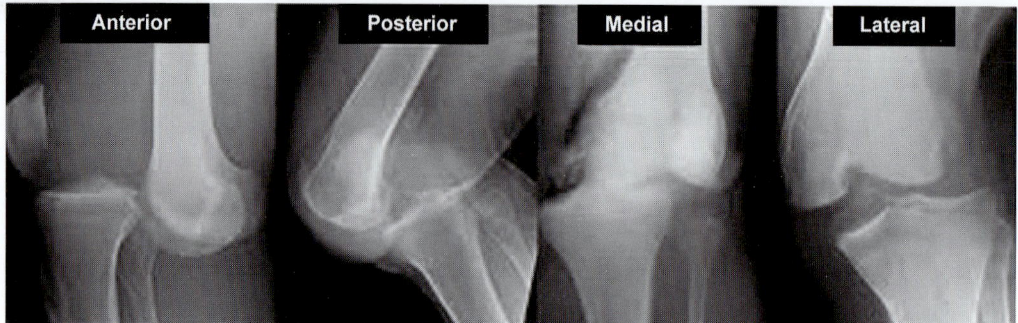

FIG. 1: Various types of knee dislocation.

- Anterior cruciate ligament (ACL) and PCL tears both are commonly involved.

- *Medial type*:
  - 3%
  - Occurs due to varus or valgus force
  - Posterolateral corner (PLC) and PCL injuries are common.
- *Rotational type*:
  - 4%
  - It is the most commonly irreducible type due to buttonholing of the femoral condyle through the capsule.
  - The posterolateral type is the most common rotational dislocation.

Modified Schenck classification ***(Table 1)***.

TABLE 1: Modified Schenck classification.

Type	Injury description
Knee dislocation 1 (KD 1)	PCL intact knee dislocation with a functioning PCL and variable collateral involvement (usually lateral)
Knee dislocation 2 (KD 2)	Complete bicruciate injury with both collaterals intact (uncommon)
Knee dislocation 3 (KD 3)	An injury to both cruciate ligaments and one collateral ligament, either medial or lateral
Knee dislocation 4 (KD 4)	An injury to both cruciate ligaments and both collateral ligaments
Knee dislocation 5 (KD 5)	A knee dislocation with periarticular fracture

(PCL: posterior cruciate ligament)

CLINICAL EVALUATION

- *Presentations*:
  - Dislocated or reduced
  - Early or late

  Prompt reduction of the dislocation is necessary and should be performed immediately, without delay for radiographic confirmation. The top priority is ensuring the integrity of the arterial supply to the knee, followed by a thorough assessment of neurologic function to identify any potential nerve impairment.
- *Signs and symptoms*:
  - *Thorough history taking*: History taking is very important as 20–50% were spontaneously reduced and usually, it is misdiagnosed.
  - *Deformity*: In case of true dislocation, the deformity is well visible, and buttonholing of the medial femoral condyle through the medial capsule leads to irreducible KD. The sign is known as the "dimple sign". Commonly seen in posterolateral dislocation. There is also limb length discrepancy.
  - *Vascular examination*: Vascular examination is very important and if missed it can lead to limb loss in case of the absent pulse. The distal pulse should be checked in a series before and after reduction and comparison is

a must with the opposite normal side. The popliteal artery is at the highest risk of getting injured during traumatic KD across the popliteal fossa secondary to proximal and distal tethering.

Mechanism of popliteal artery injury:
- Anterior dislocation—traction injury
- Posterior dislocation—complete artery tears

Neurological examination:
- Peroneal nerve is the most common nerve injury associated with Knee dislocation.
- 10–35%
- Commonly associated with posterolateral dislocations

Investigatory evaluation:
- *X-rays*: Although it is advisable to immediately reduce the KD even before getting radiographs taken. However, postreduction X-rays are taken to comment on congruency of joint.
    - Anteroposterior (AP) and lateral views
    - 45° oblique view
    - *X-ray findings*:
        - Dislocation—incongruency of joint
        - Irregular joint space—widened joint space signifies soft tissue interposition
        - Lateral capsular sign signifies Segond avulsion fracture.
        - Osteochondral defects
- *Angiogram*: ABI < 0.9, indicated for angiogram
- *CT*: To rule out fractures such as tibial eminence, tibial tubercle, and tibial plateau fractures that may not be seen on plan X-rays.
- *MRI*: To rule out cruciate ligament injury, meniscal tears, collateral injury

TREATMENT

- *Nonoperative*:
    - Closed reduction immediately followed by immobilization in extension using long knee brace or above knee cylindrical cast for 4–6 weeks, followed by MRI and then subsequent reconstruction or repair of ligaments or meniscus injuries
- *Operative*:
  Indications:
    - Irreducible knee
    - Posterolateral dislocation
    - Open fracture dislocation
    - Obese patients
    - Vascular compromise

In case of irreducible knee, medial parapatellar arthrotomy is used to reduce buttonholing followed by *external fixator application or two cross K wires application* **(Fig. 2)**.

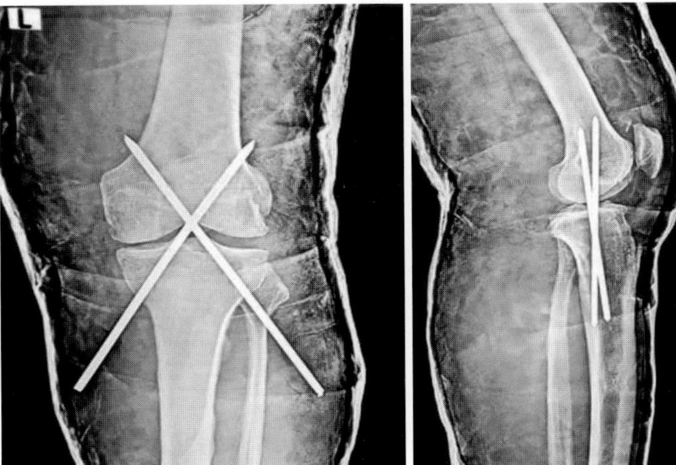

FIG. 2: Knee dislocation managed with K-wires.

Rehabilitation:

- *Physical therapy*:
  - *Goals*: Focus on restoring range of motion, strength, and functional mobility. The rehabilitation program typically includes exercises for knee flexibility, muscle strengthening, and proprioception training.
  - *Phases*: The rehabilitation process is often divided into phases—acute (focused on pain management and swelling reduction), subacute (emphasis on regaining range of motion and strength), and chronic (functional training and return to activities).
  - *Follow-up*:
    - *Monitoring*: Regular follow-up visits are essential for tracking recovery progress, managing complications, and adjusting the rehabilitation plan as needed. Imaging may be required to assess healing and identify any residual issues.

COMPLICATIONS

- *Vascular injury*: Popliteal artery injury
- Multiligament injuries
- Peroneal nerve injury
- Knee stiffness

BIBLIOGRAPHY

1. Bernstein J, Ahn J. Management of multi-ligamentous knee injuries: Surgical versus non-surgical approaches. Orthop Clin North Am. 2023;54(2):253-68.
2. Mutsuzaki H, Matsushita T, Masunari A. Two-stage ligament reconstruction with remnant preservation as treatment of knee dislocation. BMC Surg. 2023;22(1):1-13.
3. Lee D-Y, Kang D-G, Ho-Seung Jo, Se-Joon Heo, Ji-Ho Bae, Sun-Chul Hwang. A systematic review and meta-analysis comparing conservative and surgical treatments for acute patellar dislocation in children and adolescents. Knee Surg Relat Res. 2023;35(1):24-31.
4. Robertson A, Curry EJ, Gardner EC. Acute knee dislocation: An evidence-based approach to the management of traumatic knee dislocations. Injury. 2023;54(3):555-66.

CHAPTER 11.4

Acute Ligamentous and Meniscal Injuries of Knee

Pankaj Vir Singh, Gurpreet Kour

Acute injuries to the knee's ligaments, menisci, and soft tissues are common, particularly among athletes and individuals engaged in high-impact activities.

APPLIED ANATOMY OF THE KNEE JOINT

Ligaments

The knee joint is supported by four primary ligaments:

1. *Anterior cruciate ligament (ACL)*: Key stabilizer preventing anterior translation and controlling rotational movement
2. *Posterior cruciate ligament (PCL)*: Limits posterior translation and assists with rotational control
3. *Medial collateral ligament (MCL)*: Resists valgus stress, aiding medial stability
4. *Lateral collateral ligament (LCL)*: Counters varus stress and supports lateral stability

Menisci

The knee contains two menisci (medial and lateral), which are crescent-shaped cartilage structures providing shock absorption, load distribution, and joint stability. The medial meniscus is more commonly injured due to its restricted mobility and attachment to the MCL, whereas the lateral meniscus is more mobile and less frequently injured.

MECHANISMS OF ACUTE KNEE INJURIES

Ligamentous Injuries

- *ACL injuries*: Often occur via noncontact mechanisms, such as sudden changes in direction, deceleration, or pivoting. Contact injuries can also result from a direct blow to the knee.
- *PCL injuries*: Commonly result from a posterior force to the tibia, such as a fall on a bent knee or a direct impact to the anterior tibia
- *MCL injuries*: Typically caused by valgus stress due to lateral impacts, such as a blow to the outer knee
- *LCL injuries*: Result from varus stress and are often associated with other ligamentous injuries due to their relative rarity as isolated injuries

Meniscal Injuries

Meniscal injuries frequently occur in combination with ligamentous injuries, particularly ACL tears. They are often due to twisting or pivoting motions on a loaded knee, leading to different tear patterns such as longitudinal, radial, bucket-handle, or horizontal tears.

CLINICAL EVALUATION AND DIAGNOSIS OF ACUTE KNEE INJURIES

- *History*: Understanding the mechanism of injury, the presence of audible sounds (such as a "pop"), and immediate symptoms (e.g., swelling, instability, or inability to bear weight) provides critical information.
- *Physical examination*:
  - *Inspection*: Assess for swelling, deformity, and signs of hemarthrosis
  - *Palpation*: Identify tenderness, particularly over ligaments and menisci
  - *Range of motion*: Determine any limitations or pain during flexion and extension
  - *Special tests*:
    - *ACL*: Lachman test and anterior drawer test
    - *PCL*: Posterior drawer test and posterior sag sign
    - *MCL/LCL*: Valgus and varus stress tests at both 0° and 30° of knee flexion
    - *Meniscus*: McMurray and Thessaly tests to assess for meniscal injury

IMAGING FOR ACUTE KNEE INJURIES

- *X-ray*: Useful for ruling out fractures and detecting any joint space changes or bone avulsions
- *MRI*: The preferred modality for evaluating soft tissue injuries in the knee, with high sensitivity for ligamentous and meniscal injuries
- *Ultrasound*: A supplementary tool for visualizing superficial structures such as the MCL and joint effusion, and can assist in aspiration if needed.

MANAGEMENT OF ACUTE LIGAMENTOUS INJURIES

Acute Anterior Cruciate Ligament Injuries

- *Nonsurgical management*:
  - Suitable for patients with lower activity levels or minimal instability.
  - Initial management includes rest, ice, compression, and elevation (RICE) to reduce swelling.
  - Physical therapy focuses on regaining range of motion, strengthening, and proprioception to aid stability.
- *Surgical management*:
  - Recommended for young, active individuals or those with significant instability. Early ACL reconstruction can help prevent secondary knee injuries.
  - Rehabilitation typically spans 6–9 months, with a progression through pain control, range of motion exercises, and gradual strengthening.

Acute Posterior Cruciate Ligament Injuries

- *Nonsurgical management*: Appropriate for isolated low-grade injuries. Initial treatment involves RICE, bracing, and physical therapy targeting quadriceps strengthening.
- *Surgical management*: Indicated for high-grade injuries or those associated with other ligament injuries. Surgery often involves reconstruction using autografts or allografts, followed by a structured rehabilitation program.

Acute Medial and Lateral Collateral Ligament Injuries

- *Nonsurgical management*: Most acute MCL injuries are managed conservatively, as the MCL has a good healing capacity. LCL injuries, if isolated and low-grade, may also be treated nonsurgically with bracing and physical therapy.
- *Surgical management*: MCL surgery is rare in isolated acute injuries but may be considered in multiligament cases. LCL injuries that are severe or involve other ligaments often require surgical intervention and subsequent rehabilitation.

MANAGEMENT OF ACUTE MENISCAL INJURIES

Nonsurgical Management

Small, stable meniscal tears, particularly those located in the vascularized "red-red" zone, may heal without surgery. Initial treatment includes RICE, NSAIDs for pain control, and physical therapy to restore function.

Surgical Management

- *Partial meniscectomy*: Removal of damaged tissue can provide rapid symptom relief but may contribute to joint degeneration over time.
- *Meniscal repair*: Preferred for tears in the outer third of the meniscus, especially in younger, active patients. Repair preserves meniscal tissue and is generally associated with better long-term outcomes.

ABSOLUTE INDICATIONS FOR SURGICAL TREATMENT IN LIGAMENTOUS INJURIES

- *Multiligament knee injuries (MLKI)*:
  - Injuries involving more than one ligament (e.g., ACL, PCL, MCL, and/or LCL) are generally considered absolute indications for acute surgical repair, especially if there is significant instability.
  - These injuries are often associated with knee dislocations, which can pose a risk to neurovascular structures, necessitating urgent surgery.
- *Complete PCL avulsion fractures*: When the PCL is torn and avulsed along with a bony fragment from the tibia, surgical fixation is typically required to reattach the bone fragment and restore joint stability.
- *Unstable ACL injuries in high-demand athletes*: Although many ACL injuries are managed nonacutely, young athletes who require an immediate return to high-level activities may undergo early surgical reconstruction to prevent further injury and expedite rehabilitation.

ABSOLUTE INDICATIONS FOR SURGICAL TREATMENT IN MENISCAL INJURIES

- *Locked knee from bucket-handle meniscal tear*:
  - A displaced bucket-handle tear can cause mechanical locking, where the patient is unable to fully extend the knee.
  - This situation requires urgent arthroscopic surgery to reposition or repair the meniscus and restore knee motion.
- *Acute meniscal root tears*: Meniscal root tears, particularly in young patients or those with high functional demands, are often treated surgically. Acute repair is necessary to prevent rapid joint degeneration and loss of meniscal function.
- *Meniscal tears associated with ACL reconstruction*: When significant meniscal damage accompanies an ACL injury, meniscal repair or partial meniscectomy may be performed simultaneously during ACL reconstruction.

APPROPRIATE TIMING OF ACUTE SURGICAL INTERVENTION

Early surgical repair can prevent complications and the timing of surgical intervention for acute ligamentous and meniscal injuries of the knee depends on several factors, including the type and severity of the injury, the presence of joint swelling, and the risk of further complications. Here is a breakdown of the optimal timing for surgery based on current guidelines and evidence:

- *Immediate surgery (within 24 hours)*: Immediate surgery is recommended for—
  - *Knee dislocations with neurovascular compromise*: Urgent intervention is needed to address potential damage to blood vessels or nerves. This requires prompt assessment and

surgical repair to restore blood flow and prevent ischemic injury.
  - *Locked knee due to meniscal tear*: A locked knee caused by a displaced bucket-handle meniscal tear may necessitate immediate surgery to relieve mechanical obstruction and restore joint motion.
- *Early surgery (within 1–2 weeks)*: Early surgical intervention is generally preferred for—
  - *Multiligament knee injuries*: Surgery is often recommended within 1–2 weeks for severe ligament injuries involving multiple ligaments, provided there is no excessive swelling or other contraindications.
  - *Meniscal root tears in active individuals*: Timely intervention, ideally within a few days to 2 weeks, helps prevent rapid degeneration and maintains meniscal function.
  - *Complete PCL avulsion fractures*: If surgery is needed to reattach a bony fragment, early repair can be beneficial before significant bone resorption occurs.
- *Delayed surgery (3–6 weeks post injury)*: In some cases, delaying surgery for a few weeks is advantageous, especially for—
  - *ACL injuries with significant swelling or stiffness*: Waiting for 3–6 weeks allows time for swelling to subside and for prehabilitation to restore range of motion. This reduces the risk of arthrofibrosis (scar tissue formation) post surgery.
  - *Nonurgent meniscal tears*: In cases where there is no mechanical locking, some meniscal tears can be managed conservatively at first. If symptoms persist, surgery can be performed after 3–6 weeks.

General Considerations for Timing

- *Prehabilitation*: Presurgical physical therapy to reduce swelling and restore knee motion is often recommended. Improved preoperative strength and range of motion are associated with better postoperative outcomes.
- *Swelling and inflammation*: Operating on a knee with significant swelling or stiffness increases the risk of complications, such as poor wound healing and arthrofibrosis. Therefore, waiting for acute swelling and inflammation to settle down will lead to better and smoother postsurgical recovery.

MANAGEMENT OF ACUTE SOFT TISSUE INJURIES

- *Acute tendon injuries*: Partial tears of the quadriceps or patellar tendon are initially managed with immobilization and RICE. Surgical repair is often indicated for complete ruptures.
- *Bursitis and synovitis*: Acute inflammation of bursae and synovium is managed conservatively with NSAIDs, RICE, and activity modification. Aspiration may be performed if effusion is significant.

Absolute indications for acute surgical treatment in cases of ligamentous and meniscal injuries are based on the severity and type of injury, as well as the presence of concurrent injuries.

Absolute indications for immediate surgical intervention in such cases include:
- *Knee dislocation (multiple ligament injuries)*:
  - Risk of vascular injury (e.g., popliteal artery injury) or nerve injury (e.g., peroneal nerve).
  - Immediate reduction and surgical repair or reconstruction are often required to restore joint stability and prevent long-term complications.
- *Irreducible locked knee*:
  - Typically caused by a displaced bucket-handle tear of the meniscus that prevents full knee extension.
  - Requires urgent arthroscopic intervention to unlock the knee and repair the meniscus.

- *Associated vascular injury*:
  - Identified by absent distal pulses, a cold extremity, or Doppler studies showing arterial compromise.
  - Vascular repair often requires immediate surgical intervention, along with stabilization of the knee joint.
- *Open knee injuries*:
  - High-energy trauma with open wounds exposes the knee joint to contamination.
  - Immediate debridement and stabilization are required to prevent infection and maintain function.
- *Acute septic arthritis (if suspected in trauma setting)*:
  - Rare but critical; requires immediate arthroscopic lavage and antibiotic therapy to prevent joint destruction.
- Many other ligamentous or meniscal injuries (e.g., ACL or isolated meniscal tears) do not require immediate surgery and can be addressed after appropriate evaluation and planning.
- Careful clinical examination and imaging (e.g., MRI, angiography) are essential to identify these critical indications

REHABILITATION FOLLOWING ACUTE KNEE INJURIES

Phases of Acute Rehabilitation

- *Immediate phase (0–2 weeks)*: Focus on reducing swelling and pain, while initiating range of motion exercises and isometric strengthening.
- *Subacute phase (2–6 weeks)*: Progresses to more advanced range of motion exercises, closed-chain strengthening, and proprioceptive training
- *Functional phase (6 weeks to 3 months)*: Emphasis on regaining full strength and stability with dynamic exercises and activities aimed at preparing the patient for return to daily activities or sport.

BIBLIOGRAPHY

1. American Academy of Orthopaedic Surgeons. Clinical practice guideline on the management of anterior cruciate ligament injuries. AAOS Clinical Practice Guidelines. Rosemont, IL: American Academy of Orthopaedic Surgeons; 2020.
2. Ardern CL, Webster KE, Taylor NF, Feller JA. Return to sport following anterior cruciate ligament reconstruction surgery: a systematic review and meta-analysis of the state of play. Br J Sports Med. 2011;45(7):596-606.
3. Fu FH, Schulte KR. Biomechanical evaluations of knee stability. In: Proceedings of the American Orthopaedic Society for Sports Medicine Annual Meeting; 1996 Jul 6-9; Orlando, FL. Rosemont, IL: American Orthopaedic Society for Sports Medicine; 1996. p. 55-60.
4. Griffin LY, Albohm MJ. Rehabilitation of the knee after ligamentous injury. In: DeLee JC, Drez D, editors. Orthopedic Sports Medicine: Principles and Practice. 2nd ed. Philadelphia, PA: Saunders; 2003. p. 1785-805.
5. Noyes FR. Noyes' Knee Disorders: Surgery, Rehabilitation, Clinical Outcomes. 2nd ed. Philadelphia, PA: Saunders; 2016.
6. Pujol N, Panarella L, Selmi TA, Neyret P, Fithian D. Meniscal healing after repair: a review. Clin Orthop Relat Res. 2007;455:166-71.
7. Shelbourne KD, Gray T. Anterior cruciate ligament reconstruction with autogenous patellar tendon graft followed by accelerated rehabilitation. A two-to-nine-year follow-up. Am J Sports Med. 1997;25(6):786-95.

Tibial Plateau Fracture

Ravi Chauhan

Tibial plateau fractures are complex intra-articular injuries with the potential to damage surrounding structures such as vasculature, nerves, ligaments, menisci, and adjacent compartments.

APPLIED ANATOMY

The tibial plateau comprises the medial (larger, concave) and lateral (smaller, convex) plateaus. The medial plateau bears more weight, while the lateral is more prone to fractures due to its smaller surface area. Surrounding structures like the menisci and ligaments are crucial for knee stability and are often involved in injuries.

BIOMECHANICS AND MECHANISM OF INJURY

These fractures usually result from axial loading combined with varus or valgus stress. High-energy trauma causes impaction or splitting fractures, while low-energy mechanisms in osteoporotic patients lead to joint surface depression.

TYPICAL FRACTURE PATTERNS

- *Lateral plateau fractures*: Common due to compressive valgus forces during the impact
- *Medial plateau fractures*: Less frequent but more severe
- *Bicondylar fractures*: Involve both plateaus, often from high-energy trauma
- *Depression fractures*: Caused by axial loading, leading to joint instability

CLASSIFICATION

The most commonly used classification systems include:

- *Schatzker classification*: It categorizes fractures based on fracture morphology and location **(Fig. 1)**.

In 1974, *Schatzker et al.* introduced a classification for tibial plateau fractures based on AP X-rays, evaluating fragment displacement, articular depression, and condylar involvement. Later, in 1990s, the *AO/OTA* **(Fig. 2)** classification expanded on this by considering partial versus total articular involvement and fracture fragmentation. In 2018, AO updated the system to address previous limitations.

Despite their widespread use, both classifications have limitations, particularly with posterior column fractures. The *CT-based three-column classification* **(Fig. 3)** emerged to fill these gaps, offering higher reliability, especially for complex, posterior comminuted fractures. These systems guide treatment strategies and predict outcomes, though plain radiographs often miss soft tissue injuries and finer fracture details, leading to potential over-simplifications. CT-based systems provide a more comprehensive approach.

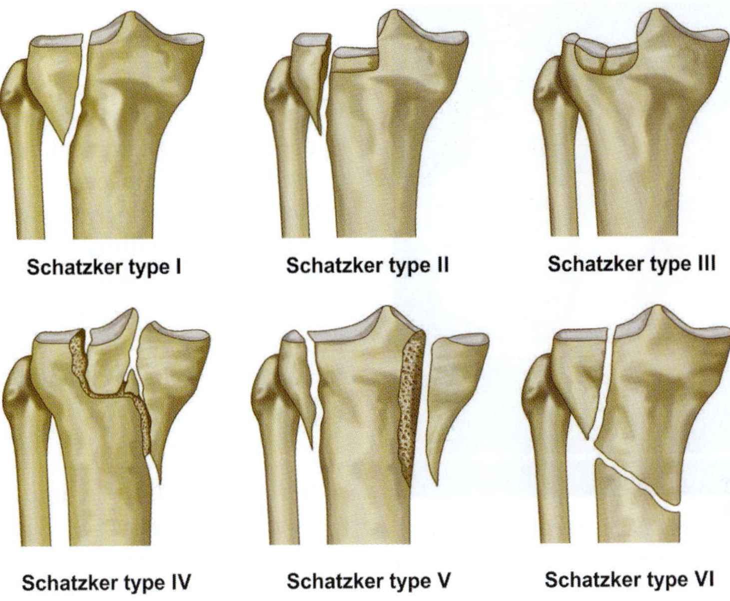

FIG. 1: Schatzker classification.

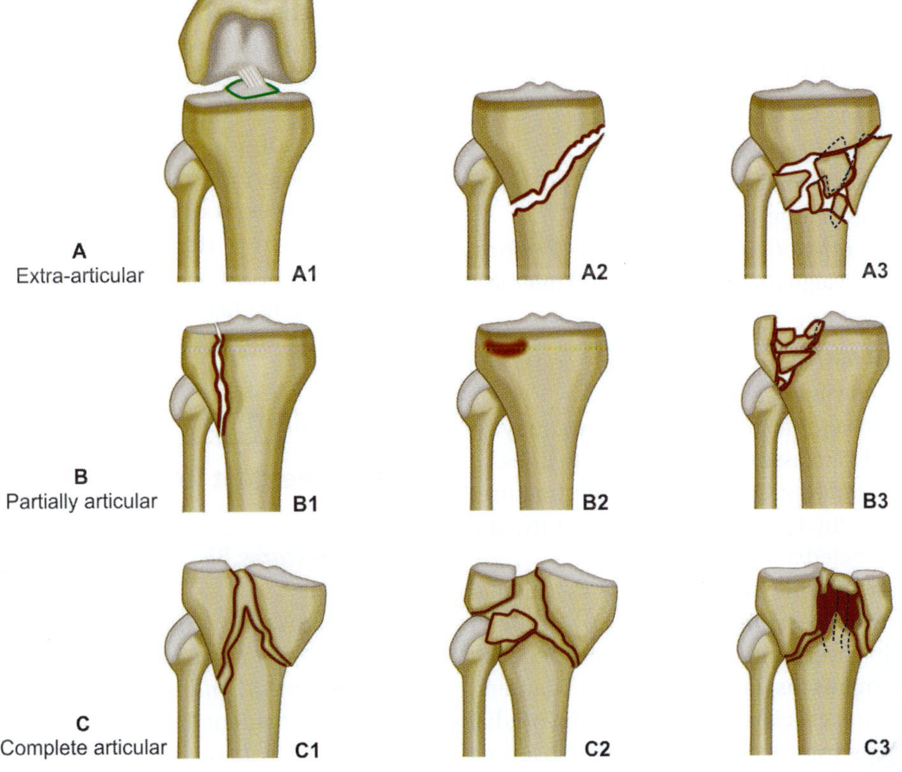

FIGS. 2A TO C: AO/OTA classification: A comprehensive system based on fracture type and severity.

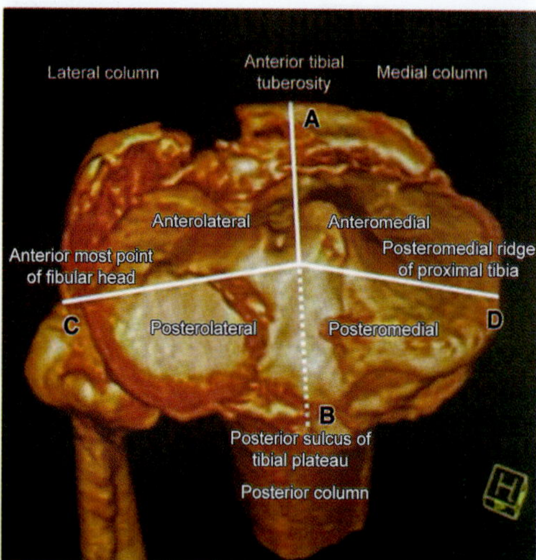

FIG. 3: CT-based classification: Offers detailed insights into fracture patterns using cross-sectional imaging for more precise management.

EVALUATION

- Swelling, bruising, deformity, blisters, or open wounds
- Rule out vascular injury (e.g., popliteal artery) and nerve damage

Special considerations:
- *Compartment syndrome*: Watch for severe pain, swelling, and paresthesia
- *Associated ligament injuries*: Perform gentle valgus/varus stress tests if tolerable

X-rays:
- *Standard views*: AP (anteroposterior) and lateral views of the knee
- *Additional views*: Oblique views may be needed to assess specific fracture lines.
- *Key findings*: Depressed or split fractures of the tibial plateau, joint incongruity, and associated fractures.

Radiographic indicators such as articular surface depression greater than 6 mm or widening over 5 mm are often associated with lateral meniscus, lateral collateral ligament, or posterior cruciate ligament injuries. Medial meniscus injuries are frequently observed when depression and widening exceed 8 mm.

CT scan:
- It is must and crucial for surgical planning.
- Precise visualization of fracture patterns, depression, displacement, and involvement of the articular surface
- *Preferred sequences*: Thin slices with 3D reconstructions to visualize bone fragments and fracture lines

A CT scan can modify the initial fracture classification and influence the treatment plan established from the initial radiographs **(Figs. 4A and B)**.

MRI:
- *Indication*: Used primarily to assess soft tissue injuries (e.g., meniscal tears, cruciate or collateral ligament injuries)
- *Pathognomonic findings*: Ligament tears, meniscal damage, or bone marrow edema. It also helps in detecting occult fractures not visible on X-rays.

The prognosis of tibial plateau fractures is significantly influenced by soft tissue injuries, making MRI essential for comprehensive evaluation.

Note: CT angiography and Doppler examination are vital tools for assessing vascular injuries in tibial plateau fractures, especially when there is suspicion of arterial compromise. Early detection of vascular damage helps guide timely surgical intervention and prevent complications.

MANAGEMENT

Urgent/Emergent Treatment

Indications:
- *Open fractures*: Risk of infection and tissue damage
- *Neurovascular injury*: Compromised blood flow or nerve function
- *Compartment syndrome*: Severe swelling, risk of permanent damage
- *Severe displacement/instability*: To prevent further joint or tissue harm

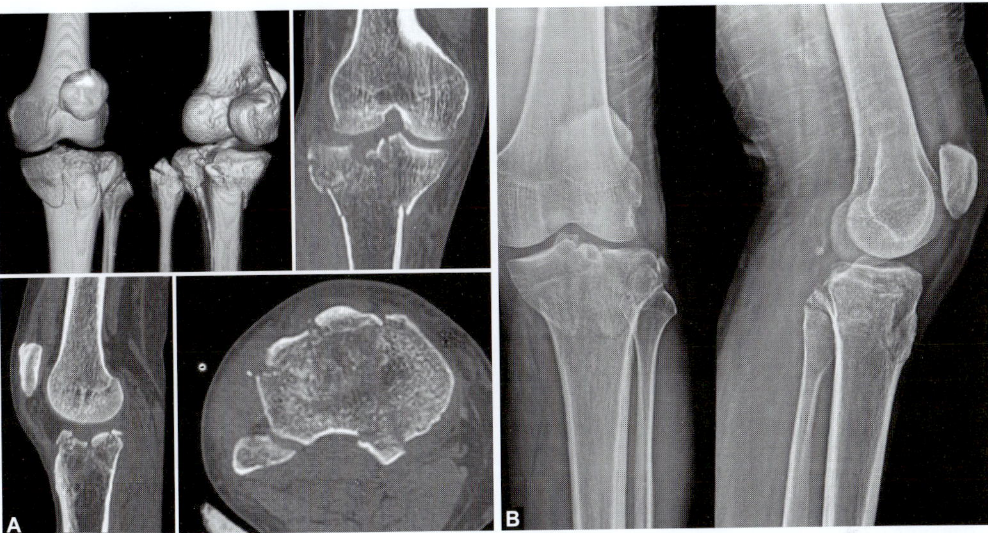

FIGS. 4A AND B: X-rays and CT scan of proximal tibia plateau fracture (3D imaging, coronal, sagittal, and axial views).

Strategy:
- *Early stabilization*: Immobilize with splint/external fixation; analgesia and elevation **(Fig. 5)**
- *Neurovascular assessment*: Immediate evaluation for vascular issues and repair or reconstruction when required
- *Compartment syndrome*: Perform fasciotomy if present
- *Surgical planning*: Urgent debridement and irrigation for open fractures, followed by definitive fixation once soft tissues heal

Nonsurgical Management

Indications:
- Minimally displaced fractures (<2 mm depression)
- Stable fractures with intact soft tissues and no ligamentous injury
- Patients with low functional demands (e.g., elderly or those with comorbidities)

Techniques:
- *Immobilization*: Use of a hinged knee brace or cast to maintain joint stability
- *Weight-bearing restrictions*: Nonweight bearing for initial 6 weeks followed by partial weight bearing for 6–8 weeks thereafter full weight bearing as tolerated
- *Physical therapy*: Early range of motion exercises once pain and swelling subside

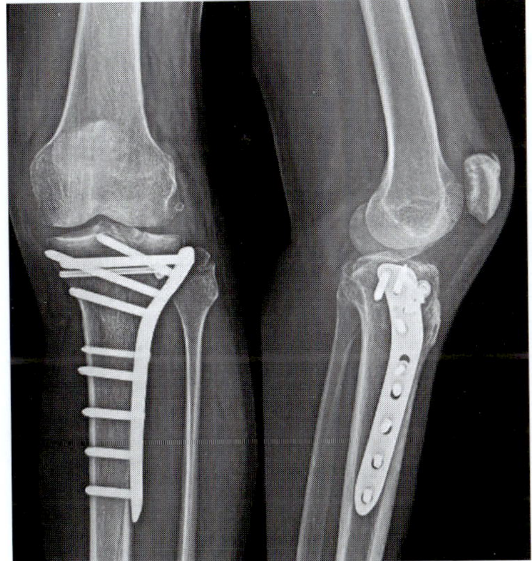

FIG. 5: Open reduction and internal fixation with lateral plating for tibial plateau fracture.

Follow-up:
- *Regular X-rays*: Monitor fracture alignment and healing every week initially for 3 weeks

Surgical Treatment

Indications:
- Displaced fractures (>3 mm articular step-off)
- Fractures with instability or joint incongruity
- Open fractures or those involving neurovascular injury
- Fractures with associated ligamentous or meniscal injuries

Contraindications:
- Medically unfit patients with severe comorbidities
- Poor soft tissue condition (relative contraindication for early surgery)

Surgical techniques:
- *Closed reduction and percutaneous fixation (CRPF)*:
  - *Indication*: Minimally displaced fractures
- *Open reduction and internal fixation (ORIF)*:
  - *Indication*: Complex, displaced fractures with joint surface disruption

Technique: The surgical approach for tibial plateau fractures is determined by the fracture pattern. A lateral approach with an anterolateral incision is standard, while posteromedial incisions are used for medial plateau fractures. Bicondylar fractures may require dual medial and lateral incisions, with posterior approaches reserved for posterior shearing fractures.

Fixation techniques based on Schatzker classification:
- *Type I (wedge split)*: Lag screws or a buttress plate may be required.
- *Type II (split wedge depression)*: Buttress plate fixation is necessary.
- *Type III (pure depression)*: Bone grafting and raft screws are typically used.
- *Type IV (medial condyle)*: Anteromedial or posteromedial buttress plates (sometimes both) are needed.
- *Type V (bicondylar fracture)*: Anterolateral and posteromedial buttress plates are used.
- *Type VI (bicondylar with shaft dissociation)*: A combination of buttress and bridge plating is required to address both articular incongruity and shaft instability.

External fixation:
- *Indication*: Polytrauma patients, open fractures, or fractures with significant soft tissue compromise
- Temporary stabilization using an external fixator to allow soft tissue recovery before definitive surgery. In cases where internal fixation is not feasible due to soft tissue damage, *the Ilizarov/hybrid frame can be used as a definitive external fixation method.* It provides stable fixation, facilitates fracture healing, and allows for early weight bearing while minimizing the risk of soft tissue complications.

Arthroscopic-assisted reduction:
- Arthroscopic visualization for accurate joint surface reduction is often combined with other fixation methods like screws or plates.

Replacement (knee arthroplasty):
- *Indication*: Elderly patients with severe comminution, poor bone quality, or pre-existing osteoarthritis

Surgical access to the proximal tibia can be achieved through anterolateral, posterolateral, medial or posterior approaches, depending on fracture morphology. Combining approaches often enhances visualization and fracture reduction, improving functional outcomes. The optimal surgical approach should be determined by a thorough analysis of the fracture pattern to minimize complications and ensure effective treatment.

COMPLICATIONS

Early Complications

Presurgery:
- *Compartment syndrome*: Infection (open fractures): Risk of contamination and soft tissue damage.
  - *Management*: Urgent debridement, antibiotics, and wound care

- *Neurovascular injury*:
  - *Management*: Immediate surgical repair or vascular reconstruction, with careful monitoring

Postsurgical:
- *Loss of reduction*: Failure to maintain proper alignment after fixation
  - *Management*: Re-evaluate with imaging; may require revision surgery for stabilization
- *Deep vein thrombosis (DVT)*: Blood clot formation in leg veins
  - *Management*: Anticoagulation therapy and early mobilization
- *Acute infection*: Infection at the surgical site
  - *Management*:
    - *Fracture healed*: Hardware removal, lavage, debridement, and antibiotic therapy
    - *Fracture not healed*: Retain hardware, perform lavage and debridement with antibiotic therapy until the fracture heals. Fracture stability is essential for both healing and resolving infection.

Late Complications

Knee stiffness:
- *Less than 3 months*: Managed with mobilization under anesthesia (MUA)
- *3-6 months*: Treated with arthroscopic release, with early MUA if needed
- *More than 6 months*: Requires open release for refractory or long-standing cases

Malunion:
- *Young, active patients without significant joint damage*: Managed with intra articular or extra-articular osteotomy to correct alignment.
- *Malunion with joint involvement or osteoarthritis*: Total knee arthroplasty (TKA) is recommended for joint replacement.

Nonunion: Nonunion may require revision surgery, including bone grafting or further internal fixation, to achieve union.

Post-traumatic osteoarthritis: In cases of advanced arthritis, TKA is the preferred treatment for restoring joint function.

REHABILITATION

Rehabilitation is influenced by factors such as age, bone quality, fracture type, associated soft tissue injuries, and fixation method.

Range of motion:
- *0–30°*: First 2 weeks
- *0–60°*: Weeks 2–4
- *0–90°*: Weeks 4–6
- *Free motion*: After 6 weeks

Weight bearing:
- *Full weight bearing*: As soon as possible with a circular external fixator or knee arthroplasty
- *No weight bearing*: Minimum of 10–12 weeks for CRIF or ORIF

Strengthening and functional training: Exercises are introduced to restore mobility and muscle function, aiming for full recovery within 6–9 months.

Orthotic support: In cases of associated ligament injuries, orthoses can protect against sagittal or coronal plane instability.

BIBLIOGRAPHY

1. Court-Brown CM, Caesar B. Epidemiology of adult fractures: A review. Injury. 2006;37(8):691-7.
2. Donovan RL, Smith JRA, Yeomans D, Bennett F, Smallbones M, White P, et al. Epidemiology and outcomes of tibial plateau fractures in adults aged 60 and over treated in the United Kingdom. Injury. 2022;53(6):2219-25.
3. Gosling T, Schandelmaier P, Muller M, Hankemeier S, Wagner M, Krettek C. Single lateral locked screw plating of bicondylar tibial plateau fractures. Clin Orthop Relat Res. 2005;439:207-14.
4. Kellam JF, Meinberg EG, Agel J. Introduction: fracture and dislocation classification compendium-2018: International Comprehensive Classification of

Fractures and Dislocations Committee. J Orthop Trauma. 2018;32 Suppl 1:S1-S170.
5. Kfuri M, Schatzker J. Revisiting the Schatzker classification of tibial plateau fractures. Injury. 2018;49(12):2252-63.
6. Luo CF, Sun H, Zhang B, Zeng BF. Three-column fixation for complex tibial plateau fractures. J Orthop Trauma. 2010;24(11):683-92.
7. Marsh JL, Buckwalter J, Gelberman R, Dirschl D, Olson S, Brown T, et al. Articular fractures: Does an anatomic reduction really change the result? J Bone Joint Surg Am. 2002;84(7):1259-71.
8. Schatzker J. Compression in the surgical treatment of fractures of the tibia. Clin Orthop. 1974;105:220-39.
9. Zhu Y, Yang G, Luo CF, Smith WR, Hu CF, Gao H, et al. Computed tomography-based three-column classification in tibial plateau fractures: introduction of its utility and assessment of its reproducibility. J Trauma Acute Care Surg. 2012;73(3):731-7.

SECTION

12

Tibia

Fracture of Tibia

Sumeet Singh Charak, Nitin Choudhary

Tibia is the most common long bone fracture.
- Accounts for 17% of lower extremity fractures
- *Bimodal age distribution*:
  - *Young patients*: High-energy trauma (e.g., accidents, sports)
  - *Older patients*: Low-energy injuries (e.g., falls)

PATHOANATOMY

- Proximal third fractures account for 5–10% of tibial shaft fractures.
- The proximal tibia has a triangular shape with a wide metaphyseal region that narrows distally.

Various deforming forces and muscle responsible **(Fig. 1)**:
- *Patellar tendon (1)*: Pulls the proximal fragment into extension, creating apex anterior or procurvatum deformities
- *Gastrocnemius (2)*: Pulls the distal fragment into flexion
- *Pes anserinus (3)*: Pulls the proximal fragment into the varus
- *Anterior compartment muscles*: Cause valgus deformity

Distal third extra-articular/junctional fracture:
- Increased risk of associated ankle injuries, especially posterior malleolus fractures, which may impact syndesmotic stability.

These fractures are considered to be inherently unstable and frequently associated with complications like delayed union, malunion, soft tissue complications, and infection.

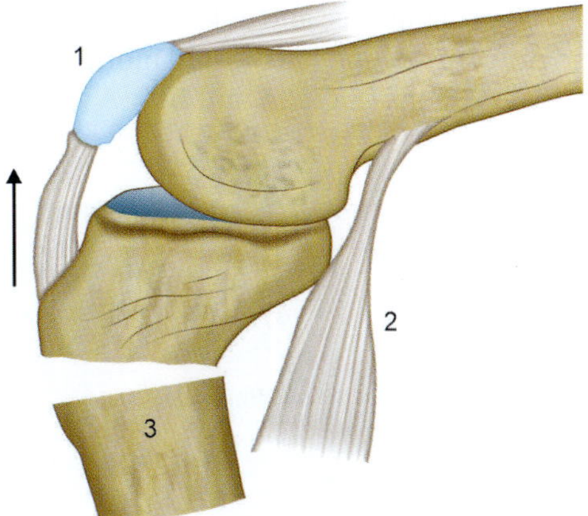

FIG. 1: Various deforming forces and muscle responsible.

Other Associated Injuries

- Tibial plateau fractures
- Tibial plafond fractures
- Femoral shaft fractures
- Floating knee injuries
- Associated fibula fractures (seen in approximately 80% of cases)
- *Musculature*:
  - Divided into four compartments—anterior, lateral, superficial posterior, and deep posterior
- *Biomechanics*:
  - Tibia bears 80–85% of lower extremity weight; stability maintained by

the interosseous membrane and tibiofibular syndesmosis
  - Fibula weight-bearing contribution is approximately 7%.

ASSESSMENT

Skin condition assessment is also of paramount importance and is a deciding factor for further management.

RADIOLOGY

- Full-length anteroposterior (AP) and lateral views of the tibia, with additional views of the knee and ankle
- Anteroposterior, lateral, and mortise view radiographs **(Figs. 2A and B)**
- *CT*: Used for assessing intra-articular extensions tibial plateau/plafond and suspected complications like nonunion

CLASSIFICATION

Classification of proximal tibia:

- *AO classification* ***(Fig. 3)***:
  - *Type A*: Simple fracture pattern
  - *Type B*: Wedge fracture pattern
  - *Type C*: Comminuted fracture pattern
- *Fracture classification of mid third tibia*:
  - Based on fracture pattern and location:
- *OTA classification* ***(Fig. 4)***:
  - *42A*: Simple fractures
  - *42B*: Wedge patterns
  - *42C*: Complex/comminuted patterns

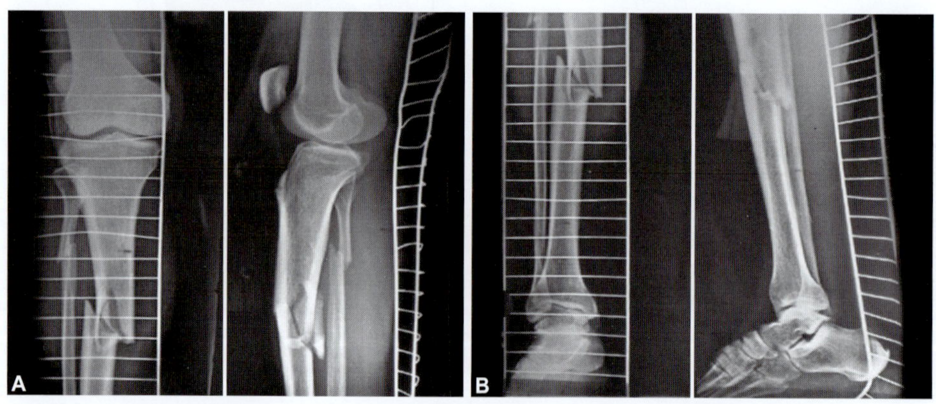

FIGS. 2A AND B: Full-length anteroposterior (AP) and lateral views of the tibia.

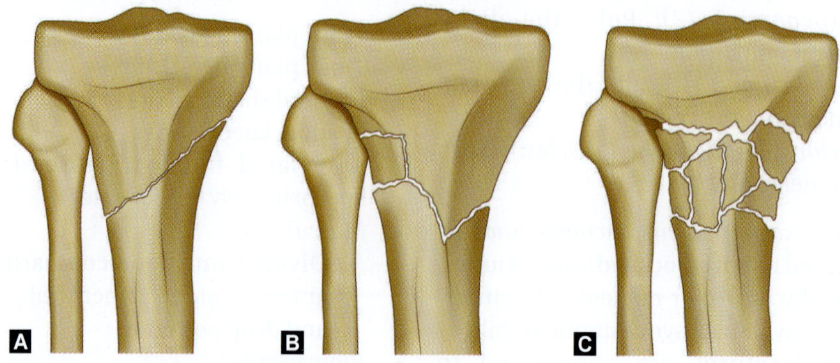

FIGS. 3A TO C: AO classification.

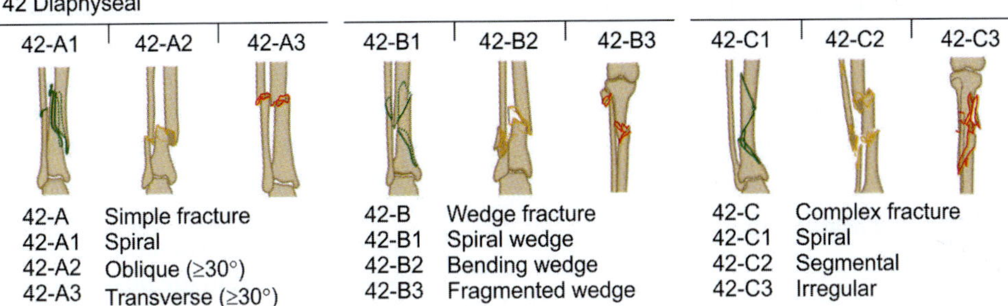

FIG. 4: OTA classification.

- *Soft tissue injury (Oestern and Tscherne classification)*:
  - Grades 0-III based on the severity of soft tissue damage
- *Open fracture classification (Gustilo-Anderson)*:
  - Types I-III-C, depending on wound size, soft tissue damage, and vascular involvement

Classification distal third:
- *The AO/OTA classification system*:
  - *43-A1*: Distal tibial extra-articular fractures which are simple metaphyseal fractures
  - *43-A2*: Distal tibial extra-articular fractures having wedge fracture fragments
  - *43-A2*: Distal tibial extra-articular fractures which are complex/communicated metaphyseal fractures

MANAGEMENT

Management includes both operative and conservative methods.

Nonoperative Management

However, these patients should be subjected to serial radiographs as these fractures tend to displace.
- *Nonoperative*:
  - *Indications*: Closed, low-energy fractures with acceptable alignment
  - *Nonoperative management*: Closed reduction/cast immobilization
- *Acceptable alignment criteria*:
  - <5° varus-valgus angulation
  - <10° anterior/posterior angulation
  - >50% cortical apposition
  - <1 cm shortening
  - <10° rotational malalignment
- *Outcomes*:
  - Associated with risks of malunion, particularly in fractures with intact fibulas
  - Managing shortening, angulation, and rotational control is challenging with nonoperative methods, especially in proximal and distal third fractures

Operative Management

- *Indications*:
  - Unacceptable alignment with closed reduction and casting
  - Soft tissue injury that precludes casting
  - Segmental or comminuted fractures
  - Ipsilateral limb injury (e.g., floating knee)
  - Polytrauma, bilateral tibial fractures, or morbid obesity

Various modalities used for the fixation of these fractures include:
- Intramedullary nailing (IMN) is the mainstay of the management of these fractures.
- *IMN is like an expert nail* with multiple locking options for distal third and proximal third tibia fractures

Nailing is used when there is sufficient proximal bone for locking screws. With use of

IM nail in junctional fracture, there was risk of varus/valgus malunion, however, with use of *poller screws* enabling proper guidewire placement and nails with multiplanar screw fixation slots the incidence of malunion has reduced.

Various nailing techniques:

Nail insertion:

- *Infrapatellar*: Through the mid-patellar tendon/paratendon approach, most commonly used technique
  - This is the standard insertion with the knee in flexion.
- *Suprapatellar*: Allows for nailing in a semiextended position, which aids in reduction which helps prevent apex anterior (procurator) deformity by neutralizing the extensor mechanism's deforming forces

Entry point:

- Located proximal to the anterior edge of the articular margin, just medial to the lateral tibial spine
- A more lateral starting point can help reduce the risk of valgus deformity, while a medial starting point may increase this risk **(Fig. 5)**.
- *Suprapatellar versus infrapatellar nailing*: Suprapatellar nailing often provides better alignment, particularly in proximal tibial fractures.
- *Provisional reduction techniques (proximal tibia)*:
  - *Blocking (poller) screws*: "*Thumb rule*" always puts poller screws on the concave side of the angular deformity **(Fig. 6)**.
  - *Coronal blocking screw (A)*: Prevents apex anterior (procurvatum) deformity by being placed in the posterior half of the proximal fragment
  - *Sagittal blocking screw (B)*: Prevents valgus deformity when placed on the lateral concave side of the proximal fragment
  - Blocking screws can enhance construct stability if left in place.
- *Unicortical plating* **(*Fig. 7*)**:
  - A short one-third tubular plate placed anteriorly, anteromedially, or posteromedially across the fracture
  - Secured proximally and distally with two unicortical screws
- *Universal distractor*: Schanz pins are inserted from the medial side, parallel to the joint, and can be used as blocking screws to assist in reduction.
- *Locking screws*:
  - Proximally and distally placed screws provide rotational stability by statically locking the construct.
  - At least 3–4 proximal/distal locking screws in shorter segment are required

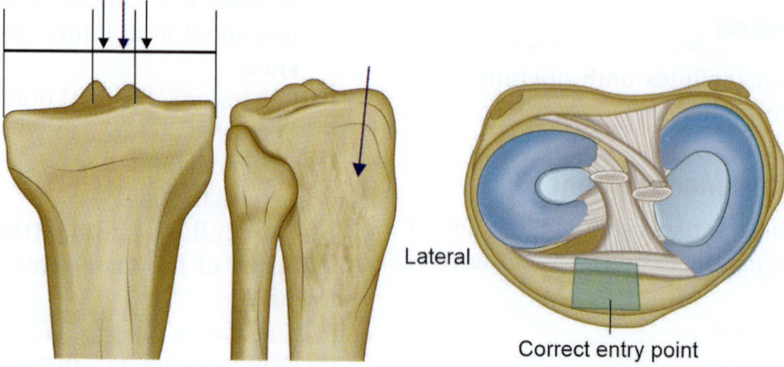

FIG. 5: A more lateral starting point.

in cases of junctional fractures; dynamic locking is not indicated in the acute phase **(Fig. 8)**.

- *Reamed versus unreamed nailing*:
    - Reamed nailing allows for a larger diameter nail and is associated with potentially higher union rates and shorter time to union compared to unreamed nailing in closed fractures.
    - Reamed nails are considered safe for open fractures, with no increased risk of nonunion, infection, or embolism.
    - Unreamed nailing is associated with a higher incidence of locking screw breakage.

Open reduction and internal fixation (ORIF):

- Once used for management for the majority of proximal and distal third

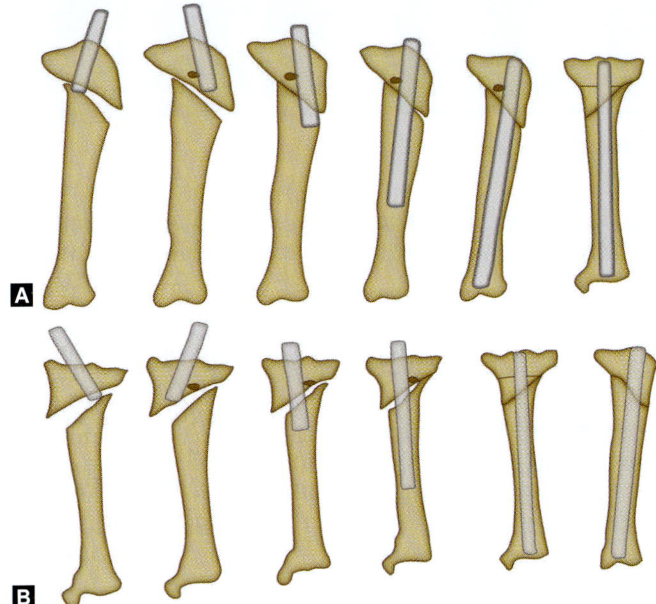

FIGS. 6A AND B: Blocking (poller) screws.

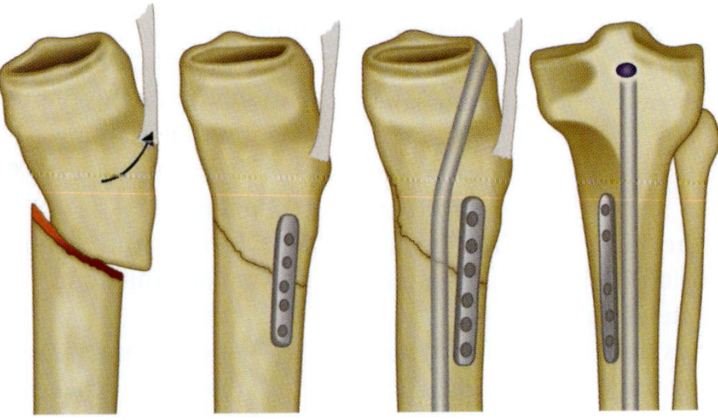

FIG. 7: Unicortical plating.

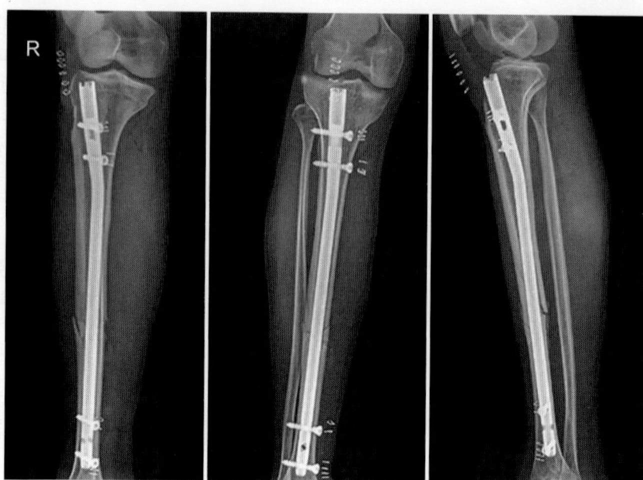

FIG. 8: Locking screws.

of tibia fractures, nowadays used less commonly due to IMN being the superior method of fixation.

Indications:

- Proximal tibial fractures with inadequate fixation with IM nailing
- Distal tibial fractures with insufficient distal fixation from IM nails
- Fractures adjacent to existing hardware, such as after a total knee arthroplasty

Various plating techniques:

Percutaneous locking plate: Suitable for extremely proximal fractures, transverse or oblique patterns, and minimal soft tissue damage. Has a higher infection rate compared to IM nailing for open fractures. Can be placed medially or laterally; lateral placement is preferred due to better soft tissue coverage.

- Anterolateral, using a straight or hockey stick incision extending from just proximal to the joint line (for intra-articular extension) to just lateral to the tibial tubercle, and distally as needed

Fibula fixation is helpful to aid in tibial plafond reduction or augment external fixation.

- *Outcomes*:
    - ORIF involves larger incisions and carries a higher risk of wound complications and hardware irritation compared to IM nailing. Wrinkle sign along with minimal invasive techniques reduces these complications dramatically.
    - Union rates for closed fractures are similar between ORIF and IM nailing, but ORIF may pose less risk of angular deformity.
    - May need hardware removal which can be difficult
    - There is a risk of superficial peroneal nerve injury during percutaneous screw insertion, especially near holes 11-13 on a 13-hole.

External fixation ***(Figs. 9A to D)***:

- *Indications*:
    - Selected cases where severe bone or soft tissue injury precludes definitive internal fixation
    - Used as damage control in polytrauma patients
    - Open fractures with soft tissue defects or contamination
- *Techniques*:
    - Various fixators are available, including uniplanar, circular, and hybrid systems.
    - Ideally, external fixation should be converted to intramedullary nailing within 7–21 days, preferably within 7 days.

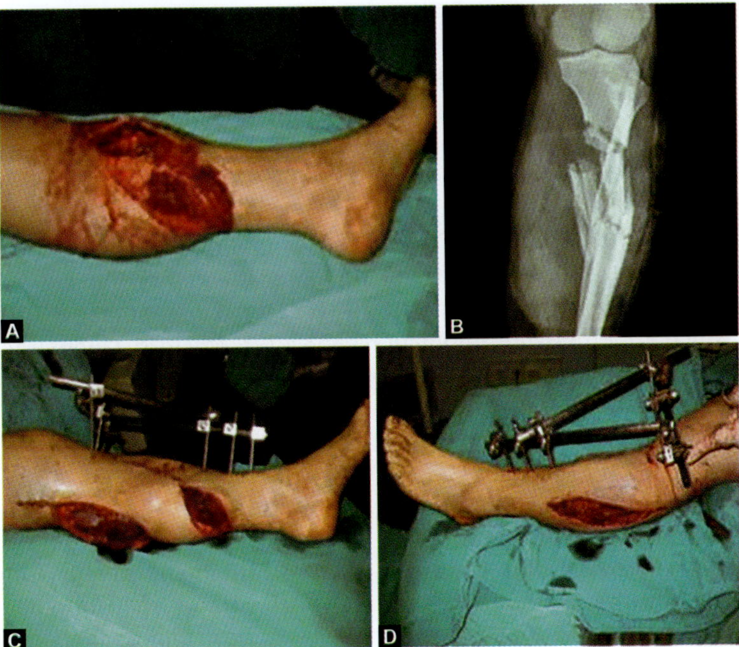

FIGS. 9A TO D: External fixation.

- *Outcomes*:
  - Definitive external fixation in type III open tibia fractures is associated with longer healing times and poorer functional outcomes compared to IM nailing.
  - Intra-articular pin placement should be avoided due to the risk of septic arthritis.
  - High rates of pin tract infections, therefore, should be converted to definitive fixation as soon as possible.
  - Rare cases of proximal or distal metaphyseal fractures. May be managed definitively with ring/hybrid fixators allowing for simultaneous soft tissue care.
  - Has a higher risk of malalignment compared to IM nailing

FRACTURE OF TIBIA WITH OR WITHOUT FIBULA FRACTURE

Isolated tibial fractures, where the tibia is fractured without an associated fibula fracture, present unique implications for management compared to fractures involving both bones. Isolated tibial fractures without fibula involvement may allow for more conservative treatment options due to relative stability, but they often have longer healing times and specific considerations for surgical alignment.

SURGICAL IMPLICATIONS OF INTACT FIBULA

The intact fibula can sometimes complicate aligning the tibial fracture fragments during nailing. Careful attention to alignment is needed to prevent valgus or varus deformities, as the fibula may limit the ability to reduce and align the tibia during surgery properly. It may lead to distraction at the fracture site.

When both the tibia and fibula are fractured, the injury tends to be less stable than an isolated tibial fracture, impacting the management approach, healing, and potential complications. Here are the key implications of tibia and fibula fractures together.

FRACTURE OF TIBIA WITH FIBULAR FRACTURE

The combination of tibia and fibula fractures generally results in a more unstable fracture pattern, often necessitating surgical intervention.

- There is a general dictum that fibular fractures which are suprasyndesmotic should not be fixed while fibular fractures which are transsyndesmotic or infrasyndesmotic require fixation.
- The fibula may also require fixation, particularly when the tibia is severely comminuted (fixation of fibula first will help in restoration of length), if it is fractured near the ankle (distal third) where stability is essential for weight bearing. Fixation of both bones can improve alignment and aid in recovery. When the fibula is to be fixed, it should be done before IMN.

Fractures involving both the tibia and fibula can experience delayed union or nonunion due to the disruption of blood supply and increased bone and soft tissue injury. Patients with both bones fractured are at a higher risk of complications like compartment syndrome, especially in high-energy trauma cases, as the injury can cause significant swelling and compression within the leg compartments.

Combined tibia and fibula fractures also often require a more extended period of immobilization and recovery compared to isolated fractures. Weight bearing may need to be delayed until there is evidence of sufficient healing on radiographs.

COMPLICATIONS OF TIBIA FRACTURE

- *Anterior knee pain*:
  - *Incidence*: Occurs in >30–50% of cases following intramedullary (IM) nailing
  - *Risk factors*:
    - Infrapatellar nailing using a patellar tendon-splitting or paratendon approach
    - Suprapatellar nailing may result in a lower incidence of anterior knee pain.
    - More common if the proximal end of the nail is left proud; a lateral radiograph is the best view to assess nail position.
- *Nonunion*: Requires ruling out infection and potential dynamization if stable
  - *Incidence*: Estimated at 2–10%
  - *Risk factors*: Open fractures, <50% cortical contact, and transverse fracture patterns
- *Malunion*:
  - Occurs in 8–10% of all tibial shaft fractures
  - Higher rates (up to 50%) in proximal third fractures with common valgus/procurvatum deformities
  - *Varus collapse* if a lateral only plate is used in the presence of medial comminution
  - Distal third fractures have a higher incidence of valgus malunion with IM nailing compared to plating.
  - *Risk factors*: Nonsurgical management with casting or external fixation
- *Compartment syndrome*:
  - *Incidence*: Estimated between 1 and 9%, occurring in both closed and open tibial fractures
  - *Risk factors*: High-energy trauma and significant soft tissue injury
- *Nerve injury*:
  - *Risk factors*:
    - Less invasive stabilization system (LISS) plate placement near screw holes 11-13 may endanger the superficial peroneal nerve.
    - Saphenous nerve risk during locking screw placement
    - Transient peroneal nerve palsy may occur post nailing, with symptoms like EHL weakness and sensory loss in the first dorsal webspace.
    - Deep peroneal nerve risk with posterolateral proximal external fixator pin placement.

- *Infection*:
  - *Incidence*: Approximately 5%
  - *Risk factors*: Open fractures, severe soft tissue damage with contamination, and delayed definitive soft tissue coverage

  Infection incidence has decreased due to the use of IMN and minimal invasive techniques (ORIF) while fixing these fractures. Proper handling of soft tissue is of paramount importance.
- *Stiffness*: This complication is mainly restricted to patients who are managed conservatively in casts for a long time.
- Complex regional pain syndrome

BIBLIOGRAPHY

1. Chan DS, Serrano-Riera R, Griffing R, Steverson B, Infante A, Watson D, et al. Suprapatellar Versus Infrapatellar Tibial Nail Insertion: A Prospective Randomized Control Pilot Study. J Orthop Trauma. 2016;30(3):130-4.
2. Cole PA, Zlowodzki M, Kregor PJ. Treatment of proximal tibia fractures using the less invasive stabilization system: surgical experience and early clinical results in 77 fractures. J Orthop Trauma. 2004;18(8):528-35.
3. Hiesterman TG, Shafiq BX, Cole PA. Intramedullary nailing of extra-articular proximal tibia fractures. J Am Acad Orthop Surg. 2011;19(11):690-700.
4. Kulkarni SG, Varshneya A, Kulkarni S, Kulkarni GS, Kulkarni MG, Kulkarni VS, et al. Intramedullary nailing supplemented with Poller screws for proximal tibial fractures. J Orthop Surg (Hong Kong). 2012;20(3):307-11.
5. Lee C, Zoller SD, Perdue PW Jr, Nascone JW. Pearls and Pitfalls with Intramedullary Nailing of Proximal Tibia Fractures. J Am Acad Orthop Surg. 2020;28(2):66-73.

Pilon Fracture

Nitin Choudhary

Etienne Destot first introduced the French word "pilon," which means pestle, in 1911 to describe the mechanical function of the talus on distal tibia. Because of the tibia's high intensity axial compression force acting as a pestle and pressing vertically into the talus, fractures of the distal tibial plafond are also known as pilon fractures. Pilon fractures are associated with a considerable insult to the soft tissue envelope, and the soft tissue status usually defines the type and timing of surgery and the risk of acute complications.

EPIDEMIOLOGY

- Most pilon fractures are a result of high-energy mechanisms; thus, concomitant injuries are common (25–40%) and should be ruled out.
- Pilon fractures have a bimodal age distribution, peaking in incidence between the ages of 25 and 50.
- More than 20% of cases are compound injuries.

CLINICAL PRESENTATION

- Swelling is often massive and rapid, necessitating serial neurovascular examinations as well as assessment of skin integrity, necrosis, and fracture blisters.
- It is critical that soft tissue injury be carefully assessed. As the impact pressure dissipate, significant injury occurs to the thin soft tissue envelope around the distal tibia. If left untreated, this could lead to insufficient healing of surgical incisions with skin slough and wound necrosis. Some recommend delaying surgery plans for 7–10 days as soft tissue heals.

RADIOLOGY

- Anteroposterior (AP), lateral, and mortise ankle radiographs
- *CT scan*: This is invaluable for preoperative planning. Coronal and sagittal reconstruction is helpful to evaluate the fracture pattern and articular surface.

CLASSIFICATION

Two main classification systems used for pilon fractures are:

1. Ruedi-Allgower classification system
2. AO classification system

- *Ruedi-Allgower* classification is based on the severity of comminution and the displacement of the articular surface. Once commonly used, however, this classification is of minimal relevance today.
  - *Type I*: Nondisplaced cleavage fracture of the ankle joint
  - *Type II*: Displaced fracture with minimal impaction or comminution
  - *Type III*: Displaced fracture with significant articular comminution and metaphyseal impaction

Prognosis correlates with increasing grade.

- The AO/OTA classification system **(Figs. 1A to C)**.

MANAGEMENT

Nonoperative Management

Though with advanced approaches and better understanding of the anatomy, most cases are managed operatively, still nonoperative management with use of plasters finds its role in cases of completely undisplaced fractures and in elderly/debilitated patients.

However, patients managed in plasters should be followed up regularly as these fractures have a high tendency of displacement.

Operative Management

Operative intervention is required in almost all cases of tibial pilon fractures except for a few cases as described above.

The main aim while fixing these fractures are:

- Restoration of the tibial articular surface
- Maintenance of fibula length and stability

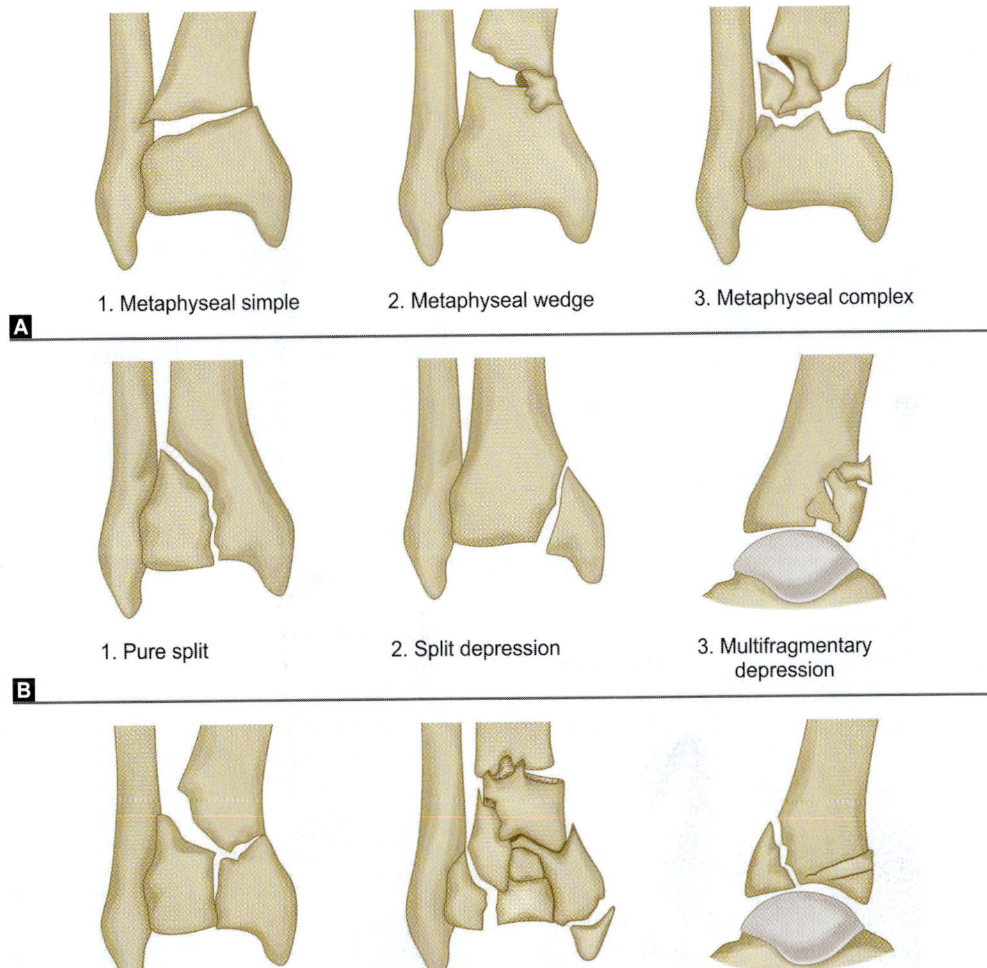

FIGS. 1A TO C: The AO/OTA classification system.

- Bone grafting of metaphyseal defects (because of metaphyseal impaction)
- Protect the soft tissue envelope

The timing of surgery is a very crucial factor in the management of these fractures. Soft tissue must be normal and not be tensed/swollen/excessively bruised which increases the risk of wound complications manifold. The *wrinkling sign* must be waited for before contemplating any surgery.

Various modalities used in operative fixation of pilon fractures are:

- *Temporary spanning external fixation across ankle joint*:
  - *Indications*:
    - Acute management of most length unstable fractures with compromised soft tissue cover
      - Provides stabilization to allow for adequate soft tissue healing
      - Capsuloligamentotaxis tends to reduce the fracture fragments indirectly
      - Keeps fracture fragments out to the length
      - Leave until swelling resolves (generally 10–14 days)

Techniques: The placement of pins should be meticulous keeping in mind the surgical incision required for definitive fixation.

- *Open reduction and internal fixation (ORIF)*:
  - *Indications*:
    - Definitive fixation for a majority of pilon fractures **(Fig. 2)**

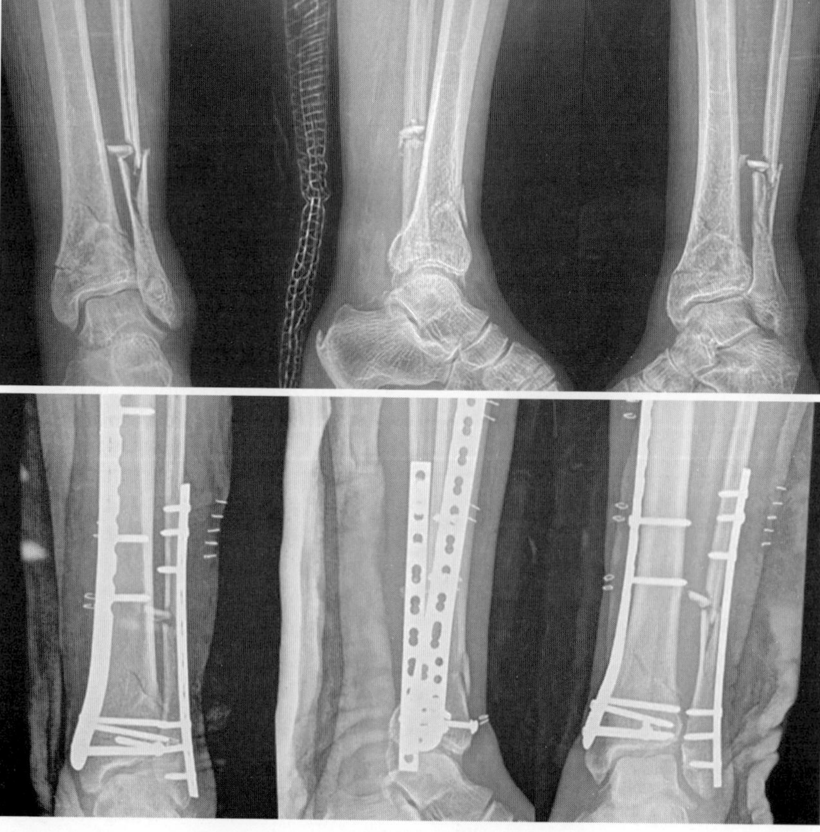

FIG. 2: Definitive fixation for a majority of pilon fractures.

- Minimally invasive ORIF with fluoroscopy-guided incisions can give excellent results in terms of both functional as well as clinical outcomes.
- Fibula fixation is helpful to aid in tibial plafond reduction or augment external fixation.

- *Outcomes*:
  - Usually have good outcomes. Skin complications pose a great threat and wrinkle signs along with minimal invasive techniques reduce these complications dramatically.

Common Surgical Approaches

- *Anterolateral approach*:
  - Often used for fractures involving the anterior aspect of the distal tibia
  - Provides good visualization for joint surface reduction
- *Medial approach*:
  - Typically employed for fractures involving the medial malleolus or the medial tibial plafond
- *Posterolateral approach*:
  - Useful for fractures involving the posterior aspect of the tibia
  - Allows for better visualization and fixation of posterior malleolar fractures
  - Can be performed with the patient in a prone or supine position
- *Two-incision technique*:
  - In cases of complex fractures, surgeons may use a combination of the anterolateral and posteromedial or posterolateral approaches.
  - This method minimizes soft tissue compromise and allows for comprehensive fracture reduction and fixation.
- *Minimally invasive plate osteosynthesis (MIPO)*:
  - Used in specific cases to reduce soft tissue trauma
  - Involves small incisions and indirect reduction techniques
  - Appropriate for fractures that can be reduced without direct visualization
- *External fixation/circular frame fixation alone*:
  - *Indications*:
    - Selected cases where bone or soft tissue injury precludes internal fixation
- *Intramedullary nailing*:
  - *Indications*:
    - Alternative to ORIF for fractures with simple intra-articular components (type A)
    - Minimal soft tissue stripping useful in patients with compromised soft tissue
    - High union rates
    - Increased valgus and recurvatum were seen in this subset as compared to plate osteosynthesis.
- *Primary ankle arthrodesis*:
  - *Indications*:
    - Severely comminuted, non-reconstructable plafond fractures
    - Elderly people who cannot tolerate multiple surgeries/prolonged immobilization in their beds
    - Manual laborers
  - *Techniques*:
    - Plate and screw fixation
    - Retrograde intramedullary TTC nail

COMPLICATIONS

- *Soft tissue slough, necrosis, and hematoma*: These come from the original trauma with inappropriate management of the soft tissues. Excessive stripping and skin closure under tension should be avoided. For appropriate closure, one may need muscle flaps, skin grafts, or secondary closure. With use of mitigation techniques of mitigation techniques (such as minimally invasive surgery and external fixation), these have been reduced.

- *Nonunion*: Reported in 5% cases. Significant comminution along with bone loss as well as hypovascularity and infection are major contributory factors.
- *Malunion*: Frequently associated with premature weight bearing, nonanatomic reduction, and insufficient buttressing (early fixator removal followed by collapse). When external fixation is used, the incidence has been found to reach 25%.
- *Infection*: Infection rate is directly proportional to the devitalization of soft tissues and open wounds. When early surgery is performed in unfavorable soft tissue circumstances, the incidence is high. Osteomyelitis, malunion, or nonunion is possible late-stage infection consequence.
- *Post-traumatic arthritis*: Increasingly common as intra-articular comminution gets worse. Highlights the necessity of articular surface anatomic repair

BIBLIOGRAPHY

1. Egol KA, Tejwani NC, Capla EL, Wolinsky P, Koval KJ. Staged management of high-energy proximal tibia fractures (OTA types 41). J Orthop Trauma. 2005;19(7):448-55.
2. Rüedi TP, Allgöwer M. The operative treatment of intra-articular fractures of the lower end of the tibia. Clin Orthop Relat Res. 1979;(138):105-10.
3. Tang X, Liu L, Tu CQ, Li J, Qin L. Soft-tissue injury management in pilon fracture. Foot Ankle Int. 2014;35(7):657-64.
4. Topliss CJ, Jackson M, Atkins RM. Anatomy of pilon fractures of the distal tibia. J Bone Joint Surg *Br*. 2005;87(5):692-7.
5. Watson JT, Moed BR, Karges DE, Cramer KE. Pilon fractures of the distal tibia. Orthop Clin North Am. 1994;25(4):871-87.

CHAPTER 12.3

Fibula Fracture

Abhai Singh Bhadwal, Shafiq Hackla

Fibula has a Latin source of derivation which means a pin. It is the slender bone which helps to form the ankle mortice and the proximal end and shaft of the fibula serve as a bone graft whenever required and neck is in proximity with the common peroneal nerve. Both fibulae bear about 7% of total body weight. The fibula helps serve as a lateral stabilizer of the ankle and knee due to the insertion of lateral collateral ligament and the biceps femoris tendon in proximal end. Most of the injuries are due to pronation and external rotation or due to a direct blow on the lateral aspect of the leg. Both bone fractures in leg at the same level indicate a high-velocity trauma and usually warrant looking for other injuries.

ANATOMY AND CLASSIFICATION OF FIBULA FRACTURES

The fibula can be divided into three main segments—the proximal end, the shaft, and the distal end (near the ankle). Each segment's location and function contribute to the unique challenges and considerations in managing fractures in that area.

Common peroneal nerve (CPN): The common fibular nerve, also called the common peroneal nerve, external popliteal nerve, or lateral popliteal nerve, is a key nerve in the lower leg. It supplies sensation to the posterolateral region of the leg and the knee joint. At the knee, it splits into two main branches—the superficial fibular nerve and the deep fibular nerve. These branches innervate the muscles of the lateral and anterior compartments of the leg, respectively. It then winds around the neck of the fibula to pierce the fibularis longus. Damage or compression of the common fibular nerve (especially due to displaced proximal fibula fractures) can lead to foot drop.

Fibula as bone graft:

- Entire two-thirds can be removed proximally without disturbing leg function.
- Proximal end is rounded and has partial covering of hyaline cartilage that can be used to replace distal end of radius.
- Middle one-third used a vascularized graft based on peroneal artery.
- Most practical bone graft for replacing diaphyseal bone loss of upper limb bones

Classification

Distal fibula is classified by Weber classification: This classification is based on the relationship of the fracture to the syndesmosis:

- *Type A*: Fracture below the syndesmosis
- *Type B*: Fracture at the level of the syndesmosis
- *Type C*: Fracture above the syndesmosis, commonly with syndesmotic injury

AO/OTA classification:
- 4F denotes fibula

Proximal end ***(Table 1)***:

Example:
4F1B3 = 4F (fibula) + 1 (proximal end) + B (partial articular) + 3 (fragmentary)

Shaft ***(Table 2)***:

Example:
4F2B3: 4F (fibula) + 2 (shaft) + B (wedge) + 3 (fragmentary)

MAISONNEUVE FRACTURE

The Maisonneuve fracture **(Figs. 1A to C)** is a spiral fracture of the upper fibula, often linked to tears in the distal tibiofibular syndesmosis, interosseous membrane, and either a medial malleolus fracture or a deltoid ligament rupture. It is caused by excessive external rotation, classifying it as a pronation-external rotation injury (Lauge-Hansen system) and a Type C ankle fracture (Danis-Weber system). Like the Galeazzi fracture, it

TABLE 1: AO classification for the proximal end of the fibula.

A: Extra-articular	B: Partial articular	C: Complete articular
A1: Avulsion	B1: Simple	C1: Simple articular, simple metaphysis
A2: Simple	B2: Split depression	C2: Simple articular, multifragmentary metaphysis
A3: Multifragmentary	B3: Fragmentary	C3: Multifragmentary articular, multifragmentary metaphysis

TABLE 2: AO classification for the shaft of fibula.

A: Simple	B: Wedge	C: Multifragmentary
A1: Spiral		
A2: Oblique	B2: Intact	C2: Intact segmental
A3: Transverse	B3: Fragmentary	C3: Fragmentary segmental

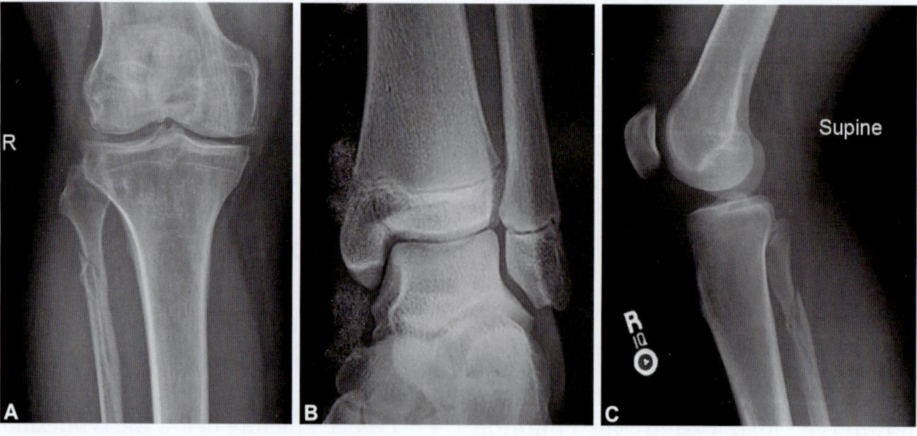

FIGS. 1A TO C: Radiograph showing Maisonneuve fracture.
Courtesy: Radiopaedia.

involves significant ligament disruption. The injury is named after French surgeon Jules Maisonneuve.

MANAGEMENT

Conservative

The mainstay of treatment is conservative in case of isolated fibular fractures without syndesmotic disruption and isolated avulsion fractures without knee instability.

- *Treatment*: Immobilization using a functional brace or short leg cast for 4–6 weeks, with early weight bearing as tolerated.
- *Proximal fibula*: Immobilization in a knee brace to provide healing for up to 6–8 weeks

Operative

Distal fibula (Weber B or C) with >2 mm displacement:

- *Syndesmotic instability (Weber C or confirmed syndesmotic injury)*: Instability in the syndesmosis requires surgical stabilization, typically with syndesmotic screws or suture button constructs.
- *Open fractures*: Open fractures demand urgent surgical debridement and stabilization to reduce infection risk and promote healing.

Relative indication: Proximal or shaft fractures with significant displacement—restoring limb alignment through surgery is critical in these cases to avoid functional impairment.

Fractures of distal one-fourth fibula are discussed separately in great detail in the chapter on ankle fractures of this book.

Combined tibia-fibula fractures: In distal tibia fractures accompanied by fibular fractures, fixation of the fibula can help maintain alignment and reduce malrotation. This is especially relevant for fractures in the distal third of the leg, and with stabilizing the fibula can assist in healing and may reduce complications.

Treatment modalities include open reduction and internal fixation (ORIF) with plating, intramedullary interlocking nailing.

Intramedullary nailing versus plate fixation: Intramedullary nails are becoming a more common alternative to plates, particularly for elderly patients. This method has been associated with reduced surgical site complications, though it is generally chosen based on fracture characteristics and patient needs. Overall, the decision for fibular fixation is based on fracture type, location, stability, and patient factors **(Figs. 2A and B)**.

COMPLICATIONS

- *Common peroneal nerve injury*: Nerve can lead to foot drop, mainly due to displaced fibular neck fracture.
- Ankle joint instability
- *Knee instability*: Due to damage to lateral collateral ligament

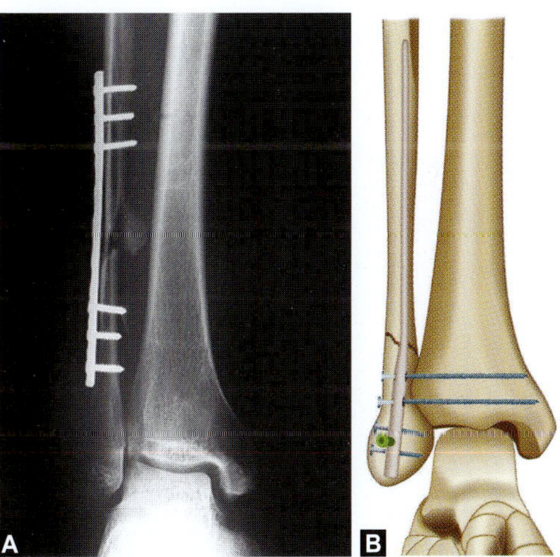

FIGS. 2A AND B: Radiograph showing fibula plating and schematic photograph of intramedullary fibular nail.

Courtesy: AO Foundation and Radiopaedia.

BIBLIOGRAPHY

1. Azar FM, Beaty JH. Campbell's Operative Orthopaedics, Volume 1, 14th edition. Amsterdam: Elsevier; 2022.
2. Buckley RE, Moran CG, Apivatthakakul T. AO Principles of Fracture Management, 3rd edition. Stuttgart: Thieme; 2017.
3. Chaurasia BD. Human Anatomy, Volume 2, 6th edition. New Delhi: CBS Publishers and Distributors; 2013.
4. CR Orthopedics. Foot drop. [online] Available from https://www.crortho.com/patient-resources/education/ankle-and-foot-library/foot-drop/ [Last accessed November, 2024]
5. Rahman S. (2021). Don't Forget the Bubbles. Fibula fractures. [online] Available from https://dontforgetthebubbles.com/fibula-fractures/ [Last accessed November, 2024]

SECTION

13

Ankle

Ankle Sprain

Sumeet Singh Charak

These sprains most frequently involve the lateral ligament complex, particularly the anterior talofibular ligament (ATFL) due to the mechanism of inversion injuries. While some ankle sprains resolve with minimal intervention, up to 40% of cases can develop into chronic ankle instability (CAI) if not managed appropriately, underscoring the importance of effective and evidence-based treatment strategies.

CLINICAL EVALUATION

The initial assessment involves a detailed history and physical examination to determine the mechanism of injury, identify symptoms, and evaluate for ligamentous involvement. Key elements include palpation of the ligaments, assessment for swelling and ecchymosis, and functional tests like the anterior drawer and talar tilt tests, which help gauge the integrity of the lateral ligaments.

IMAGING TECHNIQUES

Although physical examination remains the cornerstone of diagnosis, imaging is essential when there is a suspected fracture, syndesmotic injury, or in cases of severe swelling. The Ottawa Ankle Rules are commonly used to determine the necessity of X-rays.

The Ottawa Ankle Rules are a set of guidelines developed to help clinicians decide when X-rays are needed for patients with acute ankle injuries. These rules are used to minimize unnecessary radiography in patients who are unlikely to have a fracture. The Ottawa Ankle Rules recommend X-rays if there is:

- *Bone tenderness* at the posterior edge or tip of the lateral or medial malleolus
- *Bone tenderness* at the base of the fifth metatarsal (for foot injuries) or the navicular bone
- *Inability to bear weight* both immediately after the injury and in the emergency department for four steps

These criteria apply specifically to adults and be highly sensitive for detecting fractures, with sensitivity rates of nearly 100%. As a result, they are widely used in emergency and primary care settings to prevent unnecessary imaging, reduce costs, and minimize patient exposure to radiation.

Advanced imaging, such as ultrasound or MRI, can provide detailed insights into ligamentous damage, with MRI being particularly useful for assessing partial and complete tears in Grade II and III injuries. Ultrasound is increasingly favored for its accessibility and ability to dynamically assess soft tissue structures in real time.

CLASSIFICATION OF SPRAINS

Ankle sprains are classified into three grades based on severity:

- *Grade I (mild)*: Ligament stretching without tears. Patients experience mild tenderness and swelling but with minimal functional impairment.
- *Grade II (moderate)*: Involves partial tearing of the ligaments with moderate pain, swelling, and some joint instability
- *Grade III (severe)*: Complete ligament tear with significant instability, swelling, and bruising. These cases often require a more prolonged treatment and rehabilitation period.

Accurate classification guides the management plan and can predict the recovery trajectory and potential for recurrence.

IMMEDIATE MANAGEMENT AND ACUTE PHASE

The PRICE Protocol

Initial management of ankle sprains focuses on the PRICE (Protection, Rest, Ice, Compression, Elevation) principles, aimed at reducing pain and controlling inflammation. Protection involves the use of splints or braces to stabilize the joint and prevent further injury, particularly in Grade II and III sprains.

Early Mobilization

Recent studies have suggested that while immobilization helps protect against further damage, prolonged immobilization may hinder recovery by contributing to stiffness and muscle atrophy. Therefore, early mobilization is advocated once acute inflammation subsides, typically within the first 48–72 hours. Active range of motion (ROM) exercises, such as ankle circles and dorsiflexion/plantarflexion movements, can be initiated as soon as they are tolerable to promote ligament healing and maintain mobility.

Pharmacological Management

Nonsteroidal anti-inflammatory drugs (NSAIDs) are frequently used to alleviate pain and reduce swelling during the acute phase. However, clinicians should consider patient-specific factors, such as history of gastrointestinal issues, before prescribing NSAIDs. Some evidence also supports the use of topical anti-inflammatory agents, which may offer localized relief with fewer systemic effects.

REHABILITATION STRATEGIES

Phased Rehabilitation Approach

Rehabilitation is typically divided into three phases:

- *Phase 1 (acute phase)*: During the first week, the primary goals are to control inflammation, limit further injury, and maintain mobility. ROM exercises are emphasized, with a gradual progression to weight-bearing activities as tolerated.
- *Phase 2 (subacute phase)*: This phase focuses on restoring strength, balance, and proprioception. Proprioceptive training, including exercises on wobble boards or balance mats, is crucial for retraining the body's ability to stabilize the ankle. Resistance exercises can be introduced to target the peroneal muscles, which play a critical role in preventing ankle inversion injuries.
- *Phase 3 (return to activity)*: This phase prepares the patient for the functional demands of their specific activities. Sport-specific exercises, agility drills, and plyometric training help ensure that the ankle can withstand dynamic movements. High-impact activities are gradually reintroduced, with a focus on observing any signs of instability or pain.

Functional Rehabilitation

Functional rehabilitation is the cornerstone of successful recovery, aiming to mimic the movements and stresses that the patient will encounter postrecovery. Emphasis is placed on neuromuscular control to prevent recurrent sprains and foster long-term stability.

SURGICAL MANAGEMENT

Indications for Surgery

While conservative treatment is successful in most cases, surgical intervention may be necessary for patients with persistent instability, those who fail to improve with rehabilitation, or athletes who require full stability for high-impact sports. Common surgical options include direct ligament repair, such as the Broström-Gould procedure, which involves tightening and repairing the ATFL and CFL ligaments.

Postoperative Rehabilitation

Postsurgical rehabilitation typically mirrors the conservative phased approach but with a more cautious progression. Initial immobilization is followed by gradual mobilization and strengthening. Patients are advised to avoid high-impact activities until they achieve full functional recovery, which can take up to 6–12 months depending on the severity of the injury and the procedure performed.

PREVENTION OF RECURRENT ANKLE SPRAINS

Proprioceptive Training

Proprioceptive deficits are a significant factor in recurrent ankle sprains. Incorporating balance and coordination exercises into rehabilitation has been shown to reduce the recurrence rate by improving neuromuscular control.

Use of Bracing and Taping

Bracing and taping provide additional support and are particularly beneficial during high-risk activities. Evidence suggests that bracing is effective in reducing the risk of reinjury, and while taping can also be beneficial, it may lose effectiveness over time as it stretches. Braces are often preferred for long-term use due to their cost-effectiveness and ease of application.

Strengthening Exercises

Targeted strengthening of the peroneal muscles and other stabilizing muscles around the ankle can help mitigate the risk of recurrence by enhancing joint stability and functional strength. Programs focusing on eccentric loading have shown promise in reducing injury recurrence.

BIBLIOGRAPHY

1. Bleakley CM, O'Connor SR, Tully MA, Rocke LG, Macauley DC, Bradbury I, et al. Effectiveness of the PRICE protocol for acute ankle sprain. BMJ Open Sport Exerc Med. 2016;2.
2. Kerkhoffs GM, van den Bekerom M, Elders LA, van Beek PA, Hullegie WA, Bloemers GM, et al. Diagnosis, treatment and prevention of ankle sprains: an evidence-based clinical guideline. Br J Sports Med. 2012;46(12):854-60.
3. van Rijn RM, van Os AG, Bernsen RM, Luijsterburg PA, Koes BW, Bierma-Zeinstra SM. What is the clinical course of acute ankle sprains? A systematic literature review. Am J Med. 2008;121(4):324-31.e6.
4. Vuurberg G, Hoorntje A, Wink LM, van der Doelen BFW, van den Bekerom MP, Dekker R, et al. Diagnosis, treatment and prevention of ankle sprains: update of an evidence-based clinical guideline. Br J Sports Med. 2018;52(15):956.

Ankle Fracture

Amarjeet Singh

Ankle fractures are common and could be the result of either a trivial twisting injury in the elderly or high-energy trauma in the young population.

ANATOMY

The distal tibia, distal fibula, and talus combine to form the ankle, which is a hinge synovial joint. Together, the distal tibia and fibula form the ankle mortise that contains the body of talus bone. The muscles, ligaments, and mortise structure surrounding the ankle joint provide stability.

The anterior inferior tibiofibular ligament (AITFL), the posterior inferior tibiofibular ligament (PITFL), and the interosseous tibiofibular ligament (ITFL) form the fibrous complex known as syndesmosis.

The deltoid ligament (DL) is the structure that stabilizes ankle in eversion. It is situated medially, extending from medial malleolus to talus and to the calcaneum. However, stability on the lateral side is provided by lateral ligament complex that is formed up of the calcaneofibular ligament (CFL), posterior talofibular ligament (PTFL), and anterior talofibular ligament (ATFL).

The peroneal, posterior, and anterior tibial arteries supply blood and nerve supply is the articular branches of tibial nerve along with superficial as well as deep peroneal nerves **(Fig. 1)**.

BIOMECHANICS

The ankle's range of motion (ROM) is 30° in dorsiflexion (DF) to 45° in plantarflexion (PF); motion analysis research has demonstrated that a normal gait requires at least 10° in DF and 20° in PF.

A Talar shift of 1 mm laterally lowers surface contact by 40% whereas a 3-mm shift on the other hand can decrease it to >60%.

A 2–3-mm lateral talar displacement can result from syndesmotic injury, even in cases when the deltoid ligament is intact. A lateral shift of more than this usually implies a medial injury as well.

EPIDEMIOLOGY

The most prevalent kinds (70%) of fractures are isolated lateral/medial malleolar fractures, bimalleolar fractures, trimalleolar, and open ankle fractures representing 20%, 7%, and 2%, respectively.

CLASSIFICATION SYSTEMS

Anatomical

According to the anatomical location:

- Lateral malleolus fracture
- Medial malleolus fracture
- Bimalleolar fracture; medial and lateral malleoli (less commonly posterior as well as lateral malleoli)
- Trimalleolar fracture; medial, lateral, and posterior

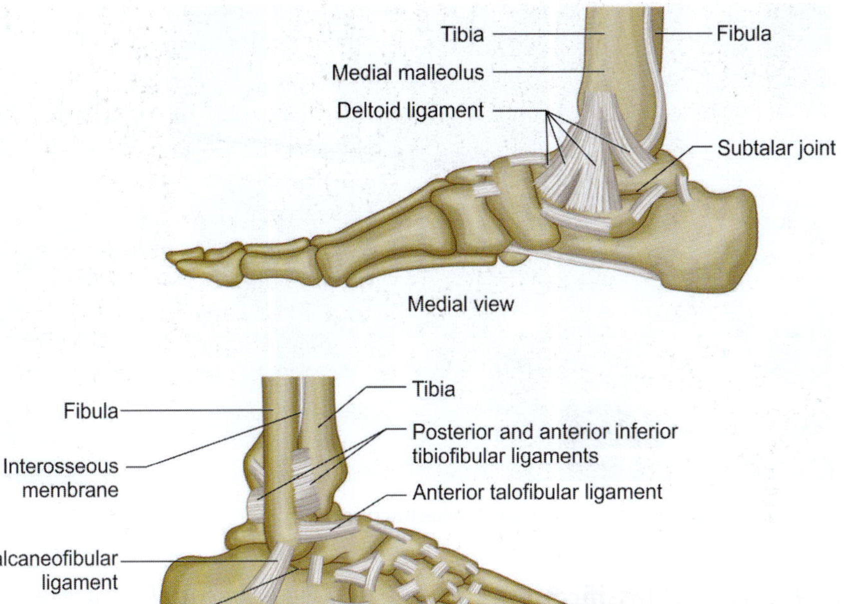

FIG. 1: Ankle anatomy.

Danis–Weber Classification

Considering fibula fracture line's location in relation to the syndesmosis:

- *Weber type A; below the level of the syndesmosis*:
    - Avulsion injury carried on by the foot's supination. It may be associated with a vertical or oblique medial malleolus fracture. Comparable to the Lauge-Hansen injury caused by supination and adduction. Usually stable and treated conservatively.
- *Weber type B; same level of the syndesmosis*:
    - Fibula fracture, oblique or spiral. Half of the patients experience anterior syndesmotic ligament rupture at the level of the syndesmosis, while the posterior syndesmotic ligament remains connected to distal fibular fragment. There may also be associated damage to the posterior malleolus or medial tissues, similar to Lauge-Hansen eversion-supination injuries. If the injury is stable, treat it conservatively (on weight-bearing X-rays). Surgical fixation is needed for unstable Weber B.
- *Weber type C; above the level of the syndesmosis*:
    - The fracture occurs above the syndesmosis but is invariably associated with corresponding medial damage. Incorporates *injuries* of the *Maisonneuve type* and is comparable to stage III Lauge-Hansen pronation-eversion or pronation-abduction injuries. Needs to be surgically fixed because it is unstable **(Figs. 2A to C)**.

AO/OTA Classification

- *44a*: Infrasyndesmotic
- *44b*: Trans-syndesmotic
- *44c*: Suprasyndesmotic

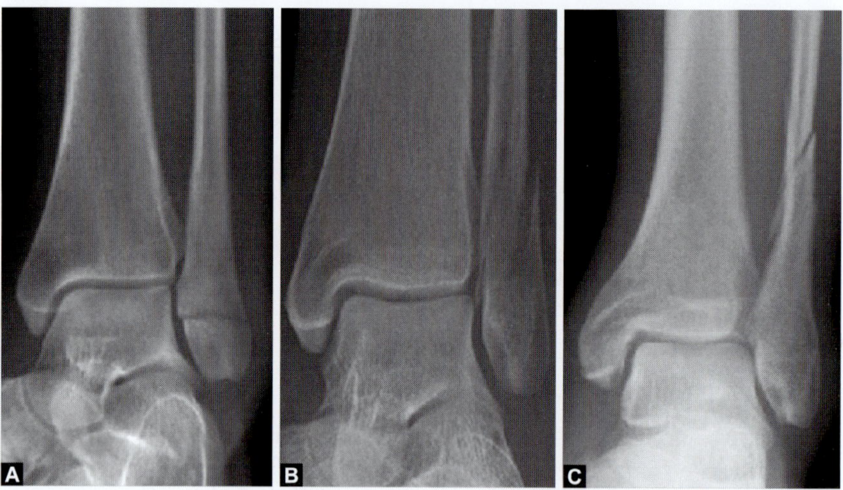

FIGS. 2A TO C: Weber classification of ankle fractures.

The Lauge–Hansen Classification

The Lauge-Hansen classification is based on the force that caused the damage and the foot's orientation. The foot position at the location of the injury is described by the first term, and movement of talus in the ankle mortise with respect to the tibia is described by the second.

Four types:

1. *Supination-adduction (SA)*:
    - Lateral ligament injury and transverse fracture of the lateral malleolus
    - Vertical fracture of the medial malleolus
2. *Supination-external rotation (SER)*—most common mechanism ~60%:
    - AITFL injury is a avulsion of tibia or fibula
    - *Distal fibula fracture*: Spiral (or oblique) fracture from anteroinferior to posterosuperior
    - PITFL injury or avulsion of posterior malleolus
    - Avulsion fracture of the medial malleolus or injury to the DL **(Fig. 3)**
3. *Pronation-external rotation (PER)*:
    - Medial malleolus fracture or DL injury
    - AITFL injury is a avulsion fracture at insertion sites
    - Fibula fracture (spiral or oblique) from anterosuperior to posteroinferior, at or above the level of syndesmosis
    - PITFL injury or avulsion of posterior malleolus
4. *Pronation-abduction (PA)*:
    - Medial malleolus transverse or avulsion fracture is a DL injury
    - AITFL injury or avulsion at insertion sites
    - At or above the level of syndesmosis, transverse or comminuted fibula fractures might result in lateral comminution or a butterfly fragment **(Fig. 4)**.

Every injury mentioned follows a pattern; e.g., SER4 injuries also include SER1, SER2, and SER3.

EVALUATION

- Uncontrolled diabetes raises the risk of Charcot's joint and has an impact on fracture and surgical wound healing. Peripheral vascular disease and peripheral neuropathic diseases further increase this risk.
- *Mobility and social history*: Because smoking and excessive alcohol consumption can impede the healing of

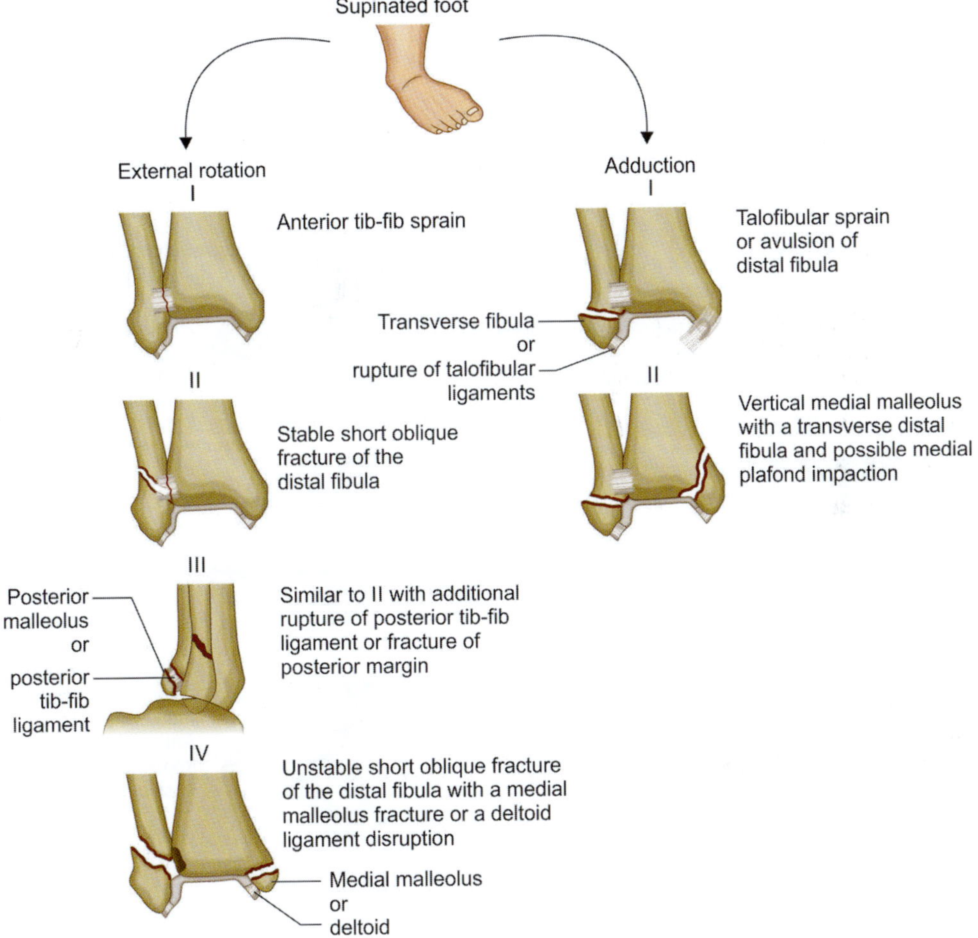

FIG. 3: Supination–external rotation (SER).

wounds and fractures, a thorough history taking is necessary.

- Greater energy mechanism associated with a higher risk of more serious injuries such as a pilon fracture (axial loading) or compartment syndrome in the leg.

Soft Tissue Assessment

The degree of swelling and the condition of soft tissue decide the choice and the timing of surgical fixation. Any skin tenting or obvious threat of soft tissue breakdown warrants an immediate attempt at reduction.

Proximal Fibula and Syndesmosis

- It is important to palpate the proximal fibula so as not to miss a proximal fibula fracture—*Maisonneuve fracture.*
- A positive squeeze test, done about 5 cm above the ankle joint, indicates a syndesmotic injury.

IMAGING

Ottawa Ankle Rules

X-rays should be requested if:

- Bony tenderness at either malleoli's posterior edge or tip (within 6 cm)

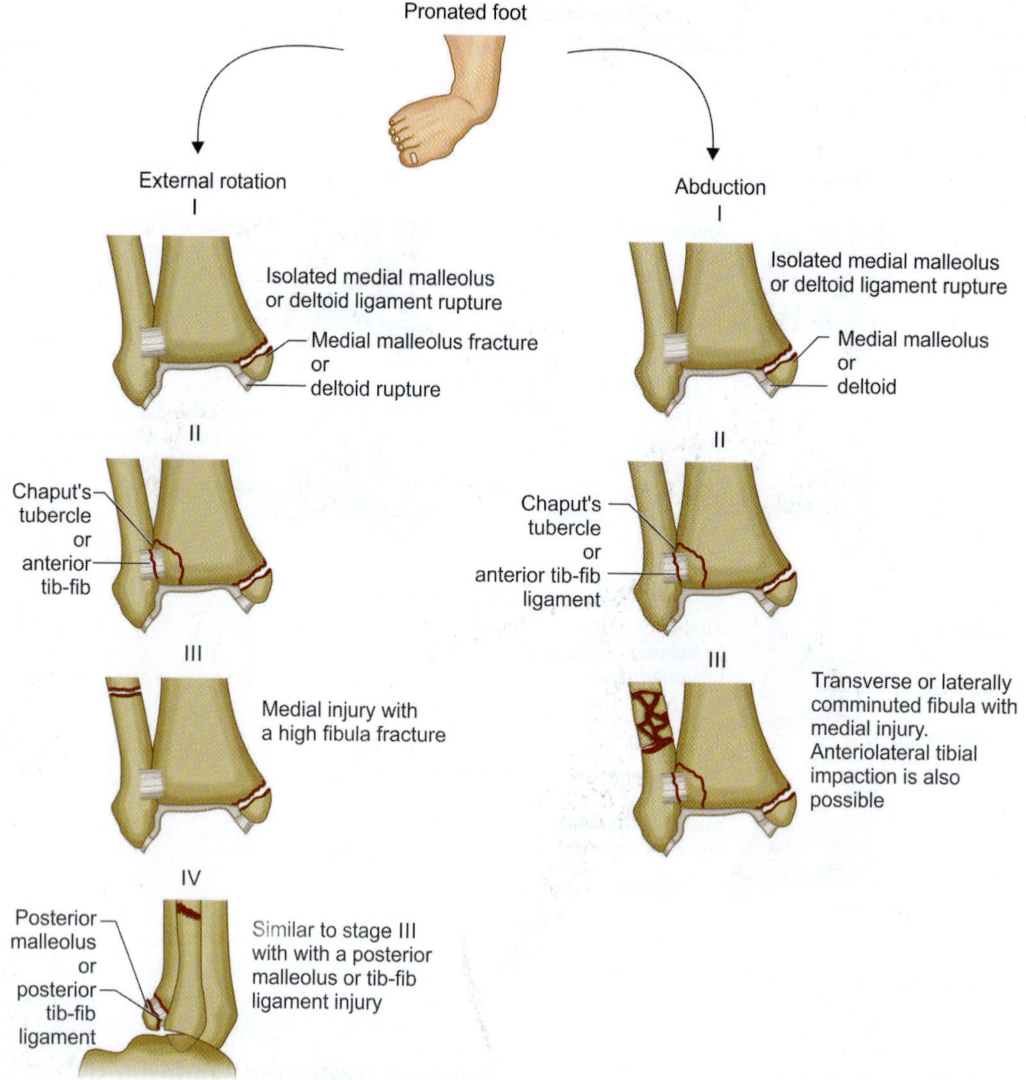

FIG. 4: Pronation–abduction.

- Inadequate weight bearing during the injury and during the evaluation, as determined by the patient's gait.

Getting X-rays must not delay the urgent reduction of an obvious deformed ankle.

Standard X-rays that are taken include—AP, lateral, and mortise views.

- *Lateral view*: Useful for posterior malleolus and seeing the relationship of talus to the distal tibia
- *Mortise view* (AP with leg internally rotated 15–20° and ankle in dorsiflexion): To evaluate the talar dome, medial malleolus, lateral malleolus, and tibial plafond of the ankle mortise

What to look for in an ankle X-ray (see Fig. 5)?

Syndesmotic injury:

- *Decreased tibiofibular overlap (C)*:
  - Measure at the most overlapping point
  - Overlap <10 mm on AP indicates syndesmotic injury.

- *Enlarged medial clear space (A) as in* **Figure 5**:
  - When seen on mortise or stress view, the medial clear space is < 4 mm.
  - In a dorsiflexed ankle, a clear area more than 5 mm combined with external rotation stress is symptomatic of a deep deltoid ligament injury.
- *Enlarged tibiofibular clear space (B)*:
  - 1 cm above the joint, measure the clear space
  - >5 mm on both AP, and mortise views, is abnormal **(Fig. 5)**.

Lateral malleolus fractures:

- *Talocrural (TC) angle*:
  - Intersection between the tibial plafond line with the line that connects both tips of the two malleoli
  - Shortening in lateral malleolus fractures increases the TC angle **(Fig. 6)**
  - Normal 83° ± 4°

Posterior malleolus fractures:

- Spur sign **(Fig. 7)**
- Misty mountains sign **(Fig. 8)**
- Double contour sign **(Fig. 9)**

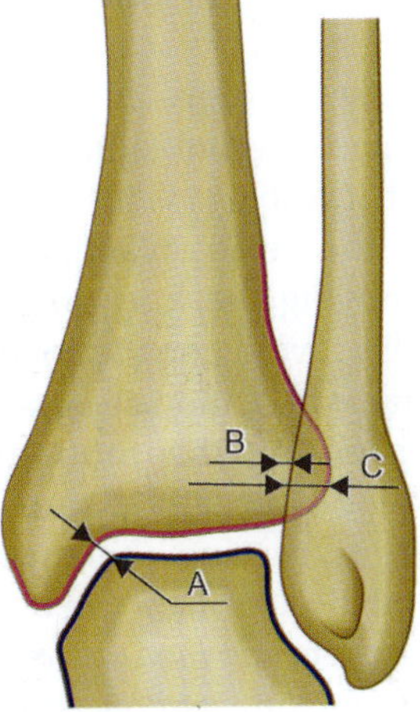

FIG. 5: Syndesmotic injury.

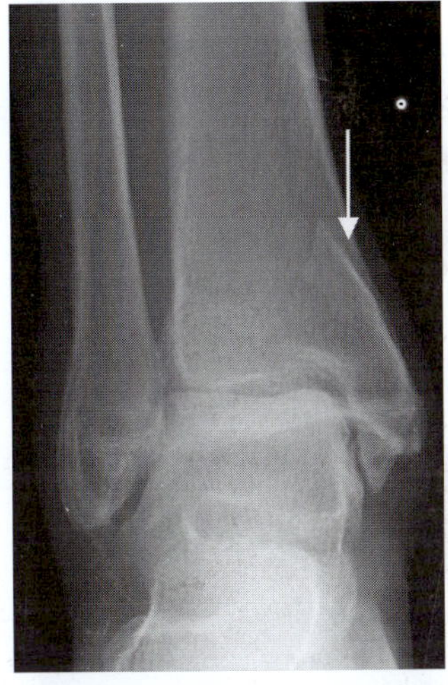

FIG. 7: Spur sign.

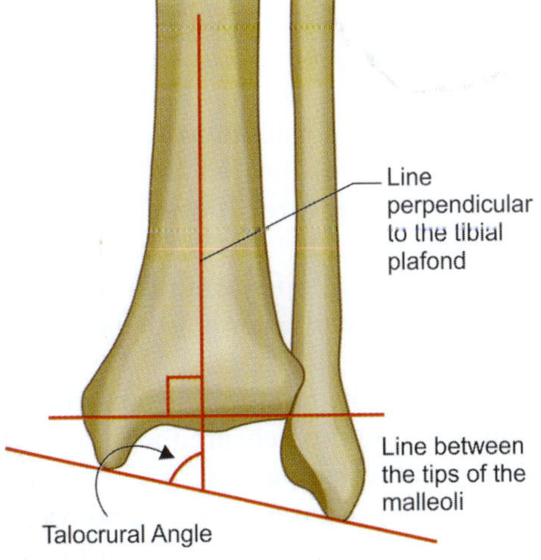

FIG. 6: Lateral malleolus fractures.

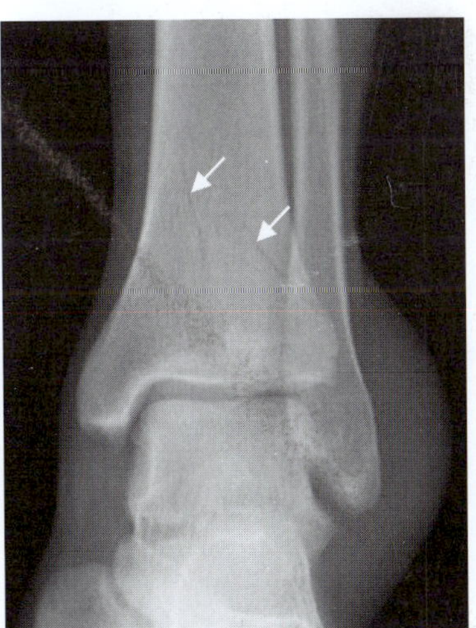

FIG. 8: Misty mountains sign.

Computed Tomography Scan

- Imperative role in surgical planning particularly in complex fractures, to analyze fracture geometry
- Plays an extremely important role in guiding management planning for posterior malleolus fractures **(Fig. 10)**.

TREATMENT/MANAGEMENT

Immediate Emergency Treatment

Any ankle fracture dislocation must be reduced in the emergency room as soon as possible. The patient's lower leg should hang off the end of the examination table when they lie supine on it. This renders gravity able to help with reduction.

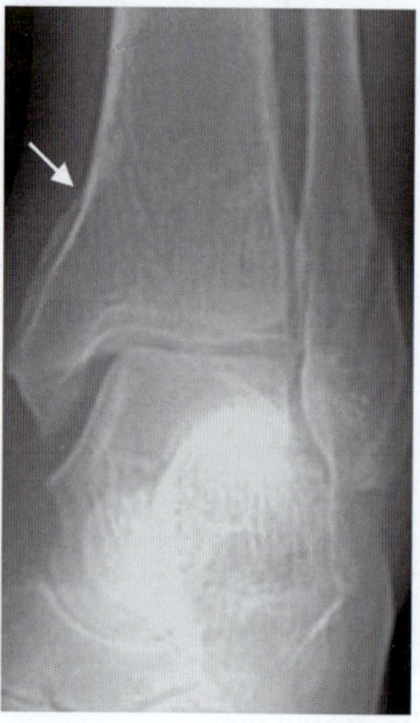

FIG. 9: Double contour sign.

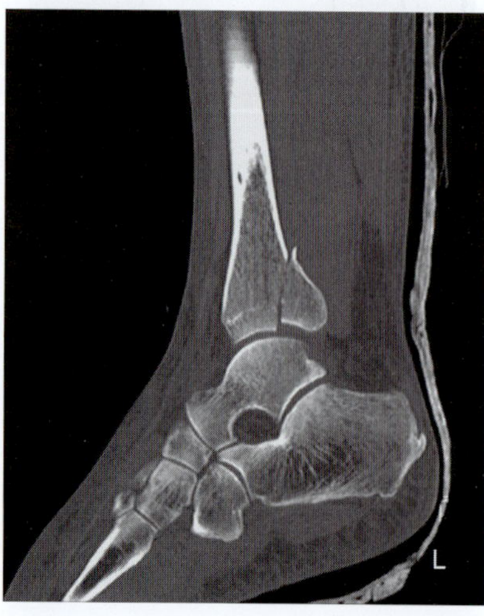

FIG. 10: Posterior malleolus fractures.

- *Reduction of a fracture with a lateral fibular buttress*:
  - Reduce anterior-posterior displacement, if present.
  - Grab the hindfoot and pull both anteriorly and distally to lessen posterior displacement.
  - To buttress the talus against the lateral malleolus, push the heel both proximally and laterally.
- *Reduction of a fracture with a medial shoulder*:
  - The first two steps same as above
  - Reduce external rotation displacement, if visible
  - Place the foot in a plantigrade position by moving the heel anteriorly and distally; avoid dorsiflexion to prevent the talus from moving posteriorly.
  - By pressing the midfoot as well as heel from lateral to medial and counterpressing the medial tibia, lateral displacement can be corrected.
- *Reduction of a medial and lateral malleolar fracture without the presence of a medial or lateral shoulder fracture*:
  - To prevent applying pressure on the malleoli, apply pressure on the midfoot, heel, or distal tibia.
  - Care not to overcorrect medially or laterally
  - Prevalent dorsiflexion of foot

If possible, dislocated ankles should be reduced before being evaluated radiographically.

Abrasions and open wounds should be cleaned and treated according to the severity of the injury.

Any apparent fracture blisters that are left intact should be covered with a sterile covering that is well-padded.

A well-padded posterior slab with U-shaped stirrups needs to be positioned to provide stability as well as comfort following reduction.

Postreduction X-rays should be documented.

The ultimate goal is to stabilize and repair the ankle mortise; nonoperative or surgical methods may be used to accomplish this.

Nonoperative Treatment

Indications:

- *Stable ankle fractures*: On weight-bearing ankle X-rays, there is an isolated unimalleolar ankle fracture without talar displacement.
- Patient unfit for surgery

Nonoperative treatment:

- Below knee cast
- Walking boot/CAM boot

If a patient cannot have surgery, reducing and applying a close contact cast with imaging guidance is a treatment option for an unstable ankle fracture.

Operative Treatment

Ankle dislocation: Urgent open reduction if there is a neurovascular deficiency or if closed reduction measures have failed.

In order to promote soft tissue healing and lower the risk of wound complications, ORIF is done either during the first 24 hours or several days following surgery in patients with unstable injuries who are medically stable and in good soft tissue health.

Indications:

- Unimalleolar fractures in weight-bearing ankle X-rays with talar shift
- Bimalleolar ankle fractures
- Trimalleolar ankle fractures
- Pilon fracture
- Maisonneuve fracture

Fibula fractures: ORIF with plate and screws or fibular nails. Comminuted fractures and patients with poor bone quality can also be managed with fibular nailing.

Transverse medial malleolus: ORIF by partially threaded screws or tension band wiring.

Vertical medical malleolus: ORIF by an antiglide plate or parallel screws.

Posterior malleolus fracture: When over 25% of the articular surface is affected, when there is a displacement of >2 mm, or when there is persistent posterior subluxation of the talus, fixation of posterior malleolus fractures is suggested.

Considering that the PITFL is still linked to the fragment, many surgeons contend that posterior malleolus fixation could be a better option than syndesmotic fixation.

A posteriorly positioned antiglide plate and/or screws through a second incision, or reduction as well as placement of an anterior to posterior lag screw, can accomplish fixation.

Ankle syndesmosis is measured via intraoperative stress views in external rotation or the Cotton test (Hook test).

Employing a bone hook beneath the image intensifier, the fibula is pulled laterally to perform the cotton test. If the fibula moves >2 mm, the test is likely positive.

Using a pointed reduction clamp to the medial as well as lateral malleoli and fixing it with screws or tight ropes minimized syndesmosis. 1 versus 2 syndesmotic screws/tight ropes are under debate but most foot and ankle surgeons prefer 2 screw/tight rope fixation in a divergent fashion.

OTHER TYPES OF ANKLE FRACTURES

Maisonneuve injury:

Pronation external rotation injury: This ankle injury is unstable and may or may not have a medial malleolus fracture. It involves an injury to the deltoid ligament, a tibiofibular syndesmosis, as well as a proximal fibular fracture.

It is critical to differentiate this from fibula fractures caused by direct impact.

Management:

- Surgical fixation; Screw +/- tight rope

- Fixation of the syndesmosis without the need to fix the fibula fracture itself. Assessment of fibular length and rotation should be made and corrected before syndesmotic fixation.
- Associated medial malleolar fractures are fixed according to the type of fracture.

Bosworth fracture-dislocation: Ankle fracture dislocation where the poster tibial border prevents the fibula from being reduced and the fibula is posteriorly dislocated. It requires ORIF.

Explanation of the surgical approaches and the techniques of fixation is beyond the scope of this chapter.

Spanning external fixator: For unstable ankle fractures with swelling, external fixators might be utilized as a temporary fixing technique.

They are particularly helpful in allowing the soft tissue to recover while maintaining ankle stability in cases of severe soft tissue edema or open fractures.

Postoperative protocol and prognosis: For stable fractures that are managed conservatively, the prognosis is excellent.

They can be allowed to weight bear in a boot immediately.

As soon as 6 weeks following the initial injury, these patients resume baseline (full weight bearing without aids).

Unstable fractures: After being in a B/K slab for a minimum of 2 weeks, these patients undergo 4 weeks of nonweight-bearing mobilization in a boot, assisted by crutches or a walker.

Full weight bearing in 6–8 weeks but return to preinjury level takes a longer time after rehabilitation.

The incidence of post-traumatic arthritis in ankle fractures even after anatomical reduction is 14% probably due to cartilage damage.

COMPLICATIONS

Complications can be both conservative and operative management.

Complications as a consequence of conservative management include:

- Ankle stiffness → Physiotherapy and surgical release
- Deep vein thrombosis (DVT) and pulmonary embolism → Pharmacotherapy
- Loss of reduction after manipulating an ankle dislocation → Further ankle manipulation or ORIF/external fixator
- Skin ulceration due to cast pressure → Wound dressing and antibiotics
- Fracture delayed union → Watchful wait
- Fracture nonunion → Surgical intervention
- Fracture malunion → Corrective osteotomy
- Ankle chronic instability → Soft tissue procedures
- Delayed return to functional activity → Guided rehabilitation
- Ankle arthritic changes → Further evaluation and surgery (fusion/TAR)

Operative management complications may include:

- Infection
- Painful scar
- Wound dehiscence
- Metalwork failure (e.g., broken plate and loose screw)
- Malpositioned metal work (e.g., screw protrusion into the joint)
- Fracture delayed union
- Prominent screws
- Vascular damage
- Fracture nonunion
- Nerves damage

The management of each complication is dealt with on an individual basis and is beyond the scope of this chapter.

BIBLIOGRAPHY

1. Brockett CL, Chapman GJ. Biomechanics of the ankle. Orthop Trauma. 2016;30(3):232-8.
2. Court-Brown CM, McBirnie J, Wilson G. Adult ankle fractures--an increasing problem? Acta Orthop Scand. 1998;69(1):43-7.
3. Daly PJ, Fitzgerald RH, Melton LJ, Ilstrup DM. Epidemiology of ankle fractures in Rochester, Minnesota. Acta Orthop Scand. 1987;58(5):539-44.
4. Ebraheim NA, Taser F, Shafiq Q, Yeasting RA. Anatomical evaluation and clinical importance of the tibiofibular syndesmosis ligaments. Surg Radiol Anat. 2006;28(2):142-9.
5. Golanó P, Vega J, de Leeuw PA, Malagelada F, Manzanares MC, Götzens V, et al. Anatomy of the ankle ligaments: a pictorial essay. Knee Surg Sports Traumatol Arthrosc. 2010;18(5):557-69.
6. Manganaro D, Alsayouri K. (2023). Anatomy, Bony Pelvis and Lower Limb: Ankle Joint. [online] Available from https://www.ncbi.nlm.nih.gov/books/NBK545158/ [Last accessed November, 2024]
7. Ugbolue UC, Robson C, Donald E, Speirs KL, Dutheil F, Baker JS, et al. Joint Angle, Range of Motion, Force, and Moment Assessment: Responses of the Lower Limb to Ankle Plantarflexion and Dorsiflexion. Appl Bionics Biomech. 2021;2021:1232468.

SECTION

14

Foot

Calcaneum Fracture

Zubair Ahmad Lone, Mohammad Farooq Butt, Tanveer Ahmed Bhat, Tahir Afzal

The calcaneus is the most common tarsal bone to fracture, constituting around 60% of all the tarsal bone fractures. It is predominantly observed in young working men, due to forceful axial loading mostly because of fall from height or motor vehicle accidents. >75% calcaneal fractures are displaced intra-articular. One-tenth of the patients have associated spine injuries, which must be looked for on clinical examination.

APPLIED ANATOMY

The calcaneum articulates with the talus to form the subtalar joint **(Figs. 1A and B).** There are three articulating facets on the superior aspect of the calcaneus: Posterior, middle, and anterior. The posterior facet is most important with respect to fracture anatomy since it is the largest of the three and is involved in more than three-quarters of the calcaneal fractures. A medial projection of the calcaneus, which lies just beneath the talar neck, is called "sustentaculum tali". The middle facet lies anteromedially over the sustentaculum tali and merges with the anterior facet. In addition to the involvement in the formation of the subtalar joint, the calcaneus, through its anterior articular surface, forms the calcaneocuboid

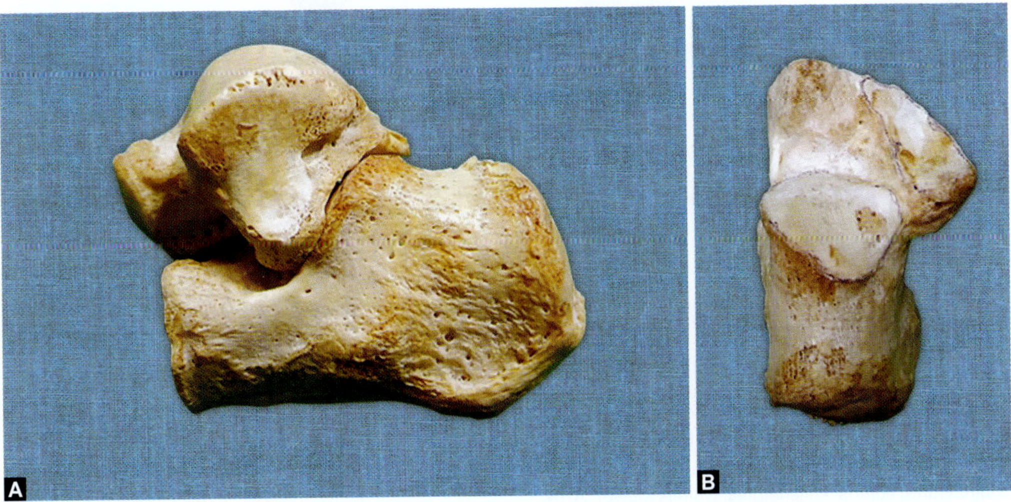

FIGS. 1A AND B: (A) A side view of the talocalcaneal articulation at the subtalar joint. (B) View of the superior surface of the calcaneus with appreciable posterior facet and sustentaculum tali with overlying middle and anterior facets.

joint. Calcaneal tuberosity is located on the posterosuperior aspect and provides attachment to the tendoachilles.

MECHANISM OF INJURY

Most calcaneal fractures result due to falls from height and high-velocity road traffic accidents. Although rare, cases secondary to sports injuries have also been encountered. Following trauma, a forceful axial loading occurs in the calcaneus's articular area, with the talus's lateral process acting as a wedge. According to Essex-Lopresti, the axial loading produces a primary fracture line through the posterior facet and if the force continues, a secondary fracture line may be produced, depending on which the fracture can be a joint depression type or tongue type **(Figs. 2A to F)**.

CLASSIFICATION

Broadly, calcaneal fractures may either be extra-articular or intra-articular. The extra-articular fractures may involve posterior process, sustentaculum tali, anterior process, body of calcaneum, medial process, or calcaneal tuberosity. Intra-articular fractures are more common, accounting for >70% of calcaneal fractures. Two, well-known, classification systems propounded for intra-articular fracture include the Essex-Lopresti classification **(Figs. 2A to F)** and Sanders classification **(Fig. 3)**. The fracture may be classified as "tongue type" or "joint depression type", depending upon where the secondary fracture line exits. Sanders classification is by far the most widely used and is based on the orientation and number of fracture lines involving the posterior facet

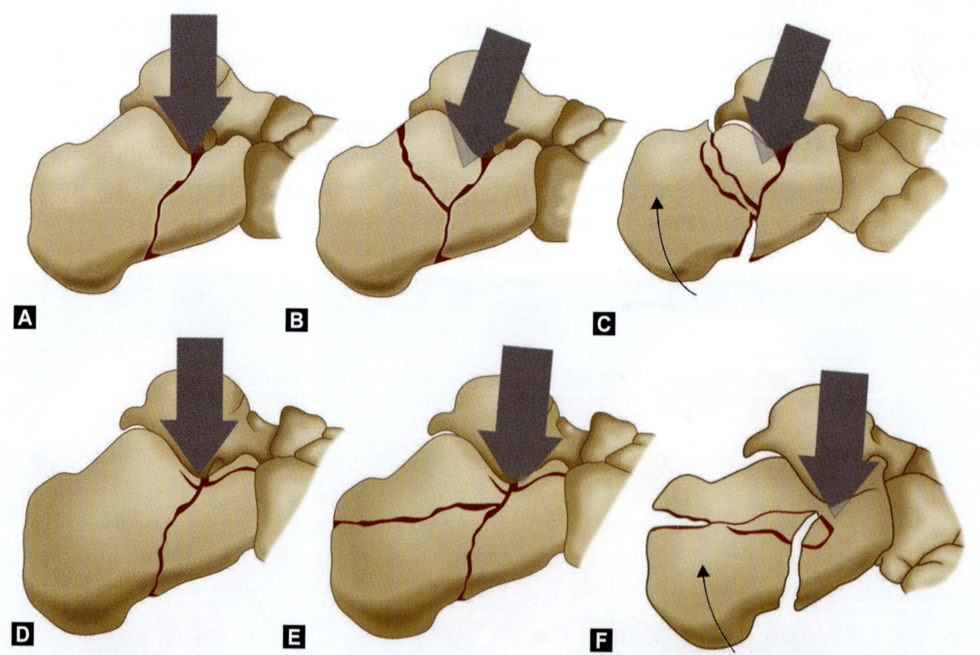

FIGS. 2A TO F: Mechanism of calcaneal fractures as explained by Essex-Lopresti. (A to C) Joint depression fracture; and (D to F) Tongue-type fracture.

Source: Court-Brown C, Heckman JD, McKee M, McQueen MM, Ricci W, Tornetta P (Eds). Rockwood and Green's, Fractures in Adults, Eighth edition. Philadelphia: Wolters Kluwer; 2014.

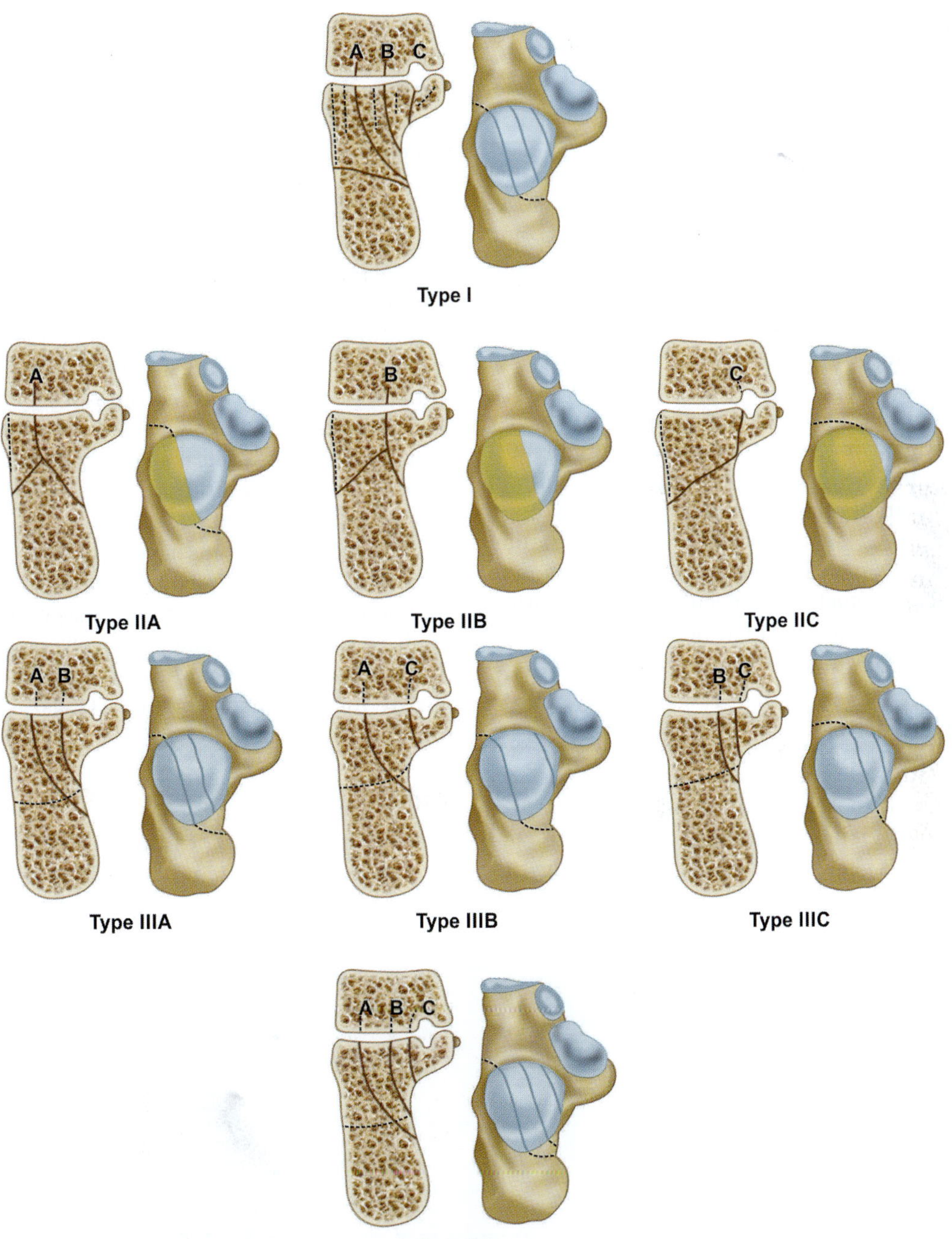

FIG. 3: CT-based Sanders classification takes into account the number of fracture lines passing into the posterior facet of the calcaneus and the displacement of the fragments. Four types of fractures have been described on this basis.

Source: Azar FM, Canale ST, Beaty JH. Campbell's Operative Orthopaedics, fourteenth edition. Amsterdam, Netherlands: Elsevier; 2021.

of calcaneum on semicoronal computed tomography (CT) cuts.

CLINICAL PRESENTATION

Most patients present with a painful heel after trauma with noticeable swelling, ecchymosis, loss of skin wrinkles, gross tenderness, and inability to bear weight. Sometimes, obvious heel widening and reduced heel height in comparison with the normal side may be noted. Blister formation and compartment syndrome are not rare. In displaced tuberosity avulsion tongue-type fractures, compromise of overlying soft tissue is common and must be looked for early. Less than one-tenth of calcaneus fractures may present as open injuries, with a classical dirty laceration, mostly medially. Spine injury, in addition to other associated musculoskeletal injuries, must always be ruled out on examination, especially during the secondary survey.

IMAGING

Plain radiographs are enough to confirm the diagnosis. Recommended radiographic views include a lateral view and an axial (Harris view) view of the calcaneus **(Figs. 4A and B)**. An anteroposterior (AP) view of the foot helps rule out extension of the fracture into the calcaneocuboid joint. Broden's views are useful intraoperatively in assessing the articular reduction of the posterior facet.

On a lateral view, primary and secondary fracture lines can be visualized. A fair idea about the displacement and orientation of fracture fragments is provided by measuring Böhler's tuber angle and the critical angle of Gissane **(Figs. 5A to C)**. The Böhler's angle normally measures around 20–40° and is reduced in displaced intra-articular calcaneus fractures involving the posterior facet. Similarly, the critical angle of Gissane, which is normally around 115–145°, is increased in these fractures.

The advent of CT scans has revolutionized the understanding of fracture anatomy and pre-operative planning. Semi-coronal cuts of CT give a fair idea regarding the involvement of the posterior facet and make it easy to classify the calcaneus fractures **(Figs. 6A and B)**.

Management

After confirmation of a calcaneal fracture, the foot is elevated, icing is advised, and

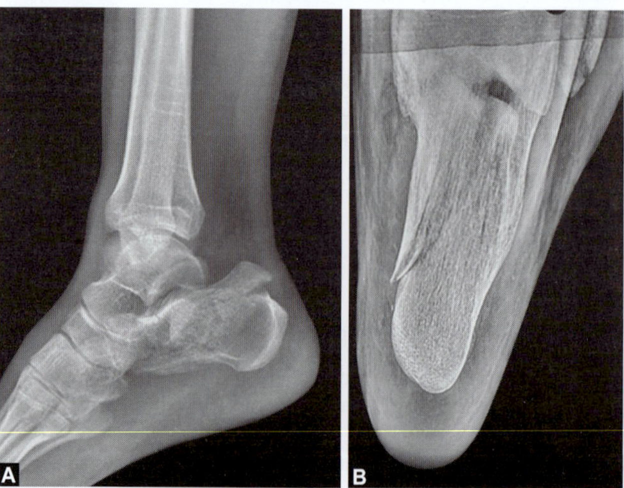

FIGS. 4A AND B: (A) Lateral and (B) axial radiographic views of a patient with a tongue-type intra-articular fracture of calcaneus.

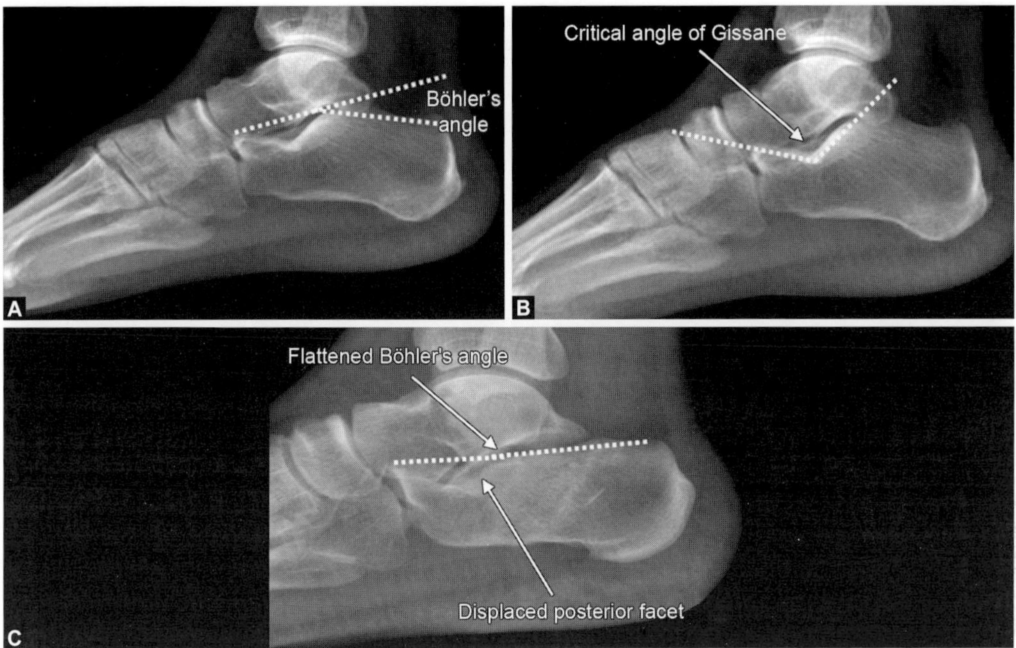

FIGS. 5A TO C: (A) Böhler's angle; (B) Critical angle of Gissane; and (C) Reduced Böhler's angle and increased angle of Gissane indicates an intra-articular calcaneus fracture.

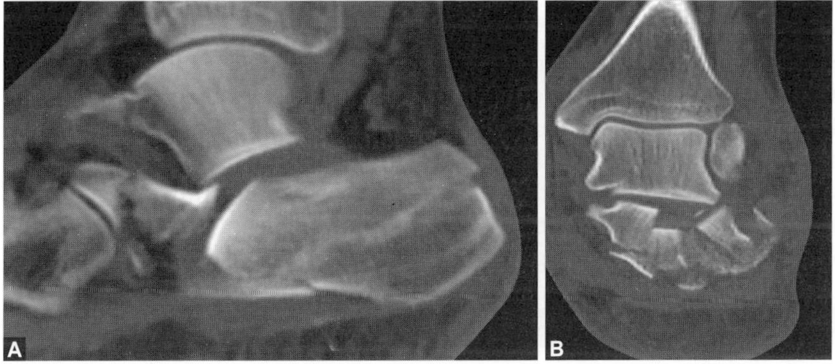

FIGS. 6A AND B: (A) Saggital and (B) semi-coronal CT cuts of a patient with intra-articular calcaneus fracture.

adequate rest is given. Depending upon the pattern and type, a calcaneal fracture may be treated either conservatively or surgically.

Conservative management is indicated for all the minimally displaced extra-articular fractures, minimally displaced intra-articular fractures (Sanders type I), anterior process fractures involving not more than one-fourth of the calcaneocuboid joint, and high-risk anticipated complication group of patients like having peripheral vascular disease, diabetes mellitus, and nonambulators. The patient has to be non-weight-bearing for around 8–12 weeks. Some surgeons prefer to manage with an initial below-knee splint or brace. However, early movements at the ankle and subtalar joint are encouraged, which gives better results in the long term.

Evidence suggests that Sanders types II and III fractures should be managed with surgical fixation **(Figs. 7A and B)**. Some

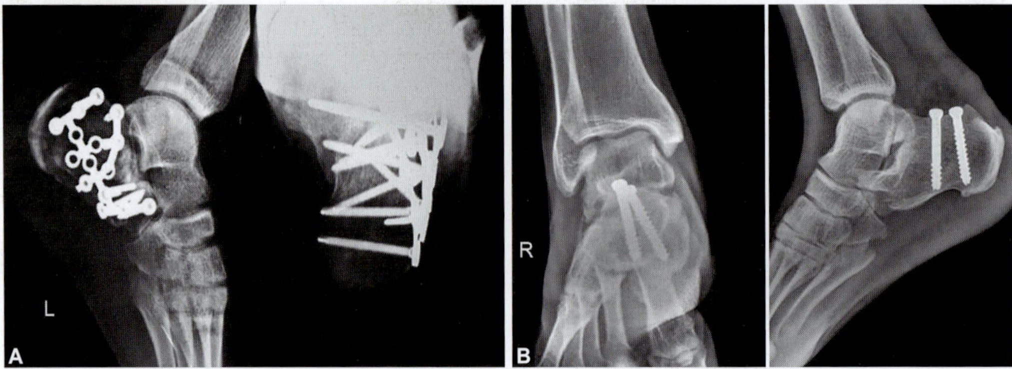

FIGS. 7A AND B: Sanders types II and III calcaneum fractures should be managed with open/closed reduction with internal fixation. (A) Calcaneus locking plate and (B) Cannulated screws.

surgeons use open reduction and internal fixation using locking plates through an extensile lateral approach, while others avoid it in view of possible soft-tissue complications. For this purpose, some researchers have worked on the sinus tarsi approach and observed good results. Many surgeons also prefer percutaneous reduction of fracture and fixation using screws. Whatever the choice of surgery or approach, the goal is to achieve a congruent reduction of the posterior facet, maintain the Böhler's angle, correct varus, and avoid heel widening or shortening.

Sanders IV fractures have the worst prognosis, and it is recommended to make an attempt to fix the fracture to restore the posterior facet. However, the surgeon may decide intraoperatively on table and go ahead with a subtalar arthrodesis in case the posterior facet is not reconstructable.

Tongue-type fractures that are not grossly displaced or do not pose a threat to the vascularity of the overlying skin are managed with Essex-Lopresti maneuver and later fixed with either pins or screws. Displaced tongue-type fractures have a propensity to compromise the soft tissue posteriorly and should be managed urgently with reduction of the fracture surgically. The reduction may be achieved with percutaneous reduction or in a few cases by open reduction. Anterior process fractures involving more than one-fourth of the calcaneocuboid joint should also be managed with surgical fixation.

BIBLIOGRAPHY

1. Cao Z-y, Cui B-h, Wang F, Zhou X-g. Robot-assisted surgery vs traditional fixation for calcaneal fractures: A retrospective study. BMC Musculoskelet Disord. 2023;24(1):123.
2. Leigheb M, Codori F, Samaila EM, Mazzotti A, Villafañe JH, Bosetti M, et al. Current concepts about calcaneal fracture management: A review of meta-analyses and systematic reviews. Appl Sci. 2023;13(22):12311.
3. Lv Y, Zhou Y-F, Li L, Yu Z, Wang Q, Sun Y-Y, et al. Comparative efficacy of minimally invasive sinus tarsi and extended lateral approaches in calcaneal fracture: a systematic review and meta-analysis. J Orthop Surg Res. 2023;18(1):459.

CHAPTER 14.2

Talus Fracture

Omeshwar Singh

- Talus fractures are common in young active and mobile individuals.
- Mostly talus fractures occur in high-velocity trauma injuries.
- The common mechanism of injury includes hyperdorsiflexion of foot.

APPLIED ANATOMY

- *The talus articulates with four bones*: Tibia, fibula, calcaneus, and navicular bones.
- 60% of talus surfaces are covered by articular cartilage.
- Talus has only ligamentous and capsular attachments with no muscular attachments.

Parts of Talus Bone (Fig. 1)

- Head
- Neck
- Body
- Lateral process
- Posterior process

Blood Supply of Talus

- *Posterior tibial artery:* Major blood supply via artery of the tarsal canal and deltoid branches—supplies most of the talar body
- Anterior tibial artery via dorsalis pedis artery—supplies talar head and neck

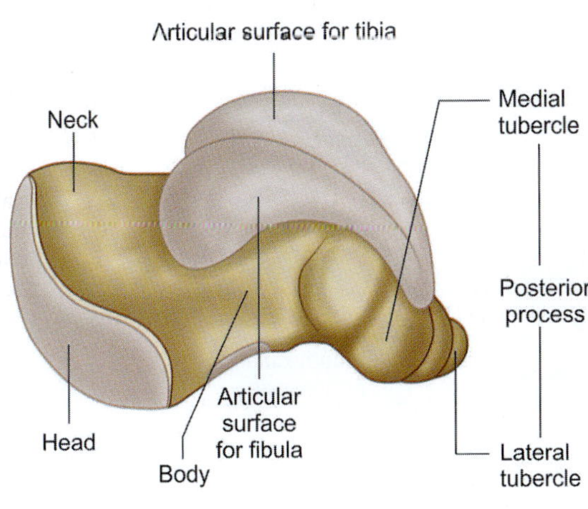

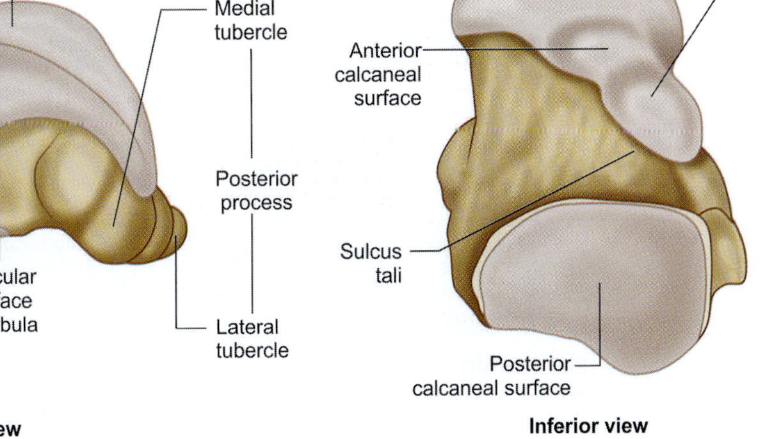

FIG. 1: Anatomy of talus.

- Perforating peroneal artery via artery of tarsal sinus—supplies talar head and neck

DIAGNOSTIC IMAGING

X-rays: Baseline investigation for initial screening of talus fractures includes:
- Anteroposterior view
- Lateral view
- Canale view **(Fig. 2)**—for better visualization of neck of talus

This view is achieved by internal rotation of the plantigrade foot on X-ray film and angling the beam at 75° to the perpendicular.

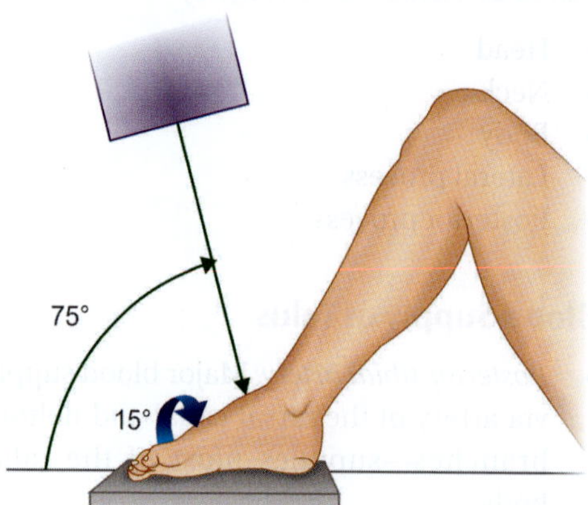

FIG. 2: Canale view of talus fracture.

Computed tomography (CT) scan is the gold standard investigation for accurate description and preoperative surgical planning of talus fractures.

ANATOMICAL CLASSIFICATION

The talar fractures can be of the following types:
- Talar head fractures
- Talar neck fractures
- Talar body fractures
- Lateral process fractures
- Posterior process fractures

TALAR HEAD FRACTURES

It can lead to talocalcaneonavicular joint disruption, shortening of the medial column, and loss of the medial longitudinal arch **(Flowchart 1)**.

TALAR NECK FRACTURES

- Fractures anterior to the lateral process of the talus are defined as talar neck fractures.
- These are the most common fractures of talus (50%).

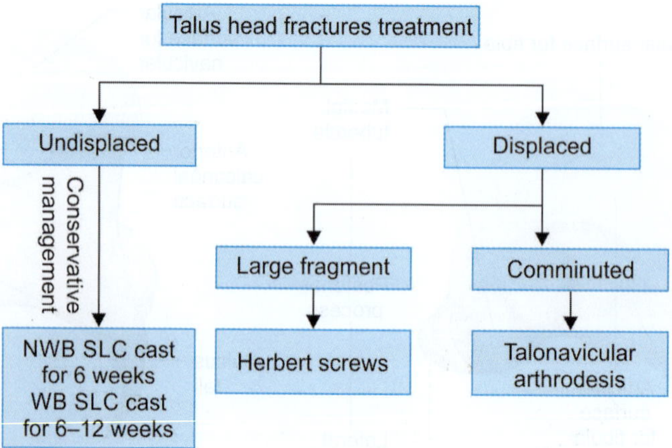

FLOWCHART 1: Talus head fracture treatment.
(NWB: no weight-bearing; SLC: short leg cast; WB: weight-bearing)

- These are also known as aviator astragalus, a term coined by Henry Graeme Anderson in 1919 due to his observation of injury patterns secondary to crashing planes.

Hawkins Classification for Talus Neck Fractures

The Hawkins classification for talus neck fractures is given in **Table 1**.

- Widely used **(Flowchart 2)**
- Predictive of avascular necrosis (AVN) rate

Internal Fixation

- Anatomic reduction and rigid fixation of articular talus fractures remain the mainstay of treatment.
- Lag screw fixation provides rigid stability.
- Screws can be inserted in both antegrade or retrograde directions.
- Antegrade direction is biomechanically stronger but difficult to place.
- Usually, two combined surgical approaches, anteromedial and anterolateral approaches, provide maximal exposure to assess reduction.

The anteromedial approach is a commonly used approach:

- Between tibialis anterior and tibialis posterior
- It exposes the medial talar neck and the anterior tibiotalar articulation
- It preserves soft-tissue attachments, especially deep deltoid ligament (blood supply)
- Medial malleolar osteotomy may be done to preserve deltoid ligament and for better visualization

Anterolateral approach:

- Extends from the tip of the lateral malleolus down the fourth ray, terminating at the talonavicular joint.
- Elevates extensor digitorum brevis and removes debris from subtalar joint.

TABLE 1: Hawkins classification for talus neck fractures.

Type	Feature	Risk
I	Undisplaced	0–13% risks of avascular necrosis
II	Displacement with subtalar subluxation or dislocation	20–50% risks of avascular necrosis
III	Displacement with subtalar and tibiotalar subluxation or dislocation	20–100% risks of avascular necrosis
IV	Displacement with subtalar–tibiotalar and talonavicular subluxation or dislocation	70–100% risks of avascular necrosis

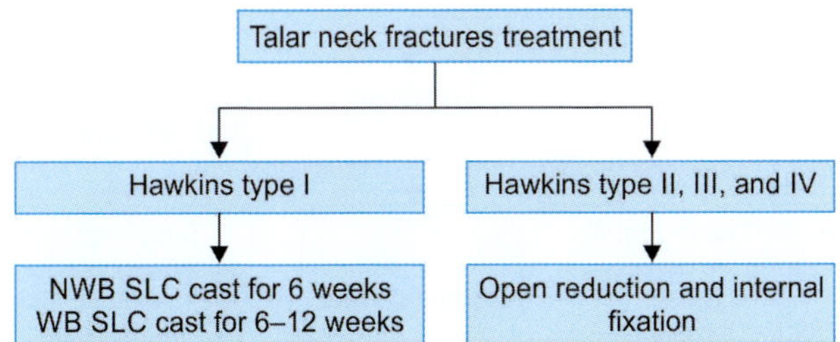

FLOWCHART 2: Talar neck fracture treatment.

(NWB: non-weight-bearing; SLC: short leg cast; WB: weight-bearing)

TALAR BODY FRACTURES

- These fractures lie proximal to the lateral process of the talus.
- Axial compression between tibial plafond and calcaneum **(Flowchart 3)**

LATERAL PROCESS OF TALUS FRACTURE

- *Mechanism of injury*: Fall on everted and dorsiflexed foot
- Commonly seen in snowboarding injuries.
- V-sign for radiographic diagnosis

Hawkins Classification for Lateral Process Fracture

The Hawkins classification for lateral process fracture is given in **Table 2**.

TALAR POSTERIOR PROCESS FRACTURE

- Uncommon fracture
- Mostly treated conservatively
- Excision of fracture fragment maybe required if pain persists despite appropriate conservative treatment

COMPLICATIONS

The complications include the following:
- *Post-traumatic arthritis:*
    - *Subtalar arthrosis:* Most common complication
    - Tibiotalar arthrosis is also common.
- *AVN* of the talus is most common complication of talar neck fracture, the rate of osteonecrosis increases with fracture grade.

TABLE 2: Hawkins classification for lateral process fracture of talus.

Type 1	• Simple fracture • *Treatment:* Fixation
Type 2	• Comminuted fracture • *Treatment:* Excision
Type 1	• Chip or avulsion fracture • *Treatment:* Conservative

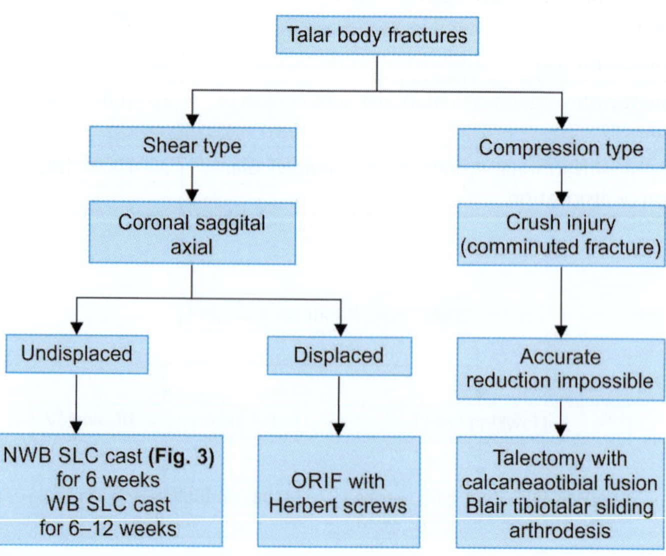

FLOWCHART 3: Classification of talar body fracture.

(NWB: non weight-bearing; ORIF: open reduction and internal fixation; SLC: short leg cast; WB: weight-bearing)

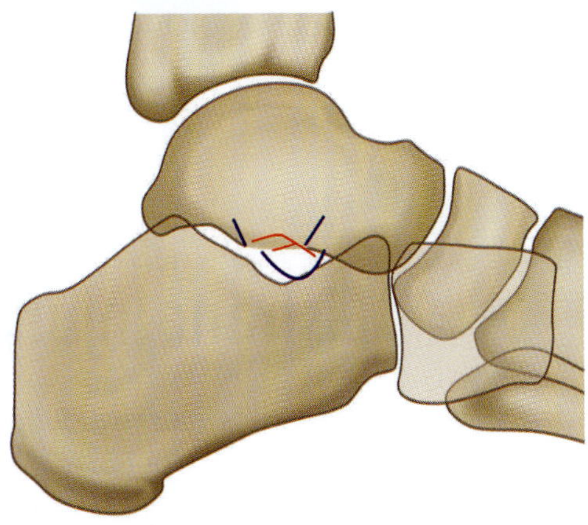

FIG. 3: Undisplaced fractures are managed conservatively with a non-weight-bearing cast for 6–8 weeks.

- *Infection:* There is a high risk of infection because of soft-tissue tripping and contamination.
- *Malunion and nonunion:* The most common malunion is varus through the talar neck, which can be treated with a medial-based opening wedge osteotomy of the talar neck.
- *Foot compartment syndrome:* Rare

HAWKINS SIGN

The Hawkins sign is indicative of diffuse osteopenia with vascular congestion and suggests continuity of blood supply.

- Radiographic sign in anteroposterior (AP) view of the ankle joint
- Thin linear subcortical radiolucency, appreciated on post-treatment images between 6–8 weeks
- Progress from medial to lateral due to vascular re-establishing from the medial side of dome through the deltoid ligament.

BIBLIOGRAPHY

1. Coltart WD. Aviator's astragalus. J Bone Joint Surg Br. 1952;34-B(4):545-66.
2. Dale JD, Ha AS, Chew FS. Update on talar fracture patterns: A large level I trauma center study. AJR Am J Roentgenol. 2013;201(5):1087-92.
3. Early JS. Management of fractures of the talus: Body and head regions. Foot Ankle Clin. 2004;9(4):709-22.
4. Gelberman RH, Mortensen WW. The arterial anatomy of the talus. Foot Ankle. 1983;4(2):64-72.
5. Hawkins LG. Fracture of the lateral process of the talus. J Bone Joint Surg Am. 1965;47:1170-5.
6. Melenevsky Y, Mackey RA, Abrahams RB, Thomson NB 3rd. Talar fractures and dislocations: A radiologist's guide to timely diagnosis and classification. Radiographics. 2015;35(3):765-79.
7. Mulfinger GL, Trueta J. The blood supply of the talus. J Bone Joint Surg Br. 1970;52(1):160-7.
8. Pastore D, Cerri GG, Haghighi P, Trudell DJ, Resnick DL. Ligaments of the posterior and lateral talar processes: MRI and MR arthrography of the ankle and posterior subtalar joint with anatomic and histologic correlation. AJR Am J Roentgenol. 2009;192(4):967-73.
9. Paulos LE, Johnson CL, Noyes FR. Posterior compartment fractures of the ankle. A commonly missed athletic injury. Am J Sports Med. 1983;11(6):439-43.
10. Pennal GF. Fractures of the talus. Clin Orthop Relat Res. 1963;30:53-63.

CHAPTER 14.3

Lisfranc Injury

Omeshwar Singh

- Tarsometatarsal (TMT) joint complex injuries include a wide spectrum of injuries ranging from mild sprains or subtle subluxations to high-energy comminuted fracture patterns.
- The term Lisfranc injury originates from Jacques Lisfranc de Saint Martin, a French military surgeon and gynecologist who described midfoot injuries and midfoot amputation.
- It is often misdiagnosed and mismanaged and up to 20% injuries are initially missed.
- Delayed or missed diagnoses have poor prognosis, which can lead to stiffness, chronic pain, and foot and ankle complex dysfunction.

APPLIED ANATOMY

The Lisfranc joint is formed by three cuneiform bones and cuboid bone proximally with the five metatarsal bases distally joined together by capsule and ligamentous structures. The osseous structure of the midfoot makes it inherently stable.

Lisfranc joint complex includes:

- Tarsometatarsal joint articulation
- Intertarsal articulations
- Intermetatarsal articulations

The second metatarsal base acts as a keystone in which it is recessed between the medial and lateral cuneiforms.

Three-column concept **(Fig. 1)** of the midfoot bony anatomy was proposed by *Chiodo and Myerson (2001).*

- *Medial column:* Articulation between the first metatarsal and the medial cuneiform
- *Middle column:* Articulation of the second and third metatarsals with the middle and lateral cuneiforms, respectively
- *Lateral column:* Articulation of the fourth and fifth with the cuboid

Ligamentous structures are critical in stabilizing the Lisfranc joint and comprise:

- TMT plantar and dorsal ligaments, which cross every TMT joint; dorsal displacement in Lisfranc injuries occurs as the dorsal ligaments are weaker.

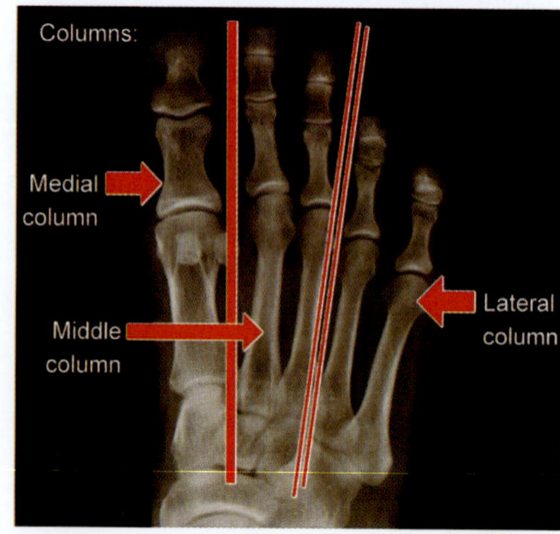

FIG. 1: Various columns of foot.

- Intermetatarsal ligaments, which connect the second to fifth metatarsals
- Lisfranc ligament is the plantar interosseous ligament connecting the medial aspect of the second metatarsal to the lateral aspect of the first cuneiform bone; this "Y" shaped interosseous ligament is a plantar structure that extends from the lateral aspect of the medial cuneiform to the medial aspect of the second metatarsal base.

FRACTURES ASSOCIATED WITH LISFRANC FRACTURE DISLOCATIONS

Fractures associated with Lisfranc fracture dislocations are as follows:

- Base of second metatarsals
- Shaft of metatarsals
- Navicular
- Cuboid

CLASSIFICATION

- *Quenu and Kuss (1909) classification*:
  - Commonly observed pattern of injury
  - Only descriptive classification, no prognostic value
  - Divided injuries into three groups **(Fig. 2)** based on anteroposterior radiographic findings:
    - *Homolateral:* All five metatarsals displaced in one direction
    - *Isolated:* One or two metatarsals displaced from others
    - *Divergent:* Displacements of metatarsals in both the sagittal and coronal planes
- *The Nunley-Vertullo classification (2002) for Lisfranc injuries* ***(Fig. 3)***:
  - Based on clinical symptoms, radiograph findings, and height of the medial longitudinal arch
  - Useful in classifying more subtle and low-energy Lisfranc injuries. This classification has prognostic value.

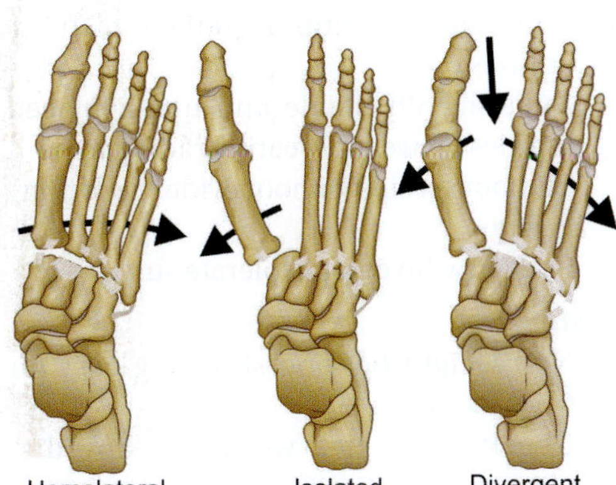

FIG. 2: Various types of Lisfranc injuries.

MECHANISM OF INJURY

The three most common mechanisms [Caused by both high-energy (direct) and low-energy (indirect) trauma]—axial loading on plantar flexed foot, twisting, and crush injury

CLINICAL EXAMINATION

- Midfoot pain with difficulty in weight bearing
- Point tenderness around the TMT joint region
- Swelling across dorsum of midfoot
- Variable deformity due to possible spontaneous reduction
- *Plantar ecchymosis:* Pathognomonic sign for Lisfranc injuries
- *Provocative maneuvers* to evaluate for instability and subtle injuries—squeezing of the midfoot, pronation, supination, abduction, and piano key test
- *Piano-key sign*: The metatarsals are grasped and passive dorsiflexion and plantar flexion are performed at the TMT joint.
  - Subluxation or pain suggests injury.
  - It can be elicited in acute injury.

IMAGING

- *Radiographs:* X-rays should be weight bearing and ideally bilateral for comparison. About 20% of the subtle

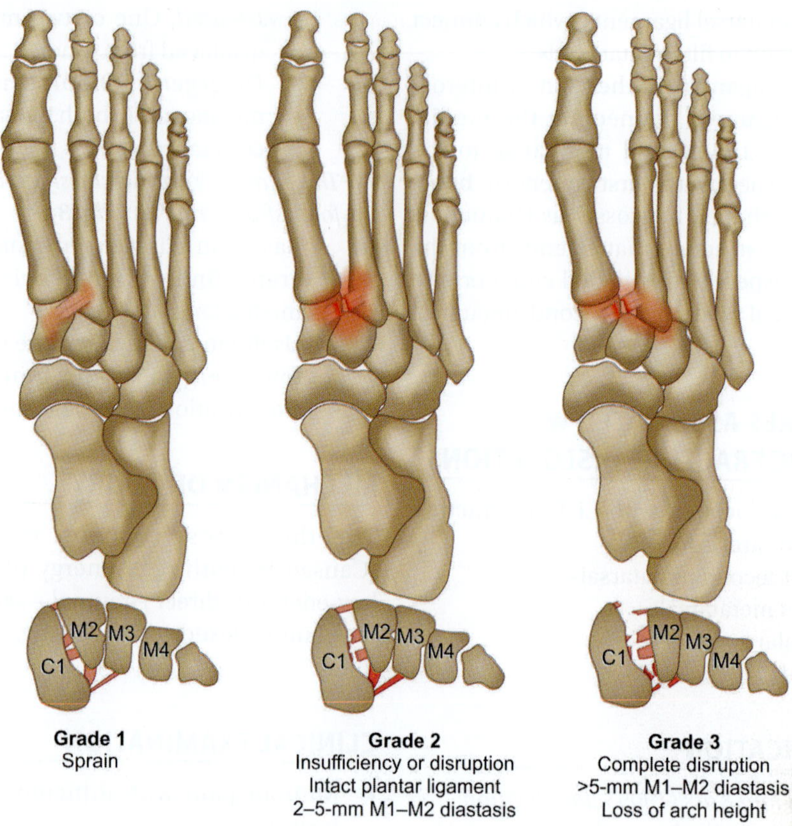

FIG. 3: Nunley-Vertullo classification.

Lisfranc injuries are missed by non-weight-bearing views **(Flowchart 1)**.

- *Dynamic stress radiographs are* indicated in case of persistent midfoot pain despite no finding on weight-bearing X-rays **(Figs. 4 and 5)**.
- *Computed tomography (CT) scan*:
  - Ideal for detecting subtle fracture and persistent displacement not evident on plain radiographs
  - Useful for preoperative planning in the setting of comminuted bony injuries
  - CT scan allows for better visualization of fracture patterns and comminution of joint surfaces.
  - CT scan is non-weight bearing and nondynamic, so it is less useful in identifying pure ligamentous injuries.
- Magnetic resonance imaging (MRI) is indicated especially in cases of ligament injuries, occult fractures, or edema.

TREATMENT

Lisfranc injuries can be managed by conservative or operative methods.

Conservative Management

Indications of conservative treatment

- The Nunley-Vertullo grade 1 Lisfranc injuries
- Anatomically stable and nondisplaced injuries on weight-bearing radiographs
- Midfoot sprains without evidence of bony injury
- Patients who cannot tolerate surgery

Treatment:

- Non-weight-bearing short leg cast for 6 weeks
- Check X-ray at 2 weeks for any displacement
- Weight-bearing short leg cast for further 4–6 weeks

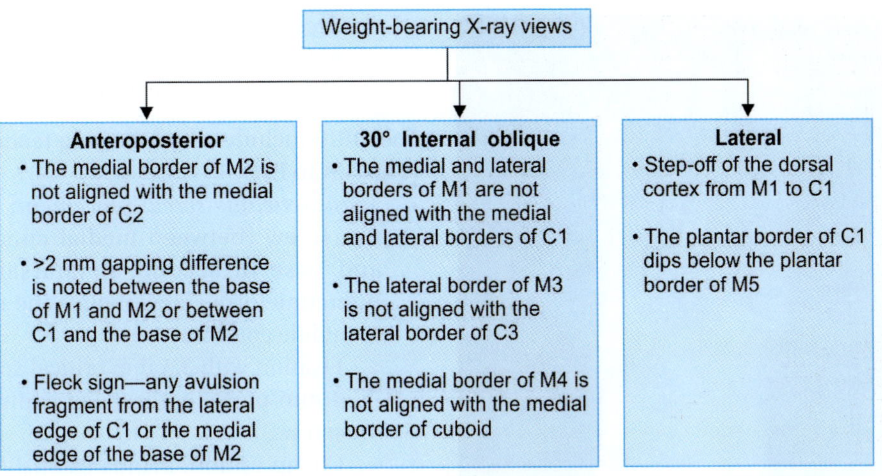

FLOWCHART 1: Various findings on X-ray suggestive of Lisfranc injuries.

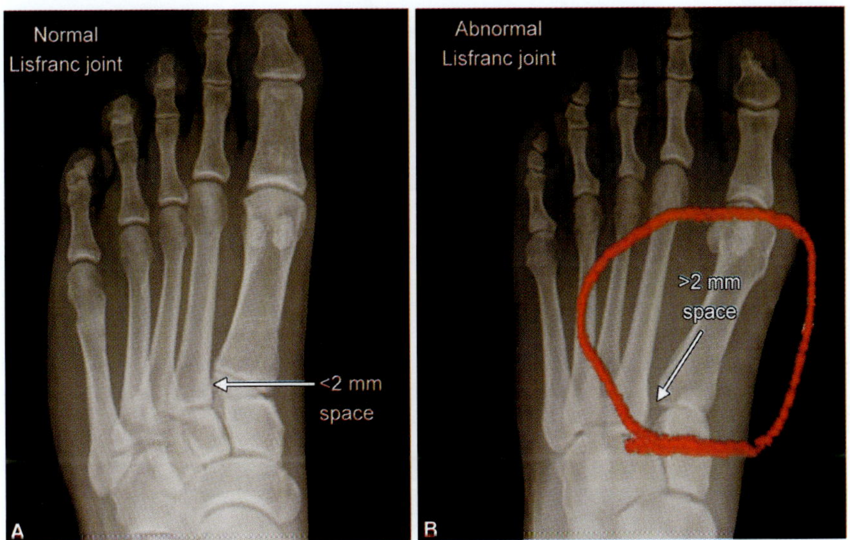

FIGS. 4A AND B: (A) Normal and (B) abnormal Lisfranc, respectively.

Operative Management

Indications: The Nunley-Vertullo grade 2 and 3 Lisfranc injuries—

- Lisfranc joint instability
- Compartment syndrome
- Open fracture

Functional outcomes after surgery depend upon anatomical reduction and stable fixation. Optimal timing of surgery is sooner the better, whenever the swelling is manageable. Poor outcomes of surgery are noticed if delayed >6 weeks

- Bony unstable Lisfranc injuries are managed by open reduction and internal fixation (ORIF).
- Pure ligamentous injuries are generally managed by primary arthrodesis (PA).
- *Approaches:* Dorsal double incision separated by a margin of 4–5 cm.
  - *First incision:* Dorsal 5 cm longitudinal incision from navicular to first metatarsal space; extensor hallucis longus (EHL) retracted medially and dorsalis pedis artery and deep peroneal nerve retracted laterally

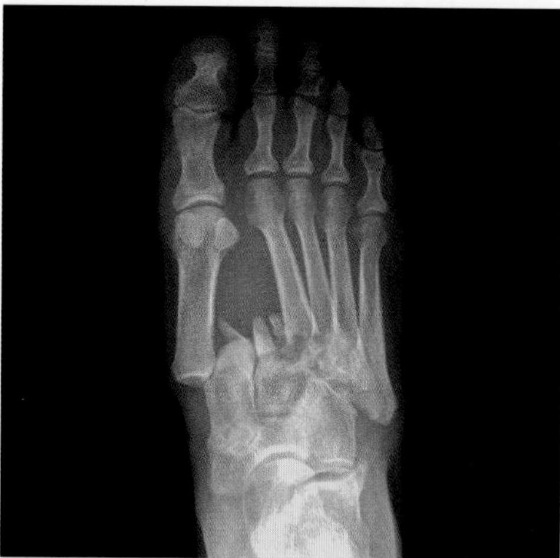

FIG. 5: Severe Lisfranc injury.

- *Second incision* is done from cuboid to third web space distally. Superficial peroneal nerve is protected.

The ORIF includes the following techniques **(Figs. 6A to E)**:

- *Transarticular-screw placement:* Home run screw (between medial cuneiform and base of second metatarsal) and Intercunieform screw reduce the medial to middle column.
  - Fixation with 3.5 mm critical screw or 4 mm partially threaded cannulated screws
  - Cheap option, avoids extensive soft-tissue stripping

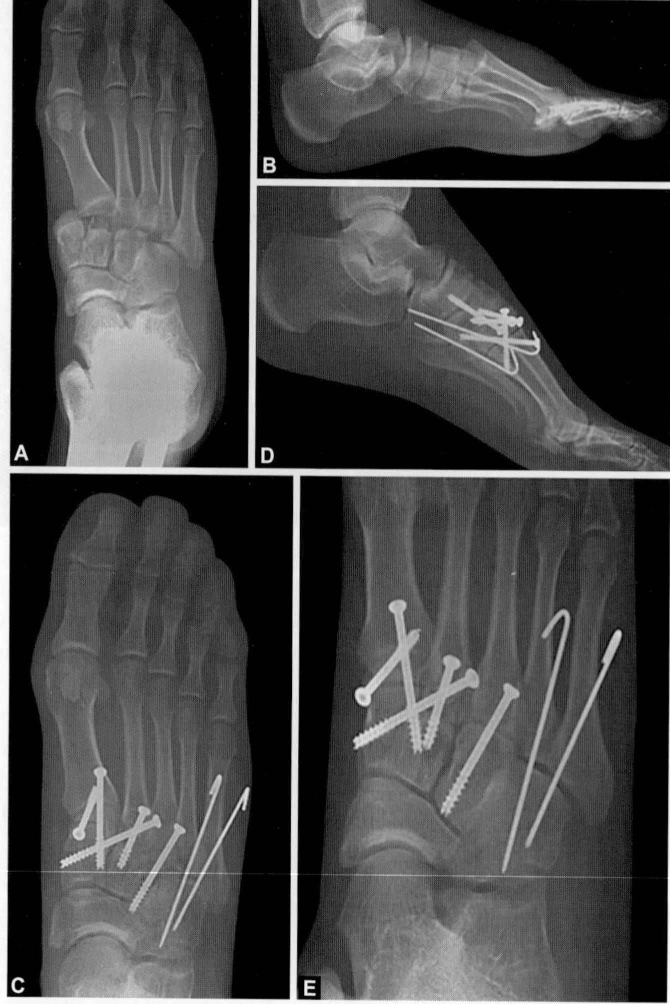

FIGS. 6A TO E: X-rays showing various methods of internal fixation of Lisfranc injury.

- Lateral column, mostly fixed with Kirschner wire (K-wires) or Steinmann pin.
- *Dorsal-bridge plating:* It is useful in repairing highly comminuted injuries.
- *Suture button:* This newer technique has promising results but needs more evidence.

Primary arthrodesis:

- Indicated for pure Lisfranc ligamentous injuries because 40–95% of ORIF for ligament injuries leads to post-traumatic osteoarthritis.
- PA is preferred for injuries older than 6 weeks.

Postoperative Management and Rehabilitation

- Short leg non-weight-bearing cast for 6 weeks followed by partial weight bearing for next 6 weeks
- Cast is removed once painless full weight bearing is achieved.
- Implant removal is done at around 6 months.

The nonoperative algorithm for management of Lisfranc injuries is given in **Flowchart 2**.

The type of operative procedure and implant of choice are given in **Flowchart 3**.

COMPLICATIONS

- *Early complications*:
  - Compartment syndrome
  - Neurovascular injury
  - Surgical site infection
- *Late complications*:
  - Post-traumatic osteoarthritis—most common complication
  - Delayed union
  - Nonunion
    - Chronic pain
    - Hardware symptoms
    - Flat foot

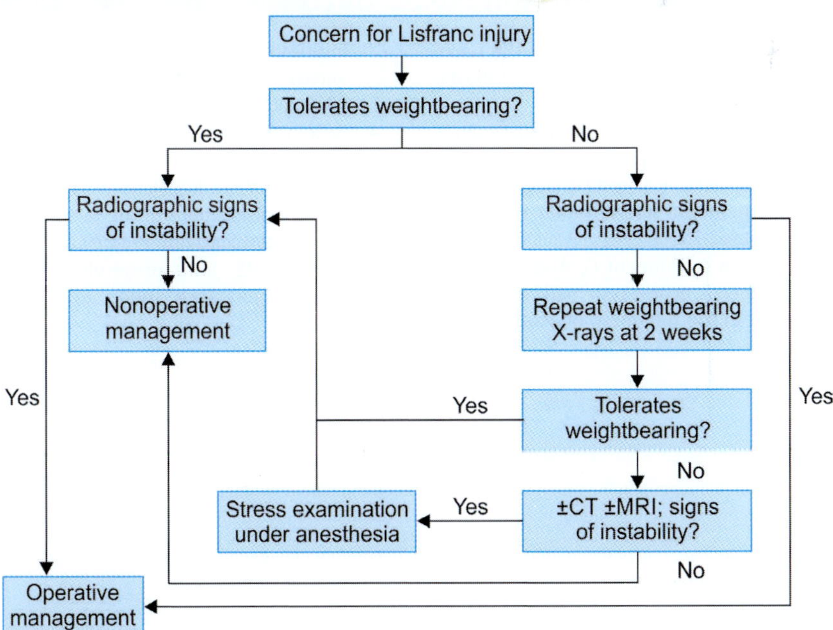

FLOWCHART 2: Nonoperative algorithm for management of Lisfranc injuries.
(CT: computed tomography; MRI: magnetic resonance imaging)

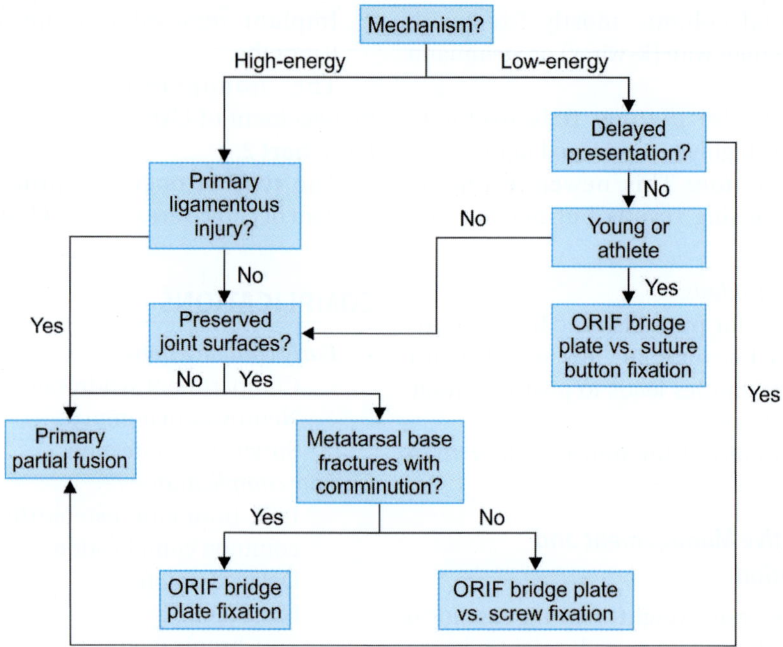

FLOWCHART 3: Type of operative procedure and implant of choice.
(ORIF: open reduction and internal fixation)

BIBLIOGRAPHY

1. Aitken AP, Poulson D. Dislocations of the tarsometatarsal joint. J Bone Joint Surg Am. 1963;45-A:246-60.
2. Alberta FG, Aronow MS, Barrero M, Diaz-Doran V, Sullivan RJ, Adams DJ. Ligamentous Lisfranc joint injuries: A biomechanical comparison of dorsal plate and transarticular screw fixation. Foot Ankle Int. 2005;26(6):462-73.
3. Alcelik I, Fenton C, Hannant G, Abdelrahim M, Jowett C, Budgen A, et al. A systematic review and meta-analysis of the treatment of acute Lisfranc injuries: Open reduction and internal fixation versus primary arthrodesis. Foot Ankle Surg. 2020;26(3):299-307.
4. Ardoin GT, Anderson RB. Subtle Lisfranc injury. Tech Foot Ankle Surg. 2010;9(3):100-6.
5. Arntz CT, Veith RG, Hansen ST Jr. Fractures and fracture-dislocations of the tarsometatarsal joint. J Bone Joint Surg Am. 1988;70(2):173-81.
6. Aronow MS. Joint preserving techniques for Lisfranc injury. Tech Orthop. 2011;26(1):43-9.

CHAPTER 14.4

Tarsal and Metatarsal Fractures including Fifth Metatarsal

Sajad Ahmad Wani, Akash Narangyal

APPLIED ANATOMY AND BIOMECHANICS OF THE TARSAL BONES

Apart from talus and calcaneum, the navicular, cuboid, and three cuneiform bones form a complex articulating structure that supports the longitudinal and transverse arches of the foot, contributing to stability, balance, and load transmission during ambulation.

- *Navicular bone:* It is situated on the medial side of the midfoot and articulates with the talus proximally, three cuneiform bones distally, and the cuboid laterally. The navicular plays a pivotal role in maintaining the medial longitudinal arch of the foot.
- *Cuboid bone:* It is present on the lateral side of the foot, it articulates proximally with the calcaneus, medially with lateral cuneiform, and distally with fourth and fifth metatarsal bones. It is essential for lateral column stability and facilitates the locking mechanism of the midfoot during toe-off in the gait cycle **(Fig. 1)**
- *Cuneiform bones:* The medial, middle, and lateral cuneiforms are situated between the navicular bone and the bases of the first three metatarsals. They play a crucial role in maintaining the transverse arch of the foot and distributing weight across the forefoot **(Fig. 2)**.

MECHANISMS OF INJURY

Tarsal bone fractures are mostly the result of either direct trauma, which is a heavy object falling on the foot or indirect trauma, which is twisting injury during sports. High-energy mechanisms are more likely to cause multiple fractures or complex fractures and dislocations or associated injuries. Low-energy injuries can happen to athletes because of very large stress put on cartilage and bones. The injuries that are most common for athletes are repetitive strains including ankle injuries and stress fractures.

IMAGING

- Standard weight-bearing anteroposterior (AP), lateral, and oblique views of the foot
- A computed tomography (CT) scan is highly sensitive and specific for detecting tarsal fractures, which are not obvious on plain X-rays.
- Magnetic resonance imaging (MRI) detects stress fractures or fractures with a suspected ligament injury.

MANAGEMENT STRATEGIES

Conservative Management

Conservative management is used for nondisplaced/minimally displaced fractures.

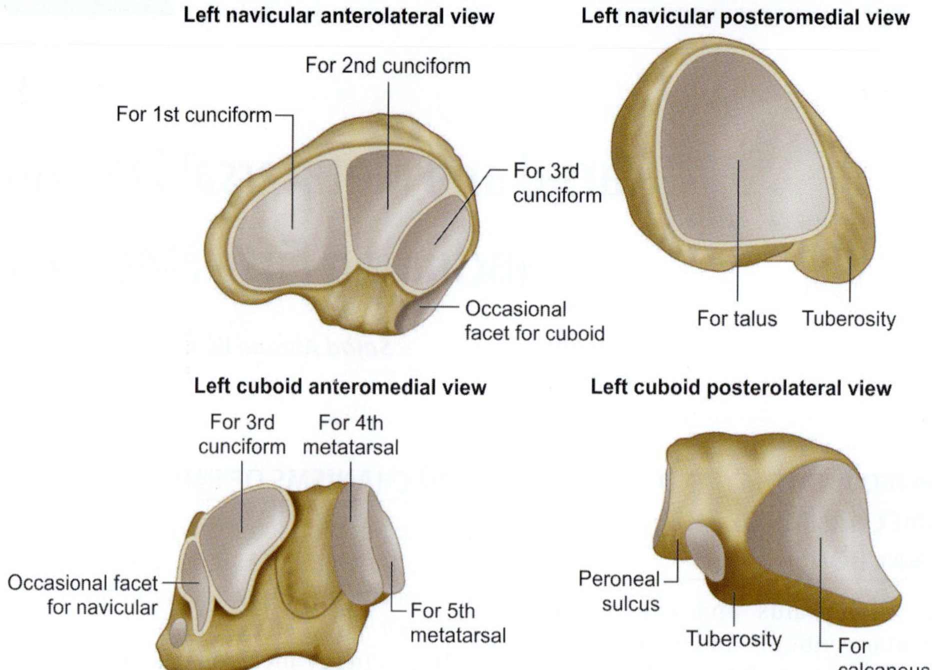

FIG. 1: Naviculum and cuboid bone.

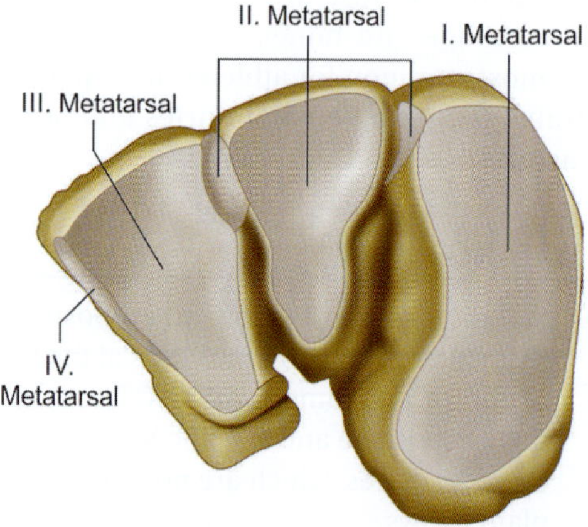

FIG. 2: Cuneiform.

Source: Cunningham DJ, Robinson A. Cunningham's Textbook of Anatomy. New York: W. Wood; 1902.

Treatment: Nondisplaced fractures are typically managed with a short leg cast or a removable boot for 4–6 weeks. Weight-bearing is usually restricted initially, followed by progressive weight-bearing as tolerated.

Surgical Management

Indications for surgery:

- Displacement of >2 mm in the navicular, cuboid, or cuneiform fractures
- Comminuted fractures
- Intra-articular fracture
- Associated soft-tissue or ligamentous injuries requiring repair

Surgical Techniques

- Open reduction and internal fixation (ORIF) is the most common surgical approach for displaced tarsal fractures. It involves realignment of the bone fragments and stabilization with screws, plates, or wires. For navicular fractures, fixation may involve screws placed percutaneously or through a dorsal approach.
    - Cuneiform fractures may also require screw fixation or wiring, depending on the fracture complexity.

- ○ *Cuboid fractures: "Nutcracker" fracture*—results from a high-energy lateral compression injury, often requiring ORIF due to the risk of lateral column shortening.
- *Minimally invasive surgery:* For certain fractures, such as those with minimal displacement but at high risk for non-union or malunion, minimally invasive techniques using percutaneous screws/wires may be appropriate.
- *Bone grafting:* In cases of nonunion, bone defects, or comminuted fractures, it provides structural support and enhances healing.

Postoperative Care

- Patients typically require immobilization in a non-weight-bearing cast or boot for 6–8 weeks, depending on the fracture type and surgical fixation.
- Gradual weight-bearing is introduced based on radiographic evidence of healing.

Complications

Potential complications of surgical management include—wound infection, hardware irritation, malunion, nonunion, avascular necrosis, and post-traumatic arthritis.

Nonunion and avascular necrosis are significant risks in navicular bone due to its tenuous blood supply.

METATARSAL FRACTURES

Applied Anatomy of Metatarsals

- *First metatarsal:* Thickest, strongest, and supports the majority of body weight during walking
- *Second, third, and fourth metatarsals:* Act as stabilizers and help distribute weight
- *Fifth metatarsal:* Most common to injury, especially at its base, where the Jones fracture occurs **(Fig. 3)**

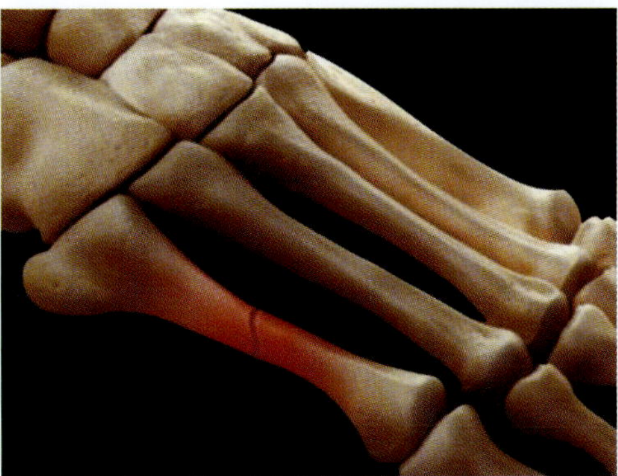

FIG. 3: Metatarsal fractures.

Types of Metatarsal Fractures

- Traumatic (acute) fractures
- Stress fractures

Diagnosis

- X-rays
- *CT scan:* In complex fractures

Management

Management depends upon the type, location, and severity of the fracture.

Conservative

Conservative management is used for non-displaced or minimally displaced fractures.

Treatment:

- The use of a slab, cast, or walking boot may be recommended to immobilize the foot.
- *Ice and elevation:* To reduce swelling and pain
- *Gradual return to activity:* After the initial healing phase, a gradual return to weight-bearing activities is allowed, along with physical therapy exercises to restore strength and flexibility.

Surgical Treatment

The surgical treatment is used for displaced fractures, open fractures, or fractures that do not heal with conservative treatment.

- *Internal fixation:* Metal pins, screws, K-wire, or plates may be used to stabilize the bones, ensuring proper healing.
- *External fixation:* For compound fractures and complex fractures

Rehabilitation

- *Nonsurgical recovery:* Typically, it takes 6–8 weeks for bones to heal.
- *Surgical recovery:* Healing may take longer due to the complexity of the injury and the need for hardware removal in some cases.

FRACTURE OF FIFTH METATARSAL BONE

Fractures of the base of the fifth metatarsal are among the most common injuries encountered in orthopedics, particularly in the context of sports and high-impact activities. Among these fractures, the Jones fracture—a transverse fracture occurring at the metaphyseal-diaphyseal junction—is particularly notorious for its high risk of nonunion and prolonged recovery.

Clinical Anatomy

The proximal section of fifth metatarsal is categorized into three parts: The tuberosity (or styloid), the intermetatarsal zone (metaphysis), and the proximal diaphysis. The tuberosity is the most proximal portion of the fifth metatarsal and connects with the cuboid bone (zone 1). The intermetatarsal zone, or metaphysis (referred to here as the "intermetatarsal zone"), is located just distal to the tuberosity and connects medially with the fourth metatarsal and is the area of true Jones fracture (zone 2). The proximal diaphysis is defined as a separate zone located just distal to the intermetatarsal zone and is the area where stress fractures occur usually (zone 3).

Three muscles are inserted at the base of the fifth metatarsal, making it a complex anatomical location. The proximal metaphyseal-diaphyseal junction is where the peroneus tertius attaches to the dorsal side, while the tubercle of the fifth metatarsal is where the peroneus brevis attaches. The abductor digiti quinti muscle is the third one. Additionally, the plantar fascia is firmly attached to the tubercle's plantar aspect.

Fractures located beyond the tuberosity have the potential to interfere with the retrograde blood flow of the nutrient artery, impeding the healing process and raising the possibility of delayed or nonunion of intermetatarsal zone fractures.

Types of Fifth Metatarsal Base Fractures with Mechanism of Injury

- *Zone 1 (avulsion fractures—93%)* ***(Figs. 4A and B)***:
    - Zone 1 injuries at the base of the fifth metatarsal are typically caused by indirect loads.
- *Zone 2 (Jones fracture—4%)* ***(Figs. 5A to C)***:
    - True Jones fractures occur in zone 2.
    - The fracture extends from the lateral aspect of the proximal metatarsal to the 4th and 5th metatarsal articular surfaces.
- *Zone 3 (3%):*
    - A proximal diaphyseal stress fracture is the third type of fracture in the proximal fifth metatarsal.

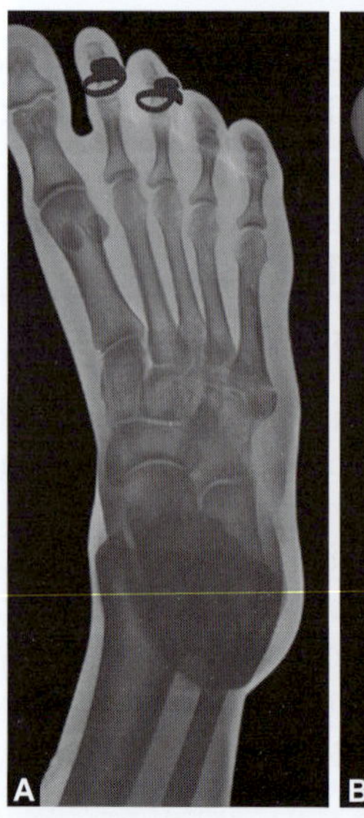

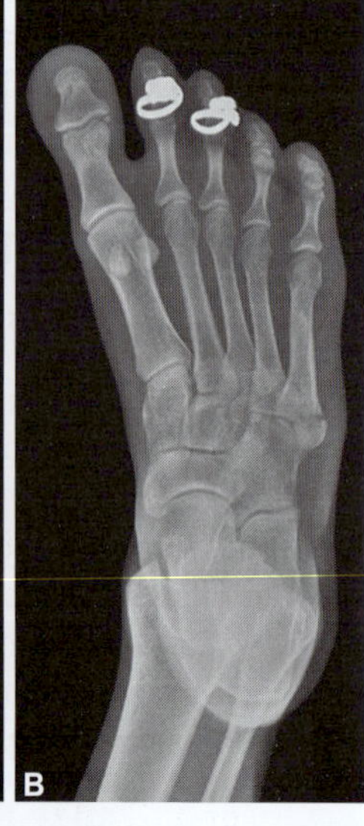

FIGS. 4A AND B: Zone 1 injury.

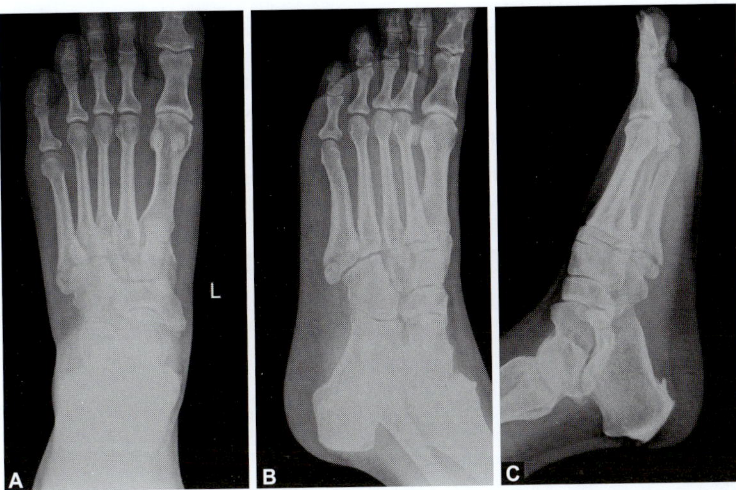

FIGS. 5A TO C: Zone 2 injury.

- Common in high-level athletes but relatively rare
- Located in the first 1.5 cm of the metatarsal shaft
- Caused by repetitive cyclic stresses in athletes

Apart from descriptive classification other classifications include:

- *Torg's classification:* According to the healing status, clinical, and radiological evaluation
- *Stewart's classification*: Based on the relationship of the fracture line to the articular surface, the fracture type, and the fracture site.

Clinical Presentation

If there are several metatarsal fractures together with significant swelling, the foot may have acute compartment syndrome.

Treatment

- *Zone 1 (avulsion fractures):*
  - Fractures in zone I, generally, are treated satisfactorily in a postoperative shoe, walking boot, or short-leg walking cast for 2–4 weeks, followed by gradual weight-bearing as tolerated.
  - For fractures with gross displacement or articular involvement in young active patients, ORIF can be considered (plating, screws, and tension band wiring) **(Figs. 6A to D)**.
- *Zone 2 (Jones fracture)/Torg type 1:*
  - An initial non-weight-bearing short leg cast is worn for 6–8 weeks followed by a weight-bearing cast until the union has been achieved.
  - Even with non-weight-bearing immobilization for 6–8 weeks, Jones fractures have a reported nonunion rate of 7–28%.
  - In competitive athletes, consideration should be given to early ORIF to decrease disability time.
  - The current gold standard for surgical management is intramedullary screw fixation. This procedure involves inserting a cannulated screw centrally along the axis of the fifth metatarsal to provide stable internal fixation and promote bone healing through compression.
  - For nonunion cases or when bone quality is poor, adjunctive bone grafting may be considered.
  - Alternative surgical techniques, such as tension band wiring or plate fixation, may be employed in specific cases where screw fixation is not feasible. However, these methods are

generally associated with a higher complication rate and less favorable outcomes **(Figs. 7A to D)**.

- *Zone 3:*
    - Fractures with clinical or radiographic evidence of chronic injury manifested by partial or complete canal obliteration and sclerosis, non-weight-bearing casting may yield satisfactory results. Generally, the period of immobilization and non-weight bearing is approximately 8 weeks.

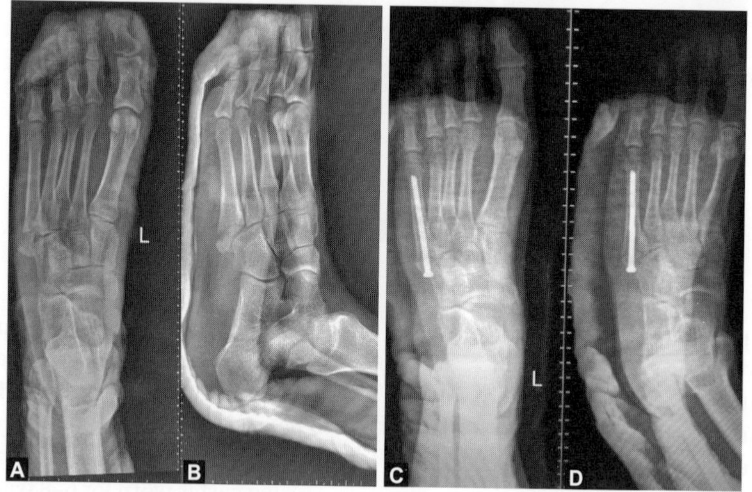

FIGS. 6A TO D: (A and B) Zone I fifth metatarsal fracture; (C and D) After screw fixation.
Source: Dr Sukhil Raina.

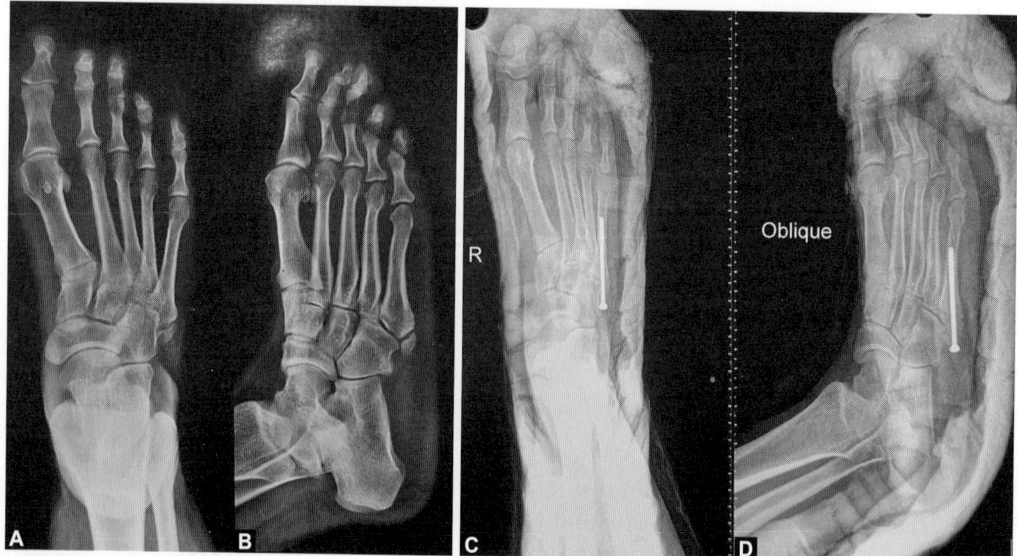

FIGS. 7A TO D: (A and B) Torg type 3; (C and D) After screw fixation with iliac crest grafting.
Source: Dr Azhar Ud Din.

- Surgery should be considered for acute fractures in competitive athletes and other individuals whose occupational demands prevent lengthy non-weight bearing immobilization, as well as for fractures that are not healing clinically after 8–12 weeks.

BIBLIOGRAPHY

1. Boden BP, Osbahr DC, Jimenez C. Low-risk stress fractures. Am J Sports Med. 2001;29(1):100-11.
2. Ding BC, Weatherall JM, Mroczek KJ, Sheskier SC. Fractures of the proximal fifth metatarsal: Keeping up with the Joneses. Bull NYU Hosp Jt Dis. 2012;70(1):49-55.
3. Glasgow MT, Naranja RJ Jr, Gleis GE, Latta LL. Tension band wiring versus intramedullary screw fixation of fifth metatarsal fractures: A biomechanical study. Am J Orthop (Belle Mead NJ). 1996;25(6):455-9.
4. Kavanaugh JH, Brower TD, Mann RV. The Jones fracture revisited. J Bone Joint Surg Am. 1978;60(6):776-82.

Toes Fractures including Tuft Toe, Turf Toes and Sesamoid Bones Fractures

Akash Narangyal, Neeraj Mahajan

Toes fracture occur most commonly in the second to fifth toes; however, fractures in the big toe (hallux) can cause a more significant impact on function **(Figs. 1A and B)**.

TREATMENT

- *Conservative treatment:* Buddy taping/strapping, rest, ice, elevation, and anti-inflammatory medications.
- *Surgical treatment:* For displaced or severe fractures and open fractures, stabilization with Kirschner wire (k-wire), pins, screws, or plates is done.

TUFT FRACTURE

Tuft fracture is defined as a fracture of the distal phalanx, most commonly the big toe. It involves break or crush injury of the very tip of the toe, resulting from direct trauma, like slamming a toe on a hard surface.

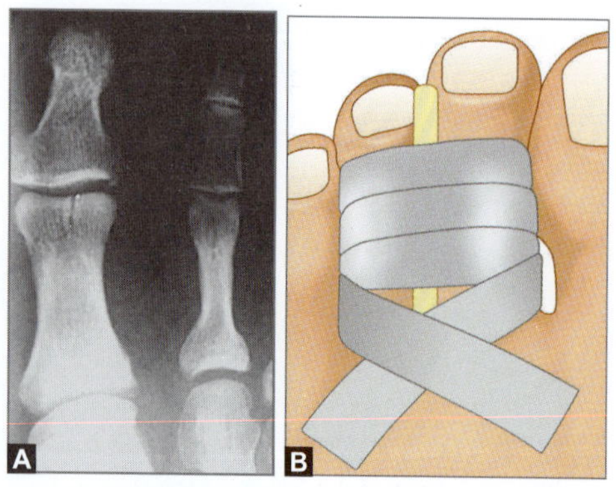

FIGS. 1A AND B: (A) Undisplaced intra-articular fracture of proximal phalanx (PP) of greater toes and (B) Buddy strapping.

Diagnosis and Imaging

X-rays are used to differentiate between simple and complicated fractures and to check the involvement of the nail bed.

Treatment of Tuft Fracture

- *Nonsurgical treatment:* Hard-soled shoe or buddy taping; drainage of subungual hematoma if needed
- *Surgical treatment:* Surgery is done in case of significant displacement or if there is an infection risk. The process involves removal of the nail or repairing the bone.

TURF TOE

Turf toe is the hyperextension injury of the big toe, mostly seen in athletes. Sprains occur at the main joint (metatarsophalangeal joint) of the big toe. It affects ligaments, tendons, and sometimes the bone **(Fig. 2)**.

Causes

It may occur when the toe is forcibly bent upwards, beyond its normal range of motion. This may be (acute) or due to repetitive stress (chronic).

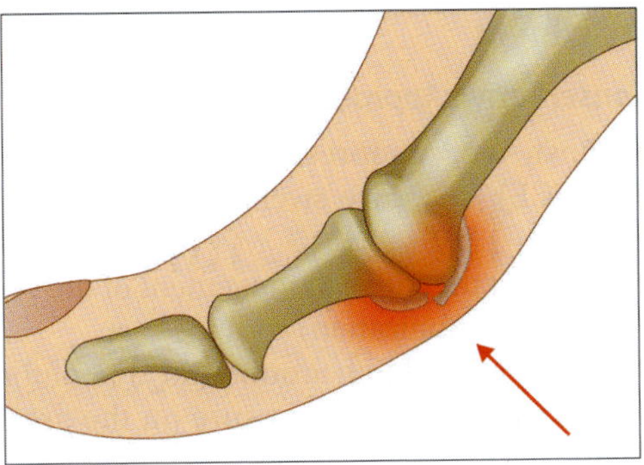

FIG. 2: Turf toe.

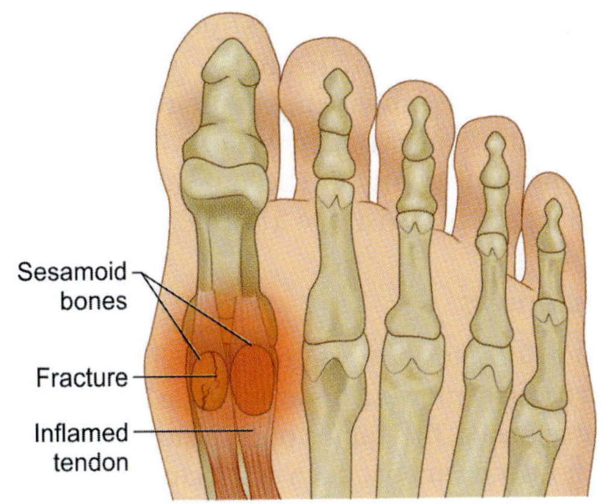

FIG. 3: Fracture of the sesamoid and inflammation of the tendon surrounding the sesamoid (sesamoiditis).

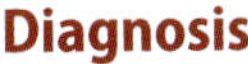

Diagnosis

- Physical examination
- *X-rays:* To rule out fractures
- *Magnetic resonance imaging (MRI)/ ultrasound:* To evaluate soft-tissue damage, such as ligament tears.

Treatment

- Rest, immobilization, ice, and compression
- Physical therapy
- *Surgical treatment:* Surgery is needed where ligaments are torn, or the joint is unstable.

Complications of Untreated Toe Injuries

- Chronic pain or stiffness
- Joint instability or deformity
- Arthritis, mostly with untreated turf toe
- Difficulty walking or while wearing certain footwear

SESAMOID BONE FRACTURES OF THE FOOT

Mostly, bones connect at joints. But some bones are not connected to any other bone. Instead, they only connect to tendons or are embedded inside muscle. These bones are sesamoids. Foot sesamoids, named for their resemblance to sesame seeds, are found in tendons of the foot's flexor hallucis brevis muscle just beneath the first metatarsal head. They endure significant pressure and stress, especially in activities like toe-off movements, running, or dancing.

Anatomy and Function of Sesamoid Bone

The two sesamoid bones are located under the first metatarsal head (big toe joint). The first metatarsal flexor tendons are attached to both of the sesamoid bones and functionally, this is similar to pulleys, increasing the leverage of the tendons and muscles that control the first metatarsal (hallux). This position allows the sesamoids to decrease friction, absorb impact, and facilitate smooth toe-off phases during gait. In addition, they also stabilize the metatarsophalangeal (MTP) joint and protect the plantar surface of the first metatarsal head. The sesamoid bones are connected to each other with very strong plantar plate and ligaments **(Fig. 3)**.

Causes of Sesamoid Fractures

- Acute fractures result from a direct injury.
- Stress fractures develop slowly due to repetitive small injuries.

- Other factors include structural abnormalities like high arches (pes cavus), excessive pronation, or a first metatarsal that is longer than normal. Wearing high heels or poorly fitting footwear can also increase the risk of a fracture.

Diagnosis

Look for signs of tenderness, swelling, or restriction of movements around the first metatarsal head. The pain is often exacerbated by toe-off movements, such as walking, running, or jumping.

The *various radiographic views* for detecting a *sesamoid bone fracture* are:

- *Dorsoplantar (DP) view*
- *Tangential (axial) view:* This is the most useful view for sesamoid fractures. It is taken with the toes dorsiflexed and the X-ray beam aimed tangentially at the sesamoids, allowing for a clear view of these bones.
- Oblique views
- *Lateral view:* Though less commonly used for detecting sesamoid fractures, this view can help evaluate the relationship of the sesamoid bones to the metatarsal and the rest of the foot.

Among these, the *tangential view* is often considered the best for detecting sesamoid bone fractures because it provides more direct and clear image of the bones.

However, sometimes sesamoid fractures may not be visible on X-rays, especially in the case of stress fractures. Other imaging, such as a bone scan, MRI, or computed tomography (CT) scans, may be needed.

Treatment

Conservative Approach

- Rest, ice, compression, and elevation (RICE) to reduce swelling and alleviate pain
- Restrict the range of movement of the big toe (immobilization) with the cast.
- J-shaped padding around the area of the sesamoid relieves pressure on the great toe.
- Analgesics
- A stiff-soled shoe or short leg-fracture braces

Surgery

Indications:

- Significantly displayed sesamoid fracture
- Nonunion

Surgery for a displaced sesamoid fracture may involve repairing the broken fragments using heavy suture (stitching).

Surgery for sesamoid fracture often involves partial or complete removal of fracture fragments of the sesamoid bone (sesamoidectomy).

Complications of surgery: Altered gait patterns or hallux valgus deformity

Recovery

Physical therapy restores strength, flexibility, and range of motion of the foot. Slowly start weight-bearing exercises. Custom orthotics or padding prevent recurrence. Recovery can take from several weeks to several months, depending on the type and severity of the fracture, also on the treatment approach.

BIBLIOGRAPHY

1. Beahrs T, Throckmorton TW. Orthoinfo. (2023). Sesamoiditis and sesamoid fracture. [online] Available from https://orthoinfo.aaos.org/en/diseases--conditions/sesamoiditis [Last accessed November, 2024].
2. Braig ZV, Beahrs T, Throckmorton TW. Orthoinfo. (2022). Stress fractures of the foot and ankle. [online] Available from https://orthoinfo.aaos.org/en/diseases–conditions/stress-fractures-of-the-foot-and-ankle [last accessed November, 2024].
3. Hatch RL, Hacking S. American Family Physician. (2003). Evaluation and Management of Toe Fractures. [online] Available from https://www.aafp.org/pubs/afp/issues/2003/1215/p2413.html [Last accessed November, 2024].

SECTION

Other Specific Fractures and Special Situations

CHAPTER 15.1

Management of Open Fractures

Khalid Muzzafar, Tejpal Singh

Open fractures pose a significant challenge in orthopedic trauma, requiring an urgent and multidisciplinary approach to minimize complications such as infection, nonunion, and limb loss.

Open fractures, characterized by the exposure of the fracture site to the external environment through a breach in the skin and soft tissues, account for approximately 2–5% of all fractures. Tibial fractures are the most common, owing to their subcutaneous location, which makes them more vulnerable to high-energy trauma. These injuries are not only associated with a higher risk of infection but also present a challenge in terms of union and functional outcomes.

CLASSIFICATION OF OPEN FRACTURES

The Gustilo–Anderson classification is the most widely used system, providing a practical framework based on the extent of soft-tissue damage, contamination, and the mechanism of injury.

Gustilo–Anderson Classification

- *Type I:* A clean wound <1 cm in length with minimal soft-tissue damage. These fractures are typically low-energy injuries, such as simple transverse or short oblique fractures.
- *Type II:* A laceration greater than 1 cm without extensive soft-tissue damage, flaps, or avulsions. The fracture is usually moderately comminuted.
- *Type III:* Extensive soft-tissue damage, often with severe contamination. This type is further subdivided into:
    - *Type III-A:* Adequate soft-tissue coverage of the fractured bone despite extensive soft-tissue laceration or high-energy trauma.
    - *Type III-B:* Extensive soft-tissue injury with periosteal stripping and bone exposure, typically requiring soft-tissue coverage procedures.
    - *Type III-C:* Associated with arterial injury requiring repair, regardless of the extent of soft-tissue injury.

Despite its widespread use, the Gustilo-Anderson classification has limitations, particularly regarding interobserver variability and its focus on the initial assessment rather than the ongoing clinical course.

Orthopaedic Trauma Association and AO Classification

The Orthopaedic Trauma Association (OTA) and AO classification systems provide a more detailed and anatomically based approach, incorporating descriptors for the type of bone injury, the degree of contamination, and the presence of segmental bone loss.

INITIAL ASSESSMENT AND STABILIZATION

The management of open fractures begins with a thorough initial assessment following the principles of advanced trauma life support (ATLS). Once the patient is stabilized, attention shifts to the injured limb, with a focus on neurovascular status, wound contamination, and soft-tissue damage.

Immediate, thorough washout:

- *Fluid type:* Normal saline (0.9% NaCl)
- *Quantity:*
  - 3–6 liters for less severe fractures
  - 6–9 liters or more for severe, highly contaminated fractures

WOUND MANAGEMENT AND DEBRIDEMENT

Wound management, particularly thorough debridement, is a cornerstone of open-fracture care. Debridement involves the meticulous removal of all devitalized tissue, foreign material, and contaminants to reduce the bacterial load and prevent infection. The timing of debridement has traditionally followed the "6-hour rule/golden hours", advocating for surgical intervention within 6 hours of injury. However, recent evidence suggests that this timeframe can be extended to 12 hours without significantly increasing infection risk.

Key Steps

The key steps are as follows:

- Administer broad-spectrum antibiotics upon diagnosis of the open fracture, even before debridement.
- Take cultures (though the role of intra-operative cultures is debated in some protocols).
- Irrigate the wound using large volumes of *normal saline* (typically 3–9 liters, depending on the severity) to reduce bacterial load before debridement.
- *Surgical technique:*
  - *Thorough inspection:* Identify the extent of bone, soft-tissue, muscle, and neurovascular injuries.
  - *Removal of devitalized tissue:* All *necrotic, devitalized,* and *contaminated tissue* (including muscle, skin, bone, and foreign material) is excised to reduce infection risk. The "four Cs" are used to assess muscle viability: *Color, consistency, contractility, and capillary bleeding.*
  - *Bone debridement:* Any bone that is *completely devoid of soft-tissue* attachments should be removed as it may act as a nidus for infection.
  - *Preservation of critical structures:* Attempt to preserve nerves, tendons, and vascular structures if they appear viable.
- *The extent of debridement:*
  - *Type I and II fractures:* Minor debridement is needed if contamination is low and tissue viability is good.
  - *Type III fractures:* More aggressive debridement is needed due to the severity of soft-tissue and bone damage, and the higher risk of contamination.
- *Temporary wound closure*: *Delayed primary closure* or *temporary coverage* with a sterile dressing or *vacuum-assisted wound closure* (VAC) is preferred to allow for further inspection and prevent infection. Avoid primary closure if there is extensive contamination or tissue loss.

Relook (Second-look) Surgery

A second-look surgery, often referred to as a *relook procedure,* is performed to reassess the wound after the initial debridement. This is particularly important in severe fractures (e.g., *Gustilo–Anderson type III* fractures) where soft-tissue and bone contamination or necrosis may not be fully apparent during the initial procedure.

Timing of Relook Surgery

- Relook surgery is typically performed *within 24–72 hours* after the initial debridement.
- In some cases, especially when there is significant soft-tissue damage or high contamination, *multiple relook surgeries* may be necessary until the wound is clean and free from necrotic tissue.

Objectives of Relook Surgery

- *Assessment of wound status:* To determine if further debridement is required or if the wound is ready for closure or reconstruction
- *Further debridement:* If any devitalized tissue or infection is observed, additional debridement should be performed.
- *Irrigation:* Additional wound irrigation is carried out to further reduce bacterial load.
- *Wound closure or coverage:* If the wound is clean and there are no signs of infection, the surgeon can proceed with wound closure or *soft-tissue reconstruction* (e.g., skin grafts, local, or free flaps).
    - If the wound remains contaminated or there is a risk of infection, *delayed primary closure* or additional *negative pressure therapy* may be continued, and another relook surgery may be scheduled.

Frequency of Relook

Relook procedures may be repeated every *24–48 hours* until the wound is sufficiently clean and stable for definitive closure or coverage.

Techniques and Strategies in Relook Surgery

- *Negative pressure wound therapy (NPWT):* Also known as *VAC therapy*, NPWT is often used between debridements. It helps remove exudate, reduces bacterial colonization, and promotes granulation tissue formation. VAC can be left in place between relook surgeries.
- *Tissue culture assessment:* In some cases, cultures are taken during each debridement to monitor bacterial load, though this is not universally recommended as cultures can be misleading.
- *Antibiotic beads or spacers:* In cases of high contamination, antibiotic-impregnated beads (e.g., gentamicin or vancomycin beads) can be placed in the wound to provide localized infection control until the next relook or definitive closure.

Definitive Wound Closure or Coverage

Once the wound is free of necrotic tissue and infection risk is minimized, the surgeon can proceed with *definitive wound closure* or coverage.

- *Direct primary closure:* Suitable for small, clean wounds with adequate soft-tissue coverage.
- *Flaps:* In large wounds, particularly *Gustilo-Anderson type IIIB and IIIC fractures*, soft-tissue reconstruction may require *local or free flaps* for coverage. Muscle flaps are often used to cover exposed bones, as they provide good vascularity and help reduce the risk of infection.
- *Skin grafts*: If the wound is granulating well but large, a skin graft may be considered.

Indications for Amputation

In some extreme cases, especially with *Type IIIC fractures* involving vascular injuries, severe contamination, and extensive tissue damage, amputation may be considered if:

- The wound cannot be adequately debrided.
- The limb is nonviable or the functional outcome will be extremely poor.
- There is a high risk of systemic infection (e.g., sepsis).

STABILIZATION OF THE FRACTURE

Stabilization of the fracture is critical not only for the protection of soft tissues but also for pain control and early mobilization.

Choice of Fixation Method

- *Type I and II fractures:* Internal fixation (intramedullary nails preferred over plates/screws)
- *Type IIIA fractures:* Intramedullary nails, temporary external fixation, or internal fixation depending on soft-tissue status
- *Type IIIB fractures:* External fixation initially, internal fixation after soft-tissue recovery.
- *Type IIIC fractures:* External fixation is preferred due to vascular injury management.

Guidelines for Conversion from External to Internal Fixation

The guidelines are as follows:

- *Early conversion (within 7–14 days):*
  - Suitable for *Gustilo-Anderson type I and II* fractures or *type IIIA* fractures with minimal contamination and good soft-tissue coverage.
  - Indicated when there is stable soft-tissue healing without infection
- *Delayed conversion (2–4 weeks or more):*
  - It is required for *type IIIB and IIIC fractures* where soft-tissue injury is more severe and may need reconstructive surgery (e.g., flap coverage).
  - Conversion is delayed until adequate soft-tissue healing is confirmed, and infection risk is eliminated.
  - *Type IIIC fractures,* in particular, may need a much longer delay due to the complexity of vascular injuries.
- *Indications for permanent external fixation:*
  - In some cases, particularly in severely contaminated wounds or where infection risk remains high, *external fixation* may be used for a prolonged period or even definitively, rather than converting to internal fixation. In such a situation, it is preferably better to use a more stable fixator like a hybrid fixator/circular fixator/rail fixator rather than a simple Hoffman fixator only.
  - This might also apply in cases where the soft-tissue envelope remains insufficient for safe internal hardware placement.

A *multidisciplinary approach* involving orthopedic surgeons, plastic surgeons, and wound-care specialists is essential to determine the ideal timing for conversion based on the patient's specific needs and injury severity.

ANTIBIOTIC THERAPY

Prophylactic antibiotic administration is a critical component of open-fracture management. Current guidelines recommend the administration of a first-generation cephalosporin (e.g., cefazolin) as soon as possible after injury. For Gustilo-Anderson type III fractures, additional coverage with an aminoglycoside (e.g., gentamicin) is advised due to the higher risk of infection from gram-negative organisms. The duration of antibiotic therapy is typically 24–72 hours but may be extended in cases of severe contamination or ongoing infection.

COMPLICATIONS AND THEIR MANAGEMENT

Complications in open fractures are common and can include infection, nonunion, malunion, osteomyelitis, and chronic pain.

Infection

Infection is the most feared complication, with rates ranging from 5–50% depending on the severity of the fracture and the adequacy of initial management. Early identification and aggressive management of infection are crucial. This may involve repeat debridement, the use of local antibiotic delivery systems (e.g., antibiotic-laden cement beads), and prolonged systemic antibiotic therapy.

Nonunion and Malunion

Nonunion and malunion can result from inadequate stabilization, infection, or severe soft-tissue injury. The Masquelet technique, involving the use of an induced membrane and staged bone grafting, has shown promise in managing segmental bone defects and atrophic nonunions.

Osteomyelitis

Chronic osteomyelitis remains a significant challenge, often requiring long-term antibiotic therapy and surgical debridement. The use of biofilm-disrupting agents and local antibiotic delivery systems are emerging strategies in the management of this complex complication.

REHABILITATION AND LONG-TERM OUTCOMES

Rehabilitation is integral to the recovery process, with a focus on restoring function, strength, and mobility. Early mobilization, guided by a multidisciplinary team of physiotherapists, occupational therapists, and mental health professionals, is essential. Rehabilitation should be individualized, taking into account the severity of the injury, and the surgical interventions performed.

BIBLIOGRAPHY

1. Court-Brown CM, Caesar B. Epidemiology of adult fractures: A review. Injury. 2006;37(8):691-7.
2. Gustilo RB, Anderson JT. Prevention of infection in the treatment of one thousand and twenty-five open fractures of long bones: Retrospective and prospective analyses. J Bone Joint Surg Am. 1976;58(4):453-8.
3. Gustilo RB, Mendoza RM, Williams DN. Problems in the management of type III (severe) open fractures: A new classification of type III open fractures. J Trauma. 1984;24(8):742-6.
4. Keating JF, Simpson AH, Robinson CM. The management of fractures with bone loss. J Bone Joint Surg Br. 2005;87(2):142-50.

CHAPTER 15.2

Crush Injuries, Mangled Extremity and Amputation in Trauma

Pardeep Singh

CRUSH INJURIES

Crush injuries occur when a body part is subjected to a significant amount of pressure or force, often resulting in severe damage to muscles, bones, blood vessels, and other tissues. These injuries are typically seen in accidents such as falls, industrial accidents, car crashes, or natural disasters like earthquakes.

Types of Crush Injuries

The crush injuries are of the following types:

- *Soft-tissue injuries:* These include damage to muscles, tendons, ligaments, and skin. This can result in contusions, lacerations, and abrasions.
- *Bone injuries:* These include fractures or dislocations due to the intense pressure. Bones may be shattered into multiple pieces.
- *Vascular injuries:* Damage to blood vessels can cause hemorrhage, leading to severe blood loss or compartment syndrome.
- *Nerve injuries:* Compression of nerves can result in loss of sensation, motor function, or both, depending on the severity.

Immediate Effects

- *Pain and swelling:* The affected area often becomes extremely painful and swollen due to the accumulation of fluids and inflammatory response.
- Bruising
- Compartment syndrome

Systemic Effects

- *Crush syndrome (or rhabdomyolysis):* A serious condition that occurs when muscle tissue breaks down and releases myoglobin into the bloodstream, which can lead to kidney damage and failure. Symptoms include muscle pain, weakness, dark urine, and fever.
- *Shock:* Severe blood loss and internal injury can result in hypovolemic shock, characterized by low blood pressure, rapid heartbeat, and organ failure.

Diagnosis

- *Physical examination:* Assessment of the injured area, including checking for pulses, sensation, and movement
- *Imaging:* X-rays, computed tomography (CT) scans, or magnetic resonance imaging (MRI) may be used to evaluate bone fractures, soft-tissue damage, and the extent of internal injuries.
- *Laboratory tests:* Blood tests can assess kidney function, electrolyte imbalance, and the presence of myoglobin.

Treatment

- *Immediate care:* First aid includes removing the source of compression if

possible, applying cold packs to reduce swelling, and immobilizing the injured area.
  - *Surgical intervention:* Necessary in severe cases to relieve compartment syndrome, repair damaged tissues, or perform debridement
  - *Medications:* Pain management with analgesics and anti-inflammatory drugs; antibiotics to prevent infection
  - *Fluid resuscitation:* To manage shock and prevent kidney damage in cases of crush syndrome
  - *Supportive care:* Monitoring and supporting kidney function and addressing any systemic complications

Long-term Management

- *Rehabilitation:* Physical therapy may be required to restore function and strength in the affected area.
- *Psychological support:* Dealing with trauma and long-term disability can require psychological support and counseling.
- *Monitoring for complications:* Ongoing evaluation is required for potential complications such as chronic pain, disability, or psychosocial issues.

Prognosis

The outcomes depend on several factors, including the severity of the injury, the promptness of treatment, and the overall health of the patient. Minor crush injuries may heal with appropriate care, while severe cases may lead to long-term disabilities or complications.

MANGLED EXTREMITY INJURY

Mangled extremity injuries refer to severe trauma affecting the arms or legs, typically resulting from high-energy impacts or accidents. These injuries can involve a combination of fractures, dislocations, soft-tissue damage, and vascular compromise. They pose significant challenges for medical professionals due to their complexity and the potential for serious complications.

Mechanism of Injury

Mangled extremity injuries often result from:

- *Motor vehicle accidents:* Collisions or rollovers can lead to severe limb trauma due to the force of impact and entrapment.
- *Industrial accidents:* Machinery or heavy equipment can cause extensive damage to limbs when safety protocols are not followed.
- *Fall from height:* High-energy impacts can result in severe limb injuries upon landing.
- *Crush Injuries:* These are caused in situations where extremities are compressed or trapped under heavy objects, leading to severe tissue damage.

Types of Injuries

- *Soft-tissue damage:* Includes lacerations, avulsions, and contusions affecting the skin, muscles, tendons, and ligaments
- *Bone injuries:* Often characterized by complex fractures such as comminuted (shattered into multiple pieces), compound (bone protrudes through the skin), or open fractures
- *Vascular injuries:* Damage to blood vessels that can lead to significant bleeding, impaired blood flow, and potential limb ischemia
- *Nerve injuries:* Compression or transection of nerves can result in loss of sensation, motor function, or both.

Trauma Scoring Systems

Several trauma scoring systems are widely used, each with its own focus and methodology. Here are some of the most commonly employed systems:

- Glasgow Coma Scale (GCS)
- Injury Severity Score (ISS)

- Abbreviated Injury Scale (AIS)
- Trauma and Injury Severity Score (TRISS)
- Revised Trauma Score (RTS)
- Mangled extremity severity score (MESS) (will be described in detail later in this chapter)

Purpose of Trauma Scoring

- *Severity assessment:* Trauma scores help in quantifying the extent of injuries and their impact on the patient's overall condition.
- *Triage and resource allocation:* Scoring systems assist in prioritizing patients based on the severity of their injuries, ensuring that those in greatest need receive prompt attention.
- *Predicting outcomes:* Trauma scores can estimate the likelihood of recovery or complications, aiding in decision-making and counseling.
- *Quality improvement:* By analyzing trauma scores and outcomes, healthcare facilities can identify areas for improvement in trauma care and protocols.

Mangled Extremity Severity Score

The MESS is a scoring system used to assess the severity of injuries to a limb and guide treatment decisions, particularly regarding the need for limb amputation or salvage.

Components of Mangled Extremity Severity Score

The MESS evaluates three main components:

1. Mechanism of Injury
2. Limb vitality
3. Age of patient

Each component is scored and the total score helps to determine the likelihood of limb salvage versus amputation.

- *Mechanism of injury*:
    - *High-energy trauma:* 2 points
        - *Examples:* Motor vehicle accidents, falls from height, and crush injuries
    - *Low-energy trauma:* 1 point
        - *Examples:* Simple fractures and minor injuries
    - *Penetrating trauma:* 1 point
        - *Examples:* Gunshot wounds and stab wounds
- *Limb vitality*:
    - *Good perfusion (normal color, temperature, and capillary refill):* 0 point
    - *Questionable perfusion (decreased capillary refill and color changes):* 1 point
    - *Poor perfusion (cold, pale, or absent pulses):* 2 points
- *Age of the patient*:
    - *<30 years:* 0 point
    - *30–50 years:* 1 point
    - *>50 years:* 2 points

Scoring System

- Mechanism of injury (1–2 points)
- Limb vitality (0–2 points)
- Age of the patient (0–2 points)

Total Score and Interpretation

- *0–4 points:* Suggest a higher likelihood of limb salvage.
- *5–6 points:* Indicate a more complex injury; limb salvage is still possible but requires careful consideration.
- *7–8 points:* Suggest a high likelihood of amputation due to severe injury, poor perfusion, and/or advanced age.

Immediate Management

Initial stabilization:

- *Immobilization:* Stabilize the injured limb to prevent further damage and reduce pain.
- *Hemorrhage control:* Apply direct pressure to control bleeding and use tourniquets if necessary.
- *Pain management:* Administer analgesics to manage pain and discomfort.

Surgical Management

Surgical intervention is often required and may include:

- *Debridement:* Removal of necrotic or contaminated tissue to prevent infection and promote healing.
- *Fracture repair:* Mostly, external fixators are used to stabilize fractured bones.
- *Vascular repair:* Surgical reconstruction or bypass of damaged blood vessels is done to restore circulation.
- *Nerve repair:* Surgical intervention to repair or graft damaged nerves is done, if feasible.

Postsurgical Care

- *Wound care:* Regular cleaning, dressing, and monitoring for signs of infection
- *Pain management:* Continued use of analgesics and potentially nerve blocks for chronic pain
- *Rehabilitation:* Physical therapy may be required to regain function, strength, and mobility. This includes exercises to improve joint range of motion and muscle strength.
- *Psychosocial support:* Counselling and support for patients dealing with trauma and potential long-term disability

Complications

Mangled extremity injuries can lead to several complications:

- *Infection:* Risk of wound infection, osteomyelitis (bone infection), or systemic infection
- *Compartment syndrome:* Increased pressure within a muscle compartment that can lead to muscle and nerve damage
- *Amputation:* In severe cases where the limb cannot be salvaged, amputation may be necessary.
- *Chronic pain and disability:* Long-term issues including chronic pain, reduced function, and psychological impact

Prognosis

The outcomes depend on various factors such as the severity of the injury, the promptness of treatment, and the overall health of the patient. While some patients may experience full recovery, others might face long-term challenges including functional impairment and chronic pain.

AMPUTATION IN TRAUMA

Surgical removal of a limb or extremity is a crucial intervention in trauma care that is sometimes encountered due to massive trauma injuries or grievous complications. In traumatic scenarios, amputation may be required to save a patient's life, prevent infection, or preserve overall function.

Indications for Amputation

Amputation in trauma is considered in cases of:

- *Severe tissue damage:* Extensive injuries that involve significant loss of muscle, skin, and bone, making limb salvage impossible or impractical
- Irreparable vascular injury
- *Compartment syndrome:* When severe pressure within a muscle compartment threatens limb function and survival, and fasciotomy (surgical release of pressure) is not sufficient
- *Infection:* Severe, uncontrollable infections, such as necrotizing fasciitis or osteomyelitis, that do not respond to antibiotics and threaten systemic health
- *Crush injuries:* Extreme cases of crush injuries where limb function cannot be restored, and removal is necessary to prevent systemic complications.

Types of Amputation

Amputations can be classified based on the level of amputation and the method used:

Methods of amputation:

- *Open amputation:* The wound is left open to allow for the removal of all infected or necrotic tissues, followed by subsequent closure or skin grafting. An open amputation is sometimes referred to as a guillotine amputation. This technique is often used in emergency or trauma settings where infection control is critical or when the amputation needs to be done quickly. The open wound allows for drainage and monitoring for infection before a more definitive closure can be done in a later surgery.
- *Closed amputation:* The wound is immediately closed after the removal of the limb, typically using sutures or skin flaps.

Preoperative Considerations

Before performing an amputation, several factors are considered:

- *Assessment of viability:* Evaluation of the injured limb's viability through physical examination, imaging studies, and vascular assessments
- *Patient's overall health:* Consideration of the patient's comorbid conditions, such as diabetes or cardiovascular disease, which may affect surgical outcomes
- *Patient and family counselling:* Discussion of the implications of amputation, including potential functional limitations and prosthetic options

Postoperative Care

Effective postoperative care is crucial for recovery and rehabilitation:

- Wound management
- *Pain management:* Use of analgesics and, if necessary, medications for phantom pain or residual limb pain
- *Physical therapy:* Early mobilization and rehabilitation to strengthen muscles, improve mobility, and prepare for prosthetic fitting
- *Prosthetic fitting:* Customization and fitting of a prosthesis to restore function and support mobility; this involves physical therapy to adapt to the prosthetic limb.

Complications

Amputation can be associated with several complications, including:

- *Infection:* Risk of wound infection, which can delay healing and require further treatment
- *Phantom limb pain:* Sensation of pain or discomfort in the amputated limb, which can be managed with medications and therapy
- *Compartment syndrome:* Although rare, it can occur in the residual limb if not managed properly
- *Prosthetic issues:* Challenges related to fitting, comfort, and function of the prosthesis

Psychological Impact

The psychological impact of amputation can be significant, affecting the patient's mental and emotional well-being:

Rehabilitation focuses on maximizing functional recovery and quality of life:

- *Physical therapy:* Continued therapy to enhance strength, flexibility, and mobility
- *Occupational therapy:* Assistance with daily living activities and adaptation to new routines
- *Vocational rehabilitation:* Support for returning to work or finding new employment opportunities
- *Support groups:* Participation in support groups and counseling for emotional and psychological adjustment.

BIBLIOGRAPHY

1. Bhandari M, Swain A. Management of crush injuries: A review of current practices. J Trauma Acute Care Surg. 2018;85(5):943-51.
2. Kumar V, Clark M, Feather A, Randall D, Waterhouse M (Eds). Clinical Medicine. 10th edition. London: Elsevier; 2020.
3. Meyer RA. Trauma and Acute Care Surgery: A Comprehensive Approach. New York: Springer; 2015.
4. Miller AN, Roper J. Long-term outcomes of crush injuries: A systematic review. Injury. 2020;51(4):721-30.

Stress Fractures

Nitin Choudhary, Archi Gupta

Stress fractures of bone, also known as fatigue fractures or march fractures, were originally described by Breithaupt in unconditioned Prussian military recruits in 1855; they typically occur in individuals who perform repetitive tasks and, therefore, result from an overuse mechanism. Stress fractures are not a single entity but rather a spectrum of severity that can impact treatment and prognosis.

PATHOPHYSIOLOGY

Stress fractures are caused by an accumulation of microdamage in the bone caused by repeated tension. There are three phases to bone fatigue failure: Initial crack formation, propagation of cracks, and total fracture. Any load or stress induces some bone deformation or strain, and any bone strain leads to some microdamage. In response to microcrack repair, bone metabolic units (BMUs), also referred to as "cutting cones", activate. A fatigue failure occurs if the healing reaction is unable to halt the propagation of cracks. It is thought that a microcrack can propagate to a size of 1–3 mm, which is significant enough to cause symptoms.

RISK FACTORS

Risk factors consist of but are not restricted to genetics, age, race, sex, hormones, nutrition, and neuromuscular function. Other predisposing factors to consider include incorrect bony alignment, wrong technique/biomechanics, bad running form, insufficient blood flow to certain bones, improper or worn-out footwear, and hard training surfaces.

STRESS FRACTURE VERSUS INSUFFICIENCY FRACTURE

There is a subtle difference between stress fractures and insufficiency fractures. Both stem from an imbalance between the formation and healing of microscopic bone damage. A stress fracture is generally felt to be the result of high loads placed on relatively normal bone, whereas an insufficiency fracture is the result of normal loads placed on bone with impaired healing capacity. Insufficiency fractures are typically seen in elderly females.

DIAGNOSIS

Clinical Presentation

Patients with stress fracture frequently experience pain that is first felt only during activity. Symptoms are usually subtle, and most patients are unable to recall a specific injury or trauma to the affected area. If activity is not reduced or altered, the symptoms either remain the same or get worse. People who train without changing their activities run the risk of developing pain with everyday activities and possibly suffering a complete fracture. Physical examination reveals point tenderness upon direct palpation of the affected bone site.

Radiology

Plain X-rays are usually negative early on in the course of a stress fracture, especially in the first 2–3 weeks. Two-thirds of initial X-rays are negative, but half ultimately prove positive once healing begins to occur making standard radiographs specific but not sensitive.

Bone scintigraphy has been shown to be nearly 100% sensitive for stress injuries of bone but with lower specificity than magnetic resonance imaging (MRI). In the clinical setting, the greatest value of bone scintigraphy is to allow early diagnosis of stress injuries.

Computed tomography (CT) delineates bone well and is useful when the diagnosis of a stress injury is difficult, particularly in the case of tarsal navicular stress fractures as well as those of the vertebral pars interarticularis or linear stress fractures.

Magnetic resonance imaging is the most sensitive and specific imaging study available to evaluate stress injuries of bone. This imaging modality has demonstrated superior sensitivity and specificity over bone scan and CT for associated soft-tissue abnormalities and edema and may delineate injury earlier than bone scan. MRI has been used more frequently recently as the primary diagnostic tool for stress fractures.

CLASSIFICATION

Majority of authors have classified stress fractures into high-risk versus low-risk stress fractures. Another major classification system for stress fractures has been proposed by Kaeding–Miller.

TABLE 1: Kaeding–Miller stress fracture classification.

Grade	Pain	Radiographic findings (CT, MRI, X-ray)
I	–	• Imaging evidence of stress fracture • No fracture line
II	+	• Imaging evidence of stress fracture • No fracture line
III	+	Nondisplaced fracture line
IV	+	Displaced fracture
V	+	Nonunion

High- versus Low-risk Stress Fractures

Low-risk stress fractures include the femoral shaft, medial tibia, ribs, ulnar shaft, and first through fourth metatarsals, all of which have a favorable natural history. These sites tend to be on the compressive side of the bone and respond well to activity modification. A low-risk stress fracture is less likely to reoccur, develop nonunion, or have a significant complication should it progress to complete fracture.

High-risk stress fracture locations include femoral neck (tension-side), patella (tension-side), anterior tibial cortex, medial malleolus, and talar neck. Not only do fractures at these anatomical sites have a predilection to progress to complete fracture, delayed union, or nonunion, but they can also refracture, or have significant long-term consequences if there is a delay in diagnosis **(Table 1)**.

MANAGEMENT OF STRESS FRACTURES

Stress Fractures of Upper Extremity

Upper-extremity stress fractures account for <10% of all stress fractures, and are commonly found in throwing athletes and rowers. The great majority of these stress injuries are considered low-risk and usually require only activity modification to heal. One of the few stress fractures of the upper extremity that may require surgical intervention is the olecranon stress fracture in a competitive thrower. Though this injury has the potential to heal with conservative management, when a stress fracture line (grade 3 injury) is discovered in a throwing athlete's olecranon process, internal fixation is the ideal treatment.

VERTEBRAL, SACRAL, AND PELVIC STRESS FRACTURES

Spondylolysis, or a stress fracture of the pars interarticularis region of the posterior elements of the vertebrae, occurs most commonly in patients performing repetitive hyperextension of the spine (gymnasts, cheerleaders, divers, and weightlifters) and is a common cause of pediatric low back pain. The L4 and L5 levels are most commonly affected. Anteroposterior (AP), lateral, and bilateral oblique views should be obtained. If positive, the classic defect of a "collar" on the neck (pars interarticularis) of the "Scotty dog" is seen on oblique views. The treatment protocol for stress fractures of the pars interarticularis is somewhat controversial. Initially, activity modification and avoidance of lumbar hyperextension are recommended. If symptoms persist, a nonrigid brace such as a corset may be applied. After 2–4 weeks of rest and bracing, patients should begin a regimen of physical therapy, which includes trunk stabilization, core strengthening, and lumbar spine flexibility exercises. Complete healing, however, may take as long as 3–6 months, and a repeat axial-cut CT scan may be considered to assess the amount of healing.

Stress fractures of the pelvis and sacrum are uncommon and typically involve the pubic rami. These injuries occur most often in women, military recruits, long-distance runners, or joggers after increases in duration, frequency, or intensity of impact-loading exercise. These patients usually will have normal hip and spine range of motion but complain of deep groin pain at the extremes of hip motion. X-rays are initially negative in most cases of both pelvic and sacral stress fractures. Bone scan or MRI is usually necessary for early diagnosis. Treatment requires cessation of running and jumping activities, protected weight bearing, and relative rest lasting from 6 weeks to 8 months.

Stress Fractures of Lower Extremity

- *Femoral neck* A femoral neck stress fracture is often delayed for 5–13 weeks. Femoral neck fractures are high-risk injuries. Tension-sided femoral neck stress fractures possess the greatest risk for fracture progression. The diagnosis requires a high degree of suspicion and usually occurs in runners with vague hip or groin pain. Examination will likely reveal an antalgic gait, pain with palpation in the groin, hip, or anterior thigh as well as pain at the extremes of hip range of motion. The radiographic appearance lags behind symptoms and may not be evident until some healing has occurred. X-rays have a high false-negative rate. Bone scan or single-photon emission computed tomography (SPECT) scans have proven useful for early diagnosis, but false negatives have been reported up to 12 days after symptom onset. MRI is becoming more popular and is a sensitive study identifying early marrow edema, which typically resolves in 8–12 weeks. Femoral neck stress fractures require aggressive management with inferior cortex fractures requiring restricted weight bearing for 6 weeks or longer. Serial radiographs should be obtained initially. Tension-sided stress fractures are an indication for surgical fixation with parallel screws or a sliding hip screw device.
- *Femoral shaft stress fractures* are most frequently found at the junction of the proximal and middle thirds of the femoral

shaft, and they are most frequently diagnosed in runners, especially in female runners. Initial discomfort while running eventually develops into discomfort during daily activities and functional limitation. Antalgic gait with normal knee and hip range of motion is confirmed by examination. Plain X-rays are negative in the early stages. 2–6 weeks following the onset of symptoms, a fracture callus and a radiolucent fracture line typically develop. An MRI or bone scan can be required for a prompt diagnosis. Femoral shaft stress fractures are typically successfully treated nonoperatively. Protected weight bearing with crutches for 1–4 weeks is a first-line strategy, depending on the severity of the symptoms and the radiologic grade of the damage.

- *Patellar stress fractures* are rare but troublesome injuries occurring most often in basketball players, soccer players, and high jumpers. Risk factors for a tension-sided (anterior cortex) stress fracture of the patella are flexion contracture and/or harvest of a patellar tendon graft for anterior cruciate ligament (ACL) reconstruction. Radiographic studies may show fracture lines in longitudinal or transverse directions, but these must be differentiated from a bipartite or tripartite patella. A bone or MRI scan identifying bone edema can clarify the diagnosis. Due to the distractive forces of the extensor mechanism, transverse fractures are prone to displacement. Nondisplaced fractures are treated in a hinged knee brace with the knee in full extension for 4–6 weeks, followed by progressive range of motion and quadriceps rehabilitation. Displaced fractures should be treated with open reduction and surgical fixation. Fractures in a longitudinal direction occur most often at the lateral patellar facet, and if displaced, the lateral fragment may be excised.
- *Tibial shaft stress fractures* account for 20–75% of all stress fractures in athletes. To effectively treat stress injuries at this anatomical site, a distinction must be made between medial tibial stress syndrome (shin splints), a compression-sided stress fracture and a tension-sided stress fracture. The most predominant type is a low-risk posteromedial cortex (compression side) stress fracture with the much less common type being the high-risk "dreaded black line" of the anterolateral cortex of the central shaft. Most commonly occurring in running sports such as soccer, track and field, basketball, or ballet, the pain occurs initially after activity. On examination, there is localized pain with point tenderness at the anterior or medial tibia. X-rays may be positive if symptoms have persisted for 4–6 weeks. Bone scan often demonstrates focal fusiform uptake, which differs from the linear uptake seen with medial tibial stress syndrome. MRI is more useful for grading and providing a prognosis for return to play. Treatment should initially involve steps to control pain and limit, if not completely discontinue, running or jumping activities. The use of crutches, immobilization, and limited weight bearing may be necessary depending on symptom severity and fracture classification. Compression-sided injuries may take 2–12 weeks to heal. Tension-sided injuries achieve faster return to play with intramedullary (IM) rod fixation. The options for treatment of injuries in this location include 4–6 months of rest, bone grafting, electrical stimulation, or IM nailing. If a patient or athlete desires to resume training for sports at the same or increased intensity, IM nailing is usually recommended.
- *Medial malleolus stress* fractures are relatively rare and are usually associated with running and jumping sports. They

are inherently unstable and prone to nonunion. A high index of suspicion is the key to their early recognition as patients typically present with the insidious onset of medial ankle pain that is increased with exercise and relieved by rest. Treatment of an incomplete fracture requires non-weight bearing and immobilization with gradual rehabilitation in low-demand individuals. In high-demand athletes and those who wish early return to sports participation, a more aggressive approach may be warranted. Complete fractures require treatment with open reduction and malleolar screw fixation.

Metatarsal Stress Fractures also Known as March Fractures

First through fourth metatarsals stress fractures are generally considered low-risk injuries. Second and third are most commonly involved metatarsals. Stress injuries to these bones are associated with running over 20 miles/week. In runners, most injuries occur in the distal shaft. However, in ballet dancers, fractures may occur proximally and often involve the medial border of the second metatarsal due to weight bearing in the *en pointe* position. Weight-bearing AP, lateral, and oblique radiographs should be obtained. In dancers with second metatarsal pain, internal and external oblique radiographs of the foot may be necessary to fully evaluate the involved bone. Treatment involves rest and the use of a stiff-soled shoe or fracture boot to decrease bending stresses across the midfoot. Once the fracture has healed, orthotic devices should be prescribed if abnormal bony alignment or foot biomechanics are present. In dancers, proximal second metatarsal stress fractures may progress to nonunion and must be aggressively managed with casting or fracture bracing until radiographic healing is present (usually 6–8 weeks).

The proximal fifth metatarsal is considered a high-risk site for stress fracture. Because of the poor blood supply to the affected area, both stress injuries and traumatic injuries are prone to nonunion. Occurring commonly in basketball players and runners, these injuries present with the insidious onset of lateral foot pain that is worse during and after running or jumping activity. Plain X-rays usually show sclerotic change around the fracture site. Bone scans are only occasionally necessary for diagnosis, but bone scan or MRI may be employed if an occult fracture is suspected. Treatment for stress fractures of the proximal fifth metatarsal, as with all high-risk anatomical sites, should be aggressive. In nonathletes, a short-leg non-weight-bearing cast or fracture brace for 6–8 weeks is recommended. Because of the potentially prolonged healing time and risk of refracture or nonunion following conservative treatment, there is now a greater tendency to use surgical fixation as the primary treatment. In high-demand athletes, IM screw fixation with a 4- or 4.5-mm cannulated screw permits faster return to play since casting alone in this population has been shown to have a high failure rate.

In addition to the previous mentions, distal fibula, calcaneum, navicular, and sesamoids of foot (very rare) are also prone to sustain stress fractures.

A general treatment algorithm for stress injuries of bone based on high-risk versus low-risk stress injuries and using Kaeding–Miller classification system **(Flowchart 1)** has been developed.

If appropriate imaging studies are done and a high index of suspicion is maintained, the diagnosis of a stress fracture is typically uncomplicated. The best way to manage stress-related bone damage is prevention. Preparticipation evaluations should include an assessment of the athlete's risk, particularly for those who have a history of stress

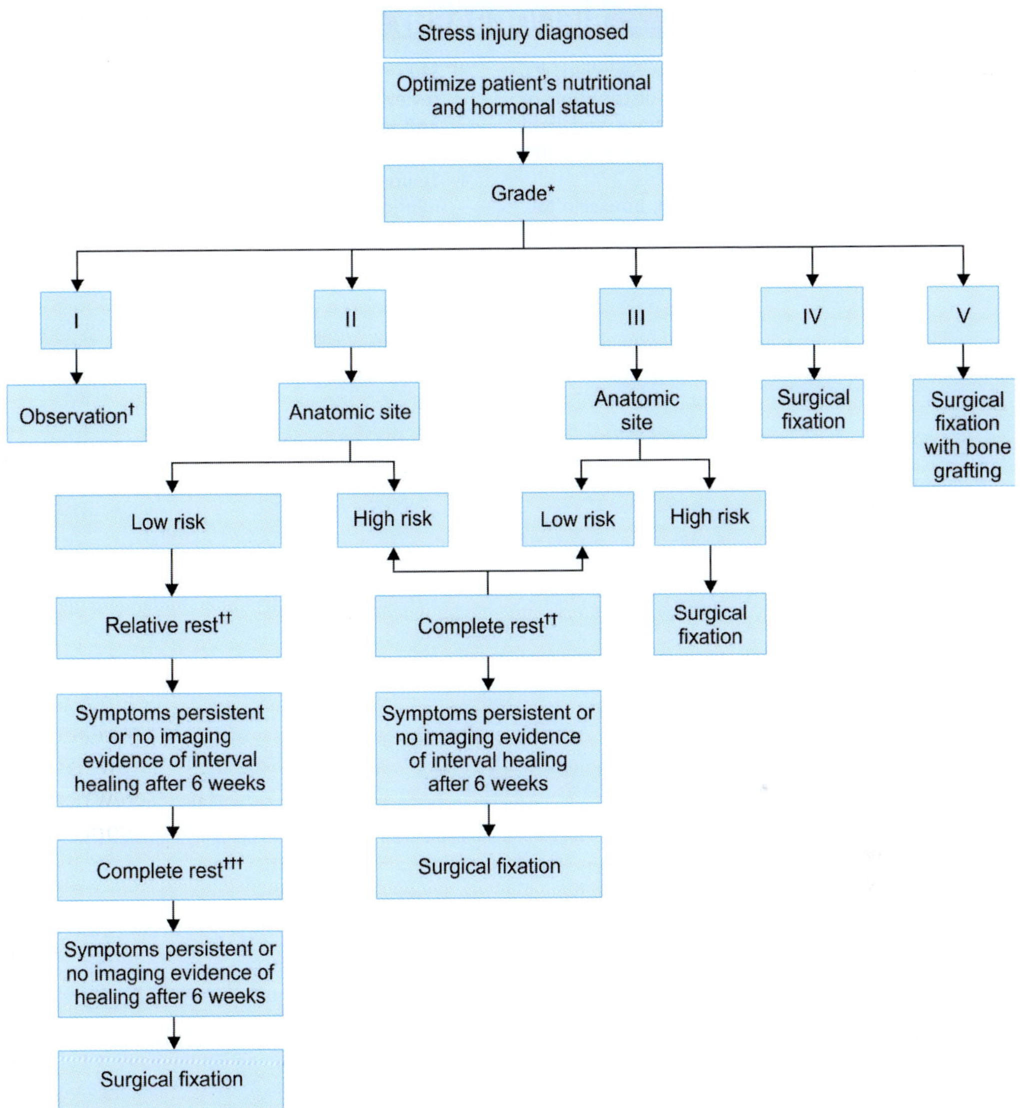

*Grade: Based on the Kaeding–Miller classification system.
†Observation: Return to activity with close-up. Consider relative rest and cross-training.
††Relative rest: Decreased frequency or intensity of inciting activity. May cross-train gradual return to full pain-free.
†††Complete rest: Discontinuation of any activity that place stress at fracture site. May include immobilization.

FLOWCHART 1: Treatment for stress injuries of bone using Kaeding–Miller classification system.

fractures. In addition to basic nutritional optimization, it is advised that females with amenorrhea correct their condition and take supplements of calcium and vitamin D. First corrective action should be taken with the use of adequately designed orthotic devices if biomechanical anomalies are found. To avoid further injuries, gait analysis, proper running form, and technique adjustments could be required.

BIBLIOGRAPHY

1. Bennell KL, Malcolm SA, Thomas SA, Wark JD, Brukner PD. The incidence and distribution of stress fractures in competitive track and field athletes: A twelve-month prospective study. Am J Sports Med. 1996;24(2):211-7.
2. Hoenig T, Ackerman KE, Beck BR, Bouxsein ML, Burr DB, Hollander K. Bone stress injuries. Nat Rev Dis Primers. 2022;8(1):26.
3. Sharma J, Heagerty R. Stress fracture: A review of the pathophysiology, epidemiology, and management options. J Fract Sprains. 2017;1(1):1006.
4. Tenforde AS, Kraus E, Fredericson M. Bone stress injuries in runners: Etiology, classification, and management. Sports Health. 2021;13(4):363-72.

CHAPTER 15.4

Pathological Fractures

Sachin Kudyar

A pathological fracture is defined as a break in a bone that occurs in the context of an underlying disease that has compromised the structural integrity of the bone.

These fractures are associated with a wide range of pathologies, including metastatic bone disease, primary bone tumors, metabolic bone disorders like osteoporosis, and infections such as osteomyelitis. Pathological fractures present significant challenges to orthopedic surgeons due to their complexity, the need for urgent intervention, and the potential for significant morbidity and mortality. Management requires a multifaceted approach that addresses both the fracture itself and the underlying disease.

The primary etiologies include:

- *Malignancies:* These can be primary bone cancers, such as osteosarcoma, Ewing's sarcoma, and chondrosarcoma and multiple myeloma or secondary bone metastases originating from other cancers like breast, prostate, lung, renal, and thyroid cancers. Metastatic bone disease is the most common cause of pathological fractures in adults, with up to 80% occurring in patients with advanced cancers. Malignant lesions can cause both osteolytic (bone destruction) and osteoblastic (bone formation) changes, which significantly compromise the bone's mechanical strength.
- *Metabolic bone diseases:* Conditions such as osteoporosis, osteomalacia, and Paget's disease of bone mainly lead to fractures in the spine, hip, and wrist.
- *Infections* like chronic osteomyelitis.
- *Benign bone lesions:* Benign tumors and tumor-like conditions, such as unicameral bone cysts, aneurysmal bone cysts, fibrous dysplasia, and giant cell tumors, can cause localized bone weakness and predispose to fractures.

DIAGNOSTIC APPROACH

A comprehensive diagnostic approach is essential for accurate diagnosis, appropriate management, and improved outcomes. This involves clinical evaluation, imaging studies, and, where necessary, histopathological confirmation.

Clinical Evaluation

- *History:* Obtain a detailed history, including the onset and duration of symptoms, pain characteristics, functional limitations, any known diagnosis of bone disease, history of malignancy, or metabolic bone disorders. Assess risk factors such as age, prior fractures, steroid use, and family history. Look for systemic signs, such as weight loss, fever, night sweats, or prior radiation therapy, that could suggest malignancy or infection.

- *Physical examination:* Evaluate for signs of an underlying systemic disease, such as skin lesions, palpable masses, or lymphadenopathy.

Imaging Studies

- *Plain radiography (X-rays):* The first step in imaging, radiographs help confirm the presence of a fracture and reveal characteristic signs of underlying pathology, such as lytic or blastic lesions, cortical thinning, and periosteal reactions.
- *Computed tomography (CT) scans:* These provide detailed cross-sectional images, particularly useful in assessing the extent of bone destruction, fracture configuration, and cortical integrity. CT is invaluable for complex anatomical regions like the pelvis or spine. Also, use high-resolution computed tomography (HRCT) chest and ultrasonography (USG) abdomen to rule out metastasis and also to detect any primary pathology.
- *Magnetic resonance imaging (MRI):* MRI is the gold standard for evaluating bone marrow involvement, soft-tissue extension, and neurovascular encasement. It is essential in assessing spinal cord compression or identifying early osteomyelitis.
- *Bone scintigraphy and positron emission tomography (PET) scans:* Bone scintigraphy is useful for detecting areas of increased bone metabolism, such as multiple metastases or multifocal disease. PET-CT scans are highly sensitive and specific for identifying metabolically active tumors and can guide biopsy and treatment planning.
- The probability of fracture for the next 6 months can be predicted by Mirels' score on X-rays, and it also helps in determining if preventive fixation of long bones is necessary.
  Mirels' score is described in **Tables 1 and 2**.

Blood investigation: All routine investigations such as serum protein electrophoresis, free light chains, and bone marrow biopsy (wherever there is a clinical suspicion of multiple myeloma).

Biopsy

When imaging suggests a malignant etiology, a biopsy is necessary to establish a definitive diagnosis:

- *Image-guided core needle biopsy:* Preferred initial method, providing sufficient tissue for histopathological and molecular analysis with minimal invasiveness
- *Open biopsy:* Reserved for cases where needle biopsy is nondiagnostic or when a larger tissue sample is required.

TABLE 2: Assessment of Mirels' scoring.

Total Mirels' score	Risk of fracture	Treatment
>9	Impending	Prophylactic fixation
8	Borderline	Consideration of fixation
<7	Not impending	Nonoperative treatment

Score: >9 = High risk of fracture; <7 = Low risk of fracture.

TABLE 1: Mirels' scoring system.

Score	Site	Pain	Lesion	Site
1	Upper limb	Mild	Blastic	<One-third
2	Lower limb	Moderate	Mixed	One-third to two-third
3	Peritrochanteric	Functional	Lytic	>Two-third

MANAGEMENT

Initial Management and Stabilization

The initial management of a pathological fracture aims to stabilize the fracture, alleviate pain, and prepare the patient for definitive treatment:

- *Pain management:* Effective pain control is essential for patient's comfort and mobilization:
    - *Pharmacological measures:* Opioids for severe pain, nonsteroidal anti-inflammatory drugs (NSAIDs) for inflammation, and adjunctive therapies like gabapentin for neuropathic pain. Pain management must be balanced with the patient's overall condition, considering potential side effects.
    - *Nonpharmacological measures:* Temporary stabilization using splints or casts reduces pain by immobilizing the fracture. Regional anesthesia or nerve blocks may be considered for intractable pain.
- *Fracture stabilization:* Temporary immobilization using splints is necessary in the acute phase, particularly for long bone fractures or in situations where definitive surgery is delayed.

Surgical Intervention

Surgical intervention is often required to stabilize the fracture, alleviate pain, and restore function. The choice of procedure depends on the fracture characteristics, patient factors, and underlying pathology. *Before undergoing final fixation, a biopsy should always be taken*, especially for a single bone lesion and in patients without any previous history of primary or metastatic malignant pathology.

Contraindications

- General health insufficient to withstand anesthesia
- A lower state of consciousness that eliminates the need for pain relief techniques that are localized
- Life expectancy < 1 month

Tumor-related Pathological Fractures

Management of fractures associated with bone tumors must be individualized based on the tumor's type, location, and the patient's overall prognosis:

- *Surgical techniques:*
    - *Wide resection and reconstruction:* For primary bone tumors, wide or radical resection with clear margins is necessary to prevent local recurrence. Reconstruction may involve:
        - *Joint replacement (arthroplasty):* It is indicated when a joint is extensively involved or when the patient has a reasonable life expectancy. Hip and shoulder arthroplasties are common in proximal femoral and humeral lesions.
        - *Endoprosthetic replacement:* Modular or custom prostheses can replace large bone segments (e.g., proximal femur or humerus).
        - *Bone grafts:* Autografts (from the patient) or allografts (from a donor) can be used to fill bone defects.
        - *Cement augmentation:* Polymethyl methacrylate (PMMA) bone cement can provide additional stability, especially in vertebral or pelvic fractures.
- *Surgical stabilization:*
    - *Indications for surgical intervention:* Surgical stabilization is recommended for fractures in weight-bearing bones, unstable fractures, or fractures causing severe pain or neurological deficits (such as in vertebral compression fractures with spinal cord compression).
        - *Internal fixation:* Intramedullary nails are preferred over plates for

long-bone fractures. Techniques should provide durable stabilization to withstand the mechanical forces of daily activities.
  - *Timing of surgery:* Surgery should be performed as soon as possible if the patient is medically stable to reduce morbidity and mortality associated with prolonged immobility and pain.

Adjuvant Therapy

Radiation therapy is typically used postoperatively to control local disease and reduce the risk of recurrence. Systemic therapies, including bisphosphonates (e.g., zoledronic acid) or denosumab, are used to manage bone resorption and reduce skeletal-related events.

Indications for radiation therapy: Localized radiation may be used for:
- Persistent pain after surgical stabilization
- Areas with high disease burden not amenable to surgical intervention
- Solitary plasmacytoma or impending fractures where surgical stabilization is not feasible

Timing and dosage: Radiation is typically administered at a dose of 20–30 Gy in 5–10 fractions, depending on the location and clinical indications. Lower doses may be sufficient for pain relief in palliative settings.

Early initiation of systemic therapy: After fracture stabilization, systemic therapy should be initiated promptly to control myeloma and reduce the risk of additional skeletal-related events.

Multidisciplinary Approach

Effective management of pathological fractures requires a collaborative approach:
- *Orthopedic surgeons:* Responsible for surgical intervention, fracture stabilization, and coordination of immediate postoperative care
- *Oncologists:* Manage the systemic treatment of malignant diseases, coordinate adjuvant therapies like chemotherapy and radiation, and monitor for recurrence or metastasis
- *Radiologists:* Provide diagnostic imaging and interventional support, such as image-guided biopsies or ablations
- *Rehabilitation specialists and physical therapists:* Develop individualized rehabilitation programs to restore function, strength, and mobility, and ensure that patient achieves optimal recovery.
- *Palliative care teams:* Offer symptom management, psychological support, and guidance in cases where curative treatment is not an option, ensuring quality of life for the patient.

The management approach should be individualized, and regular updates from clinical trials and guidelines should be reviewed to ensure adherence to the latest evidence-based practices.

BIBLIOGRAPHY

1. Coleman RE, Lipton A. Metastatic bone disease: Pathogenesis and therapeutic options. Nat Rev Clin Oncol. 2019;16(6):341-52.
2. Ruggieri P, Angelini A, Mavrogenis AF. Surgical treatment of metastatic bone disease. Orthop Surg. 2018;10(2):93-9.
3. Zaikowski RJ, Saraf AJ. Current approaches to the management of osteoporotic fractures. JBMR. 2020;35(4):671-81.
4. Chow E, Hoskin P, Mitera G. Radiation therapy for bone metastases. Clin Oncol. 2015;27(3):137-44.
5. Nguyen L, Bouxsein ML. Systematic approaches to osteoporosis management. Osteoporos Int. 2019;30(10):2131-46.

Periprosthetic Fractures

Simran Preet Singh, Neelam V Ramana Reddy

PERIPROSTHETIC FRACTURES AROUND THE FEMUR

Periprosthetic fractures are common complications seen after primary and revision hip arthroplasty.

These fracture are classified as per Vancouver classification **(Fig. 1)**:

- *A:* Around trochanteric region
  - A_G: Involving greater trochanter
  - A_L: Involving lesser trochanter
- *B:* Around the femoral stem
  - *B1:* Stable implant
  - *B2:* Loose implant with good bone stock
  - *B3:* Loose implant with inadequate bone stock
- *C:* Distal to the femoral stem

Modified Vancouver classification: Divides B2 into further four subtypes:

1. *Burst:* Community fracture around the stem
2. *Clamshell:* Fracture involving the medial neck and calcar region
3. *Reverse clamshell:* Fracture involving the lateral cortex in a reverse-oblique pattern
4. *Spiral:* Fracture with loose bone-cement or cement-stem interface

Treatment

Nonoperative Treatment

Indications include:

- Undisplaced diaphyseal fracture with a stable femoral stem
- Proximal fracture related to osteolysis with adequate distal stem fixation
- Minimally displaced trochanteric fracture

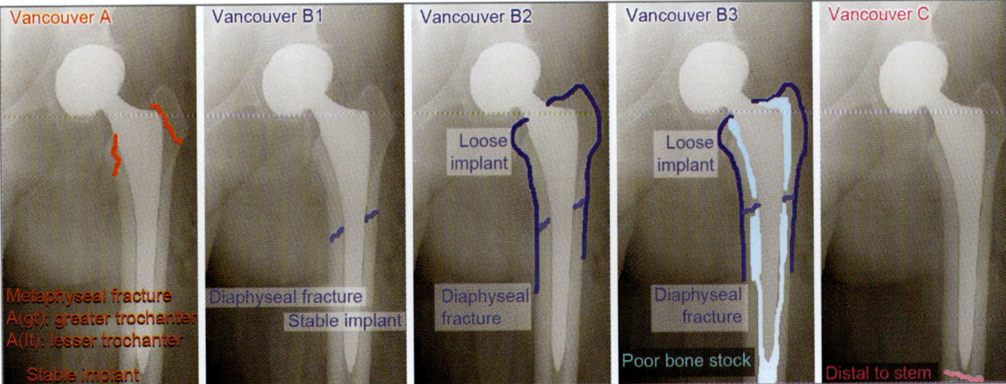

FIG. 1: Vancouver classification.

Operative Treatment

- *Type A:*
  - A_G: Undisplaced (<2 cm)—conservative treatment
    - Displaced—fixation with wires, cables, or claw plate **(Fig. 2)**
  - A_L: Usually conservative, but if posteromedial calcar is involved cerclage is done.
- *Type B:*
  - *B1:* Open reduction and internal fixation (ORIF) with plate and cable construct (Ogden construct) **(Figs. 3A and B)**
  - *B2*: Removal of loose prosthesis with long stem; revision ± plate/cerclage wiring
  - *B3*: Long stem revision + plating or allograft prosthesis composite or proximal femur replacement (mega prosthesis)
- *Type C*: ORIF with distal femoral locking plate (DFLP) **(Figs. 4A and B)**

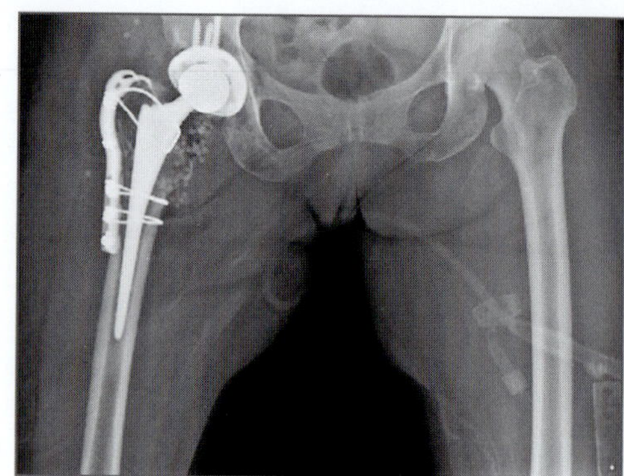

FIG. 2: Vancouver Type A_G fracture is managed by claw plating and cerclage.

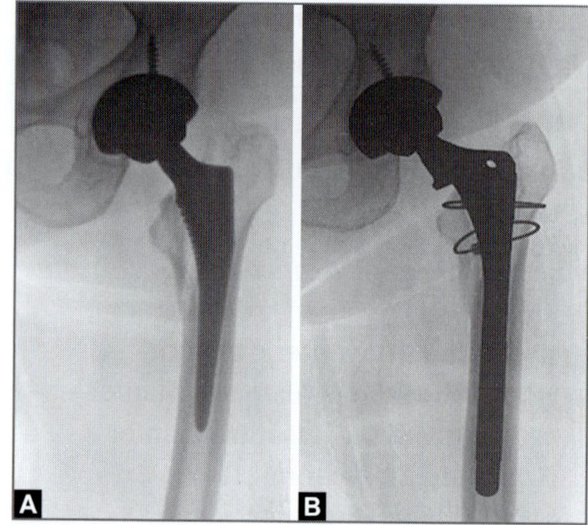

FIGS. 3A AND B: Vancouver type B is managed by long stem revision and cerclage wires.

Tips and Tricks

Some important tips and tricks are as follows:

- Passing cables below the lesser trochanter helps to reduce the opposite pull of abductors.

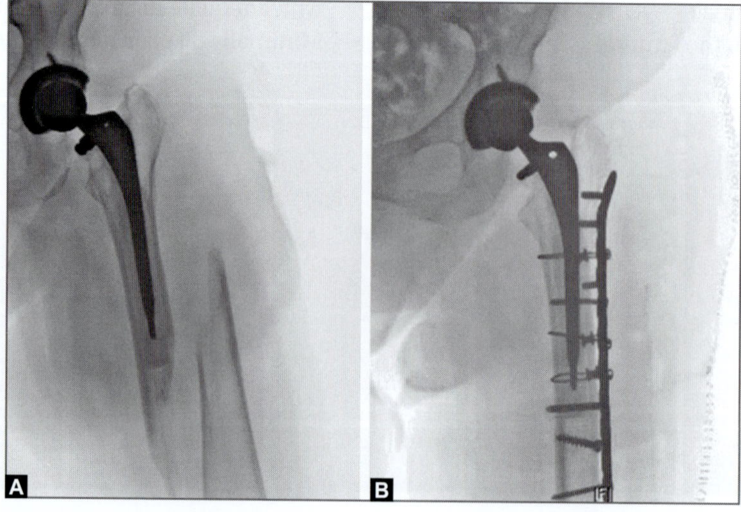

FIGS. 4A AND B: Vancouver type C fracture managed by plating and cerclage wires (Ogden construct).

- If the integrity of the abductor mechanism is compromised, dual mobility and constrained liners should be used.
- *For B1 fractures:*
    - Span the entire length of the femur, if possible.
    - The proximal portion should span the femur by 2.5 cortical diameter.
    - A combination of locking and non-locking screws should be used for distal femoral fixation.
    - Stabilization with bicortical screws has a greater load to failure and stiffness than unicortical screws.
- The minimal invasive plate osteosynthesis (MIPO) technique can reduce morbidity and avoid large incisions.
- Cable and plate systems are insufficient for the treatment of fractures and should be supplemented with intramedullary or screw fixation.
- If allograft strut is used, it must not end at the same level as plate.

Current Trends

- Intramedullary nailing has been advocated for Vancouver Type C fractures in Europe, especially in elderly and low-demand patients for early mobilization.
- Orthogonal plates (one lateral and one anterior) have statistically higher repetitive load to failure and greater torsional and bending stiffness than lateral plates alone.

PERIPROSTHETIC FRACTURES AROUND KNEE

The most common periprosthetic fractures around total knee arthroplasty (TKA) are distal femur fractures.

Classification

Fractures around the femoral component: Lewis and Rorabeck **(Fig. 5)**—

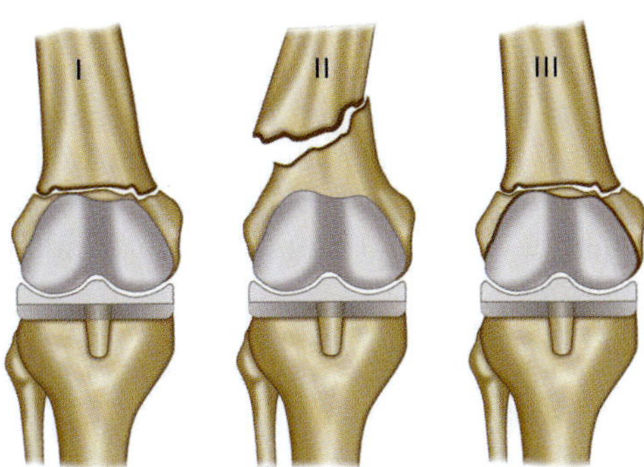

FIG. 5: Lewis and Rorabeck classification.

- *Type I:* Undisplaced fracture with stable prosthesis
- *Type II:* Displaced fracture with stable prosthesis
- *Type III:* Loose component irrespective of fracture configuration

Treatment

Nonoperative Treatment

Historically, treatment included prolonged traction with subsequent bracing.

Indications:

- Nondisplaced fracture in patients with severe comorbidities
- Patient with malignancy undergoing palliative treatment
- Nonambulatory status (paraplegia)

Complications

- Deep vein thrombosis (DVT)
- Pulmonary embolism
- Bed sores
- Malalignment/malunion or nonunion

Operative Treatment

ORIF Using Locking Plates

It can be used in scenario of periprosthetic supracondylar fractures with stable femoral components and interprosthetic fractures, i.e., between a total hip arthroplasty (THA) and a total knee replacement (TKR).

Locked plates allow the screw heads to lock in the plate creating a "fixed-angle" construct. Postoperatively, early range of motion (ROM) is key to rehabilitation. Non-weight bearing for 6–8 weeks followed by protected weight bearing for 3 months is the standard protocol.

- *Surgical tips:*
    - Longer plate constructs show higher union rates. These also tend to decrease refracture and hardware failure.
    - Using multiple locking screws with the largest diameter prevents loss of distal fixation.
    - Use a long plate with at least 8 or more holes in the proximal fracture fragment.
- *Pitfalls:*
    - Malreduction, usually a valgus reduction
    - Varus collapse at the fracture site
    - Nonunion/malunion
    - Loss of distal fixation
- *Outcomes:*
    - Less-invasive stabilization system (LISS) allows an early range of motion and enhanced bone healing.
    - Union rates range from 78 to 100% with locking plate constructs.
    - Increased rates of reoperation are seen after plating.

Retrograde Intramedullary Nail Fixation

It is an excellent choice for supracondylar fracture with stable prosthesis. The benefits involve the use of a previous incision and preserving the periosteal blood supply and biology without opening the fracture site.

- *Surgical issues:*
    - Intramedullary nails (IMNs) need an open-box femoral component construct.
    - The location and size of the box can pose technical challenges often affecting the sagittal alignment of the fracture.
    - A narrow femoral box can lead to a reduction in the nail size to be used, and hence decrease its mechanical strength.
    - Poor entry point can result in malreduction, classically an apex anterior angulation or anterior translation.
- *Pitfalls:*
    - Axial shortening at the fracture site
    - Loss of fracture reduction in the middle of reaming and nail placement
    - Fracture malalignment
    - Knee pain
- *Outcomes:*
    - Increased chances of failure in osteoporotic bone and fracture with short distal fragments are seen with IMN.
    - Union rates are similar as compared to locking plate constructs.
    - Malunion is greater with IMN.

Distal Femur Replacement (also Known as Megaprosthesis)

It is considered in patients with supracondylar fractures or fractures involving femoral prostheses with loose implants or inadequate bone stock. The prosthesis usually provides stable fixation allowing early rehabilitation and faster recovery **(Figs. 6 and 7)**.

The treatment algorithm is given in **Flowchart 1**.

FRACTURES AROUND TIBIAL COMPONENT

Felix Classification (Fig. 8)

- *Type I:* Fracture of the tibial plateau
- *Type II:* Fracture around tibial stem/keel
- *Type III:* Fracture distal to stem
- *Type IV:* Fracture of tibial tuberosity
    - *Subtype A:* Well-fixed tibial stem **(Figs. 9A and B)**.
    - *Subtype B:* Loose tibial stem
    - *Subtype C:* Intraoperative fracture.

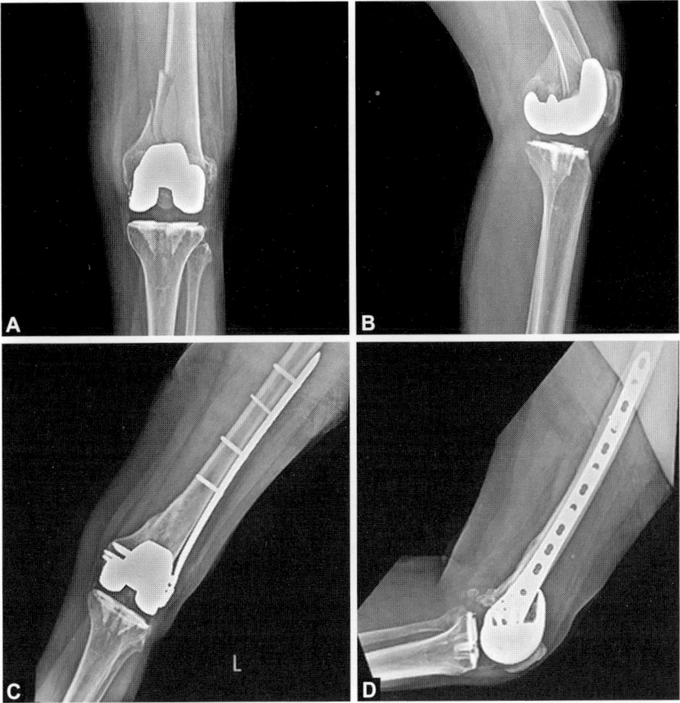

FIGS. 6A TO D: Open reduction and internal fixation using a locking plate for type 2 fractures.

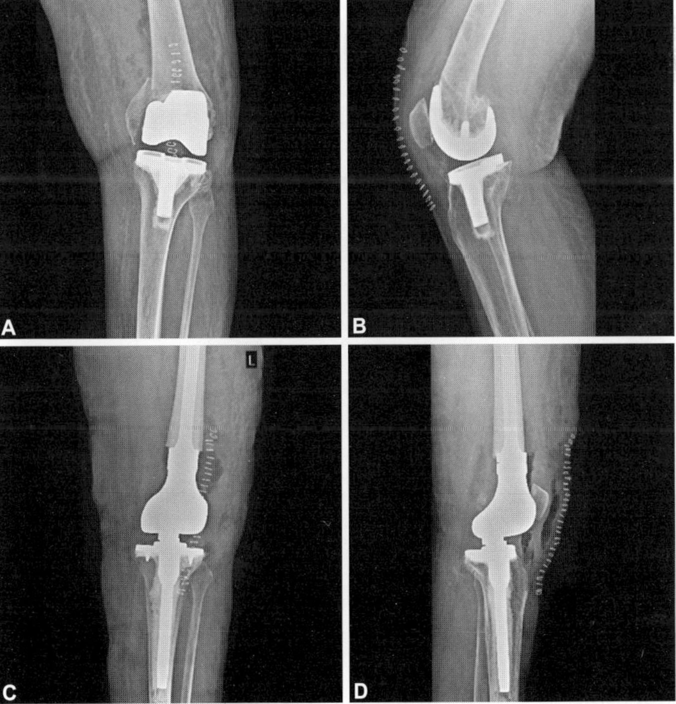

FIGS. 7A TO D: Distal femur replacement for type 3 fractures.

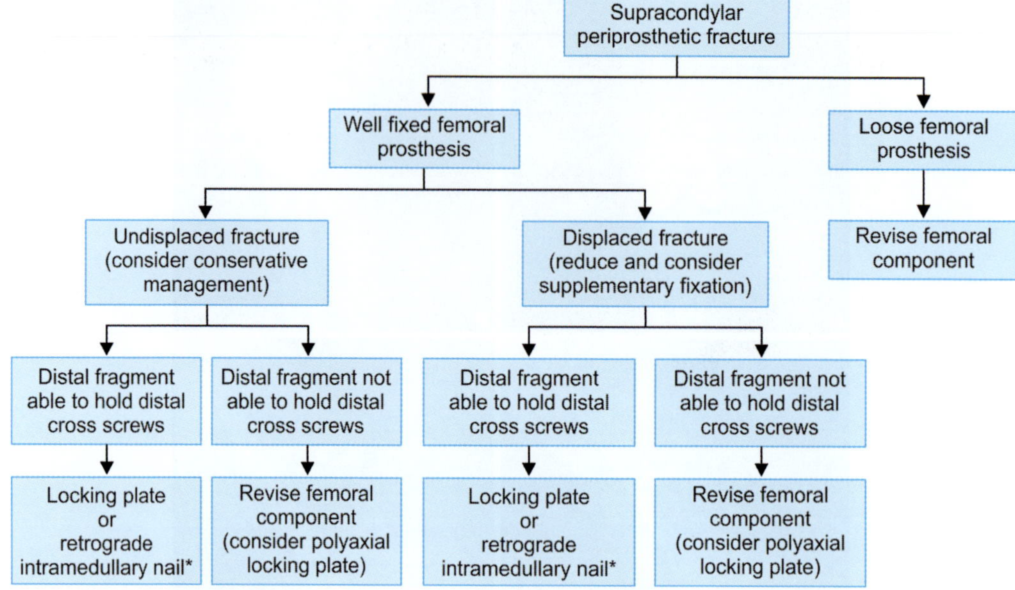

*with compatible femoral implants.

FLOWCHART 1: Management algorithm for periprosthetic fractures in the distal femur.

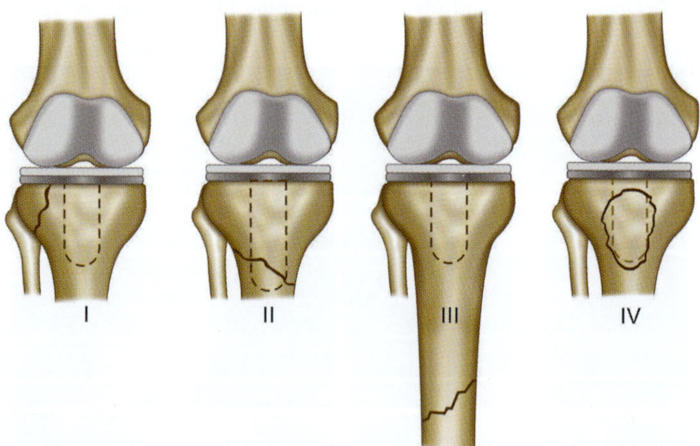

FIG. 8: Felix classification.

Treatment

The algorithm for treatment is given in **Flowchart 2**.

Nonoperative Treatment

Nonoperative treatment is indicated in nondisplaced fractures. A cast or brace is indicated for the treatment.

Operative Treatment

Indicated in displaced tibial fractures with well-fixed or loose prosthesis.

- *ORIF with plating:* Done in displaced fractures involving metaphyseal-diaphyseal junction
- *Nailing:* For type 3 fractures (midshaft tibia) **(Figs. 10A to C)**

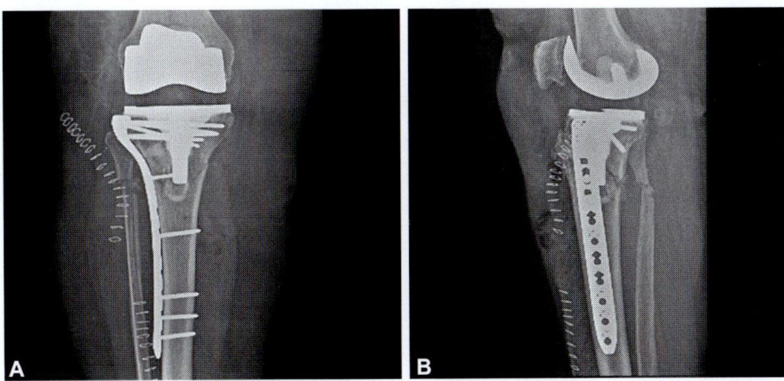

FIGS. 9A AND B: Type 2 fracture managed with open reduction and plating.

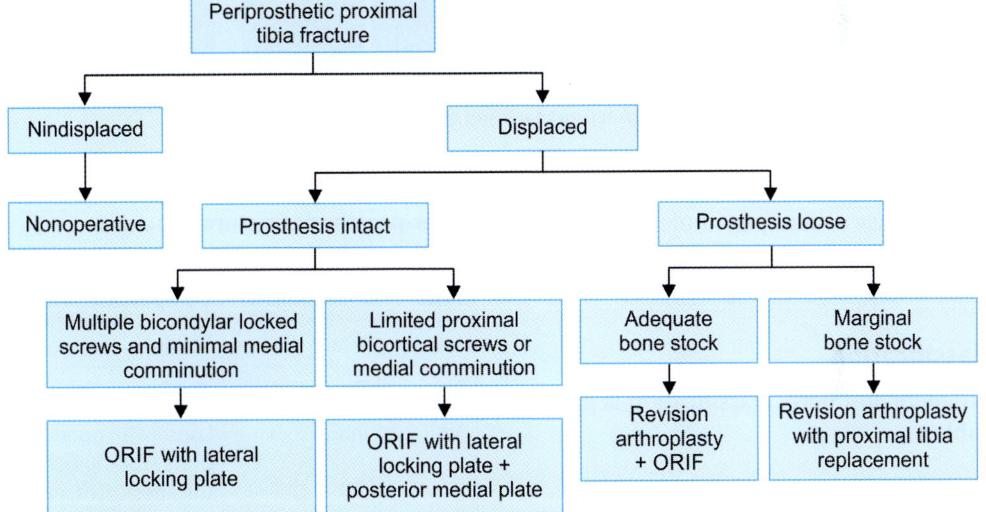

FLOWCHART 2: Periprosthetic proximal tibia fracture treatment.
(ORIF: open reduction and internal fixation)

- *Revision arthroplasty:* Tibial fractures associated with loose components
- *Surgical tips:*
    - The maximal number of locking screws should be placed in the proximal fragment.
    - Proper tissue handling techniques should be used.
    - Maintain skin bridges between incisions.
- *Pitfalls:*
    - Loss of proximal fixation
    - Skin necrosis

FRACTURES AROUND PATELLA

Incidence of per-prosthetic fractures in resurfaced patella range from 0.2 to 21% whereas incidence in unresurfaced patella are approx 0.05%.

Risk Factors

The risk factors involve:

- Avascular necrosis AVN of patella
- Asymmetric patellar resection
- Unsuitable patellar thickness

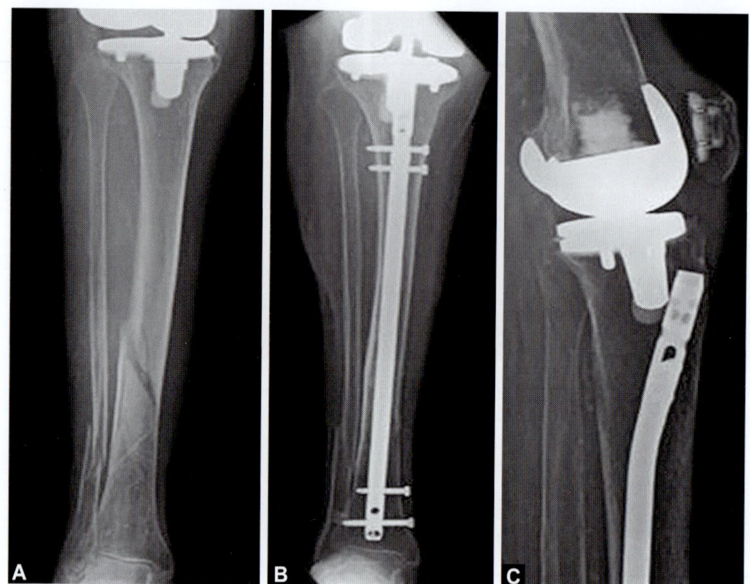

FIGS. 10A TO C: Type 3 fracture managed by interlocking nailing.

- *Prosthesis-related:*
  - Single central peg implant
  - Uncemented patellar button
  - Metal backed implant

Classification

Ortiguera and Berry classification is given in **Table 1**.

Treatment

The algorithm for treatment is given in **Flowchart 3**.

Conservative Treatment

Conservative treatment involves close treatment with immobilization in extension.

Indications:

- Type 1 fractures
- Undisplaced fractures with intact extensor mechanism

Operative Treatment

Indications:

- Loose patellar prosthesis
- Fracture with disruption of extensor mechanism

TABLE 1: Ortiguera and Berry classification of per-prosthetic fracture of patella.

Type	Extensor mechanism	Component
1	Intact	Stable
2	Disrupted	Stable or loose
3a	Intact	Loose with good bone stock (patellar thickness > 10 mm)
3b	Intact	Loose with poor bone stock (patellar thickness < 10 mm)

Techniques:

- ORIF
- Partial patellectomy with tendon repair
- Complete patellectomy
- Extensor mechanism allograft (for chronic extensor tendon disruption)

PERIPROSTHETIC FRACTURES AROUND SHOULDER ARTHROPLASTY

Periprosthetic fractures around shoulder arthroplasty include the fractures occurring around total shoulder arthroplasty and hemi-

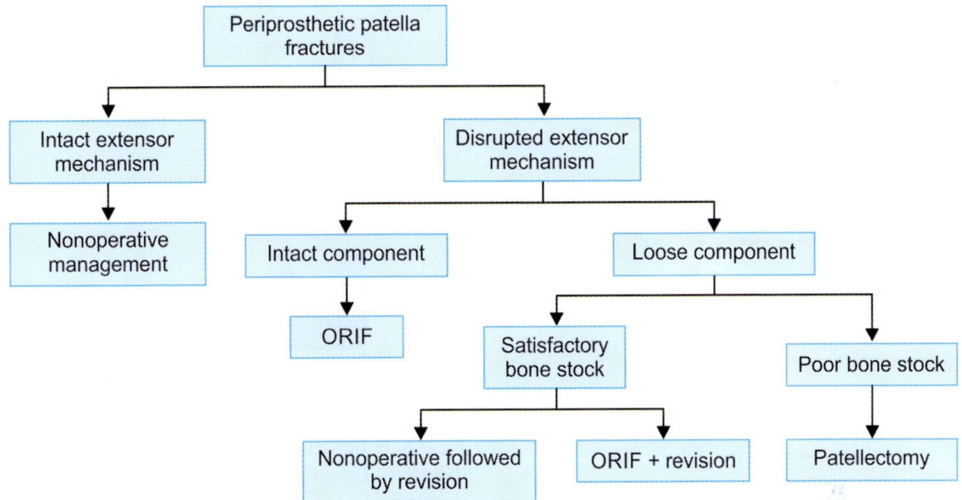

FLOWCHART 3: Periprosthetic patella fractures.
(ORIF: open reduction and internal fixation)

arthroplasty. The overall rate is approximately 0.5–3%.

Intraoperatively: Glenoid fractures > Humeral fractures

Postoperatively: Humeral fractures > Glenoid fractures

Classification

Wright and Cofield classification of periprosthetic humeral fracture **(Fig. 11)**

- *Type A:* Fracture line originating at stem tip and extending proximally
- *Type B:* Fracture line originating at stem tip and having less proximal extension
- *Type C:* Fracture distal to the tip of the prosthesis and extending into the distal humeral metaphysis

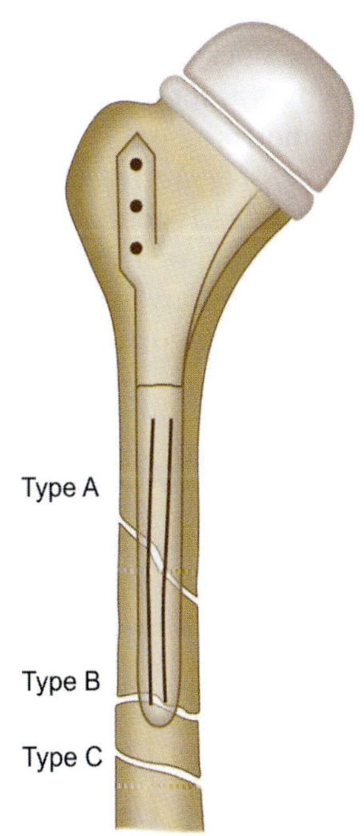

FIG. 11: Wright and Cofield classification of periprosthetic humeral fracture.

Treatment

Conservative/Nonoperative Treatment

Immobilization: Coaptation splint followed by bracing

Indications:

- Oblique or spiral type A or B fractures with a stable prosthesis
- Undisplaced type C fractures

Operative Treatment

- *ORIF:*
    - *Indications:*
        - Type A and B fractures with stable prosthesis

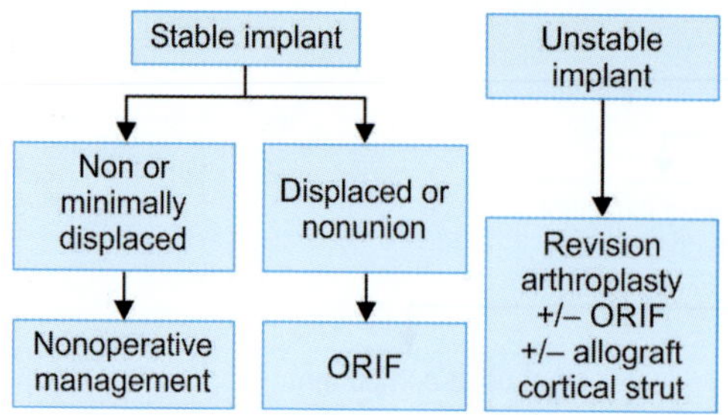

FLOWCHART 4: Treatment algorithm of stable implant and unstable implant.

(ORIF: open reduction and internal fixation)

- Type C with failed nonsurgical management

- *Revision arthroplasty:*
  - *Indications:*
    - Loose prosthesis
    - Inadequate bone stock
  - *Revision using long-stem prosthesis:*
    - Bone stock is poor.
    - Bypass fracture by two cortical diameters
  - *Revision using short-stem prosthesis:*
    - Bone stock is good.
    - Conversion to a shorter stem with supplementary fixation

The treatment algorithm is given in **Flowchart 4**.

PERIPROSTHETIC FRACTURES AROUND ELBOW

Periprosthetic fractures around elbow are the common reasons for revision after elbow arthroplasty.

Classification

O'Driscoll classification ***(Fig. 12)***:

- *Type A:* Periarticular fracture around the humeral or ulnar component
- *Type B:* Diaphyseal about the stem
  - *B1*: Well-fixed implant
  - *B2*: Loose implant with acceptable bone stock
  - *B3*: Loose implant with severe bone loss

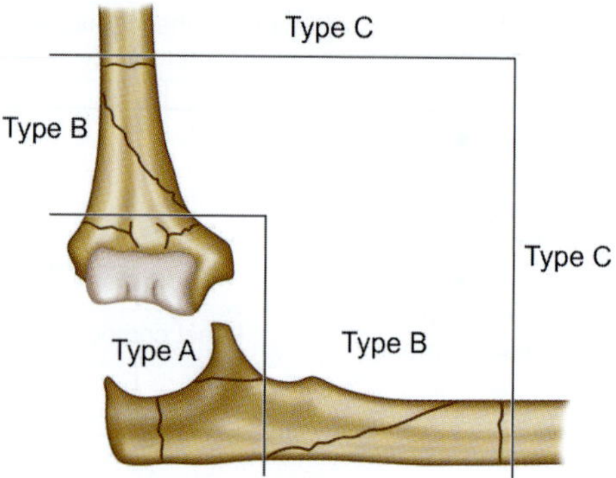

FIG. 12: Periprosthetic fractures of the humerus and ulna are classified according to the region involved. Type A: Periarticular; Type B: Involving Shaft around the stem; Type C: Involving Shaft beyond the tip of the stem.

- *Type C:* Diaphyseal outside the margins of stem

Treatment

Nonsurgical Treatment

Indications:

- Humeral condylar fractures
- Humeral shaft fractures above the prosthesis
- Undisplaced olecranon fractures with intact extensor mechanism

Treatment protocol:

- *Humeral fractures:* These require 2–3 weeks of immobilization followed by functional motion. Restrict activity until there are clinical or radiological signs of healing.
- *Ulnar fractures:* 4–6 weeks of sling or cast immobilization.

Surgical Treatment

- *Revision:* Fracture humerus/ulna with a loose prosthesis
- *ORIF:*
  - Ulnar shaft fracture with secure prosthesis
  - Displaced olecranon fracture with good bone

BIBLIOGRAPHY

1. Cameron B, Iannotti JP. Periprosthetic fractures of the humerus and scapula: Management and prevention. Orthop Clin North Am. 1999;30(2): 305-18.
2. Gliatis J, Megas P, Panagiotopoulos E, Lambiris E. Midterm results of treatment with a retrograde nail for supracondylar periprosthetic fractures of the femur following total knee arthroplasty. J Orthop Trauma. 2005;19(3):164-70.
3. Johnston AT, Tsiridis E, Eyres KS, Toms AD. Periprosthetic fractures in the distal femur following total knee replacement: A review and guide to management. Knee. 2012;19(3):156-62.
4. Khwaja A, Mahoney W, Johnson J, Trompeter A, Lowe J. Biomechanics of periprosthetic femur fractures and early weight bearing. Eur J Orthop Surg Traumatol. 2021;31(5):861-9.
5. Liporace FA, Yoon RS. Periprosthetic Fractures of Hip and Knee: Surgical Techniques and Tips. New York, US: Springer; 2018
6. Mondanelli N, Troiano E, Facchini A, Ghezzi R, Di Meglio M, Nuvoli N, et al. Treatment algorithm of periprosthetic femoral fractures. Geriatr Orthop Surg Rehabil. 2022;13:21514593221097608.

CHAPTER 15.6

Atypical Fractures

Ayaz Ali Mir

Atypical femoral fractures (AFFs) are insufficiency or stress fractures occurring at the subtrochanteric area of the femur's proximal shaft starting from the lateral cortex. AFFs are mostly but not exclusively associated with the long-term use of bisphosphonates or other antiresorptive agents. AFFs are fundamentally different from common osteoporotic fractures with different pathogenesis.

DIAGNOSTIC CRITERIA FOR ATYPICAL FEMORAL FRACTURES

According to the American Society for Bone and Mineral Research (ASBMR) 2010, revised in 2014, a fracture must meet the following conditions to be classified as an AFF.

Location

Fracture must occur in the femoral shaft, extending from just distal to the lesser trochanter to proximal to the supracondylar flare.

Major Criteria

A diagnosis requires at least four out of five of the following:

1. *Minimal or no trauma*: The fracture occurs with minimal trauma, such as a fall from standing height or less, or no identifiable trauma.
2. *Fracture line characteristics:*
   - The fracture originates in the lateral cortex and is transverse in orientation.
   - If incomplete, it involves only the lateral cortex.
3. *Short medial spike*: The fracture may exhibit a short medial spike when complete.
4. *Minimal/No comminution*: The fracture shows little to no fragmentation.
5. *Localized periosteal or endosteal thickening*: Localized cortical thickening (periosteal or endosteal) is present at the lateral cortex, often referred to as a "beaking" or "flaring" appearance.

Minor Criteria

The following features may also be observed but are not required for diagnosis:

1. *Generalized diaphyseal thickening*: Diffuse thickening of the femoral diaphysis may be present.
2. *Prodromal symptoms*: Patients may report prodromal pain in the affected limb before the fracture occurs.
3. *Bilateral fractures*: Similar fractures or cortical abnormalities may occur in the contralateral femur.
4. *Delayed healing*: These fractures often demonstrate prolonged healing times.

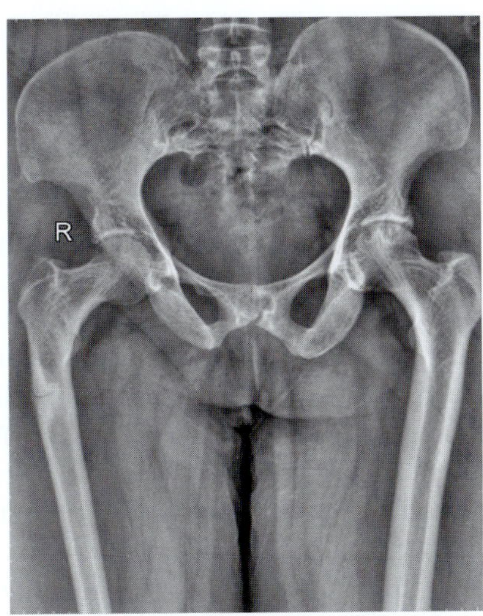

FIG. 1: Atypical femoral fracture, incomplete involving lateral cortex with typical endosteal and periosteal thickening in a 50-year-old female with groin pain receiving zoledronic acid for the last 5 years.

Exclusion Criteria

Comminuted/spiral fracture, femoral neck/intertrochanteric fracture, periprosthetic fractures, and evidence of other diseases like primary or metastatic bone tumor, Paget's disease, and fibrous dysplasia **(Fig. 1)**

PREVALENCE

The incidence of AFF after bisphosphonate use among women >50 years of age ranges from 0.07/10,000 per year in patients taking bisphosphonates for >3 months to 13.1/10,000 per year in patients on bisphosphonate for >8 years. With an average of about 4.5/10,000 on current bisphosphonate users.

PATHOGENESIS AND RISK FACTORS

Bisphosphonate-induced atypical femoral fractures are proposed to be due to accumulated microdamage, altered angiogenesis, and suppressed bone remodeling and repair mechanisms leading to increased bone mineralization, resulting in increased cortical thickness and brittleness of bone.

Differences in femoral curvature and neck-shaft angle in Asian women can explain why stress fracture is eight times more common in Asian women.

Ibandronate (a bisphosphonate) and denosumab (a monoclonal antibody) are commonly used in the management of bone metastases in breast cancer to reduce skeletal-related events (SREs) such as fractures, spinal cord compression, and bone pain, can also be the causative agents for atypical fracture.

In summary, any pharmacological agent causing decreased bone turnover can cause AFF.

Systemic bone diseases that affect bone turnover in similar ways as non-Hodgkin's lymphoma, hypophosphatemia, and osteopetrosis also cause fractures like bisphosphonate-induced AFF.

Long-term use of glucocorticoids and protein pump inhibitors also increases general fracture risk with probably no specific predilection for the specific site of AFF. Bisphosphonates are frequently used with these medications thus increasing fracture risk.

Genetic mutations: The search for the answer to the question of why only a few people on bisphosphonates are developing AFF led to finding of genetic mutations like COL1A2 (coding for collagen), GGPS1, and PLS3.

DIFFERENTIAL DIAGNOSIS

Differential diagnosis includes pathological fractures, hypophosphatasia (HPP), osteogenesis imperfecta, and stress fractures.

TREATMENT

Screening: A high degree of suspicion may help identify incomplete fractures, hence, reducing morbidity. About 40% of patients having AFF have incomplete fractures on the opposite side amenable to conservative management. Careful evaluation of unexplained groin pain and a transverse black line in the subtrochanteric region of the femur in patients receiving bisphosphonates, even for a brief period, is necessary.

Conservative Management

As recommended by ASBMR, conservative management is indicated in:

- Incomplete fracture with no groin pain
- Periosteal thickening without cortical lucency

Patients are treated with limited weight-bearing, avoiding strenuous exercises, and stopping any antiresorptive medication and vitamin D supplementation, till there is no increased activity on bone scan or edema in MRI.

Patients with a radiolucent line of >50% of the lateral cortex at the trochanteric region with functional pain have a 28% risk of progressing to complete fracture and will benefit from prophylactic fixation.

Surgical Treatment

These patients have impaired bone remodeling potential, hence fracture healing is delayed. The gold standard treatment of AFF is cephalomedullary nailing. AFF treated with plate fixation has a higher rate of reoperation compared to fractures treated with nailing. Compared to general fractures, AFF treatment is complex and demanding. There is little scope for error. Fracture reduction should be anatomically perfect with no gap and with no varus/valgus malreduction. Risk factors for delayed union include high body mass index (BMI), subtrochanteric location, postoperative gap at fracture, particularly at the anterior or lateral cortex, and failure to restore normal neck-shaft angle.

BIBLIOGRAPHY

1. Black DM, Cummings SR, Karpf DB, Cauley JA, Thompson DE, Nevitt MC, et al. A randomised trial of the effect of alendronate on risk of fracture in women with existing vertebral fractures. Fracture Intervention Trial Research Group. Lancet. 1996;348(9041):1535-41.
2. Black DM, Rosen CJ. Postmenopausal osteoporosis. N Engl J Med. 2016;374(21):2096-7.
3. Eastell R, Rosen CJ, Black DM, Cheung AM, Murad MH, Shoback D. Pharmacological management of osteoporosis in postmenopausal women: An Endocrine Society clinical practice guideline. J Clin Endocrinol Metab. 2019;104(5):1595-622.
4. Jha S, Wang Z, Laucis N, Bhattacharyya T. Trends in media reports, oral bisphosphonate prescriptions, and hip fractures 1996-2012: An ecological analysis. J Bone Miner Res. 2015;30(12):2179-87.
5. Shane E, Burr D, Abrahamsen B, Adler RA, Brown TD, Cheung AM, et al. Atypical subtrochanteric and Diaphyseal femoral fractures: second report of a task force of the American Society for Bone and Mineral Research. J Bone Miner Res. 2014;29(1):1-23.

Gunshot and Blast Injuries

Younis Kamal

Due to the complex nature of gunshot and blast injuries—characterized by high-energy impact, severe soft-tissue disruption, and risk of contamination—managing such cases presents unique challenges.

MECHANISMS OF INJURY AND INITIAL MANAGEMENT

Gunshot injuries may be classified based on the projectile's velocity, with high-velocity wounds typically resulting in extensive tissue damage and bone comminution. Blast injuries, conversely, often combine direct impact with secondary and tertiary effects, including shrapnel wounds, burns, and crush injuries. Initial management involves stabilizing the patient, controlling bleeding, and assessing the extent of musculoskeletal damage [follow advanced trauma life support (ATLS) protocol].

TREATMENT STRATEGY

Wound Debridement

Effective debridement is fundamental in managing these injuries. High-energy gunshot wounds and blast injuries are generally managed as Grade III open fractures, which necessitate aggressive surgical debridement to minimize infection risk. The primary goal is to remove all devitalized tissue, foreign materials, and bone fragments to reduce the bacterial load. Irrigation with a significant volume of saline—often with pressure-assisted delivery—is recommended to thoroughly cleanse the wound.

In cases with severe contamination or delayed presentation, debridement may need to be staged over multiple surgeries, with meticulous inspection and removal of nonviable tissue at each stage. For shotgun injuries that scatter metallic pellets, selective removal of retained pellets is generally pursued only when they are intra-articular, as aggressive removal can exacerbate soft-tissue damage.

Fracture Stabilization

External fixation: This is frequently the initial treatment of choice, especially for highly comminuted fractures or those with extensive soft-tissue damage. External fixators allow for wound access and facilitate ongoing debridement without compromising fracture alignment. They also stabilize the fracture and mitigate the risk of additional soft-tissue injury. In cases where the soft-tissue envelope improves, definitive fixation with internal methods can be considered.

Internal fixation and definitive reconstruction: Once the risk of infection is controlled and soft-tissue conditions permit, transitioning to internal fixation may be appropriate. For this purpose, intramedullary nailing and locking plates are common methods. Bone grafting, utilizing either autografts or allografts, may be necessary for managing segmental defects or extensive bone loss.

Antibiotic Administration

The administration of prophylactic antibiotics is a standard protocol in the treatment of gunshot and blast wounds involving bone. Broad-spectrum antibiotics, particularly those effective against both gram-positive and gram-negative bacteria, are initiated early. For severe injuries or those with extensive contamination, a combination therapy with aminoglycosides and beta-lactams is often recommended. The duration is usually limited to avoid antibiotic resistance but must be sufficient to address the risk of deep-seated infection.

Soft-tissue Management and Reconstruction

Soft-tissue injuries from gunshots and blasts often require complex reconstruction. Flap coverage, utilizing local or free flaps, is commonly indicated for extensive skin and muscle defects to facilitate wound healing and protect underlying structures. Negative pressure wound therapy (NPWT) is widely utilized to manage large wounds before definitive closure or grafting, as it promotes granulation tissue formation and reduces edema.

Management of Associated Neurovascular Injuries

Gunshot and blast injuries frequently involve nerve and vascular damage, particularly in the extremities. For vascular injuries, immediate repair through direct anastomosis or grafting is critical to restore perfusion and prevent ischemic complications. If primary repair is unfeasible, temporary vascular shunting may be utilized.

Nerve repair: When nerve injuries are identified, primary neurorrhaphy (direct nerve repair) is attempted whenever feasible. Nerve grafting is considered for gaps where direct repair is not possible. The timing of nerve repair is essential; delayed repair may be appropriate if extensive contamination or swelling prevents immediate intervention.

BIBLIOGRAPHY

1. Weatherford B. Gun Shot Wounds - Trauma. Orthobullets. 2024.
2. Gill R, Morris JD, Moore HJ. Gunshot and Blast Injuries of the Extremities: A Review of 45 Cases. Journal of Orthopaedic Surgery and Research. 2024.
3. Mafi J, Hashemi M, Rajabi R. Management of Extremity Injuries Caused by Gunshot Wounds: An Evolving Perspective. Journal of Orthopaedic Trauma. 2023.
4. Zielinski M, Kwiatkowski JM, Król WS. Orthopaedic Trauma and Reconstruction of Ballistic Injuries. Musculoskeletal Key. 2024.

CHAPTER 15.8

Managing Fractures in Pregnant Women

Archi Gupta, Nitin Choudhary

Trauma during pregnancy, while relatively uncommon, presents significant challenges that stem from the unique anatomical and physiological changes occurring in the maternal body, as well as the presence of the fetus within the gravid uterus. Understanding the incidence, causes, impact, and management of trauma in pregnancy is critical for healthcare providers to ensure the safety and well-being of both mother and child.

Research indicates that the severity of the injury, rather than pregnancy itself, is the primary determinant of mortality risk. As pregnancy progresses, the risk of trauma to both the fetus and mother increases, with about 15% of injuries occurring during the first trimester and up to 55% occurring during the third trimester.

RISK FACTORS FOR TRAUMA

Several risk factors have been identified that increase the likelihood of trauma in pregnant women:

- *Young age:* Younger pregnant women may be more prone to risky behaviors or hazardous situations that can lead to trauma.
- History of domestic violence
- *Substance abuse:* Drug abuse can impair judgment and increase susceptibility to accidents.

ASSESSMENT OF INJURED PREGNANT PATIENTS

General Assessment

- *Routine assessment:*
  - Follow the standard advanced trauma life support (ATLS) protocols.
  - The primary focus should be on providing optimal resuscitation to the mother while monitoring the fetus, especially if viable.
- *Multidisciplinary approach:*
  - Involve a team including an obstetrician, neonatologist, radiologist, and trauma surgeon for comprehensive care.
- *Categorization of pregnant trauma patients:*
  - *Unknown pregnancy:* All trauma patients of childbearing age should be tested for pregnancy. This is crucial as early pregnancy is highly sensitive to radiographic studies, though necessary life-saving procedures should not be delayed.
  - *Less than 26 weeks' gestation:* Focus on maternal resuscitation since the fetus is not yet viable outside the womb.
  - *More than 26 weeks' gestation:* Both maternal and fetal well-being need to be considered, presenting a more complex situation.

- *Perimortem stage:* If the mother is in a critical condition, an early cesarean section may be necessary to improve maternal resuscitation chances and potentially save the fetus.
- *Positioning and support:*
  - Avoid placing the patient supine after 20 weeks' gestation to prevent supine hypotension syndrome, caused by uterine compression of the vena cava. Instead, tilt the patient to the left side or position the patient at a 15° tilt to alleviate this issue.
  - Provide supplemental oxygen due to decreased maternal respiratory reserve.
  - The mother can tolerate blood loss up to 2,000 mL, but this can affect uterine blood flow. Avoid using vasopressors unless absolutely necessary, as they can further compromise uterine perfusion.
- *Secondary survey:*
  - Obtain a thorough medical and obstetric history, including information on pre-existing conditions like hypertension, eclampsia, and diabetes, as well as details of injury mechanism, and substance use history.
  - Conduct a full physical examination of all limbs and body systems.
  - Perform radiological examinations of suspected fractures, ensuring minimal radiation exposure.
- *Ultrasound and focused assessment with sonography for trauma (FAST) scan:*
  - Use a FAST scan to detect intra-abdominal hemorrhage.
  - Follow-up with an ultrasound of the fetus and placenta, either after the FAST scan or integrated into the trauma evaluation.
- *Additional considerations:* Administer tetanus prophylaxis as per standard guidelines (if not administered during pregnancy).

Radiological Assessment

General Considerations

- Radiographic and computed tomography (CT) scans pose risks to the developing fetus, which vary depending on the gestational age.
- Adhere to as low as reasonably achievable (ALARA) principle to minimize radiation exposure while ensuring diagnostic efficacy.

Imaging Strategies

- *Radiographs:* These are safe for extremities at any stage of pregnancy, provided adequate shielding is used to reduce fetal exposure by up to 30%.
- *Magnetic resonance imaging (MRI):* It is preferable for stable patients with suspected ligamentous injuries. MRI is less suitable for unstable patients due to time constraints and the potential teratogenic effects of gadolinium-based contrast agents.
- *Ultrasound:* It is a preferred first-line modality for abdominal trauma to detect free fluid and evaluate the fetus and placenta, ideally with obstetrician involvement.
- *CT scans:* These are essential for unstable patients or when detailed imaging of the chest, abdomen, or pelvis is required. Use low-dose protocols, and if iodine contrast is necessary, follow up with the child with thyroid and renal function post-delivery. Modern CT scanners with iterative reconstruction techniques significantly reduce radiation dose.

Imaging Protocols

Use CT scanners with the highest number of detector rows and apply iterative reconstruction methods to minimize radiation. Ensure that dose settings and imaging techniques are optimized for the pregnant patient.

An imaging strategy for pregnant trauma patients should be pre-established, considering initial assessment, follow-up imaging, and the need for specialized care.

MANAGEMENT

Managing trauma in pregnancy is complex due to the dual concern for both the mother and the fetus.

Surgical Interventions

Elective procedures should generally be deferred until after childbirth to ensure the safety of both the mother and the fetus. However, this does not apply to emergency surgical interventions, which should proceed as necessary. Fracture management, based on the severity of bone and soft-tissue injuries, often requires immediate surgical attention and cannot always be postponed. Most surgical procedures can be performed safely on pregnant patients, but specific considerations related to anesthesia, intra-operative imaging, and orthopedic techniques must be addressed to ensure optimal outcomes.

Anesthesia

Anesthesia is generally safe during pregnancy and is not associated with an increased risk of stillbirths, birth defects, or neural tube defects. However, managing the airway in pregnant patients can be challenging. The likelihood of difficult intubation increases significantly in later stages of pregnancy. Pregnant women are also at a higher risk of aspiration and hypoxia due to decreased functional respiratory reserve and increased oxygen demands. Effective ventilation aims to maintain appropriate levels of oxygen (PaO_2) and carbon dioxide ($PaCO_2$) for the stage of gestation. Frequent blood gas measurements can be crucial in these situations.

Monitoring uterine and fetal well-being is important, as signs of fetal distress may indicate maternal hypovolemia. Evaluating maternal volume status can be complex, as central venous and left ventricular filling pressures may not always correlate well. For precise hemodynamic monitoring, some experts recommend the use of a Swan-Ganz catheter.

Intraoperative Imaging

Key practices include precise positioning of the primary beam, effective use of the leaf shutter, and minimizing radiation exposure to the uterus with proper lead shielding. Lead shielding helps reduce scattered radiation from both the unit and external sources, but scatter from irradiated tissues cannot be mitigated. Minimizing irradiation time and extensively using the "last image hold" feature are essential.

Guidelines for intraoperative radiography also apply to fluoroscopy. Dose levels to the fetus can vary significantly depending on the equipment. Based on latest scientific evidence if the gravid uterus is directly exposed to the X-ray beam, a dose of 100 mSv could be reached in approximately 3 minutes with a 28 cm field of view (FOV), but only 1.5 minutes with a 20 cm FOV.

Orthopedic Surgical Management

The research on orthopedic injuries in pregnant patients is limited. Generally, fractures in pregnant patients are managed similarly to those in non-pregnant individuals. Due to the typically young age of pregnant patients, inadequate treatment of fractures can lead to significant long-term effects.

When managing fractures, it is crucial to avoid direct radiation to the uterus and use proper shielding. While intraoperative imaging is generally safe with adequate precautions, it becomes more complex with pelvic and proximal femoral fractures. Minimally invasive techniques, which rely heavily on intraoperative imaging, are not recommended. Instead, open techniques that reduce the need for imaging are preferred.

Pregnancy increases the risk of thromboembolism, which starts in the first trimester and often affects the left lower limb. The limited data on venous thromboembolism (VTE) in pregnant women suggests that recommendations are based largely on studies from non-pregnant populations. Risk factors specific to pregnant trauma patients include immobility, blood loss, transfusion, and surgical procedures. Low-molecular-weight heparins are considered safe, and anticoagulation decisions should be tailored to individual risk factors. Prompt surgical intervention to restore mobility is often beneficial despite the inherent risks.

Positioning the patient on their left side can alleviate pressure on the vena cava and prevent supine hypotension syndrome. If left lateral positioning is not feasible, manual displacement of the uterus should be attempted. Blood loss should be closely monitored and communicated with the anesthetist, as normal hemodynamic parameters might mask reduced uterine blood flow. Pelvic and acetabular fractures present particular challenges in pregnant patients. The literature mostly consists of case reports, with a trend toward conservative management. A review from a major trauma center found only seven pregnant patients with pelvic fractures, resulting in five maternal and three fetal survivors. Severe trauma cases require specialized care, as the mortality rate for mothers and fetuses can be significant. Surgical interventions carry risks of maternal blood loss and potential injury to the uterus or fetus, making cesarean sections a potentially life-saving option. Additionally, the gravid uterus in the third trimester may complicate the placement of external fixators.

Decisions regarding operative intervention must consider factors such as fetal gestational age and viability, the degree of maternal and fetal compromise, radiation exposure, and the need for fracture fixation. Each case requires a tailored approach to balance the risks and benefits effectively.

OUTCOMES

During pregnancy, trauma puts the mother and the fetus at serious risk. Unfortunately, because of the particular nature of these injuries and the difficulties in gathering data, there is little information available on the precise prognosis for patients who are pregnant. Even small injuries can result in premature labor or fetal loss; nevertheless, the majority of information currently accessible relates to severe trauma. Fetal loss may occur in 4–61% of pregnant trauma victims, according to estimates. On the other hand, there is disagreement over the association between gestational age and fetal loss; some research has not found a conclusive link. Notably, head trauma has been linked to higher preterm labor rates, albeit this is not always correlated with higher rates of fetal mortality.

BIBLIOGRAPHY

1. Ali J, Yeo A, Gana TJ, McLellan BA. Predictors of fetal mortality in pregnant trauma patients. J Trauma. 1997;42(5):782-5.
2. American College of Obstetricians and Gynecologists. ACOG Practice Bulletin No. 251: Trauma in pregnancy. Obstet Gynecol. 2022;140(2).
3. Barraco RD, Chiu WC, Clancy TV, Como JJ, Ebert JB, Hess LW, et al. Practice management guidelines for the diagnosis and management of injury in the pregnant patient: The EAST practice management guidelines work group. J Trauma. 2010;69(1):211-4.
4. El-Kady D, Gilbert WM, Anderson J, Danielsen B, Towner D, Smith LH. Trauma during pregnancy: An analysis of maternal and fetal outcomes in a large population. Am J Obstet Gynecol. 2004;190(6):1661-8.
5. Thomas H, Baskett TF. Trauma in pregnancy. Obstet Gynecol Clin North Am. 1995;22(1):69-89.

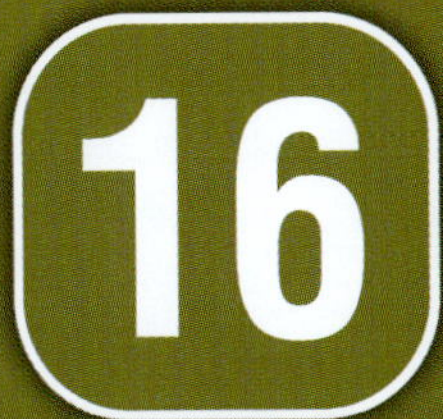

Management of Polytrauma, DCO and Various Trauma Scoring System

CHAPTER 16.1

Management of Polytrauma, DCO and Various Trauma Scoring System

Aswanikumar Singh Jamedar

The initial or emergency treatment of a polytrauma or high-velocity trauma patient is different compared to an isolated or low musculoskeletal trauma.

Therefore, the mechanism of injury is very important while managing any trauma patients. Typically high-velocity injuries include:

- Road traffic accident (RTA) (fall from significant height, i.e., >10 feet)
- Blast injuries
- Gunshot injuries
- Burns
- Facial trauma including facial injuries

Of all deaths from trauma, 30–40% are caused by bleeding. 80% of traumatic injuries are because of blunt injuries, with the majority of deaths secondary to hypovolemic shock. Intraperitoneal bleeds occur in 12% of blunt trauma; therefore, it is essential to identify the source and treat it quickly.

One of the three deaths that occurred in the hospital is a result of causes, that could have been prevented. Often these deaths occur due to factors like simple management errors in the early hours after injury *("Golden Hour")*, rather than because of a lack of complex and advanced definitive treatment.

Quick initial resuscitation, stabilization, and transport to the appropriate healthcare facility are crucial to saving lives. The chances of mortality rapidly increase after every 30 minutes of elapsed time without treatment after injury.

Deaths due to trauma can occur in three phases:

1. *Immediate*: Usually occurs at the site of accidents and is due to severe injuries like visceral injuries or severe brain injuries and not much can be done about this.
2. *Early deaths*: Occur within minutes to hours *(Golden hour)* after injuries and are usually because of problems with the airway, lung injuries, or major bleeding because of abdominal or pelvic fractures. These are the deaths, which can be potentially preventable if treated properly and timely.
3. *Late deaths*: They occur a few days to a few weeks after initial injuries and usually occur because of secondary complications such as acute respiratory distress syndrome (ARDS), sepsis, pulmonary embolism (PE), and multiorgan failure.

Therefore, there is a significant need for a protocol-based structural approach regarding managing these types of injuries. It helps to minimize early and delayed mortality.

Based on this background, all these injuries should be treated as per ATLS (Advanced Trauma Life Support) protocol.

Various important steps/aspects of ATLS protocol-based management include:

- Triage and appropriately transporting the patient
- Algorithm/protocol-based care in hospital
- Damage control measures (minimize systemic inflammation and organ failure)

- This approach is nowadays applied across the world so that all healthcare can speak the same language when it comes to managing such patient.

The ethos or the principles of ATLS-based care are:

- Treat the greatest threat to life first.
- Lack of definitive diagnosis should never impede the start of immediately indicated treatment.
- A detailed history and investigation are not the essential prerequisite to begin the evaluation and treatment of an acutely injured patient.

Musculoskeletal injuries are a significant component of trauma care (85%), often involving multiple systems and requiring prompt and accurate assessment and intervention. However, resuscitation takes priority over musculoskeletal injuries.

ADVANCED TRAUMA LIFE SUPPORT APPROACH TO MUSCULOSKELETAL INJURIES

As a rule, always consider life before limb, however, the delay in recognition and appropriate treatment of musculoskeletal injuries can result in life- or limb-threatening situations.

ATLS protocol involves:

- *Primary survey*: With simultaneous resuscitation
- *Secondary survey*: Provisional and definitive care
- *Tertiary survey*: Head to toe examination, evaluation, and management

Meanwhile, it involves simultaneously a multidisciplinary approach and treatment.

Primary survey includes:

A—Airway with *C-spine* control

B—Breathing

C—Circulation

D—Disability/*neurological/musculoskeletal*

E—Exposure/environmental control

A—Airway and cervical spine protection: The priority is to ensure a patent airway while simultaneously protecting the cervical spine.

- *Open the airway*:
  - Use the jaw-thrust or chin-lift maneuver to open the airway without moving the cervical spine.
  - If the patient is unconscious and at risk of obstruction, insert an oropharyngeal airway.
- *Clear the airway*:
  - Suction of any blood, vomit, or debris from the mouth and pharynx
  - If necessary, remove any foreign bodies that may be obstructing the airway.
- *Secure the airway*:
  - If the airway cannot be maintained, consider advanced airway management, such as endotracheal intubation.
- Maintain cervical spine protection throughout the procedure using manual in-line stabilization (MILS). In all patients with high-velocity injury, it is suspected to have a cervical spine injury. Therefore, MILS should be maintained while securing the airway. If intubation is required, techniques such as rapid sequence induction (RSI) with MILS should be employed to minimize cervical spine movement. Ideally, there should be arrangements already prepared to use adjuncts like a supraglottic airway device or video laryngoscopy if intubation proves challenging.
- Immobilization of the cervical spine (C-spine) is crucial in trauma patients to prevent further injury to the spinal cord, especially when a cervical spine injury is suspected. Here is how to properly immobilize the cervical spine:
- *Manual in-line stabilization*:
  - To maintain the head and neck in a neutral position while preventing any movement that could exacerbate a potential spinal injury.

- *Technique*:
- The rescuer should position themselves at the head of the patient.
- Use both hands to grasp the sides of the patient's head, with the palms on the ears, and thumbs pointing toward the face.
- Gently but firmly hold the head in a neutral position, aligning it with the spine, and keep the neck stable without applying traction.
- Continue manual stabilization until the cervical collar is applied.

- *Application of a cervical collar*:
  - *Technique*:
    - *Sizing*: Select the appropriate size of the cervical collar based on the patient's neck size. Measure the distance between the bottom of the chin and the top of the shoulder (trapezius muscle).
    - *Application*:
      - Ensure the patient's head is in a neutral position (not flexed or extended).
      - Slide the back portion of the collar behind the neck while maintaining manual stabilization.
      - Wrap the front portion of the collar under the chin, ensuring it fits snugly but not too tightly.
      - Secure the collar using the Velcro straps, ensuring the head remains in a neutral position.
- *Spinal motion restriction (SMR)*:
  - *Technique*:
    - *Backboard/spine board*:
      - *Log-roll the patient while maintaining manual cervical stabilization, and position them onto a backboard.*
      - *Secure the patient to the backboard using straps across the chest, hips, and legs.*
    - Additional padding may be placed under the head if necessary to maintain neutral alignment.
    - *Head immobilization*:
      - Use head immobilizers (blocks or pads) on either side of the head once the cervical collar is in place.
      - Secure the head immobilizers with a forehead strap and a chin strap, ensuring they are snug but not overly tight.
- *Considerations during immobilization*:
  - Avoid excessive movement
  - Monitor for discomfort or airway compromise
- *During transport*:
  - Keep the patient in a supine position with the head immobilized.
  - If the patient vomits or there is a need for airway management, log-roll them carefully to the side while maintaining cervical spine alignment.

These steps are crucial in preventing further spinal injury and ensuring the patient's safety during initial trauma management and transport.

B—breathing and ventilation:

- *Provide oxygen*:
  - Administer 100% oxygen via a nonrebreather mask or bag-valve-mask (BVM) if the patient is not breathing adequately.
- *Ventilate*:
  - Assist ventilation with a BVM if the patient has inadequate respiratory effort.
  - Perform needle decompression for tension pneumothorax if identified (e.g., severe respiratory distress, hypotension, tracheal deviation).
- *Seal open pneumothorax*:
  - Apply an occlusive dressing (three-sided dressing) to any open chest wound, leaving one side unsealed to act as a flutter valve.
- *Assess and treat chest injuries*:
  - Assess for flail chest and provide supportive care (e.g., positive pressure ventilation).

  - Consider chest tube insertion for significant pneumothorax or hemothorax.
- Musculoskeletal injuries can impair respiratory function, particularly in cases of rib fractures or thoracic spine injuries.
- During the primary survey, the presence of a flail chest, tension pneumothorax, or hemothorax should be quickly identified. A needle decompression should be performed immediately if tension pneumothorax is suspected, followed by chest tube insertion for definitive management. Continuous monitoring with pulse oximetry and capnography is essential to ensure adequate ventilation.

C—circulation with hemorrhage control: Hemorrhage is a leading cause of preventable death in trauma. Musculoskeletal injuries, particularly those involving long bones or the pelvis, can result in significant blood loss. Immediate bleeding control which may at times require an application of a tourniquet for extremity hemorrhage control or a pelvic binder for suspected pelvic fractures is crucial. In practice, this means assessing for signs of shock early, obtaining rapid vascular access (preferably with two large-bore IVs), and initiating fluid resuscitation as per the ATLS guidelines. A blood transfusion is often necessary especially in cases of massive hemorrhage, guided by the hemodynamic response.

- *Assess circulation*:
  - Evaluate pulse, blood pressure, and capillary refill.
- *Fluid resuscitation*:
  - Establish at least two large-bore (16–18 gauge) IV lines or intraosseous access if IV access is difficult.
  - Begin with rapid administration of isotonic crystalloid solutions (e.g., normal saline or Ringer's lactate).
  - For signs of shock, administer blood products (e.g., packed red blood cells) early if available.
- *Monitor response*:
  - Continuously monitor vital signs, urine output, and mental status to evaluate the effectiveness of resuscitation.

D—disability (neurological status) and identifying any obvious major injuries of limbs: A rapid neurological assessment is necessary to identify deficits related to spinal injuries or traumatic brain injury. The Glasgow Coma Scale (GCS) should be used as a proper assessment tool, and any decrease in GCS or new-onset focal neurological deficits should prompt urgent imaging (CT of the head and spine). Immobilization of the spine should continue until spinal injuries are ruled out.

- However, a quick assessment can be done by the *APUV score* to assess the level of consciousness which is:
  - *A*—alert, *P*—responding to painful stimuli, *U*—unresponsiveness, *V*—responding to verbal command
- Evaluate pupil size and reactivity
- *Stabilize*:
  - If there is evidence of increased intracranial pressure (ICP), consider early interventions (e.g., elevating the head of the bed, hyperventilation in certain cases, and mannitol administration).
  - Ensure continued protection of the cervical spine.
- *Splintage to fracture* after in-line alignment and restoration of gross deformity, but this should not delay the resuscitation. Meanwhile, an attempt should be made to control any hemorrhage by applying a pressure bandage. Also, do not forget appropriate and adequate analgesia.
- A quick and careful log roll is done to examine the whole spine for any tenderness, step, swelling, and per-rectal examination that has to be done during this maneuver. Meanwhile, in a patient with normal GCS, this is the time to rule out any C-spine injury by palpating for

any tenderness, gentle range of motion, and evaluating for any neurological symptoms in limbs.

E—exposure and environmental control:

- *Expose the patient*:
  - Fully expose the patient to assess for additional injuries, ensuring no life-threatening conditions are missed.
- *Prevent hypothermia*:
  - Use warming blankets, increase room temperature, and administer warmed IV fluids to prevent hypothermia, which can exacerbate shock.
- This means removing clothing and using warm blankets or a warming device to prevent hypothermia. Hypothermia can exacerbate coagulopathy and worsen outcomes, so actively warming the patient while conducting a thorough secondary survey is critical.
- *Reassess continuously*:
  - Continuously reassess the patient's condition, particularly after each intervention, to ensure ongoing management of life-threatening conditions.

Adjuncts to primary survey:

- *Monitoring equipment*:
  - *Pulse oximetry*:
    - Monitors oxygen saturation and helps assess the effectiveness of oxygenation and ventilation.
  - *Capnography*:
    - Measures end-tidal CO_2 ($ETCO_2$), which provides information about ventilation status and the effectiveness of chest compressions if CPR is in progress.
  - *Electrocardiogram (ECG/EKG)*:
    - Continuously monitors the heart's electrical activity to detect arrhythmias, ischemia, or other cardiac conditions that might influence resuscitation decisions.
  - *Blood pressure monitoring*:
    - Noninvasive or invasive (arterial line) monitoring to assess and track the patient's blood pressure in real-time, essential for evaluating circulation.
- *Primary series of imaging*:
  - *Focused assessment with sonography for trauma (FAST)*:
    - A rapid bedside ultrasound examination used to detect free fluid in the abdomen, pelvis, and pericardium, indicating internal bleeding.
  - *Chest X-ray (CXR)*: To assess for thoracic injuries such as pneumothorax, hemothorax, rib fractures, pulmonary contusions, and aortic injury. It can reveal conditions like tension pneumothorax, which may require immediate intervention, or widened mediastinum suggesting possible aortic injury.
  - *Pelvic X-ray*: To evaluate for pelvic fractures, which can be a major source of hemorrhage in trauma patients. It helps identify pelvic ring fractures or dislocations that may necessitate urgent management, including pelvic binding or angiographic embolization.
  - *Lateral cervical spine X-ray*: Ensure to see the upper border of T1 *to see the adequacy of X-rays.* To assess for cervical spine injuries, especially in patients with suspected spinal trauma. Helps identify fractures or dislocations of the cervical vertebrae. This is particularly important in maintaining spinal precautions.

These X-rays are prioritized because they can quickly detect injuries that may require immediate intervention during the primary survey. Advanced imaging, such as a full cervical spine series, CT scans, or other targeted X-rays, may follow during the secondary survey or as the patient's condition stabilizes.

- *Blood investigations*:
  - *Blood gas analysis (ABG/VBG)*:
    - Provides information on oxygenation, ventilation (pH, pCO_2),

and metabolic status (lactate levels), which are critical in assessing the severity of shock and guiding resuscitation.
- *Blood type and cross-match*:
  - Prepared for blood transfusion in case of significant hemorrhage requiring rapid administration of blood products
- *Complete blood count (CBC) and coagulation studies*:
  - Assesses hemoglobin, hematocrit, platelet count, and coagulation status (PT/INR, aPTT), providing essential information for managing bleeding and coagulopathy.
  - Pregnancy test in case of females of reproductive age group and toxicology screening if there is a suspicion of poisoning along with trauma.

- *Urinary and gastric catheters*:
  - *Urinary catheter*:
    - Insertion of a Foley catheter allows monitoring of urine output, which is a key indicator of renal perfusion and overall circulatory status. It also helps assess for potential bladder injury.
  - *Gastric tube (nasogastric or orogastric)*:
    - Helps decompress the stomach, reducing the risk of aspiration and providing insight into the presence of gastrointestinal bleeding. Orogastric tubes are preferred if there is a risk of basilar skull fracture.
  - The rule is finger and tube in every orifice, so *every orifice* must be examined and all the polytrauma patients or unconscious patients should be catheterized and may need N/G tube.
- *Pain management and sedation*:
  - *Pain management*: Adequate pain control is crucial in managing musculoskeletal injuries. In the emergency department, initial pain management often involves intravenous opioids, titrated to effect. For example, morphine or fentanyl can be administered, with careful monitoring of respiratory status. Nonsteroidal anti-inflammatory drugs (NSAIDs) can be added for their anti-inflammatory effects. However, care should be taken in patients with renal impairment or risk of bleeding. Regional anesthesia, such as a femoral nerve block for femur fractures, provides excellent pain relief and can facilitate patient comfort and cooperation during further evaluation and treatment.
  - *Sedation*:
    - If intubation is required, appropriate sedatives and neuromuscular blocking agents are administered to facilitate the procedure.
- *Consideration of additional measures*:
  - *Tranexamic acid (TXA)*:
    - Early administration of TXA can be considered in patients with severe hemorrhage to help control bleeding.
  - *Blood product administration*:
    - In cases of significant hemorrhage, consider administering packed red blood cells, plasma, and platelets early to manage shock and coagulopathy.

Secondary survey:
- *AMPLE history*:
  - *A*—History of any drug allergy
  - *M*—Medication history
  - *P*—Past medical history of any comorbidities
  - *L*vLast meal taken when?
  - *E*—Event before and after injury or incident
- *Head-to-toe examination (look, feel, and move)*: During the secondary survey, a detailed musculoskeletal examination is performed **(Flowchart 1)**.
- *Bleeding control* by direct pressure, splinting, and fluid resuscitation

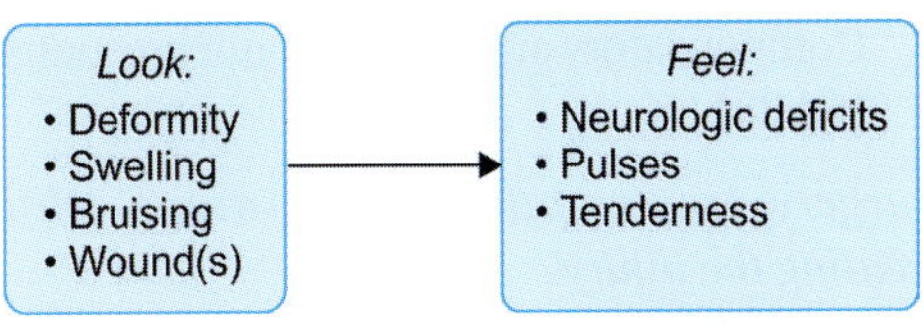

FLOWCHART 1: Head-to-toe examination.

- Meanwhile, careful documentation of findings is crucial, as is deciding on the need for further imaging or orthopedic consultation.
- *Radiological assessment*: Radiographs are essential for diagnosing fractures, dislocations, and other musculoskeletal injuries. Obtaining at least AP and lateral views of the affected area is standard and at times may be additional views. X-rays are guided by the rule of 2, which is two views, two limbs at times especially in the case of children for comparison purposes, two joints (which means one joint above and one below, especially in case of diaphyseal fracture), and two times (at times before reduction or application of splint and afterwards).
- For more complex injuries, such as those involving the spine or pelvis, CT imaging provides better detail and can guide surgical planning. MRI may be indicated for soft tissue injuries or when there is suspicion of spinal cord involvement. Knowing when to escalate from plain films to advanced imaging is key to efficient and effective patient management.

Always follow the sequence of priority as below:

- Life before limb, limb before bone, then vascularity, then neurology of limb, then soft tissues, then joint and then bony injuries and not the other way around

Common orthopedic urgencies and emergencies:

- Unstable pelvic fracture
- Fractures or dislocations associated with vascular injury
- Acute compartment syndrome
- Crush syndrome
- Unstable spinal injuries
- Fracture or dislocation associated with or potentially associated with neurological injuries
- Fracture or dislocation potentially associated with avascular necrosis
- Fracture and dislocation are associated with significant soft tissue damage or compromise.
- Open fractures
- Multiple long bone fractures, as they can generate significant bleeding like femur fracture can cause approximately 750–1,500 mL of blood loss, while a fracture tibia can cause approximately 300–750 mLs of blood loss.
- *Bilateral femur fractures*: Historical mortality rates approximately 40% and is an independent risk factor for ARDS

Orthopedic emergencies and urgencies should be treated in the overall context of polytrauma patients. Their detailed management of each of these emergencies is going to be discussed in each of the concerned section/chapter of this book.

Tertiary survey: Once the patient is stable and GCS normalizes, another complete head-to-toe survey is required. The goal is not to miss any smallest or so-called trivial injury as well and treat it appropriately. Because missing any injury even if it is a minor injury can have a significant negative impact on patient's eventual outcome in term of the full restoration of preinjury status and which should be the target of any treatment.

MULTIDISCIPLINARY TEAM APPROACH

The management of such injuries often involves a multidisciplinary team, including general surgeons, orthopedic surgeons, radiologists, anesthesiologists, and emergency specialists. Effective communication and coordination among team members are essential to optimize patient outcomes. This means regular team briefings, clear documentation of the treatment plan, and ensuring that all relevant specialists are involved in decision-making from the outset. One of the members has to be the team leader with a clearly defined role for other members and clearly communicate to the patient party about the diagnosis, treatment and likely prognosis and document this as well.

DEFINITIVE SURGERY (EARLY TOTAL CARE) VERSUS DAMAGE CONTROL ORTHOPEDICS AND DAMAGE CONTROL SURGERY

The concept of "damage control orthopedics" (DCO) and damage control surgery (DCS) is employed in patients with life-threatening injuries. This approach involves initial provisional stabilization of fractures (e.g., external fixation, traction, and appropriate splintage), hemorrhage control (abdominal visceral packing), soft tissue management, and delayed definitive fixation until the patient is hemodynamically stable. Recent studies have shown that in select patients, "early total care" (ETC) can be safely performed. The decision between DCO and ETC should be based on the patient's overall condition, injury severity, and the availability of surgical resources.

This requires close collaboration between general surgeons, orthopedic surgeons, and anesthetists to develop an individualized care plan.

The goal of DCO is to avoid the "*second hit*" because of surgery on a polytrauma patient. "*First hit*" happens due to initial trauma.

DCO involves:

- Treating polytrauma patients to minimize the *impact of the "second hit"*
- Definitive treatment was delayed until physiology improved, as the patient is *"too sick for ETC"*.
- By DCO, we try to avoid MOF (multiorgan failure) and ARDS

Physiologic response to trauma:

- Systemic inflammatory response (SIRS)
- Compensatory anti-inflammatory response (CARS)

Surgery creates additional trauma while treating the injury!

"Second hit":

- May exacerbate systemic inflammatory response
- May lead to secondary lung injury
- An inappropriately timed secondary intervention may result in crossing threshold resulting in ARDS or MOF

"First Hit": We as surgeons have no control.

"Second Hit": We as surgeons have control.

Unresolved issues with DCO:

Early total care (ETC) involves:

- Definitive, not provisional stabilization of all fractures
- Can be dangerous in under-resuscitated patients

Early definitive fixation may be considered standard of care in *stable patients.*

Potential issues with overutilization of DCO:

- Unnecessary delay in definitive treatment
- Longer ICU stays
- Longer time on ventilator
- Longer hospital stays
- Increased cost

When to use DCO?

- Which parameters?
- Problems with inflammatory markers
- Which injury types are predictive?

What about injuries other than the femur?

- Some fractures are not amenable to external fixation like the spine and acetabulum.

Indications for DCO:

- Persistent hemodynamic instability
- Persistent metabolic acidosis
- Severe head injury with cerebral perfusion pressure (CPP) < 70 mm Hg; ICP > 20 mm Hg
- Spinal cord injury with evolving neuro deficit (reduction/fixation of the spine may be a higher priority)
- Cardiac dysfunction

Indications for definitive fixation:

- *Adequate resuscitation*: Lactate < 4.0, base excess ≥ 5.5, pH ≥ 7.25
- Coagulopathy corrected
- Early definitive fixation (within 36 hours) of axial (pelvis/spine), femoral fracture, and acetabulum fractures in stable patients reduces complications, length of stay, and costs.

Predicting the "second hit":

- Which patients will be affected?

Patient risk stratification:

- Stable
- Borderline
- Unstable
- In extremis

Some controversy exists regarding acute treatment of "borderline" patients **(Table 1)**.

Algorithm for ETC versus DCO

Refer to **Flowchart 2**.

Definitive treatment in DCO:

- Patients who underwent conversion between 2 and 4 days were compared to those who underwent conversion between 5 and 8 days.

TABLE 1: Classification systems for clinical patient assessment.

	Parameter	Stable (grade I)	Borderline (grade II)	Unstable (grade III)	In extremis (grade IV)
Shock	Blood pressure (mm Hg)	100 or more	80–100	60–90	<50–60
	Blood units (2 hours)	0–2	2–8	5–15	>15
	Lactate levels	Normal range	Around 2.5	>2.5	Severe acidosis
	Base deficit (mmol/L)	Normal range	No data	No data	>6.8
	ATLS classification	I	II–III	III–IV	IV
Coagulation	Platelet count (μg/dL)	>110	90–110	<70–90	<70
	Factor II and V (%)	90–100	70–80	50–70	<50
	Fibrinogen (g/dL)	1	Around 1	<1	DIC
	D-dimer	Normal range	Abnormal	Abnormal	DIC
	Temperature	<33°C	33–35°C	30–32°C	30°C or less
Soft tissue injuries	Lung function; PaO_2/FiO_2	350–400	300–350	200–300	<200
	Chest trauma scores; AIS	AIS 1 or 2	AIS 2 or more	AIS 2 or more	AIS 3 or more
	Chest trauma scores; TTSS	0	I–II	II–III	IV
	Abdominal trauma (Moore)	≤ II	≤ III	III	III or >III
	Pelvic trauma (AO class)	A type (AO)	B or C	C	C (crush, rollover)
	Extremities	AIS I–II	AIS II–III	AIS III–IV	Crush, rollover injuries

(ATLS: Advanced Trauma Life Support; AIS: abbreviated injury scale; FiO_2: fraction of inspired oxygen; PaO_2: partial pressure of oxygen; TTSS: thoracic trauma severity score)

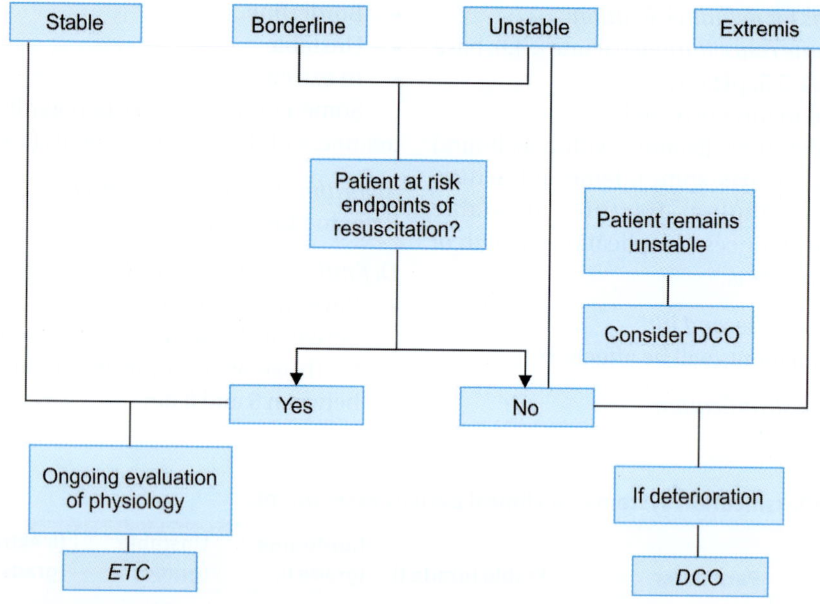

FLOWCHART 2: Algorithm for ETC versus DCO.
(ETC: early total care; DCO: damage control orthopedics)

- Multiorgan dysfunction syndrome (MODS) 46% in the early group versus 16% in the late group

Timing of definitive treatment in DCO:
- An interpretation of Pape's work→
  The majority of patients treated with DCO should probably *wait until at least postinjury day 5 (five)* before definitive treatment.

VARIOUS SCORING SYSTEMS FOR POLYTRAUMA PATIENTS

Polytrauma scoring systems are crucial in assessing the severity of injuries in patients with polytrauma patient, guiding treatment decisions, and predicting outcomes. Here is a description of some of the latest and updated polytrauma scoring systems, along with their advantages and disadvantages:
- Abbreviated injury scale (AIS)
- Injury severity score (ISS)
- New injury severity score (NISS)

Abbreviated injury scale:
- *Nine anatomic areas*:
  i. Head
  ii. Face
  iii. Neck
  iv. Thorax
  v. Abdomen
  vi. Spine
  vii. Upper extremity
  viii. Lower extremity
  ix. External
- *Each area scored from 0 to 6*:
  - 0—none
  - 1—minor
  - 2—moderate
  - 3—serious
  - 4—severe
  - 5—critical
  - 6—not survivable

Injury severity score:
- Calculated from AIS
- Highest AIS value from each anatomic area, i.e., 6
- The three highest AIS values (from different anatomic areas)
  - → Squared and → summed

$$AIS^2 + AIS^2 + AIS^2$$

Injury severity score correlates with:
- Morbidity, mortality, and length of hospital stay

Defines polytrauma when ISS ≥ 18:
- *Highest score*: 75 (not survivable)

Problem with ISS: Injuries within the same anatomic system are counted only once.
- *Advantages*:
  - Simple and quick to calculate
  - Well-validated and extensively used in research and clinical practice
  - Strong correlation with mortality risk
- *Disadvantages*:
  - Does not account for the age or physiological status of the patient
  - It may underestimate severity in patients with multiple moderate injuries.
  - It is not as effective in predicting outcomes in elderly patients.

New injury severity score:
- The three highest AIS values regardless of anatomic region are utilized.
- It may be a better predictor of morbidity and mortality.
- The NISS is a modified version of the ISS that sums the squares of the three highest AIS scores, regardless of body region. This revision addresses some of the limitations of the ISS.
- *Advantages*:
  - Provides a more accurate reflection of overall injury severity
  - A better predictor of mortality compared to the traditional ISS
  - Simple to apply, similar to ISS
- *Disadvantages*:
  - Still does not consider age, comorbidities, or physiological factors
  - Not as widely adopted as ISS, leading to less consistency in its use

Trauma and injury severity score (TRISS):
- TRISS combines the ISS, revised trauma score (RTS), and patient age to predict survival probability. It is a hybrid scoring system that incorporates both anatomical and physiological data.
- *Relevance*: TRISS is highly relevant in today's clinical practice because it combines anatomical (injury severity score) and physiological (revised trauma score) data, along with patient age, to predict survival probabilities. This hybrid approach allows for a more comprehensive assessment of trauma severity, making it particularly useful in both clinical and research settings.
- *Advantages*:
  - *Predictive power*: TRISS has a strong predictive ability for mortality, which is crucial in guiding treatment decisions and resource allocation in trauma centers.
  - *Benchmarking*: It is widely used for benchmarking trauma care and comparing outcomes across institutions, helping to improve overall trauma care quality.

The *best and most relevant polytrauma scoring system* today depends on the specific clinical context, but the *injury severity score (ISS)* remains the most widely used and accepted scoring system globally. However, for a more comprehensive and contemporary approach, the *trauma and injury severity score (TRISS)* is often considered the better option.

POSTOPERATIVE CARE AND REHABILITATION

Postoperative care is vital to the overall recovery of patients with musculoskeletal injuries. This includes effective pain management using a multimodal approach, prevention of complications such as deep vein thrombosis (DVT) with prophylactic anticoagulation, and early mobilization to prevent muscle atrophy and joint stiffness.

CONCLUSION

The initial and emergency management of musculoskeletal injuries is a critical component of trauma care. Adhering to the ATLS protocol ensures that life-threatening conditions are promptly addressed, while a systematic approach to musculoskeletal injuries facilitates accurate diagnosis and timely intervention.

- *Primary survey*:
  - *Identify* life-threatening injuries
- *Secondary survey*:
  - *Identify* limb-threatening injuries

Identifying patients with *occult hypoperfusion* is necessary to minimize morbidity and mortality.

- Identifying and treating *orthopedic urgencies and emergencies* in the *initial evaluation is critical in minimizing* morbidity and mortality.
- Knowledge of certain *scoring systems* is necessary in managing polytrauma patients.
- Knowledge of *damage control orthopedics* and when to implement methods of DCO is critical.

Always remember "Life before Limb".

BIBLIOGRAPHY

1. American College of Surgeons Committee on Trauma. Advanced Trauma Life Support (ATLS) Student Course Manual, 10th edition. Chicago, IL: American College of Surgeons; 2018.
2. Pape H-C, Giannoudis P, Krettek C. The timing of fracture treatment in polytrauma patients: relevance of damage control orthopedic surgery. Am J Surg. 2002;183(6):622-9.
3. Guerado E, Bertrand ML, Cano JR, Cerván AM, Galán A. Damage control orthopaedics: State of the art. World J Orthop. 2019;10(1):1-13.
4. Papakostidis C, Giannoudis PV. Timing of pelvic surgery in polytrauma patients: A systematic literature review. Injury. 2020;51 Suppl 3.
5. Smith JE, Greaves I. Advanced trauma life support (ATLS) and beyond. Emerg Med J. 2016;33(1):74-7.

SECTION

Common Complications and Management

CHAPTER 17.1

Management of Neurological Injuries

John Mohd, Abhimanu Kaith

Neurological injuries resulting from orthopedic trauma are complex, requiring comprehensive and multidisciplinary care to optimize recovery outcomes. The interdependence of musculoskeletal and neural structures means that trauma to one often affects the other, necessitating tailored strategies for diagnosis, treatment, and rehabilitation.

PATHOPHYSIOLOGY OF NEUROLOGICAL INJURIES IN ORTHOPEDIC TRAUMA

Neurological injuries in orthopedic trauma can be classified as direct or indirect. Direct injuries typically result from trauma that physically disrupts nerve tissue, while indirect injuries results from ischemia, edema, or compression, which can lead to secondary neuronal damage. Common types include:

- *Nerve transection:* Severe fractures or penetrating injuries often cause lacerations, leading to a discontinuity in the nerve pathway and requiring surgical intervention.
- *Crush and compression injuries:* These occur frequently in fractures or compartment syndrome, where swelling and hematoma exert pressure on nerves, potentially leading to ischemic damage.
- *Traction and stretch injuries:* Dislocations, especially of large joints like the shoulder or hip, can overstretch nerves, damaging their structural integrity and impairing function.

Vascular injury and ischemia: Vascular compromise, common in high-energy traumas, can cause neurological injuries associated with orthopedic trauma which are typically classified based on the mechanism, anatomical location, and severity of nerve damage.

A well-established classification is Seddon's classification, which categorizes nerve injuries by the extent of structural damage and potential for recovery. More recent classifications, such as Sunderland's classification, provide further detail by subdividing nerve injuries based on histological features. Here is an overview of the main classification systems.

Seddon's Classification

Seddon's classification divides nerve injuries into three types based on the degree of nerve damage:

1. *Neuropraxia:* This is the mildest form of nerve injury, where there is a temporary conduction block without structural damage to the nerve fibers. It usually results from compression or ischemia. Recovery is generally complete and occurs within days to weeks, as the nerve does not undergo Wallerian degeneration.

2. *Axonotmesis:* In this moderate form of injury, the axons are damaged, but the surrounding connective tissue structures (endoneurium, perineurium, and epineurium) remain intact. This type of injury results in Wallerian degeneration distal to the site of injury. Recovery is possible but can take several months, as axonal regeneration must occur.
3. *Neurotmesis:* This is the most severe type of injury, where there is complete disruption of the nerve, including both the axons and the surrounding connective tissue. Without surgical intervention, recovery is unlikely because spontaneous regeneration is severely limited.

Sunderland's Classification

Sunderland expanded upon Seddon's classification, breaking down nerve injuries into five degrees of severity, which provides more detail regarding the extent of structural damage:

1. *First-degree (Neuropraxia):* Equivalent to Seddon's neuropraxia, where there is no axonal or connective tissue damage, just a temporary block in nerve conduction.
2. *Second-degree:* Corresponds to axonotmesis, with axonal damage and Wallerian degeneration, but the surrounding connective tissue (endoneurium) remains intact. Axonal regrowth can occur along the original pathway.
3. *Third-degree:* Both the axon and endoneurium are disrupted, but the perineurium remains intact. Recovery is possible but less predictable, as regeneration may not follow the correct pathway, potentially leading to incomplete or misdirected recovery.
4. *Fourth-degree:* There is disruption of the axon, endoneurium, and perineurium, with only the epineurium remaining intact. This severe injury typically requires surgical repair, as axonal regeneration is blocked by scar tissue.
5. *Fifth-degree (Neurotmesis):* Complete nerve transection, including all connective tissue layers. Spontaneous recovery is highly unlikely, and surgical intervention is needed to restore continuity for potential regeneration.

Anatomical Classification Based on Location

This classification is based on the anatomical region of the nerve affected, which helps to tailor management strategies according to the specific neural structures involved:

- *Peripheral nerve injuries:* Common in extremity trauma, affecting nerves like the radial, ulnar, median, sciatic, and peroneal nerves. These injuries often result from fractures or lacerations.
- *Plexus injuries:* Affecting the brachial or lumbosacral plexus, these injuries are often associated with high-energy trauma, such as from motor vehicle accidents. Brachial plexus injuries are particularly complex due to the involvement of multiple nerve roots and trunks.
- *Spinal cord injuries:* Usually result from fractures or dislocations of the vertebral column, leading to varying degrees of neurological deficit based on the level and extent of spinal cord involvement. They may cause both motor and sensory deficits and are classified as complete or incomplete injuries.

Functional Classification

Functional classification categorizes nerve injuries based on the impact on motor and sensory functions, often used in clinical settings to guide rehabilitation:

- *Motor nerve injuries:* Predominantly affecting motor functions, leading to weakness or paralysis in the corresponding muscles. These are often associated with motor neurons or mixed nerves.
- *Sensory nerve injuries:* Resulting in loss of sensation, such as numbness or tingling,

along the distribution of the affected nerve. Sensory deficits can significantly impact quality of life by affecting balance and proprioception.
- *Mixed nerve injuries:* Involve both motor and sensory fibers, leading to a combination of motor deficits and sensory loss. Most peripheral nerves are mixed, and injuries often present with both types of symptoms.

Etiological Classification

This classification is based on the underlying cause or mechanism of injury:
- *Traumatic injuries:* Caused by direct trauma, such as lacerations, crush injuries, or penetrating wounds.
- *Compression injuries:* Result from sustained pressure on a nerve, which can occur due to fractures, dislocations, or compartment syndrome.
- *Ischemic injuries:* Due to vascular compromise, leading to reduced blood supply to the nerve. This is commonly seen in high-energy trauma where blood vessels are also damaged.
- *Iatrogenic injuries:* Nerve injuries caused by medical procedures, such as surgeries or injections. They can be accidental but are often preventable with careful surgical planning.

Imaging Techniques

- *High-resolution MRI and MR neurography:* These techniques have become gold standards for evaluating nerve injuries. MRI offers excellent soft-tissue contrast, enabling precise localization of injuries and assessment of associated edema or fibrosis. MR neurography, in particular, is valuable for visualizing peripheral nerves and detecting entrapment syndromes.
- *Ultrasound imaging:* Real-time, noninvasive, and widely accessible, ultrasound is increasingly used for peripheral nerve imaging. It can detect nerve discontinuity, monitor healing progress, and guide injections for pain management. Emerging techniques, like elastography, can also provide information on tissue stiffness and elasticity, adding another layer of diagnostic detail.
- *Three-dimensional (3D) CT and CT myelography:* For evaluating bony structures and complex fractures that may impact neural elements, 3D CT offers enhanced anatomical detail. CT myelography, meanwhile, can visualize nerve roots and spinal canal structures when MRI is contraindicated, such as in patients with metallic implants.

Electrophysiological Testing

- *Advanced nerve conduction studies (NCS) and electromyography (EMG):* NCS can now provide detailed data on conduction block and axonal damage, while EMG helps in pinpointing the location and severity of nerve dysfunction.
- *High-density surface electromyography (HD-sEMG):* A newer technique, HD-sEMG, offers a noninvasive alternative that can capture detailed muscle activity patterns, which is useful for monitoring recovery and functional outcomes.
- *Somatosensory evoked potentials (SSEPs):* Widely used in spinal cord injuries, SSEPs assess the integrity of sensory pathways, helping to gauge the severity of neural impairment and track recovery during rehabilitation.

Timing of these Studies

- *Within the first few days:* Not typically recommended, except in cases of suspected conduction block due to neuropraxia.
- *3–6 weeks postinjury:* Ideal for initial comprehensive assessment in cases of axonal injury.
- *3 months and beyond:* Follow-up studies to assess recovery, guide surgical planning, and determine long-term prognosis.

TREATMENT MODALITIES

Optimal management of neurological injuries in orthopedic trauma often requires a combination of surgical and nonsurgical treatments.

Surgical Management

- *Direct nerve repair and grafting:* Techniques like epineural and perineural repair, along with fascicular nerve grafting, are crucial for addressing nerve discontinuities. The choice of autograft or synthetic conduit is guided by factors like defect length and injury location. Research on biodegradable conduits and nerve scaffolds is showing promise, with studies indicating reduced scar formation and improved nerve regeneration.
- *Nerve transfers:* Nerve transfers are increasingly favored for severe nerve injuries, especially when direct repair is not feasible. Advances in this field have expanded indications for brachial plexus and other complex injuries, with novel transfer techniques improving outcomes in both motor and sensory functions.
- *Neurolysis and nerve decompression:* For cases involving compression, neurolysis can alleviate symptoms by freeing the nerve from scar tissue or other adhesions. Decompression surgery, including techniques for carpal and cubital tunnel syndromes, is increasingly supported by data showing significant improvements in quality of life and nerve function.

Nonsurgical Management

- *Pharmacological management:* Multimodal pain management is essential, with medications such as nonsteroidal anti-inflammatory drugs (NSAIDs), anticonvulsants, and antidepressants playing roles in neuropathic pain relief. Emerging drugs targeting specific pain receptors and pathways are showing potential in clinical trials, particularly for chronic pain management.
- *Biological therapies:* Stem cell therapies, platelet-rich plasma (PRP), and growth factor injections are being explored for their regenerative potential. Research indicates that these therapies can enhance nerve regeneration by promoting cellular repair mechanisms and reducing inflammation.
- *Physical therapy and functional rehabilitation:* Rehabilitation is pivotal for optimizing recovery. Advanced techniques like functional electrical stimulation (FES) and proprioceptive neuromuscular facilitation (PNF) are standard, but virtual reality (VR) and robotics-assisted rehabilitation are gaining traction for their ability to facilitate neural plasticity and motor learning.
- *Neuromodulation techniques:* Spinal cord stimulation (SCS), transcutaneous electrical nerve stimulation (TENS), and more recently, transcranial magnetic stimulation (TMS) are being investigated for their ability to modulate pain pathways and stimulate neural recovery.
- *Prevention* of any contracture and keeping joints supple during the recovery process, by appropriate splints and passive stretching exercises.

PROGNOSIS AND OUTCOMES

Prognostic factors such as the type and location of injury, timeliness of intervention, and patient-specific variables (e.g., age and comorbidities) play significant roles in recovery trajectories. While many patients achieve partial or complete recovery, challenges persist in managing chronic symptoms like neuropathic pain and residual deficits.

- *Predictive biomarkers and imaging:* Research into biomarkers, including serum proteins and imaging markers, is helping to predict outcomes and tailor rehabilitation strategies. Advanced imaging techniques are enabling earlier detection of changes in nerve health, informing therapy adjustments.

- *Functional outcome metrics:* Standardized scales like the DASH (*D*isabilities of the *A*rm, *S*houlder, and *H*and) and SF-36 (*S*hort *F*orm Health Survey) are commonly used to assess functional outcomes. Long-term follow-up studies reveal that personalized rehabilitation programs and patient's adherence are key determinants of success.

BIBLIOGRAPHY

1. Campbell WW, DeJong RN. DeJong's the Neurologic Examination, 8th edition. Philadelphia: Wolters Kluwer Health/Lippincott Williams & Wilkins; 2013.
2. Cho YJ, Kim YW, Oh JK, Lee SJ. Surgical management of peripheral nerve injuries in patients with extremity trauma: a clinical review. Clin Orthop Surg. 2020;12(1):1-12.
3. Khan MA, Reichert I, Stanner D, Watt J. Contemporary management of peripheral nerve injuries. Orthop Trauma. 2016;30(6):463-73.
4. Lundborg G. A 25-year perspective of peripheral nerve surgery: evolving neuroscientific concepts and clinical significance. J Hand Surg Am. 2000; 25(3):391-414.
5. Midha R. Nerve repair and grafting in brachial plexus injuries. Neurosurg Clin N Am. 2009;20(1):27-38.
6. Robinson LR. Traumatic injury to peripheral nerves. Muscle Nerve. 2000;23(6):863-73.
7. Rosén B, Lundborg G. The long term recovery pattern in neurophysiology and disability after median nerve injury. J Hand Surg Br. 2003;28(4):318-22.

Management of Vascular Injuries

Gagandeep Singh Raina

Vascular injury is one of the most dreaded injury in field of orthopedics. They amount to about 1% of all the trauma to extremities. Fractures associated with vascular injuries are complex, limb and even life-threatening injuries that require immediate diagnosis and treatment.

Vascular injury can occur because trauma, which can be penetrating, blunt, or a combination of these two. Penetrating injuries can occur with projectiles like bullets, blast fragment, etc., or stabs with knife, coat hangers, keys, etc., whereas blunt trauma occurs due to fractures or dislocations.

TABLE 1: Different definitions of hard and soft sign for Western Trauma Association (WTA) and Eastern Association for the Surgery of Trauma (EAST).

WTA	EAST
Expanding hematoma	Pulsatile bleeding
Bruit	Thrill
Thrill	Pulse deficit
External bleeding	Bruit
Pulselessness	Expanding hematoma
Pallor	
Paresthesia	
Paralysis or pain	

EVALUATION AND DIAGNOSIS

Trauma associations like Western Trauma Association (WTA) and Eastern Association for the Surgery of Trauma (EAST) have their own criteria and guidelines for the diagnosis and treatment of vascular injuries.

The diagnosis of vascular injuries is based on the presence of hard or soft signs. Both the WTA and the EAST have separate definitions of hard and soft signs **(Table 1)**.

As per the WTA, the hard signs are used only for main arteries, which includes anything proximal to the anterior tibial artery or tibioperoneal bifurcation but it excludes the profunda femoris artery.

Soft signs include a history of arterial bleeding at the scene or in transfer, neurological deficit occurring in a nerve adjacent to a name artery, proximity of the injury to name artery, or a small nonpulsatile hematoma present over an artery. The WTA and the EAST definition of soft signs is the same.

Clinical Evaluation

Signs and symptoms suggestive of a vascular injury include five Ps:

1. *P*ain: Severe pain often persistent and worsening, sometimes disproportionate to the injury,
2. *P*allor: Change of color of the limb, often pale compared to other limb.
3. *P*ulses: Absent or feeble pulses distal to the site of trauma.
4. *P*aralysis: Inability to move the affected limb.

5. *Paresthesia:* Numbness or abnormal sensations in the limb.

First step in the assessment of circulation is the bilateral palpation of the distal pulses ***(Flowchart 1)***.

Secondary survey is done after the completion of primary survey and now we look for soft signs for vascular injuries. Equal and bilaterally palpable pulses are a favorable sign indicating that no or a limited arterial injury is present. However, even with equally palpable pulses bilaterally, radiological studies should be done for a complete examination of the patient.

Imaging and Diagnostic Tests

- *Doppler ultrasound:* It is a rapid, non-invasive assessment of blood flow and can identify arterial occlusion or thrombosis.
- *CT angiography:* Detailed visualization of both arteries and veins is seen, allowing for the identification of injuries and planning of surgical interventions.
- *Conventional angiography:* Used in cases where CTA shows inconclusive result or when immediate intervention is required, offering high-resolution imaging of the vascular structures.

Management Strategies

Stabilization of the Fracture

Immediate fracture stabilization with splints or external fixation devices is crucial to prevent further vascular damage and reduce the risk of additional complications. Elevate the injured limb to reduce swelling. This reduces the pressure and improves circulation.

Vascular Consultation and Surgical Intervention

Early involvement of a vascular surgeon is imperative when a vascular injury is suspected. If vascular injury is confirmed, surgical intervention may be necessary. This involves following steps:

1. *Debridement:* All the necrotic or damaged tissue is removed.
2. *Repair:* End-to-end anastomosis is done to restore blood flow.
3. *Reconstruction:* In cases of severe injury, more complex procedures like grafting may be required to reconstruct the damaged vessel.

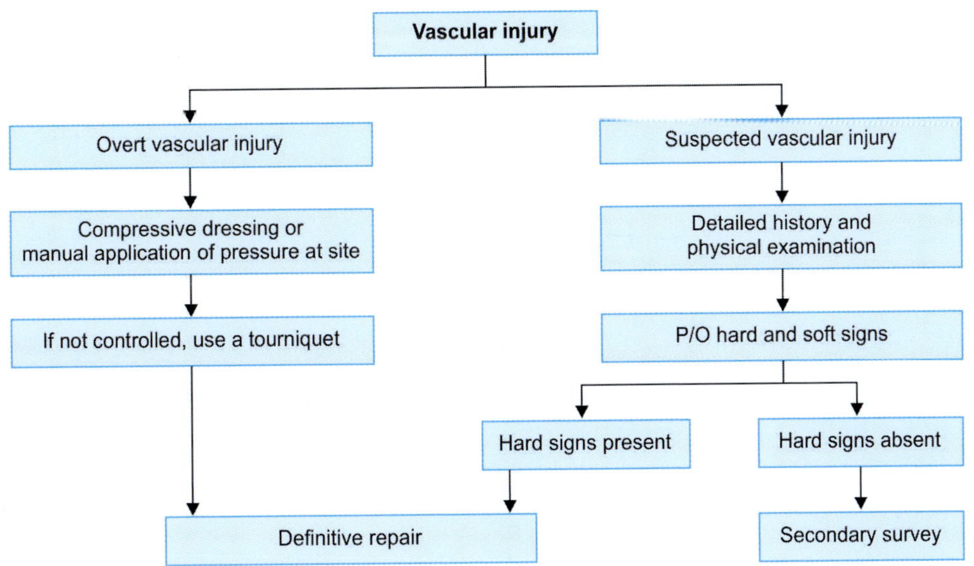

FLOWCHART 1: Vascular injury treatment.

Looking for Compartment Syndrome

Monitor for signs of compartment syndrome. Symptoms include severe pain, decreased sensation, and muscle weakness. Management involves immediate fasciotomy to relieve pressure and restore perfusion to the affected area.

Anticoagulation and Thromboprophylaxis

When a vascular repair is done, anticoagulant therapy is necessary to prevent any thromboembolic events. This should be carefully managed to balance the risk of bleeding with the benefits of preventing clot formation.

In cases of severe traumatic vascular injuries, one must decide whether the limb can be saved or not. There are various scoring systems that have been created to predict whether limb is salvageable limb. These include the Mangled Extremity Severity Score (MESS described in Chapter 15.2 in this book), Limb Salvage Index, Predictive Salvage Index, etc.

The MESS is probably the most used and known score and consists of various parameters (injury, limb ischemia shock, age, and time since trauma) which are used to determine whether an amputation is needed or not. Score ≤ 6 indicates revascularization can be done whereas score of 7 or more would require an amputation. However, in studies with larger sample size, these scoring systems have failed to prove effective in predicting the need for amputation.

BIBLIOGRAPHY

1. Feliciano DV, Moore FA, Moore EE, West MA, Davis JW, Cocanour CS, et al. Evaluation and management of peripheral vascular injury. Part 1. Western Trauma Association/critical decisions in trauma. J Trauma. 2011;70(6):1551-6.
2. Fox N, Rajani RR, Bokhari F, Chiu WC, Kerwin A, Seamon MJ, et al., Eastern Association for the Surgery of Trauma. Evaluation and management of penetrating lower extremity arterial trauma: an Eastern Association for the Surgery of Trauma practice management guideline. J Trauma Acute Care Surg. 2012;73(5 Suppl 4):S315-20.
3. Lebowitz C, Matzon JL. Arterial Injury in the Upper Extremity: Evaluation, Strategies, and Anticoagulation Management. Hand Clin. 2018;34(1):85-95.
4. Miller-Thomas MM, West OC, Cohen AM. Diagnosing traumatic arterial injury in the extremities with CT angiography: pearls and pitfalls. Radiographics. 2005;25(Suppl 1):S133-42.

Compartment Syndrome

Pardeep Singh

Compartment syndrome is a condition characterized by increased pressure within a confined anatomical space, or compartment, which compromises the function and viability of the muscles and nerves within that space. It can occur in any compartment of the body but is most commonly seen in the limbs, particularly the lower leg and forearm. It is an orthopedic emergency and needs urgent attention and treatment.

- Conservative treatment is ineffective, fasciotomy should be performed urgently.

ANATOMY OF COMPARTMENT SYNDROME

The human limbs are divided into several compartments, each surrounded by a tough and inelastic fascia. These compartments contain muscles, nerves, and blood vessels. The fascias are relatively rigid and do not stretch, so any increase in pressure within the compartment can lead to reduced blood flow, ischemia (lack of blood supply), and potential tissue damage.

- The most common compartments affected by compartment syndrome include:
  - Leg (osteofascial)
  - Forearm (osteofascial)
  - Hand (osteofascial)—the carpal tunnel is a separate compartment.
  - Foot (osteofascial)
  - Thigh (osteofascial/fascial)—three compartments, anterior (quadriceps), posterior (hamstrings and the adductor groups)
  - Upper arm—three compartments, the deltoid, the posterior (the triceps), and the anterior (biceps-brachialis)
  - Buttock (fascial)—gluteal muscles
  - Shoulder (fascial)
  - Paraspinal muscles (fascial)

TIMEFRAME

- The golden period is often considered to be within 6 *hours* of the onset of compartment syndrome.
- *Critical threshold:* Beyond this timeframe, the risk of irreversible muscle and nerve damage increases significantly. Prompt intervention within this period can help to prevent severe outcomes. *The best time to act, however, is at the time of impending compartment syndrome.*

Factors Influencing the Golden Period

- *Severity of pressure elevation*:
  - Higher pressures and longer durations of elevated pressure increase the risk of severe complications.
  - Mild pressure elevation may have a slightly extended golden period compared to severe cases.
- *Patient's factors*:
  - Younger patients may have better tissue resilience and a potentially

longer golden period compared to older individuals.
  - Patients with pre-existing conditions such as diabetes or peripheral vascular disease may experience quicker deterioration.
- *Nature of the injury*: The severity of trauma and the extent of initial injury can impact the length of the golden period. For example, crush injuries may lead to a shorter golden period due to more immediate and severe pressure effects.
- *Treatment response*: The effectiveness of initial conservative measures (e.g., elevation and immobilization) can influence the golden period.

Causes: Compartment syndrome can arise from a variety of causes, which are generally categorized into acute and chronic forms:
- *Acute compartment syndrome:* This is an emergency condition often resulting from:
  - *Trauma:* Fractures, severe bruises, or crush injuries.
  - *Surgical complications:* Postoperative swelling or hematoma formation.
  - *Reperfusion injury:* After prolonged ischemia and subsequent restoration of blood flow.
  - *External pressure:* Tight bandages, casts, or prolonged immobilization.
  - *Vascular disorders:* Conditions affecting blood flow to the compartments.
  - Burns
  - Intravenous infusion and accidental leakage.
- *Chronic compartment syndrome:* This typically develops gradually and is usually associated with:
  - *Exercise:* Particularly in activities involving repetitive muscle use, such as running or weightlifting. It is also known as exertional compartment syndrome.
  - *Overuse:* Chronic repetitive stress or overuse of the affected muscles.

Signs and symptoms: The presentation of compartment syndrome can vary but generally includes the *"Five P's"* are classic clinical signs used to identify compartment syndrome:
1. *Pain:*
   - Pain out of proportion is the pathognomic feature of compartment syndrome.
   - *Characteristics:* Severe and unrelenting pain that is disproportionate to the level of injury or trauma. Pain may worsen with passive stretching of the affected muscles.
   - *Onset:* Pain can be early and intense, often described as a deep ache or throbbing. It is persistent and may not respond well to standard analgesics.
2. *Pallor:*
   - *Characteristics:* The affected limb may appear pale or have a diminished color compared to the unaffected limb. This occurs due to reduced blood flow and possible ischemia.
   - *Onset:* Pallor is often observed in later stages of compartment syndrome, especially if the condition has progressed and resulted in significant tissue damage.
3. *Pulselessness:* It is a late sign and typically suggests severe and potentially irreversible compartment syndrome.
4. *Paralysis:* Paralysis or severe weakness is often a sign of significant nerve damage and is usually observed in more advanced cases.
5. *Paresthesia:* Abnormal sensations such as tingling, burning, or numbness in the affected limb. This occurs due to nerve compression or damage.
   - *Onset:* Paresthesia can be an early warning sign and often precedes more severe symptoms like paralysis or pulselessness.

Diagnosis: Diagnosing compartment syndrome involves a combination of clinical examination and, when necessary, measuring intracompartmental pressure. Methods include:

- *Clinical evaluation:* Careful assessment of symptoms, history, and physical examination findings.
    - *Intracompartmental pressure measurement:* This is the most definitive diagnostic tool and involves using a pressure monitor inserted into the compartment.
    - *Direct measurement using a manometer*
        - Procedure:
            - A needle or catheter is inserted into the compartment, and a pressure gauge (manometer) measures the pressure.
            - The most common sites for measurement include the anterior compartment of the leg or the forearm.
        - *Technique:* The procedure is often performed under sterile conditions, sometimes with local anesthesia. Measurements are taken at multiple points within the compartment to ensure accuracy.
    - *Indirect measurement*
        - *Device-based methods:* Devices such as the Stryker™ intracompartmental pressure monitor or other electronic sensors can be used to measure pressure noninvasively.
        - These methods are less commonly used but may offer advantages in certain clinical settings.
- *Intracompartmental pressure thresholds*:
    - Generally, a pressure of 30 mm Hg or higher is suggestive of compartment syndrome. However, thresholds can vary based on clinical guidelines and the specific situation.
    - *Differential pressures:* Sometimes, the pressure gradient between the compartment and the diastolic blood pressure is used, with a difference of 30 mm Hg or more indicating a problem.
- *Imaging:* While not primarily diagnostic, imaging (e.g., X-rays, USG, US-color Doppler) can help to identify underlying causes such as fractures or bleeding.

Treatment: Immediate treatment is crucial to prevent irreversible damage. Management strategies include:

- Immediately provide oxygen by mask, correct any hypotension, and remove the circumferential bandages. Splitting of cast reduces pressure by 30% which increases to 65% if the cast is split and spread. Complete splitting and padding the cast adds 10% to relieve pressure, and complete removal adds another 15%. There could be a total of 85–90% reduction, if the cast is fully removed.
- *Elevation of limb:* The limb should not be elevated above the heart level as this reduces the mean pressure but not the compartment pressure.
- *Surgical intervention:* The definitive treatment for acute compartment syndrome is fasciotomy, a surgical procedure that involves cutting open the fascia to relieve pressure. Timely intervention is critical to prevent long-term damage or loss of function.

INDICATIONS FOR FASCIOTOMY

Clinical Symptoms

- *Classic signs:* Severe pain that is disproportionate to the injury, pallor, pulselessness, paralysis, and paresthesia.
- *Unrelenting pain:* Pain that worsens with passive stretching of the affected muscles.

Elevated Intracompartmental Pressure

- *Measurement:* Intracompartmental pressure exceeding 30 mm Hg or a pressure gradient (difference between compartmental pressure and diastolic blood pressure) > 30 mm Hg.
- *Failure of conservative measures:* If initial conservative treatments such as elevation

and pain management are insufficient to alleviate symptoms.

Progressive Symptoms

Worsening condition: If symptoms progress despite nonsurgical management, this indicates that surgical intervention is necessary to prevent permanent damage.

SURGICAL TECHNIQUE

- *Forearm decompression*: The volar curvilinear approach of Henry and the dorsal approach.
- *Decompression of leg*: The two-incision techniques of Mubarak et al. are preferred compared to single incision.
    - Single-incision technique of Matsen et al.
- *Foot decompression*:
    - Dorsal—two incisions, overlying the second and fourth metatarsals are the gold standard.
    - Medial—one incision, along the inferior border of the first metatarsal, but superior to the abductor muscle.
    - Calcaneal (uncommonly used)—one incision, beginning medially, from the inferior border of the posterior tuberosity extending toward the inferior surface of the first metatarsal.

Compartment Syndrome of the Hand

- *Dorsal approach:* This is often preferred for the dorsal compartments as it provides access to multiple compartments at once. It involves making an incision along the dorsum of the hand to release the interosseous and adductor compartments.
- *Volar approach:* For volar compartments, an incision along the volar aspect of the hand (sometimes the radial or ulnar side) is used to decompress the thenar and hypothenar compartments.
- *Carpal tunnel release:* If there is involvement of the carpal tunnel (median nerve compression), a separate incision to release the transverse carpal ligament is typically performed.

Wound Management

- *Initial wound management:* The fasciotomy wound is often left open initially to accommodate swelling and prevent further complications. A sterile dressing or temporary closure device may be used.
- *Delayed closure:* Once the swelling has subsided and the risk of infection has been managed, the wound is usually closed at a later stage. This may involve secondary suturing, skin grafts, or flap coverage.

Complications of Fasciotomy

- Infection
- Delayed wound healing
- Functional impairment
- Recurrence

Complications of the Compartment Syndrome

Muscle necrosis: Permanent damage to the muscle tissue due to prolonged ischemia can lead to permanent functional damage.

- *Kidney damage:* Rhabdomyolysis (breakdown of muscle tissue) can lead to kidney damage and systemic complications.

PROGNOSIS

The outcome of compartment syndrome largely depends on the timeliness of treatment. Early diagnosis and intervention generally lead to a better prognosis and functional recovery. Delayed treatment may result in significant muscle and nerve damage, affecting the overall functional outcome **(Flowchart 1)**.

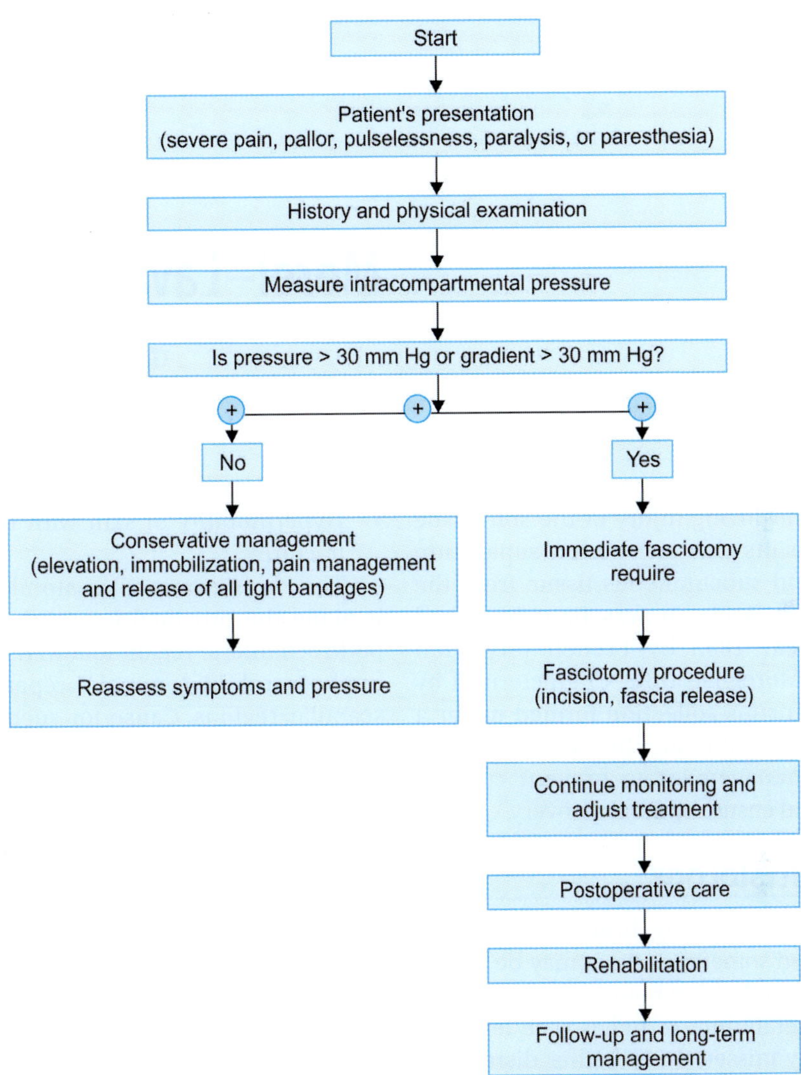

FLOWCHART 1: Showing an algorithm-based approach to the management of compartment syndrome.

BIBLIOGRAPHY

1. Matsen FA, Winquist RA, Krugmire RB. Diagnosis and management of compartmental syndromes. J Bone Joint Surg. 1980;62(2):286-91.
2. McQueen MM, Duckworth AD. Acute Compartment Syndrome. Br J Surg. 2024;111(5):295-302.
3. Mortensen SJ, Vora MM, Mohamadi A, Wright CL, Hanna P, Lechtig A, et al. Diagnostic Modalities for Acute Compartment Syndrome of the Extremities: A Systematic Review. JAMA Surg. 2019;154(7):655-65.
4. Mubarak SJ, Pedowitz RA, Hargens AR. Compartment syndromes. Curr Orthoped. 1989;3:36-40.
5. Pertsikapa M, Fyntanidou B, Limnaios P, Sidiropoulou T. Trauma Patients and Acute Compartment Syndrome: Is There an Ariadne's Thread That Can Safely Guide the Anesthesiologist/Emergency Physician Out of the Labyrinth? Medicina. 2024;60(8):1279.

Morel–Lavallée Lesion

Gagandeep Singh Raina

The Morel–Lavallée lesion is described as a closed degloving injury of the soft tissue which results due to sudden separation of skin and subcutaneous tissue from the underlying fascia. It was first described in the year 1853 by French physician Maurice Morel–Lavallée. Characterized by a subcutaneous collection formed under a necrotic layer of tissue, this lesion requires precise management to prevent complications and ensure optimal recovery.

PATHOPHYSIOLOGY

Generally caused by blunt high-energy trauma and sometimes there may be a fracture of the underlying bony like the proximal femur, acetabulum or pelvis. The lesion is commonly missed due to other distracting injuries like fractures. However, early identification is important as these lesions are a risk factor for infection of surgical site. It results due to the disruption of capillaries resulting in an effusion containing hemolymph and necrotic fat which sets off a chronic inflammatory reaction that results in the formation of a fibrous capsule encapsulating a lesion filled with blood components, fibrin, debris, and necrotic fatty tissue.

Symptoms

The lesion may present with:
- Soft-tissue swelling
- Multiple bruises
- Fluctuant and compressible swelling
- Hypermobility of skin with underlying fracture

The most common anatomic location is along the proximal lateral thigh, in the peritrochanteric region followed by gluteal, lumbosacral, abdominal, prepatellar, and scapular regions. Cause for such locations is the presence of hypermobile skin in these regions.

DIAGNOSIS

The diagnosis is usually made on clinical history and physical examination.

Imaging Studies

Plain radiograph: Morel–Lavellée lesion is not seen on a plain X-ray, but a radiograph is done to rule out any underlying fracture.

Ultrasound: USG can quickly assess the extent of the hematoma and the relationship between necrotic and viable tissue. It is predominantly echogenic in the acute phase, becoming more hypoechoic as blood products liquefy over time. A capsule of variable thickness may be seen.

CT scan (rarely used): Provides detailed cross-sectional imaging, useful for assessing deeper structures and guiding surgical planning.

MRI (rarely needed): It is able to clearly determine the relationship of the collection

TABLE 1: Six types of lesions.

Type	Shape	Description	T1W	T2W	Capsule	Enhancement
1	Laminar	Seroma like	Decreased	Increased	Occasional	Absent
2	Oval	Hematoma like	Increased	Increased	Thick	Variable
3	Oval	Chronic organizing	Intermediate	Heterogeneous	Thick	Internal and peripheral
4	Linear	Closed laceration	Hypointense	Hyperintense	Absent	Variable
5	Round	Pseudonodular	Variable	Variable	Thin or thick	Internal and peripheral
6	Variable	Infected ± sinus tract	Variable	Variable	Thick	Internal and peripheral

with the underlying fascia. The fluid is of variable signal intensity depending on makeup and may even show a fluid-fluid level.

Mellado and Bencardino **(Table 1)** gave a classification which was based on various characteristics of the lesion and as per this classification six types of lesions of Morel-Lavallée lesions are described.

Other post-traumatic injuries must be ruled out before establishing the diagnosis. This includes fat necrosis, hematoma due to coagulopathy, and early-stage myositis ossificans with diffuse subcutaneous edema which is very rare.

TREATMENT

Conservative Management

Compression is used for smaller lesions which are without a definite capsule. Percutaneous aspiration of the Morel-Lavallée lesion can also be done but the rate of recurrence is high. The presence of a capsule is a contraindication for conservative or percutaneous treatment, thus leading to recurrence if not managed surgically.

Sclerodesis can be used successfully in Morel-Lavallée lesions, especially in cases where percutaneous aspiration fails. *Commonly used sclerosing agents include doxycycline, tetracycline, vancomycin, erythromycin, absolute ethanol, and talc.* It acts by destruction within the periphery of the lesion, which causes fibrosis. The efficacy of sclerodesis has been reported as 95.7%.

Doxycycline

- *Dose:* 500 mg mixed with 10–20 mL of saline or sterile water, depending on the lesion volume.
- *Administration:* Injected directly into the lesion cavity after drainage, sometimes left in for a short time, then removed. Compression bandaging follows.

Polidocanol

- *Dose:* Typically, a 1–3% solution; the volume injected should generally match the volume of the aspirated fluid.
- *Administration:* Injected under ultrasound guidance. Some clinicians use around 10–20 mL per session, depending on lesion size.

Ethanol (Absolute Alcohol)

- *Dose:* 5–10 mL of absolute ethanol per 10 mL of aspirated fluid, depending on lesion size.
- *Administration:* Injected into the cavity for about 5–10 minutes before being aspirated. This technique requires close monitoring due to the risk of tissue necrosis and pain.

Talc

- *Dose:* 2–5 g of sterile talc, mixed into a suspension with saline.
- *Administration:* Injected into the cavity, ideally under image guidance. This method may be reserved for larger or recurrent lesions.

Tetracycline

- *Dose:* 500 mg mixed with 10–20 mL of saline or sterile water.
- *Administration:* Injected into the cavity after drainage, similar to doxycycline. Compression is recommended afterward to enhance efficacy.

Surgical Management

This includes a long single incision or multiple small incisions at the proximal and distal part of the lesion followed by curettage and removal of the fibrous capsule and placement of suction drains in cases where the overlying skin is viable. In cases with necrotic skin, the lesion needs to be debrided, followed by reconstruction of the soft-tissue envelope.

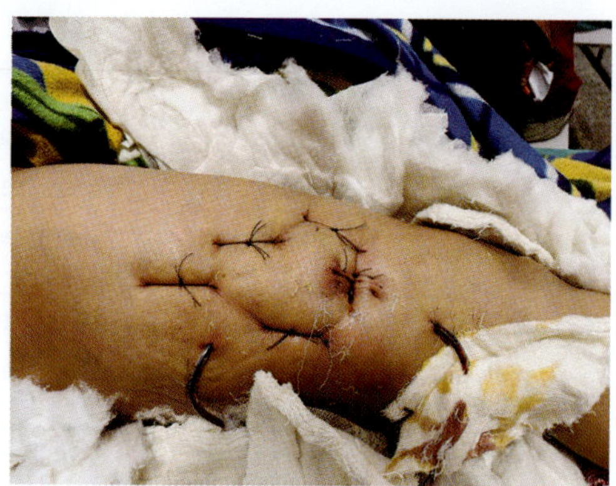

FIG. 1: Quilting suture.

The end goal in the management of Morel-Lavallée lesions is the closure of dead space within the lesion and this can be achieved in multiple ways using *a fibrin sealant, quilting sutures **(Fig. 1)** or low suction drains.*

Rehabilitation: Physical therapy may be necessary to regain function and mobility, especially if the lesion affects a joint or limb.

Follow-up: Regular follow-up appointments are crucial to monitor for complications, such as recurrence, infection, or wound dehiscence. Ongoing assessment ensures timely intervention if problems arise.

BIBLIOGRAPHY

1. Carlson DA, Simmons J, Sando W, Weber T, Clements B. Morel-lavalée lesions treated with debridement and meticulous dead space closure: surgical technique. J Orthop Trauma. 2007;21(2):140-4.
2. Gilbert BC, Bui-Mansfield LT, Dejong S. MRI of a Morel-Lavallee Lesion. AJR Am J Roentgenol. 2004;182:1347-8.
3. Hak DJ, Olson SA, Matta JM. Diagnosis and management of closed internal degloving injuries associated with pelvic and acetabular fractures: The Morel-Lavallée lesion. J Trauma. 1997;42:1046-51.
4. Harma A, Inan M, Ertem K. The Morel-Lavallee lesion: A conservative approach to closed degloving injuries. Acta Orthop Traumatol Turc. 2004;38:270-3.
5. Haydon N, Zoumaras J. Surgical management of Morel–Lavallée lesion. Eplasty. 2015;15:ic14.
6. Kottmeier SA, Wilson SC, Born CT, Hanks GA, Iannacone WM, Delong WG. Surgical management of soft tissue lesions associated with pelvic ring injury. Clin Orthop Relat Res. 1996;329:46-53.
7. Letournel E, Judet R. Fractures of the acetabulum, 2nd edition. Berlin, Germany: Springer-Verlag; 1993.
8. Mallado JM, Bencardino JT. Morel-Lavellée lesion: Review with Emphasis on MR imaging. Magn Reson Imaging Clin North Am. 2005;13:775-82.
9. Nair AV, Nazar P, Sekhar R, Ramachandran P, Moorthy S. Morel-Lavallée lesion: A closed degloving injury that requires real attention. Indian J Radiol Imaging. 2014;24(3):288-90.
10. Shen C, Peng JP, Chen XD. Efficacy of treatment in peri-pelvic Morel-Lavallee lesion: a systematic review of the literature. Arch Orthop Trauma Surg. 2013;133(5):635-40.

CHAPTER 17.5

Fat Embolism Syndrome

Anita Kour

Fat embolism syndrome (FES) is a sudden respiratory condition caused by the entry of fat and marrow particles into the bloodstream, which triggers an inflammatory reaction. The first documentation of fat embolism was in 1862 by Zenker, and Von Bergmann clinically diagnosed it in 1873. FES commonly occurs in patients with trauma, especially those with orthopedic injuries. However, fat embolism has also been reported in nonorthopedic trauma cases such as burns, lung transplants, and liposuction.

CLINICAL SIGNS AND SYMPTOMS

- *Respiratory system*: Dyspnea, ARDS (acute respiratory distress syndrome), and tachypnea
- *Neurological*: Altered sensorium, restlessness, focal neurological deficits, decreased level of consciousness
- *Cardiovascular*: Tachycardia, hypotension, myocardial ischemia, heart failure, arrythmias
- *Systemic*: Fever
- *Skin*: Petechial rash
- *Eye*: Retinopathy

The majority of patients with FES experience respiratory depression, with pulmonary circulation being the most commonly affected, affecting up to 75% of cases.

RADIOLOGICAL IMAGING FINDINGS IN FAT EMBOLISM SYNDROME

- *Chest X-ray*: Pulmonary edema, diffuse interstitial infiltrates
- *Chest CT scan*: Diffuse areas with pulmonary edema and congestion, patchy ground glass opacities, small bilateral pleural effusion
- *Cerebral MRI (for cerebral fat embolism)*: Bright spots on a dark background and microbleeding

The presence of elevated biological markers such as lipase, free fatty acids, and phospholipase A2 has been observed in patients with FES. It is essential to note that this increase is not unique to lung injury patients. Additionally, microscopic examination of blood, urine, or sputum can provide valuable insights.

DIAGNOSTIC CRITERIA

Guard and Wilson's Criteria

Major criteria:

- Respiratory distress
- Cerebral symptoms in nonhead injury patients
- Petechial rash

Minor criteria:

- Tachycardia (>110 bpm)
- Fever (>38.5°C)

- Jaundice
- Renal changes
- Drop in hemoglobin
- New onset of thrombocytopenia
- Elevated erythrocyte sedimentation rate (ESR)
- Fat microglobulinemia

Two major criteria or one major and four minor criteria is a diagnosis of FES.

Other diagnostic criteria include Schonfeld's scoring system and Lindeque's criteria. There detail description is beyond the scope of this chapter.

TREATMENT

The treatment of FES focuses on supportive care and preventing complications, as there is no specific cure.

Supportive Care (Primary Treatment)

- *Oxygen therapy:* Initial treatment often involves oxygen via nasal cannula or face mask to improve oxygenation. Severe cases may require mechanical ventilation with positive end-expiratory pressure (PEEP) to maintain adequate oxygen levels and support respiratory function.
- *Fluid management:* Fluid resuscitation is essential to maintain hemodynamic stability. However, avoid over-resuscitation to prevent worsening pulmonary edema, which could exacerbate respiratory complications.
- *Hemodynamic monitoring:* Regular monitoring of vital signs, blood gases, and hematocrit levels is crucial to assess the patient's status and tailor interventions accordingly.

Pharmacologic Interventions

- *Corticosteroids:* While the role of corticosteroids remains controversial, they may help to reduce inflammation and stabilize capillary membranes, potentially minimizing the severity of FES. Dosing and timing are still debated, with early administration typically considered more effective.
- *Anticoagulation:* This is generally avoided in FES unless indicated for other reasons, as there is no evidence it prevents or treats fat emboli.

Early Fracture Stabilization

Stabilizing long bone fractures as soon as feasible (usually within the first 24 hours) can decrease the release of fat emboli into circulation. Techniques include external fixation or internal fixation, depending on the case specifics and patient's stability.

Symptom-specific Treatments

- *Respiratory support:* Patients with significant hypoxemia may need ventilatory support. Positive pressure ventilation [such as continuous positive airway pressure (CPAP) or bilateral positive airway pressure (BiPAP)] or intubation with mechanical ventilation can help those with severe respiratory distress.
- *Neurological monitoring:* FES may cause confusion, agitation, or seizures. Neurological monitoring is essential, especially in patients with head trauma, as these symptoms can overlap with traumatic brain injury.

Prevention in High-risk Cases

Prophylactic corticosteroids are sometimes considered for patients with high-risk fractures, though this practice is still under study.

Nutritional Support

- Providing nutritional support helps to manage metabolic demands, which is vital in trauma patients.

Since there is no definitive cure, managing FES hinges on early recognition, supportive care, and minimizing complications. Prompt stabilization of fractures and addressing hypoxia are the core elements.

It is advisable to promptly perform surgical fixation for long-bone fractures to reduce the likelihood of FES. Manipulation of the fracture ends before surgical fixation can cause a temporary release of fat emboli. Patients undergoing nonsurgical treatment have consistently elevated levels of cytokines, which return to beeline levels after surgical fixation. Research has shown that immediate fixation results in a 7% occurrence of ARDS, while delayed fixation by >24 hours is associated with a 39% incidence of ARDS.

During operative fixation, increased intramedullary pressure can result in more fat emboli entering the circulation. Care should be taken to limit intramedullary pressure during operative fixation. Although reaming may elevate intramedullary pressure, it has not been linked to an increased incidence of FES.

Various surgical techniques, such as drilling holes in the cortex, lavaging bone marrow, using a bone vacuum, and employing tourniquets, have been tested to reduce embolization, but none have definitively been shown to decrease FES.

BIBLIOGRAPHY

1. Burger LW, Dines DE, Linscheid RL. Fat embolism syndrome and the adult respiratory distress syndrome. Mayo Clinic Proc. 1974;49:107-9.
2. Chastre J, Fagon JY, Soler P, Fichelle A, Dombret MC, Huten D, et al. Bronchoalveolar lavage for rapid diagnosis of the fat embolism syndrome in trauma patients. Ann Intern Med. 1990;113:583-8.
3. E Von Bergmann. Ein fall todlicher fettembolie. Berliner Klinische Wochenschrift;1873.
4. Johnson KD, Cadambi A, Seibert GB. Incidence of adult respiratory distress in patients with multiple musculoskeletal injuries: Effect of early operative stabilization of fractures. J Trauma. 1985;25:375-84.
5. Mimoz O, Edouard A, Beydon L, Quillard J, Verra F, Fleury J, et al. Contribution of bronchoalveolar lavage to the diagnosis of posttraumatic pulmonary fat embolism. Intensive Care Med. 1995;21:973-80.
6. Vedrinne JM, Guillaume C, Gagnieu MC, Gratadour P, Fleuret C, Motin J. Bronchoalveolar lavage in trauma patients for diagnosis of fat embolism syndrome. Chest. 1992;102:1323-7.

CHAPTER 17.6

Complex Regional Pain Syndrome

Ankita Khajuria, Tahir Afzal

Complex regional pain syndrome (CRPS) is a severe and chronic pain condition characterized by disproportionate pain, sensory, motor, autonomic, and trophic disturbances, typically following trauma or surgery. The condition is divided into two subtypes: (1) CRPS-I (without confirmed nerve injury) and (2) CRPS-II (with confirmed nerve injury). CRPS poses significant challenges for orthopedic surgeons due to its unpredictable course, potential for disability, and multifactorial pathophysiology. Early recognition and comprehensive management are essential to prevent chronicity and optimize patient's outcomes.

PATHOPHYSIOLOGY

Complex regional pain syndrome involves a complex network of pathological mechanisms:

- *Neurogenic inflammation:* An exaggerated inflammatory response, mediated by the release of neuropeptides (e.g., substance P, calcitonin gene-related peptide) from primary afferent neurons, leads to vasodilation, increased vascular permeability, and neurogenic edema. This inflammatory cascade sensitizes nociceptors, resulting in hyperalgesia and allodynia.
- *Peripheral and central sensitization:* Peripheral sensitization is marked by heightened sensitivity of nociceptors to both painful and nonpainful stimuli, while central sensitization involves the abnormal amplification of pain signals in the spinal cord and brain. This process is driven by N-methyl-D-aspartate (NMDA) receptor activation, which lowers the pain threshold and perpetuates chronic pain.
- *Autonomic dysregulation:* Dysfunction of the sympathetic nervous system may manifest as altered blood flow, sweating abnormalities, and temperature changes. This dysregulation contributes to the hallmark vasomotor and sudomotor symptoms of CRPS.
- *Immune system involvement:* Recent studies suggest the involvement of autoantibodies and an exaggerated immune response, indicating that CRPS may have an autoimmune component. Elevated levels of proinflammatory cytokines [e.g., tumor necrosis factor-alpha (TNF-α) and interleukin (IL)-6] and mast cell activation have been implicated in sustaining pain and inflammation.

DIAGNOSIS

Complex regional pain syndrome is primarily a clinical diagnosis based on the Budapest criteria, which require:

1. Continuing pain disproportionate to any inciting event.

2. Presence of at least one symptom in three of the following four categories:
   i. *Sensory:* Hyperesthesia or allodynia.
   ii. *Vasomotor:* Temperature asymmetry, skin color changes, or asymmetry.
   iii. *Sudomotor/Edema:* Edema, sweating changes, or asymmetry.
   iv. *Motor/Trophic:* Decreased range of motion, motor dysfunction (weakness, tremor, and dystonia), or trophic changes (hair, nail, and skin).
3. At least one sign in two or more of the above categories during clinical examination.
4. No other diagnosis that better explains the signs and symptoms.

MANAGEMENT

Effective management of CRPS requires a multimodal and multidisciplinary approach tailored to the individual patient's presentation and disease stage. The primary goals are to relieve pain, restore function, and improve quality of life.

Pharmacological Management

- *Nonsteroidal anti-inflammatory drugs (NSAIDs):* Useful in the early stages to manage mild pain and inflammation. While NSAIDs can provide initial relief, their role is limited in long-term management.
- *Anticonvulsants and antidepressants:* Agents such as gabapentin, pregabalin (anticonvulsants), and tricyclic antidepressants (e.g., amitriptyline) or serotonin-norepinephrine reuptake inhibitors (SNRIs, such as duloxetine) are considered first-line for neuropathic pain. They reduce pain by modulating pain pathways and diminishing central sensitization.
- *Corticosteroids:* Short courses of corticosteroids (e.g., prednisolone) are effective in the early inflammatory phase of CRPS. They help to reduce inflammation, edema, and pain, particularly in the first few months of disease onset. Long-term use should be avoided due to potential side effects.
- *Bisphosphonates:* Bisphosphonates, such as alendronate and pamidronate, have shown efficacy in CRPS by reducing bone resorption and pain. Recent clinical trials suggest that they may be particularly beneficial in cases with osteoporotic changes or severe pain.
- *Topical analgesics:* Capsaicin patches and topical lidocaine can provide localized pain relief. Capsaicin works by depleting substance P, a neuropeptide involved in pain transmission, while lidocaine stabilizes neuronal membranes and reduces ectopic discharges.
- *Ketamine infusions:* Low-dose intravenous ketamine, an NMDA receptor antagonist, is recommended for refractory CRPS. Ketamine infusions have been shown to reduce pain intensity by blocking central sensitization. This should be administered under specialist supervision due to potential side effects, such as hallucinations and liver toxicity.
- *Opioids:* Use of opioids is generally discouraged due to the risk of dependency and the limited evidence of efficacy in neuropathic pain. However, they may be considered in carefully selected cases where other modalities have failed.

Nonpharmacological Management

- *Physical therapy and rehabilitation:* Early and sustained physical therapy is vital to prevent contractures, improve range of motion, and restore function. Techniques such as graded motor imagery, mirror therapy, and desensitization exercises can reduce pain and improve motor function. A progressive, patient-specific rehabilitation plan is essential to avoid pain exacerbation.

- *Occupational therapy:* Focuses on improving activities of daily living and enhancing the patient's functional capacity. It includes adaptive strategies, assistive devices, and ergonomic modifications to reduce pain and maximize independence.
- *Psychological interventions:* Psychological support, including cognitive-behavioral therapy (CBT), is crucial in addressing the emotional and psychological impact of CRPS. This can help to manage anxiety, depression, and pain-related fear-avoidance behaviors.
- *Interventional pain management:*
  - *Sympathetic nerve blocks:* Stellate ganglion blocks (upper extremity CRPS) or lumbar sympathetic blocks (lower extremity CRPS) can provide diagnostic and therapeutic relief. Although the effects may be temporary, these blocks can be useful in a subset of patients, particularly when there is significant autonomic dysfunction.
  - *Spinal cord stimulation (SCS):* SCS is an established modality for managing refractory CRPS. Multiple studies and randomized controlled trials have demonstrated significant pain reduction and functional improvement with SCS. It should be considered when conservative measures fail.
  - *Intrathecal drug delivery systems:* Intrathecal pumps delivering opioids, baclofen, or clonidine are reserved for severe, refractory cases where other treatments are ineffective. These systems provide targeted pain relief with lower systemic drug exposure.

Emerging Therapies

- *Neuromodulation techniques:* Noninvasive brain stimulation techniques such as repetitive transcranial magnetic stimulation (rTMS) and transcranial direct current stimulation (tDCS) are being investigated for CRPS. These techniques aim to modulate pain pathways and neuroplastic changes associated with chronic pain.
- *Immunomodulatory therapies:* Given the potential autoimmune component of CRPS, therapies such as intravenous immunoglobulin (IVIG) and monoclonal antibodies against proinflammatory cytokines (e.g., TNF inhibitors) are being explored in clinical trials.
- *Virtual reality (VR) therapy:* VR is emerging as a novel therapy for pain modulation and rehabilitation in CRPS. VR-based interventions focus on mirror therapy principles, distraction techniques, and graded exposure therapy to manage pain and improve function.

BIBLIOGRAPHY

1. Birklein F, Dimova V. Complex Regional Pain Syndrome–Up-to-Date. Pain Rep. 2017;2(6):e624.
2. Goebel A, Barker C, Turner-Stokes L. Complex Regional Pain Syndrome in Adults: UK Guidelines for Diagnosis, Referral, and Management in Primary and Secondary Care. London: Royal College of Physicians; 2018.
3. Harden RN, Oaklander AL, Burton AW, Perez RS, Richardson K, Swan M, et al. Complex Regional Pain Syndrome: Practical Diagnostic and Treatment Guidelines, 4th Edition. Pain Med. 2013;14(2):180-229.

CHAPTER 17.7

Malunion, Delayed Union and Nonunion

Ankita Khajuria

Malunion results when the normal anatomical alignment of a bone is not restored during the healing process. This can occur due to several factors, such as inadequate reduction (alignment of the fracture ends), suboptimal fixation (insufficient stability during healing), or premature removal of immobilization devices. Malunion can also result from biological factors, such as delayed or impaired bone healing due to inadequate blood supply, infection, or systemic conditions affecting bone metabolism.

The deformity resulting from malunion can be characterized by several dimensions: *Angular deformity, rotational deformity, shortening, and translation*—when there is lateral or anterior/posterior displacement of the bone fragments.

DIAGNOSIS OF MALUNION

Diagnosing malunion involves a thorough clinical examination and imaging studies:

- *Plain radiographs:* Standard X-rays in at least two orthogonal planes (anteroposterior and lateral) are the initial imaging modality of choice.
- *CT scans:* For complex fractures or malunions involving joints, CT provides detailed images that help in assessing the extent of deformity and planning surgical correction.
- *Three-dimensional (3D) reconstruction:* Advanced 3D reconstruction imaging can be helpful in preoperative planning, especially in complex deformities or when planning corrective osteotomy.
- *Magnetic resonance imaging (MRI)*: MRI is generally reserved for cases where there is a need to evaluate soft-tissue structures, including ligaments, tendons, and cartilage.

MANAGEMENT OF MALUNION

The management of malunion largely depends on the severity of the deformity, the symptom it causes, the bone involved, and the patient's functional demands and overall health status.

Nonsurgical management may be considered in cases where the deformity is mild, asymptomatic, or where the risks of surgery outweigh the potential benefits. Nonsurgical options include:

- *Physical therapy:* A tailored rehabilitation program focusing on improving strength, flexibility, and function may help to manage symptoms in patients with mild deformity or those not suitable for surgery.
- *Orthotics and bracing:* Custom orthotics or braces can be used to offload weight from the affected limb, provide support, or correct minor angular deformities. For

instance, shoe lifts may be employed to compensate for leg length discrepancy.

Surgical Management

Surgical intervention is often required for symptomatic malunion, especially if it causes significant pain, functional impairment, or aesthetic concerns. The goal of surgery is to restore the normal anatomy of the bone, correct deformities, and improve function. Surgical options include:

- *Corrective osteotomy:* The bone is then stabilized using internal fixation methods such as plates, screws, or intramedullary nails. The type and site of osteotomy depend on the location and type of deformity. For example, a closing wedge osteotomy may be used for an angular deformity, whereas a rotational osteotomy may be indicated for rotational malunions.
- *External fixation:* In cases where internal fixation is not possible or when there is a high risk of infection (e.g., in cases with poor soft-tissue coverage or compromised vascularity), external fixation may be used. External fixators can be adjusted postoperatively to gradually correct deformities.
- *Bone grafting:* If there is significant bone loss, bone grafting may be necessary. Autografts (bone harvested from the patient's body) or allografts (donor bone) can be used to fill the defect and promote healing.
- *Soft-tissue procedures:* In some cases, soft-tissue contractures or scarring may also need to be addressed to achieve optimal correction. This may involve releasing tight ligaments or tendons, removing scar tissue, or lengthening procedures.
- *Joint replacement surgery:* If the malunion has led to severe joint damage, such as posttraumatic arthritis, joint replacement (arthroplasty) may be considered, particularly for older patients or those with significant comorbidities.

DELAYED UNION OF FRACTURES

Delayed union refers to a fracture that takes an extended time to heal compared to typical bone healing timelines, without completely failing to heal (as in nonunion). In a delayed union, there is evidence of gradual bone repair, but the process is slower than anticipated. This can be influenced by various factors:

- *Blood supply:* Bones need an adequate blood supply for healing. When this supply is compromised—due to location (e.g., scaphoid or tibial shaft fractures), injury severity, or soft-tissue damage—the healing process slows down.
- *Stabilization:* Proper immobilization and stabilization are crucial. Inadequate fixation, such as from poorly fitted casts or unstable surgical implants, can allow excessive movement at the fracture site, hindering healing.
- *Patient-related factors:* Conditions such as smoking, diabetes, malnutrition, and use of corticosteroids are associated with delayed bone healing. Smoking, e.g., reduces blood flow to bone tissues, affecting their regenerative ability.

Diagnosis

Delayed union is often diagnosed through follow-up X-rays or other imaging, which reveals slow or insufficient callus (bone tissue) formation at the fracture site, compared to expected healing timelines.

Treatment Options

- *Improved fixation:* If poor stabilization is a factor, reinforcing or changing the fixation device (e.g., using plates or screws) may enhance healing.
- *Nutritional and lifestyle modifications:* Addressing nutrition, minimizing alcohol, and quitting smoking support healing. Supplementing with calcium and vitamin D may also be recommended.

- *Bone stimulators:* Electrical or ultrasound bone stimulators may be used to promote healing, especially in cases unresponsive to traditional methods.
- *Bone grafts or substitutes:* If healing remains insufficient, bone grafts or substitutes may be considered to encourage new bone formation.

With timely intervention, most delayed unions can progress to complete healing, though careful follow-up is essential to monitor and address potential complications, however, if not treated properly, delayed union can lead to nonunion of fractures.

FRACTURE NONUNION

Pathophysiology of Fracture Nonunion

The pathophysiology of fracture nonunion is multifactorial, involving a complex interplay of biological, mechanical, and systemic factors. The key factors contributing to nonunion include:

- *Mechanical factors:* Instability at the fracture site due to inadequate fixation, malalignment, or excessive motion can hinder the bone healing process. Hypertrophic nonunion is particularly associated with mechanical instability, where the biological potential for healing is present but mechanical conditions are unfavorable.
- *Biological factors:* Impaired vascularity, insufficient cellular activity, and inadequate inflammatory response can contribute to nonunion. Atrophic nonunion often results from compromised biological factors, such as poor blood supply, avascular necrosis, or soft-tissue damage.
- *Systemic factors:* Patient-related factors, such as advanced age, smoking, diabetes, malnutrition, and use of certain medications (e.g., nonsteroidal anti-inflammatory drugs), can adversely affect fracture healing.
- *Infection:* Infection at the fracture site, particularly in open fractures or following surgical fixation, is a significant risk factor for developing nonunion. Osteomyelitis can disrupt bone healing by altering the local environment and impairing cellular and vascular responses.

Classification of Nonunion

The classification of nonunion helps to guide treatment decisions by categorizing the condition based on various factors such as the biological and mechanical aspects of the nonunion **(Figs. 1A to G)**. Here is a detailed overview:

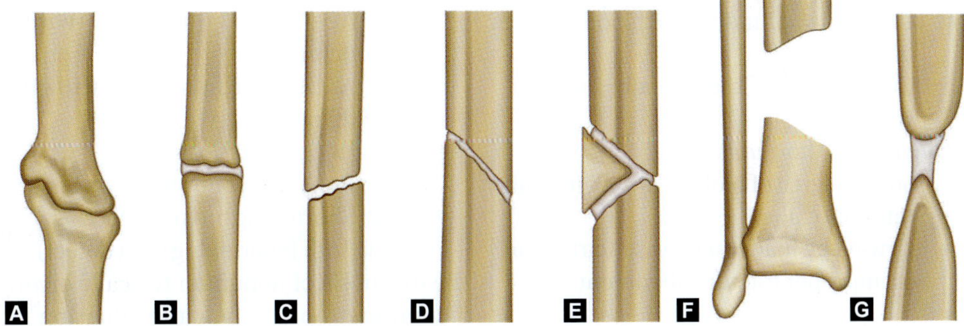

FIGS. 1A TO G: (A) Elephant foot; (B) Horsehoof; (C) Oligotrophic; (D) Torsion wedge; (E) Comminuted; (F) Gap; (G) Atrophic nonunions.

Based on Healing Status

Atrophic Nonunion

Characterized by a lack of significant bone formation and a gap filled with fibrous tissue.

- *Features:* Thin, dense, and often sclerotic edges of the fracture site with minimal callus formation.
- *Causes:* Typically, due to poor biological factors such as inadequate blood supply or infection.

Hypertrophic Nonunion

Involves excessive callus formation without adequate ossification.

- *Features:* Enlarged, well-vascularized, and often lumpy callus formation with a wide gap.
- *Causes:* Usually a result of inadequate mechanical stabilization or excessive movement at the fracture site.

Based on Cause

Biological Nonunion

Biological nonunion typically involves compromised healing potential of the bone due to factors like poor blood supply, infection, or cellular deficits.

Types of biological non-union:

- *Atrophic non-union:*
  - Minimal or no callus formation.
  - Bone ends are thin, sclerotic, and may be resorbed.
  - Often due to inadequate blood supply or infection.
  - Considered a "biologically inactive" state.
- *Oligotrophic non-union:*
  - Some degree of biological activity with minimal callus.
  - Caused by inadequate vascularization or improper fracture alignment.

Mechanical Nonunion

Due to mechanical factors.

- Mechanical nonunion can also be classified as simple and complex nonunion

Simple Nonunion

Characterized by a straightforward gap between the fractured ends with clear edges.

- *Features:* Simple appearance on X-rays or CT scans with a visible gap.

Complex Nonunion

Includes complications such as infection, malalignment, or additional fractures.

- *Features:* Complicated radiological findings with additional pathologies affecting the fracture site.

Based on Treatment History

Primary Nonunion

Occurs despite initial appropriate treatment.

- *Features:* May be related to inherent factors in the patient or fracture.

Secondary Nonunion

Develops after initial successful healing which subsequently fails.

- *Features:* These may involve complications such as hardware failure or reinjury.

  Paley classification of nonunion specifically deals with legs bones and is based on bone loss, fracture laxity, deformity and shortening **(Figs. 2A and B)**.
- *Type A (<1 cm bone loss):*
  - A1: Mobile deformity
  - A2: Fixed deformity
    - A2-I: Stiff nonunion without deformity
    - A2-II: Stiff nonunion with fixed deformity
- *Type B (>1 cm bone loss):*
  - B1: Bony defect no shortening
  - B2: Shortening but no defect
  - B3: Both (shortening with defect)

The diagnosis of nonunion typically involves a combination of clinical evaluation and imaging techniques. Clinically, patients with nonunion present with persistent pain, abnormal movement at the fracture site, and functional impairment.

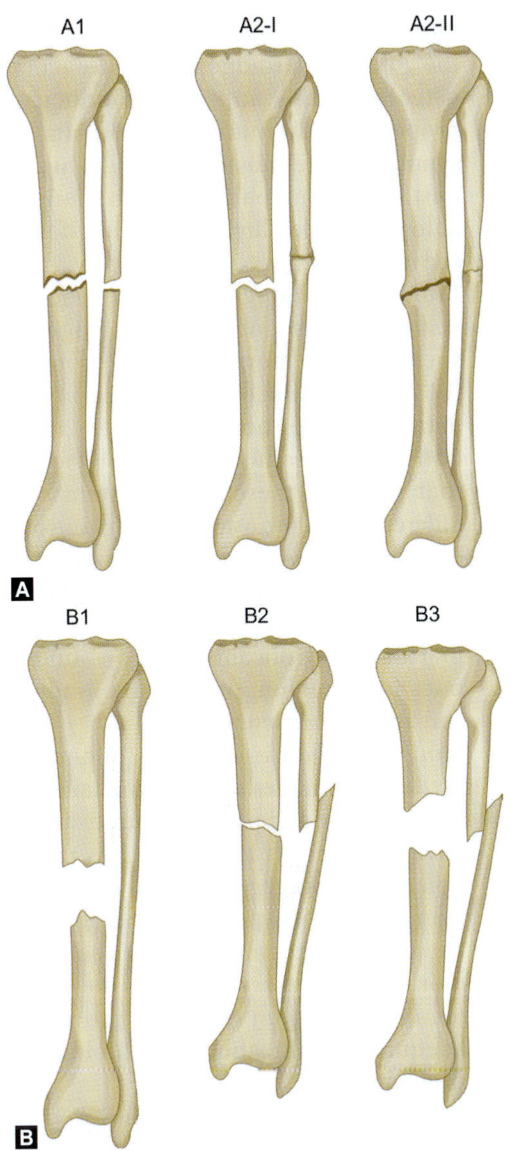

FIGS. 2A AND B: Paley classification of nonunion.

Radiographically, signs of nonunion include a lack of bridging callus on serial X-rays, a persistent fracture line, or the presence of pseudoarthrosis. Anteroposterior (AP) and lateral and oblique views and at times stress views such as valgus and varus views are necessary to confirm union or nonunion. In AP and lateral view at least three cortices need to be bridged before saying it is a united fracture. Advanced imaging modalities, such as CT and MRI, may be employed to assess bone healing, vascularity, and the presence of infection or soft-tissue involvement.

It is important to rule out infection both clinically as well as by having inflammatory markers and also to rule out any systemic modifiable cause of nonunion.

MANAGEMENT STRATEGIES FOR FRACTURE NONUNION

The management of fracture nonunion is guided by the type of nonunion, the patient's overall health, and the presence of any complicating factors such as infection or comorbidities. The primary objectives of management are to achieve bone union, restore limb function, and minimize complications. Current approaches to management can be broadly categorized into nonsurgical and surgical strategies.

Nonsurgical Management

Nonsurgical management is primarily considered in cases where the nonunion is stable, the patient is not a suitable candidate for surgery, or when the risks of surgery outweigh the benefits. Nonsurgical strategies include:

- *Extracorporeal shock wave therapy (ESWT):* ESWT can stimulate bone healing in cases of delayed union and nonunion, particularly hypertrophic nonunions. The mechanical stimulus provided by shock waves is believed to enhance local blood flow, stimulate osteoblast activity, and promote callus formation. According to a meta-analysis published in the Journal of Orthopedic Trauma (2023), ESWT demonstrated a union rate of approximately 70% in hypertrophic nonunions, making it a viable option for select patients.
- *Bone stimulation:* Electrical bone stimulation, including pulsed electromagnetic field (PEMF) therapy, low-intensity pulsed ultrasound (LIPUS), and direct current stimulation, has

been used to promote bone healing. A Cochrane review (2023) highlighted that PEMF therapy significantly improved healing rates in nonunions, particularly in patients who were poor candidates for surgery due to medical comorbidities.

- *Pharmacological agents:* Pharmacologic interventions, such as the use of bone anabolic agents like teriparatide (parathyroid hormone analog) and bisphosphonates, have been explored to enhance bone healing. Teriparatide has shown promise in small clinical trials, with evidence suggesting it may accelerate fracture healing in atrophic nonunions by stimulating osteoblast activity and increasing bone mineral density. However, larger randomized controlled trials are needed to establish definitive guidelines for its use in nonunion management.
- *Immobilization and offloading:* Prolonged immobilization and offloading using external braces, casts, or functional orthoses may be considered in select cases where surgery is contraindicated. However, this approach is generally less favored due to the prolonged duration required and the risk of joint stiffness, muscle atrophy, and further complications.

Surgical Management

Surgical intervention remains the gold standard for the treatment of nonunion, particularly in cases where nonsurgical methods have failed or are deemed inappropriate. The choice of surgical technique is guided by the type of nonunion, the bone involved, patient's factors, and the presence of infection. The primary surgical approaches include:

- *Internal fixation with bone grafting:* Internal fixation, using plates, screws, or intramedullary nails, is often combined with bone grafting to provide mechanical stability and enhance biological healing. Autologous bone grafting, typically harvested from the iliac crest, remains the gold standard due to its osteogenic, osteoinductive, and osteoconductive properties. Alternatively, allografts or synthetic bone substitutes may be used, particularly in patients with limited autograft availability or significant donor site morbidity.
- *Biological augmentation:* In recent years, the use of biological agents such as bone morphogenetic proteins (BMPs) has gained prominence in the management of nonunion. BMP-2 and BMP-7 are osteoinductive growth factors that promote mesenchymal stem cell differentiation into osteoblasts, enhancing bone healing. A systematic review and meta-analysis published in "The Bone and Joint Journal (2022)" demonstrated that BMPs significantly improve union rates in nonunion, particularly in tibial and long bone fractures.
- *Minimally invasive techniques:* Minimally invasive techniques, such as percutaneous bone grafting and percutaneous fixation, have emerged as alternatives to traditional open surgery, particularly in the management of hypertrophic nonunions. These techniques aim to reduce surgical morbidity, preserve soft tissue, and minimize infection risk while providing adequate stabilization and biological stimulation.
- *Ilizarov technique and circular external fixation:* The Ilizarov technique, which employs a circular external fixator, is particularly effective for complex nonunions, including those with bone loss, deformity, or infection. The technique allows for the gradual correction of deformities, distraction osteogenesis for bone lengthening, and stable fixation while promoting biological healing.
- *Management of infected nonunions:* Infected nonunions pose a significant challenge and require a combined approach involving debridement of

necrotic tissue, stabilization, and local and systemic antibiotic therapy. The Masquelet technique, which involves a two-stage procedure with the placement of an antibiotic-impregnated cement spacer followed by bone grafting, has shown favorable outcomes in the management of infected nonunions. According to a multicenter study published in "The Journal of Bone and Joint Surgery (2023)," the Masquelet technique achieved a union rate of over 80% in infected nonunions with a low recurrence of infection.

Emerging therapies include:
- Gene therapy
- Stem cell therapy
- Three-dimensional-printed scaffolds

BIBLIOGRAPHY

1. Anderson DE, Ellis TL. Delayed union and nonunion of fractures: Current concepts, prevention, and correction. Bioengineering. 2024;11(6):525.
2. Heckman JD, Mahoney PCJ, Court-Brown C. Rockwood and Green's Fractures in Adults. United States: Lippincott Williams & Wilkins; 2019.
3. Ekegren CL, Edwards ER, De Steiger R, Gabbe BJ. Incidence, costs and predictors of non-union, delayed union and malunion following long bone fracture. Int J Environ Res Public Health. 2018;15(12):2845.
4. Nauth A, Lane J, Watson JT, Giannoudis PV. Bone graft substitutes in the treatment of tibial plateau fractures. Injury. 2015;46(5):S16-25.
5. Varshney M. Essential Orthopedics: Principles and Practice. New Delhi: Jaypee Brothers Medical Publishers (P) Ltd.; 2022.

Fracture and Infections

Jujhar Singh, Vedant Bajaj

According to research, the infection rate after closed fractures is 1.8%, while after open fractures, it is 27%. Patients with fracture-related infections (FRIs) have a reported 70% recovery rate, a 9% recurrence rate, and a 3% amputation rate. Their expenses are 6.5 times higher than those of noninfected cases. Common causative organisms include *Staphylococcus aureus,* Group A and B *streptococcus, Escherichia coli, Pseudomonas aeruginosa, Klebsiella pneumoniae,* and *Enterobacter.*

Treatment of such fractures can be challenging because of the unpredictable nature of bone damage, the presence of associated soft-tissue injuries, and the various concomitant comorbidities. The primary complications include infection associated with fractures and impaired healing of fractures (or nonunion), both of which affect around 5% of patients. However, this rate significantly rises for specific types of fractures, particularly those accompanied by nearby open wounds.

INFECTION SEVERITY SCORE

By examining six clinical factors, the infection severity score (ISS) assigns a grade to the degree of infection. The clinical, radiological, and historical data are taken into account.

Higher scores indicate the potential of incomplete eradication or infection recurrence, as well as the necessity for a second debridement. It can advocate for the final mode of achieving union in the second stage to be external fixation as opposed to internal fixation.

Reduced scores suggest a simpler elimination of the infection, which may facilitate definitive internal fixation in the subsequent stage or external fixation within the same stage. The ISS would aid in evaluating any remaining infection **(Table 1)**.

Infections were categorized based on the criteria established by Trampuz et al. into three groups: (1) early infections (occurring within <2 weeks), (2) delayed infections (occurring between 2 and 10 weeks), and (3) late-onset hardware-related infections (occurring after >10 weeks).

WHY DOES INFECTION CAUSE NONUNION?

- Dissection of pus through the planes and periosteum
- Fragmentation and dissolution of fracture hematoma
- Inflammatory mediators promote fibrous tissue formation
- If fixation was done, then implant failure destabilizes the fragments.
- Increase catabolic response at fracture ends.

TABLE 1: Infection severity score (ISS).

Sinuses	Skin	Sequestra	Discharge	Implant	Treatment needed
Nil = 0	Supple = 0	None = 0	Nil = 0	None = 0	ABC beads = 1
Few or dried = 1	Thin/ adherent = 1	<5 mm/ single/few = 1	1–2 drops/day = 1	Ex fix only = 1	ABC rod = 3
Multiple/ active = 2	Ulcerated = 2	>5 mm/ multiple = 2	Few drops/day = 2	Plating = 2	ABC beads and Rod = 5
		> 1 cm/ multiple = 3	Daily dressing = 3	Nailing = 3	
		Whole circumference = 5	Severe soakage with foul smell = 7	Nailing and plating/ multiple surgeries = 4	

Note: Six parameters are measured and score is given of a maximum of 25 points which is then converted out of 100.

CLINICAL PICTURE AND EXAMINATION

The diagnosis of infection may be obvious or obscure. A proper history is important to diagnose a patient of infected nonunion or osteomyelitis. There may be past history of trauma/open fracture/operative intervention. Personal history is of utmost importance in patients with infected nonunion:

- Medical history such as diabetes mellitus (DM), endocrinopathy, vitamin D deficiency, etc.
- Physiologic age
- Heart disease (endocarditis), chronic obstructive pulmonary disease (COPD), renal/hepatic disorder
- Nutrition
- Intravenous (IV) drug abuse and smoking
- Chronic medication
- Current and previous ambulatory or functional status before the initial injury

Patients may present with:

1. Raised body temperature or fever, with pain and swelling
2. Discharging sinuses
3. Waxing and waning of symptoms ("The Walenkamp phenomenon" is characterized by a classic pattern of cyclical pain that escalates to a severe and deep tension, which subsequently diminishes following the rupture of pus, leading to a temporary state of healing.)

Furthermore, one must not forget to examine the following:

- Assess the range of motion in adjacent joints, as stiffness resulting from prior treatment is frequently observed.
- Evaluate the neurovascular condition distally.
- Examine the regional lymph nodes for enlargement and mild tenderness (considering tuberculosis as a potential cause for matted lymph nodes).
- Look for indications of pathological fractures.

Infected nonunions, particularly those categorized as Cierney–Madar type IV osteomyelitis, exhibit several distinct clinical features that indicate the presence of infection and complications in the healing process. The main characteristics of infected nonunion are as follows:

- *Painful nonunion:* Typically, painful unless there is a significant gap (>1 cm) filled with mature fibrous tissue, in which case the nonunion may be painless.
- Raised local temperature
- Discharging sinus
- Scar healed by secondary intention
- Tethered skin
- Irregularity of bone

DIAGNOSIS

- *Laboratory investigations:* White blood cells (WBC) count > 11,000 cells/mm^3, erythrocyte sedimentation rate (ESR) > 30 mm/h, and C-reactive protein (CRP) > 1.0 mg/dL—all these are suggestive of infection.
  - White blood cells can be elevated within the normal range, or at a borderline level, contingent upon the degree of infection activity. In cases of subclinical infection, all these parameters may appear normal.
  - The ESR and CRP are valuable tools for tracking treatment progress.
  - In pediatric infections, CRP demonstrates slightly greater sensitivity compared to ESR in identifying the presence of infection.
  - Recent studies indicate that interleukin (IL)-6 serves as a reliable marker for postoperative infection, as it exhibits a more rapid increase and a quicker return to baseline levels compared to CRP and ESR.
- *The gold standard for diagnosis of infection:* Isolating cultured tissue from the nonunion site at the time of surgical intervention. It is recommended to perform three biopsies from the nonunion area. A minimum of two specimens must yield positive results to establish the diagnosis of infection.
- *Plain radiographs:*
  - Bone destruction may manifest as periosteal new bone formation, focal bony lysis, cortical loss, endosteal scalloping, and deterioration of trabecular bone architecture, accompanied by new bone apposition and eventual peripheral sclerosis.
  - A significant late indicator is the presence of regional osteoporosis alongside a localized area of seemingly increased density. Osteoporosis reflects metabolically active, living bone, while the segment that does not exhibit osteoporosis may be metabolically inactive and potentially necrotic.
- Ultrasonography has the capability to identify a subperiosteal fluid collection during the initial phases of osteomyelitis
- *Magnetic resonance imaging (MRI):* It is the imaging modality of choice for the evaluation of infection. It offers superior anatomical detail of the medullary space, cortex, and periosteum, along with excellent soft-tissue contrast, which is essential for identifying edema and fluid. Preoperative MRI can decrease both the duration of surgery and the degree of surgical exposure needed in procedures involving surgical debridement.
- *Scintigraphic techniques:*
  - *99Tc-methyl diphosphonate (MDP) technetium bone scan* is widely utilized in the investigation of infections, effectively detecting reparative processes in the bone.
  - *111-Indium-immunoglobulin G (IgG) scan:* For assessing infections and inflammatory conditions affecting the joints.
  - *111-Indium-oxime WBC scan* along with ^{99m}Tc-sulfur colloid bone marrow scans are considered the gold standard for detecting infections in total hip arthroplasty, providing valuable insights into bone marrow activity that aid in assessing bone necrosis and musculoskeletal infections.
- *18F-fluorodeoxyglucose positron emission tomography (FDG-PET):* This method provides high accuracy in diagnosing chronic osteomyelitis. Scintigraphy imaging specificity improves with CT, whether for osteomyelitis or orthopedic implant infections. FDG-PET offers a simple method and quick results, usually within 2–3 hours, compared to traditional techniques.

TREATMENT

Treatment of infected nonunion is technically demanding, prolonged, and needs a team. There are two schools of thought in the treatment of infected nonunion:

1. *The "union-first" strategy:* The primary objective is to establish union initially, followed by addressing the issue of infection as it arises. This strategy does not prioritize the complete elimination of infection as its foremost goal. "Infection per se does not cause nonunion".
2. *The "infection-elimination first" strategy (more popular):* The primary goal is to eradicate the infection, followed by the secondary aim of achieving bone union.

Stage 1: Radical Debridement, Reconstruction of Bone and Soft Tissue, Management of Dead Space, and Control of Infection

- Loss of cover due to debridement of extraosseous soft tissue is most effectively addressed by a muscle flap. The muscle flap aids in early union, total infection elimination, and the introduction of much-needed vascularity.
- The nonunion site can be transformed into horizontal surfaces through the resection of bone from partial defects and unevenly shaped bony ends. Extensive resections may lead to considerable shortening. Regeneration in long bones may occur at a slow pace, making it challenging to attain precise limb lengths.
- Bone formation is poor in diabetics, anemic patients, and smokers.

Local Antibiotic Delivery Systems

- An antibiotic-impregnated cement block effectively fills the dead space, enabling the release of the antibiotic in significantly high concentrations at the local site.
- Cement beads mixed with gentamycin or tobramycin are placed on a stainless-steel wire in the extramedullary area. Adding antibiotic powder or liquid during polymerization enhances antibiotic release. It is essential to remove these cement beads within 6 weeks.
- The cement can be molded into a block that fills the entire bony void. Alternatively, it may be shaped into a cylinder, with "Rush" or "Ender" nails inserted through it to anchor the cement block to the bone.

Recent advances: A new research employs a large diameter nail with an antibiotic cement dual core around a metal rod, showing effectiveness in treating compound fractures and potentially infected nonunions without significant bone gaps.

For smaller gaps, absorbable carriers can eliminate the need for a second surgery. Good options are calcium sulfate cement and chitosan polymer. In mild infections, debridement and definitive fixation can be performed together in the same procedure.

Fracture Stability

- External fixator
- Ilizarov external fixation technique
- The limb reconstruction system (LRS) fixator
- *Taylor spatial frame (TSF):* Its computer adjustment system aids in realigning tibial angles and supports lengthening procedures.

Stage 2: Reconstruction of Bone Defect

Bone grafting methods for infected nonunion:

- *Papineau open bone grafting (originally described by Rhinelander)*: This procedure involves:
    1. Multiple debridements at intervals of 5–7 days, accompanied by intramedullary stabilization.
    2. *Grafting:* Once healthy granulation tissue appears use "matchstick" cancellous grafts 3–6 cm × 3 mm × 4 mm in overlapping circular fashion with or without saline irrigation and wound packing.

3. *Skin cover:* Either spontaneous or various flaps/graft for coverage.

This technique is ideal for a small defect up to 3–4 cm. Stable fixation is a prerequisite.

- Friedlander technique—thorough debridement + stabilization and closure followed by open bone grafting **(Fig. 1)**.

Bone Transport

- *External bone transport:* The treatment focuses on addressing bone loss exceeding 4 cm, along with the correction of deformities and the lengthening of limbs. This procedure may be classified as monofocal, involving a single corticotomy, or bifocal, which entails dual site corticotomy with movement directed toward each other.
- *Internal bone transport using olive/hooked wires:* It is employed for defects 7–10 cm and larger.
- *Combined bone transport:* For larger defects due to major bone loss combined with limb deformities, deep soft-tissue scars, and local blood supply insufficiency.

Union at the docking site can be enhanced using iliac crest bone grafts. If these sites are depleted, injecting bone marrow aspirate at the nonunion site is beneficial. The effectiveness of the aspirate can be improved with demineralized bone matrix (DBM), β-tricalcium phosphate, or hydroxyapatite. If budget permits, platelet concentrates with bone morphogenetic protein (BMP) may also be used. These techniques can be applied multiple times. To promote expedited

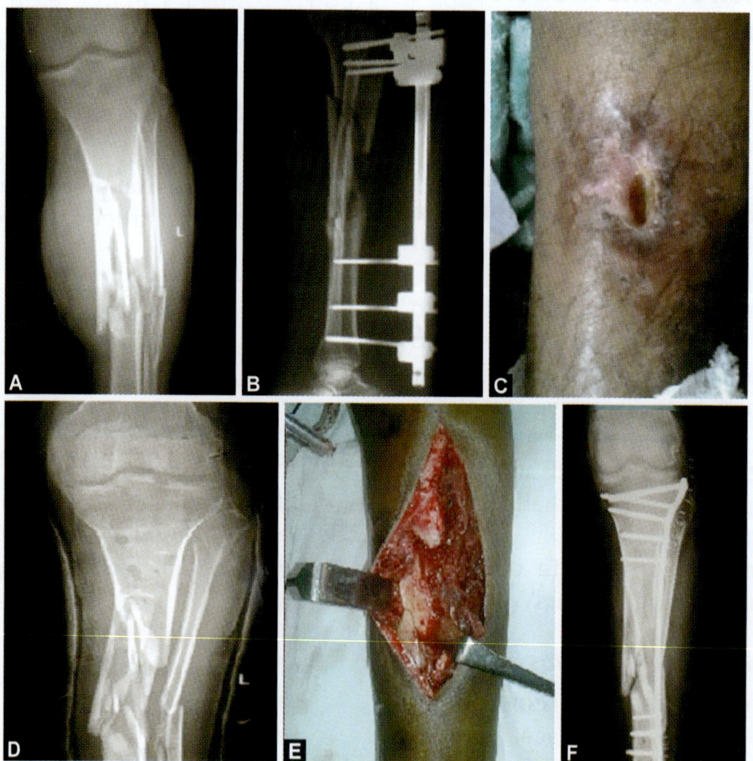

FIGS. 1A TO F: A case of open tibia fracture grade 3B managed initially with fixation followed by debridement and plate fixation as definitive management. (A) Comminuted open fracture proximal tibia, (B) Managed with initial debridement and external fixator; (C) Wound healed without any discharge; (D) Debridement of wound; and (E) Second stage surgery using a plate; (F) Subsequent plating and bone grafting.

healing at the nonunion site, the bony edges can be refreshed, and internal stability can be achieved by interlocking one end into the other.

For oblique nonunion surfaces, side-to-side compression is optimal. Fracture surfaces compress perpendicularly. To enhance vascularity at the nonunion site, drilling fine wire holes creates new channels and accelerates healing.

MASQUELET-INDUCED MEMBRANE TECHNIQUE

It is a two-stage technique:

1. *First stage: Radical debridement, cement spacer, and temporizing fixation*—the induced membrane arises from the tissue's reaction to foreign materials. This newly generated membrane is notably active. Initially, it is crucial to conduct extensive debridement and to eliminate any existing infection. The bone defect is then filled with a cement spacer.
2. *Second stage: Placement of bone graft into "induced membrane" and definitive fixation*—after several weeks, the bone graft replaces the spacer. Factors like spacer properties, bone fixation method, timing of the second stage, and graft characteristics greatly influence healing and outcomes. Larger defects can be treated with a reamer-irrigator-aspirator (RIA) graft or upper tibia material. A 6- to 8-week interval between stages, antibiotic-impregnated bone cement, and internal fixation can lower complication rates.

AN ALGORITHM BASED MANAGEMENT OF INFECTED UNION IS DESCRIBED IN FLOWCHARTS 1 AND 2

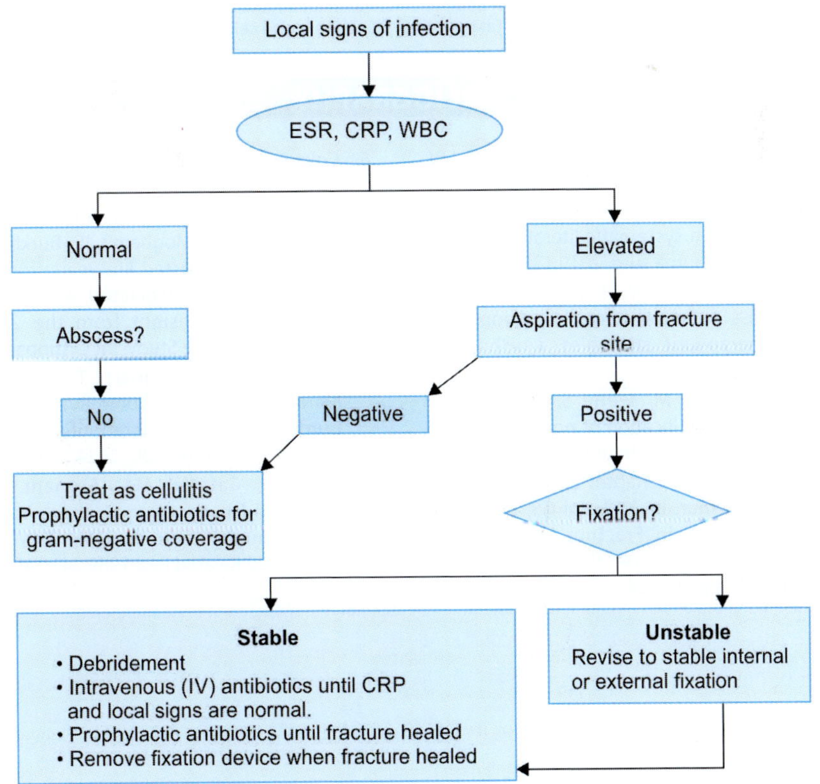

FLOWCHART 1: Early infection < 4-week postfracture.

(CRP: C-reactive protein; ESR: erythrocyte sedimentation rate: WBC: white blood cells)

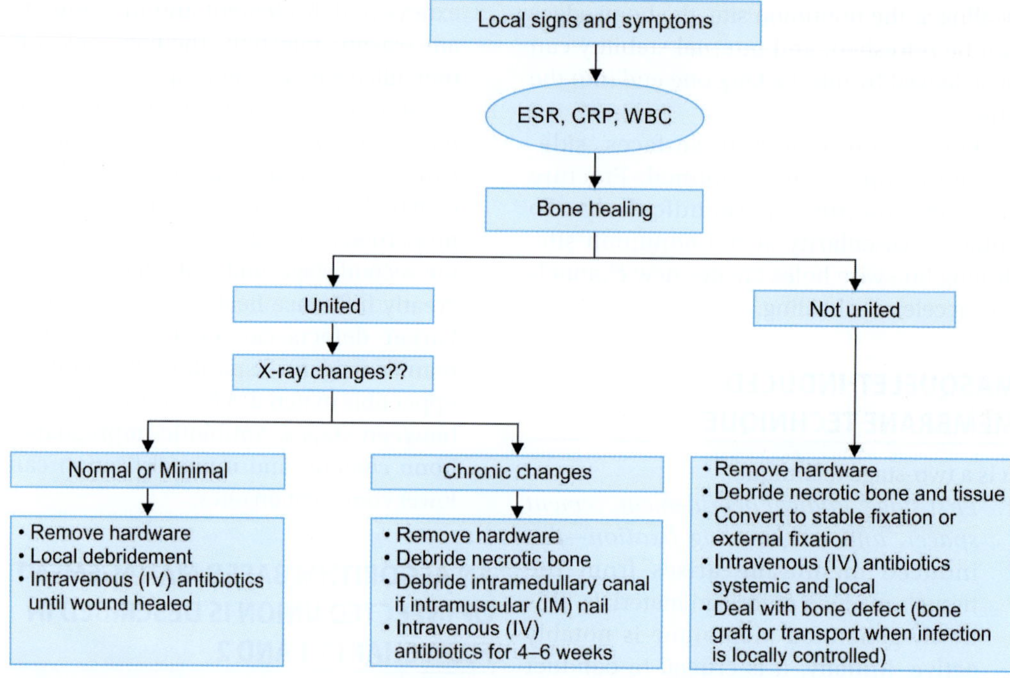

FLOWCHART 2: Late infection >4-week postfracture.
(CRP: C-reactive protein; ESR: erythrocyte sedimentation rate: WBC: white blood cells)

BIBLIOGRAPHY

1. Bezstarosti H, Van Lieshout EM, Voskamp LW, Kortram K, Obremskey W, McNally MA, et al. Insights into treatment and outcome of fracture-related infection: a systematic literature review. Arch orthopaed trauma surg. 2019;139:61-72.
2. Birt MC, Anderson DW, Toby EB, Wang J. Osteomyelitis: Recent advances in pathophysiology and therapeutic strategies. J orthopaed. 2017;14(1):45-52.
3. Calori GM, Phillips M, Jeetle S, Tagliabue L, Giannoudis PV. Classification of non-union: need for a new scoring system. Injury. 2008;39:S59-63.
4. Chaudhary Milind M. Chapter 25: Infected gap nonunions of femur. In: Kulkarni GS, Babhulkar S (eds). Guidelines in Fracture Management, Nonunion in Long Bone II. Noida: Thieme Publisher; 2016. pp. 309-24.
5. Colston J, Atkins B. Bone and joint infection. Clin Med. 2018;18(2):150-4.
6. Lewandrowski KU, da Silva RC, Elfar JC, Alhammoud A, Moghamis IS, Burkhardt BW, et al. Disability-adjusted life years from bone and joint infections associated with antimicrobial resistance: an insight from the 2019 Global Burden of Disease Study. Int Orthopaed. 2024:1-2.
7. Metsemakers WJ, Moriarty TF, Morgenstern M, Marais L, Onsea J, O'Toole RV, et al. The global burden of fracture-related infection: can we do better? Lancet Infect Dis. 2024;24(6):e386-93.
8. Paley D, Catagni MA, Argnani F, Villa A, Bijnedetti Gb, Cattaneo R. Ilizarov treatment of tibial nonunions with bone loss (1976-2007). Clin Orthopaed Related Res. 1989;241:146-65.

SECTION

18

Tendon Injuries

CHAPTER 18.1

Biceps and Triceps Tendon Rupture

Rifaaqat Ghani, Ifzal Ahmed Khan, Irfan Ahmed Poswal

Biceps tendon rupture, particularly of the long head of the biceps (LHB), is a relatively common injury among active individuals, especially those over the age of 40 years. The injury typically occurs as a result of overuse, degenerative changes, or acute trauma. While many patients may present with pain and functional limitations, the optimal treatment approach remains the subject of ongoing debate.

APPLIED ANATOMY AND PATHOPHYSIOLOGY

The biceps muscle comprises two heads: (1) the short head, which originates from the coracoid process, and (2) the long head, which originates from the supraglenoid tubercle of the scapula and inserts into the radial tuberosity in the forearm. Ruptures of the biceps tendon most commonly occur in the long head, which is more prone to degeneration due to its intra-articular course and frequent exposure to mechanical stress.

DIAGNOSIS

Patients with biceps tendon rupture often present with a sudden onset of pain, a "pop" in the shoulder or elbow, and weakness in forearm supination or elbow flexion. A characteristic "Popeye" deformity may also be observed in cases of complete rupture. Ultrasound and MRI are commonly used to confirm the diagnosis and assess the extent of the injury.

TREATMENT OPTIONS

Nonoperative Management

Nonoperative management is typically considered for:

- Older patients with minimal functional impairment.
- Patients with a rupture of the LHB but with an intact short head, preserve some elbow flexion and supination strength.
- Individuals not engaged in heavy lifting or manual labor.

Conservative treatment includes activity modification, anti-inflammatory medications, and physical therapy.

Studies have demonstrated that nonoperative treatment can result in satisfactory outcomes for pain relief and the resumption of daily activities. However, patients should be informed that residual weakness, particularly in supination strength, may persist. Functional limitations are typically well-tolerated by nonathletic individuals.

Surgical Management

Surgical management is usually recommended for younger, active patients, or those whose jobs require significant use of the biceps muscle. Surgical options include tenodesis or tenotomy, depending on patient's factors and surgeon's preference.

BICEPS TENOTOMY

In biceps tenotomy, the LHB is released from its attachment to the glenoid. This simple and minimally invasive procedure can relieve pain and restore function without the need for tendon reattachment.

Indications

- Older and less active patients
- Patients with significant degeneration of the tendon
- Individuals with high surgical risk where a less invasive procedure is preferred.

Outcomes: The primary advantage of tenotomy is rapid pain relief with a quick return to activity. However, it may lead to a cosmetic deformity ("Popeye" sign) and potential cramping, although these are usually well-tolerated.

BICEPS TENODESIS

In tenodesis, the LHB is reattached to the humerus, maintaining the tendon's length-tension relationship. This procedure is preferred in younger, more active patients who desire to maintain muscle strength and function, and it is associated with better cosmetic outcomes compared to tenotomy.

Indications

- Younger and athletic individuals.
- Patients with high demands on their biceps strength, such as those engaged in manual labor.
- Patients wishing to avoid cosmetic deformities and muscle atrophy.

Outcomes: Biceps tenodesis is associated with excellent functional outcomes, with most patients regaining near-full strength in elbow flexion and forearm supination. Postoperative rehabilitation involves protecting the repair for a period of weeks, followed by gradual strengthening exercises. Recent studies have shown that both arthroscopic and open techniques for biceps tenodesis yield comparable results, with high rates of patient satisfaction.

Hybrid Techniques and Emerging Therapies

Newer techniques, such as hybrid procedures that combine tenotomy and tenodesis, are being explored. The rationale behind these approaches is to optimize the benefits of both procedures by minimizing complications while preserving function.

Rehabilitation

Early Phase (Weeks 1–4)

- Immobilization with a sling
- Passive range-of-motion exercises to maintain flexibility
- Avoidance of resisted biceps contraction

Intermediate Phase (Weeks 4–8)

- Progressive active range-of-motion exercises
- Gradual strengthening of the shoulder and elbow, avoiding high-stress activities

Late Phase (Weeks 8–12)

- Full range-of-motion exercises
- Strengthening exercises focused on biceps, shoulder, and scapular stabilizers
- Return to sport or labor-specific training

Complications

Common complications include infection, stiffness, nerve injury, and rerupture. Cosmetic deformity is more commonly associated with tenotomy, while tenodesis carries a risk of failure of fixation. Additionally, overuse of the arm too early in the rehabilitation process may lead to reinjury or prolonged recovery.

TRICEPS TENDON RUPTURE

Triceps tendon ruptures are rare injuries, accounting for <1% of all tendon ruptures.

Anatomy and Pathophysiology

The triceps brachii muscle consists of three heads: (1) the long head, (2) lateral head, and (3) medial head. These converge into a single tendon, which inserts into the olecranon process of the ulna. The tendon serves a key role in elbow extension, especially in activities requiring pushing or overhead movements.

Triceps tendon ruptures typically occur at the osteotendinous junction, although mid-tendon and muscle belly injuries can also occur. The injury is most often seen in middle-aged individuals who engage in activities with eccentric loading of the triceps, such as weightlifting, contact sports, or heavy labor. Ruptures may also be associated with predisposing factors such as anabolic steroid use, chronic tendinopathy, or systemic diseases like diabetes or chronic renal insufficiency.

Diagnosis

Patients typically report a sudden "pop" or sharp pain at the posterior elbow, followed by weakness in elbow extension. Physical examination may reveal a palpable defect above the olecranon, swelling, and bruising. However, in partial ruptures, the clinical presentation can be more subtle.

Diagnostic imaging plays a key role, particularly in cases where the diagnosis is uncertain. Ultrasound is often the first imaging modality used, as it is readily available and can provide real-time information about the tendon. Magnetic resonance imaging (MRI) is the gold standard for confirming the diagnosis, particularly for partial tears and to assess the degree of retraction and surrounding tissue involvement.

Treatment Options

Nonoperative Management

Nonoperative management may be appropriate for patients with partial triceps tendon ruptures, elderly patients with low functional demands, or those with medical comorbidities that increase surgical risk. Conservative treatment typically involves immobilization, followed by a gradual rehabilitation program to restore function.

Surgical Management

Surgical repair is generally considered the gold standard for complete triceps tendon ruptures.

Techniques

- *Primary repair:* In acute ruptures, a primary repair is preferred. This involves direct reattachment of the tendon using nonabsorbable sutures passed through bone tunnels in the olecranon. The use of suture anchors has become more common, as they provide a less invasive method with comparable biomechanical strength.
- *Augmentation or grafting:* In cases of chronic ruptures or significant tendon degeneration, the native tendon may not provide sufficient tissue for a successful repair. In such cases, augmentation with an allograft or autograft may be required. This can restore continuity and strength to the repair.

Type of Sutures Used in Triceps Tendon Repair

The most commonly used is *nonabsorbable sutures,* such as *number 2 or number 5 FiberWire or Ethibond.*

Common suture configuration: Krackow stitch, son-Allen stitch, and Figure-of-eight.

- In some cases, *suture anchors* but commonly used sizes for triceps tendon repair range from 4.5 to 6.5 mm.

Postoperative Rehabilitation

- *Early phase (Weeks 0–4):* The elbow is typically immobilized in slight flexion (45°). Passive range-of-motion exercises may begin around 4 weeks postoperatively, but active extension is usually avoided to protect the repair.

- *Intermediate phase (Weeks 4–8):* Gradual reintroduction of active-assisted and active range-of-motion exercises, focusing on elbow flexion and extension. Strengthening exercises, including isometric contractions, are introduced gradually to improve muscle control and prevent atrophy.
- *Late phase (Weeks 8–12):* Full range-of-motion exercises and progressive resistance training to improve muscle strength and endurance. Return to sports or labor-specific training can be considered at around 3–6 months postoperatively, depending on the patient's progress.

Complications

Common complications include infection, rerupture, stiffness, and hardware-related issues such as anchor loosening. Chronic ruptures, in particular, present a challenge due to tendon retraction and fibrosis, which can complicate the repair and lead to suboptimal outcomes.

Other potential complications include:

- Residual weakness
- Heterotopic

BIBLIOGRAPHY

1. American Academy of Orthopaedic Surgeons. Clinical Practice Guideline on the Treatment of Biceps Tendon Pathologies. United States: American Academy of Orthopaedic Surgeons (AAOS); 2022.
2. American Shoulder and Elbow Surgeons. ASES Guidelines for the Management of Biceps Tendon Injuries. United States: American Shoulder and Elbow Surgeons (ASES); 2021.
3. MacDonald P, Verhulst F, McRae S, Old J, Stranges G, Dubberley J, et al. Biceps tenodesis versus tenotomy in the treatment of lesions of the long head of the biceps tendon in patients undergoing arthroscopic shoulder surgery: a prospective double-blinded randomized controlled trial. Am J Sports Med. 2020;48(6):1439-49.
4. van Riet RP, Morrey BF, Ho E, O'Driscoll SW. Surgical treatment of distal triceps ruptures. J Bone Joint Surg Am. 2003;85(10):1961-7.

CHAPTER 18.2

Wrist and Hand Tendon Injury

Nusrat Jabeen

The tendons of the wrist and hand can be divided into two categories: (1) *extensor tendons* and (2) *flexor tendons.*

Flexor Tendons

The primary flexor tendons include:

- *Flexor digitorum superficialis (FDS):* Responsible for flexion of the proximal interphalangeal (PIP) joints.
- *Flexor digitorum profundus (FDP):* Responsible for flexion of the distal interphalangeal (DIP) joints.
- *Flexor pollicis longus (FPL):* Responsible for thumb flexion.

Extensor Tendons

Key extensor tendons include:

- *Extensor digitorum communis (EDC):* Responsible for extension of the fingers.
- *Extensor indices proprius (EIP):* Provides independent extension of the index finger.
- *Extensor pollicis longus (EPL):* Extends the thumb at the interphalangeal joint.

The tendons pass through sheaths that help to reduce friction and are often constrained by retinacula and pulleys, which play critical roles in tendon gliding and function. Injury can disrupt these systems and lead to adhesions, loss of motion, and significant dysfunction.

The tendons of the wrist and hand are divided into distinct zones, each of which has clinical significance in injury and repair. The flexor and extensor tendons are categorized differently. Below is a summary of these zones and their applied anatomy.

Flexor Tendon Zones

Zone I

Location: From the insertion of the FDP on the distal phalanx to just distal to the insertion of the FDS on the middle phalanx.

Zone II (No Man's Land)

- *Location:* From the distal palmar crease to the insertion of the FDS on the middle phalanx.
- Considered a critical area for tendon injuries due to its complex anatomy. Both the FDP and FDS tendons are present here. Surgical repair in this zone is particularly challenging because of potential adhesions that could impair tendon gliding and finger movement.

Zone III

- *Location:* From the distal edge of the carpal tunnel to the distal palmar crease.
- Injuries in this zone affect both flexor tendons as well as the lumbrical muscles. Repair here is more straightforward compared to Zone II but still requires careful attention to avoid adhesion formation.

Zone IV

- *Location:* Corresponds to the carpal tunnel.
- *Applied anatomy:* Injuries in this zone often involve the tendons passing through the carpal tunnel, including both flexor tendons and the median nerve. Trauma or surgery in this zone can lead to median nerve dysfunction (e.g., carpal tunnel syndrome).

Zone V

- *Location:* Proximal to the carpal tunnel, extending to the musculotendinous junction in the forearm.
- Injuries here typically result from lacerations and can involve multiple tendons, nerves, and blood vessels. Repair must address not only tendon function but also neurovascular integrity.

Extensor Tendon Zones

Zone I

- *Location:* Over the DIP joint.
- *Applied anatomy:* Injuries here result in a mallet finger, characterized by an inability to extend the DIP joint.

Zone II

Location: Over the middle phalanx.

Zone III

- *Location:* Over the PIP joint.
- *Applied anatomy:* Injuries in this zone can cause boutonnière deformity, where the PIP joint is flexed, and the DIP is extended

PATHOPHYSIOLOGY OF TENDON INJURIES

Common tendon injuries include:

- *Tendon lacerations:* Typically caused by sharp objects, resulting in complete or partial tendon transection.
- *Ruptures:* Often associated with degenerative changes or forceful movement, as seen in rheumatoid arthritis or sports-related injuries.
- *Tendinopathies:* Chronic overuse can lead to tendinosis or tenosynovitis, causing pain, swelling, and impaired function.

DIAGNOSIS

The following techniques are commonly used:

- *Clinical examination:* Specific tests, such as the *Jersey finger test* (for FDP tendon injuries)
- *Ultrasound:* Dynamic ultrasound is useful for detecting tendon ruptures, tenosynovitis, and evaluating tendon healing postrepair.
- *Magnetic resonance imaging (MRI):* MRI provides detailed information about soft-tissue structures and is particularly useful in chronic or complex cases where the diagnosis is unclear.

SURGICAL MANAGEMENT

Flexor Tendon Injuries

Indications for Surgery

Surgical repair is indicated for complete lacerations or ruptures of flexor tendons, as conservative management alone is inadequate in restoring function. Early intervention, ideally within first 2 weeks post-injury, is crucial to minimize scarring and improve outcomes.

Extensor Tendon Injuries

Extensor tendon injuries are generally easier to manage surgically compared to flexor tendon injuries due to their more superficial location and less complex anatomy.

Techniques

- *Direct repair:* Extensor tendon lacerations are typically repaired with a figure-of-eight or running suture technique, depending on the zone of injury. In cases where the tendon is too damaged, a tendon graft or transfer may be required.

- *Tendon grafting and transfers:* In chronic or neglected tendon ruptures, especially in cases with significant tissue loss, tendon grafting or tendon transfers (e.g., using the *palmaris longus* or *plantaris* tendons) may be necessary to restore function.
- Flexor tendon injuries, especially in zone II (the so-called "no man's land"), are among the most challenging to treat due to the intricate anatomy and high risk of complications such as adhesions and contractures.

The ideal suture for tendon repair in the hand and wrist depends on several factors, including the type of tendon (flexor or extensor), the location of the injury, and the surgeon's preference. However, certain suture types and techniques are commonly recommended for optimal strength and healing.

- *Nonabsorbable sutures* are preferred for tendon repairs because they provide long-lasting tensile strength and allow for early mobilization. Examples include:
    - Prolene (polypropylene) and nylon
- *Absorbable sutures:* Sometimes used in deeper layers for soft-tissue repair, but less common in the actual tendon repair because they lose strength over time. Examples include:
    - *Polydioxanone (PDS):* It has longer absorption times compared to other absorbable sutures, but is still weaker than nonabsorbable options.

Suture Size

- Typically, *3-0* or *4-0 sutures* are used for tendon repairs in the hand. Finer sutures like *5-0* may be used for smaller tendons, but strength must be carefully considered.

Suture Technique

- *Core sutures*:
    - It is applied using modified Kessler or Strickland technique
    - *Four-strand repair:* This is a common standard for flexor tendon repair, as it offers increased strength compared to the traditional two-strand repair. More strands (such as six-strand) provide even more strength.
- *Epitendinous sutures*:
    - A continuous or interrupted epitendinous suture is often used around the outside of the tendon repair to provide added strength, improve tendon gliding, and reduce gapping at the repair site. This technique uses finer sutures like *6-0*.

CONSERVATIVE MANAGEMENT

Partial Tendon Injuries

Partial tendon injuries may be managed conservatively, especially if <50% of the tendon is affected. Splinting or bracing may be used to offload the tendon and allow for healing. Recent evidence suggests that partial flexor tendon injuries can heal with appropriate immobilization and rehabilitation.

COMPARATIVE OUTCOMES

Recent meta-analyses comparing early motion protocols versus delayed mobilization in flexor tendon repairs suggest that early controlled mobilization provides better outcomes in terms of strength, range of motion, and patient's satisfaction. For extensor tendon repairs, outcomes are generally excellent when repairs are performed early and with appropriate rehabilitation, though chronic injuries tend to have poorer outcomes.

Phases of Rehabilitation

- *Early phase (0–4 weeks):* Immobilization in a splint to protect the tendon repair is standard, though early passive or active-assisted range of motion may be allowed, depending on the repair technique.

- *Intermediate phase (4–8 weeks):* Gradual weaning from immobilization with a focus on a controlled active range of motion. Strengthening exercises are typically avoided during this phase to prevent overloading the healing tendon.
- *Late phase (8–12 weeks):* Progressive strengthening exercises and functional retraining are introduced. Resistance exercises targeting grip strength and fine motor skills help to restore full function.
- *Return to function (3–6 months):* Functional and work-specific exercises are incorporated, with the goal of returning to normal activities, including sports or manual labor.

RETURN TO WORK AND SPORTS

The timeline for returning to work and sports varies depending on the severity of the injury and the demands of the activity. For manual laborers or athletes, return to full function may take 6–12 months, depending on the nature of the injury and treatment.

BIBLIOGRAPHY

1. Hoornenborg D, van der Oest MJW, Vegter M, Bijker D, Selles RW. Effectiveness of early motion protocols after extensor tendon repair in zones V and VI: A systematic review. J Hand Surg Eur Vol. 2021;46(4):365-73.
2. Eissens MH, Schut SM, van der Sluis CK. Early active wrist mobilization in extensor tendon injuries in zones 5, 6, or 7. J Hand Ther. 2007;20(1):89-91.
3. van Velzen L, Wolff J, Schreuders TAR, Hovius SER, Selles RW. Biomechanical evaluation of flexor tendon repair techniques: A systematic review and meta-analysis. J Hand Surg Am. 2021;46(7):584-92.

CHAPTER 18.3

Quadriceps and Patellar Tendon Rupture

John Mohd, Bhat Jameel Mohd Jabbar

Quadriceps tendon rupture (QTR) is a relatively uncommon but serious injury, predominantly affecting middle-aged to elderly individuals, especially males. It is commonly associated with degenerative changes in the tendon due to aging, systemic diseases, or steroid use.

MECHANISM OF INJURY AND RISK FACTORS

Quadriceps tendon rupture often occurs following indirect trauma, such as a fall, sudden deceleration, or direct impact to the knee. Degeneration of the tendon—due to chronic conditions such as diabetes, renal failure, hyperparathyroidism, or corticosteroid use—weakens its structure and predisposes it to rupture. Additionally, localized inflammatory diseases like tendinitis may play a contributory role.

CLINICAL PRESENTATION

- Sudden onset pain and swelling around the knee
- Difficulty extending the knee or bearing weight
- A palpable gap above the patella
- Inability to perform an active straight leg raise

DIAGNOSIS

Clinical examination is often sufficient, but imaging modalities are important for confirmation:

- *X-rays:* May reveal patella baja, suggesting a rupture, but often are nondiagnostic.
- *Ultrasound:* A useful and accessible tool to confirm tendon rupture at the bedside.
- *MRI:* Gold standard for confirming diagnosis, especially in partial ruptures or when clinical suspicion is high despite negative X-rays.

TREATMENT

Nonoperative management: Nonoperative treatment is rarely indicated, usually reserved for patients with partial tears, minimal functional impairment, or those who are poor surgical candidates. This may involve immobilization in full extension and gradual physiotherapy rehabilitation. However, nonoperative management has a higher risk of poor functional outcomes and prolonged disability.

Surgical repair: It is the treatment of choice for complete ruptures and must be performed promptly—ideally within the first few weeks of injury for optimal outcomes. Delayed repair is associated with higher complication rates, including chronic weakness and joint stiffness. Surgical techniques include:

- *Direct repair:* Using transosseous tunnels or suture anchors to reattach the tendon to the patella. This is the standard technique for acute ruptures.
- *Augmentation techniques:* In cases of chronic or complex ruptures, augmentation with autografts (e.g., hamstring tendons), allografts, or synthetic materials may be necessary to enhance the repair strength.

For quadriceps tendon repair, *nonabsorbable* sutures are the standard choice due to their superior strength and durability.

For optimal results, most surgeons prefer using *heavy gauge sutures,* such as *No. 2 or No. 5 FiberWire* or *Ethibond,* due to the robust mechanical demands on the quadriceps tendon. These sutures are typically passed through *transosseous tunnels* or fixed with *suture anchors* to secure the tendon to the patella.

SUTURE TECHNIQUE

The *Krackow locking stitch* is commonly employed in quadriceps tendon repair because it allows for secure tendon-to-bone reattachment. This stitch distributes tension evenly along the tendon, minimizing the risk of repair failure.

This combination of high-strength suture material and secure suturing techniques helps to ensure a durable repair, even during early rehabilitation.

POSTOPERATIVE CARE AND REHABILITATION

Postoperative protocols typically involve passive knee range of motion movements for 4–6 weeks, followed by gradual weight-bearing and progressive active range-of-motion exercises. Early controlled mobilization can improve tendon healing and prevent joint stiffness. Return to full activity, including sports, is generally allowed 6–9 months postoperatively, depending on the extent of injury and surgical success.

COMPLICATIONS OF QUADRICEPS TENDON RUPTURE

Complications include:

- Tendon rerupture, especially in delayed repairs
- Joint stiffness or loss of motion
- Quadriceps weakness or atrophy
- Deep vein thrombosis (DVT)

PATELLAR TENDON RUPTURE

Patellar tendon rupture (PTR) is a debilitating injury typically occurring in active individuals under 40 years old.

Mechanism of Injury and Risk Factors

They typically occur after sudden and forceful knee extension, often during activities like jumping or rapid changes in direction. Risk factors include:

- *Chronic degeneration* of the tendon due to patellar tendinitis or repetitive microtrauma
- *Systemic conditions* such as diabetes, chronic renal failure, rheumatoid arthritis, and hyperparathyroidism
- *Corticosteroid injections* and long-term fluoroquinolone use, which can weaken tendons.

Direct trauma to the knee can also cause PTR, but indirect mechanisms are more common.

Clinical Presentation

- Sudden onset of pain, swelling, and inability to straighten the knee
- A palpable gap at the site of the rupture, just below the patella
- *Patella alta* (high-riding patella) on X-ray due to the loss of distal anchoring
- Inability to perform an *active straight leg raise* or extend the knee against resistance

The presence of these signs should prompt urgent diagnostic evaluation and early treatment.

- *X-rays:* Show patella alta, which is a key indicator of PTR.
- *Ultrasound:* A fast and bedside option to visualize the rupture.
- *MRI:* The gold standard for diagnosing partial or complete ruptures, particularly in cases where clinical findings are unclear.

Treatment

Nonoperative management: Nonoperative treatment is generally limited to patients with partial ruptures, minimal functional loss, or those unfit for surgery. This approach is associated with poorer outcomes, including quadriceps weakness and reduced range of motion, making it less favorable in most cases.

Surgical repair: Surgical intervention is the treatment of choice for complete ruptures. Timing is critical with early repair (within 2–3 weeks of injury) offering the best outcomes. Delayed repair can be more challenging due to tendon retraction and scar formation.

Surgical options include:

- *Primary repair:* This involves reattaching the torn patellar tendon to the inferior pole of the patella. Transosseous suture tunnels or suture anchors are commonly used for fixation. The *Krackow or Bunnell stitch* technique is often employed to reinforce the tendon and provide strong fixation.
- *Augmentation techniques:* For chronic ruptures or cases with poor tissue quality, augmentation using autografts (e.g., semitendinosus or gracilis tendons) or allografts may be necessary to enhance repair strength and prevent rerupture.
- *Suture anchors:* Modern techniques often employ suture anchors instead of transosseous tunnels. Anchors provide a reliable fixation with less bone drilling, reducing the risk of complications like patellar fracture.

Suture type: Nonabsorbable sutures such as *FiberWire®*, *Ethibond®*, or *Prolene®*.

Suture techniques: Krackow stitch (locking and strong fixation) or *Bunnell stitch* (pulley-type and figure-of-eight).

Suture diameter: No. 2 for routine repairs and *No. 5* for high-demand or complex cases.

Fixation method: Transosseous tunnels or *suture anchors* for tendon reattachment to the patella.

Postoperative Care and Rehabilitation Protocol

- *0–6 weeks:* Immobilization in full extension, nonweight bearing, or partial weight-bearing.
- *6–12 weeks:* Gradual range of motion exercises, progressing to full knee flexion.
- *3–6 months:* Focus on quadriceps strengthening, gait training, and return to functional activities.
- *6–9 months:* Return to sports and full activity, depending on strength and functional recovery.

Complications

- Tendon rerupture (especially with delayed repair)
- Patellar baja (low-riding patella) due to improper tendon tensioning
- Joint stiffness
- Quadriceps weakness
- DVT

Proper surgical technique and adherence to rehabilitation protocols are key to minimizing these risks.

BIBLIOGRAPHY

1. Arnold EP, Sedgewick JA, Wortman RJ, Stamm MA, Mulcahey MK. Acute quadriceps tendon rupture: presentation, diagnosis, and management. JBJS Rev. 2022;10(2):e21.00171.
2. Hatch RS, Daniels D, Chahal J. Contemporary management of patellar tendon rupture: A systematic review. Orthop J Sports Med. 2022;10(7):23259671221110253.
3. Jildeh TR, Young JR, Okoroha KR, et al. Clinical outcomes of patellar tendon repair with suture anchors versus transosseous tunnels. Am J Sports Med. 2023;51(5):1291-8.
4. Lighthart WA, Cohen DA, Levine RG, Bader DL, Kagen L, Beynnon BD. Functional outcomes following quadriceps tendon repair: A comparison of techniques. J Bone Joint Surg Am. 2022;104(2):128-35.
5. Rosso F, Cottino U, Bonasia DE, Bruzzone M. Patellar tendon rupture. In: Arthroscopy and Sport Injuries. Springer; 2016. pp. 87-95.
6. Shah VM, Andrews T, Rowe S, Foster W. Surgical outcomes in quadriceps tendon rupture: A systematic review. J Orthop Trauma. 2023;37(4):212-20.

CHAPTER 18.4

Tendo Achilles Rupture

Vipin Sharma, Pulkit Sharma

The Achilles tendon is the largest and strongest tendon in the human body.

ANATOMY AND FUNCTION OF THE ACHILLES TENDON

The Achilles tendon connects the gastrocnemius and soleus muscles to the calcaneus (heel bone), playing an essential role in plantar flexion of the foot. Blood supply to the tendon is limited, particularly in the watershed area located 2–6 cm proximal to its insertion, which contributes to its vulnerability to injury.

PATHOPHYSIOLOGY OF ACHILLES TENDON RUPTURE

Achilles tendon ruptures commonly occur during activities that involve sudden acceleration or deceleration, such as jumping or sprinting. The mechanism of injury often involves an eccentric loading of the tendon while the ankle is dorsiflexed. Microtrauma, overuse, and intrinsic degenerative changes within the tendon fibers are frequently implicated in spontaneous ruptures. Aging, reduced blood supply, and mechanical wear further contribute to this degenerative process.

Tendon ruptures typically occur in the avascular zone, where collagen degradation exceeds synthesis. Studies have shown that degenerative changes, such as collagen disorganization, mucoid degeneration, and neovascularization, precede many ruptures, even in asymptomatic patients.

RISK FACTORS

Several factors increase the risk of Achilles tendon rupture. These include:

- *Age:* Ruptures are most common in individuals aged 30–50 years.
- *Sex:* Men are more likely to suffer Achilles tendon ruptures than women.
- *Activity level:* Participation in high-impact sports, particularly those requiring bursts of speed or jumping, is a well-documented risk factor.
- *Previous tendon injury:* A history of tendinopathy or partial rupture increases the risk of a full rupture.
- *Medications:* Fluoroquinolone antibiotics and corticosteroids are linked with an increased risk of tendon rupture due to their detrimental effects on tendon structure and healing.

DIAGNOSIS

Common presenting symptoms include sudden pain in the posterior ankle or calf, often described as a "pop" or "snap," followed by difficulty in weight-bearing and plantar flexion.

Physical examination findings may include:

- *Thompson test:* A lack of plantar flexion when the calf is squeezed is indicative of a complete rupture.
- *Palpable gap:* A gap may be felt in the tendon, typically 2–6 cm proximal to its insertion.
- *Inability to stand on toes:* This functional test is a good indicator of rupture.

Imaging, particularly ultrasound or magnetic resonance imaging (MRI), can confirm the diagnosis, especially in cases of partial tears or in patients with equivocal clinical findings.

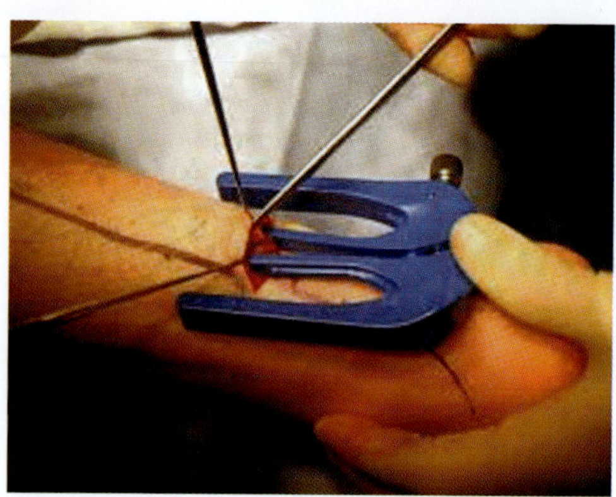

FIG. 1: Shows minimal invasive repair using Achillon jig.

MANAGEMENT

While traditional treatment options included primarily surgical repair, there is now increasing evidence supporting non-operative management in certain patient populations.

Surgical Management

Indications for Surgery

Surgical intervention is typically recommended for younger, more active patients, especially those involved in sports or occupations requiring high-demand lower limb function. Surgical repair is also favored in patients with a delayed diagnosis or those with a complete rupture and a significant gap between the tendon ends.

Techniques

There are two primary surgical approaches to Achilles tendon repair:

1. *Open repair:* The traditional open repair involves a longitudinal incision along the posterior aspect of the ankle. The tendon ends are sutured together using a strong, nonabsorbable suture. While effective, this approach is associated with risks such as wound complications and infections.
2. *Minimally invasive repair:* This technique involves smaller incisions, reducing the risk of wound complications (**Fig. 1**). Recent advancements in minimally invasive techniques have shown promising outcomes, with comparable rerupture rates and fewer complications compared to open repair.

Augmentation Techniques

To enhance the strength of the repair and reduce the risk of rerupture, augmentation techniques, such as the use of allografts, autografts, or synthetic scaffolds, may be employed in cases of chronic rupture or poor tendon quality. These techniques promote tissue healing and provide additional mechanical support.

Preferable sutures used for repair are, nonabsorbable sutures, such as *number 2 Ethibond* or *number 5 Prolene,* are widely used for Achilles tendon repairs, particularly with a strong and durable technique like the *Krackow stitch.*

Conservative Management

Indications for Nonoperative Treatment

Nonoperative management has gained popularity, particularly for patients with lower functional demands, older age, or those with medical comorbidities that make surgery risky. Recent studies indicate that, with appropriate rehabilitation protocols, nonsurgical treatment can result in functional outcomes comparable to surgical repair with a lower risk of complications such as infection.

Functional Rehabilitation

The cornerstone of conservative management is functional rehabilitation. This approach involves early weight-bearing and controlled mobilization, which stimulates tendon healing through mechanotransduction. Evidence suggests that early mobilization, as opposed to prolonged immobilization, leads to better outcomes in terms of strength, range of motion, and patient's satisfaction.

Comparative Outcomes

Several randomized controlled trials and meta-analyses have compared surgical and nonsurgical management. Recent evidence suggests that while surgery may reduce the risk of rerupture, functional outcomes, including return to activity, patient's satisfaction, and strength, are similar between the two approaches when early mobilization protocols are used. A key consideration is the trade-off between the slightly lower rerupture rate with surgery and the higher risk of wound complications compared to conservative treatment.

Phases of Rehabilitation

- *Immobilization phase (0–2 weeks):* In both surgical and conservative treatment, initial immobilization in a plantarflexed position is used to protect the healing tendon.
- *Early mobilization phase (2–6 weeks):* During this phase, controlled ankle movement is introduced using a functional brace or cast. Partial weight-bearing with the assistance of crutches is encouraged.
- *Strengthening phase (6–12 weeks):* Isometric and isotonic exercises are introduced to restore strength to the calf muscles. Gradual progression of resistance is recommended.
- *Return to activity phase (3–6 months):* At this stage, patients are encouraged to gradually return to their previous level of activity. Plyometric and sport-specific exercises are incorporated to restore agility and power.

Return to Sport

One of the primary concerns for athletes recovering from Achilles tendon rupture is the timeline for returning to sport. Studies indicate that the average return-to-sport time is around 6–9 months, although this varies depending on the individual's preinjury activity level and the type of rehabilitation program. Functional testing, such as single-leg heel raises and hop tests, is often used to assess readiness for return to sport.

BIBLIOGRAPHY

1. Del Buono A, Chan O, Maffulli N. Minimally invasive versus open surgery for acute Achilles tendon rupture: a quantitative review. Br Med Bull. 2020;136(1):45-58.
2. Maffulli N, Longo UG, Kadakia A, Spiezia F. Achilles tendon ruptures. Clin Orthopaed Related Res. 2021;479(5):1013-26.
3. Ochen Y, Beks RB, van Heijl M, Hietbrink F, Leenen LP, van der Velde D, et al. Operative treatment versus nonoperative treatment of Achilles tendon ruptures: systematic review and meta-analysis. BMJ. 2019;364:k5120.
4. Soroceanu A, Sidhwa F, Aarabi S, Kaufman A, Glazebrook M. Surgical versus nonsurgical treatment of acute Achilles tendon rupture: a meta-analysis of randomized trials. J Bone Joint Surg Am. 2020;100(20):1811-9.

SECTION

19

Pediatric Fractures: Basics

CHAPTER 19.1

Unique Considerations in Children and Interpreting Pediatric X-rays

Rashid Anjum

Children's fractures differ significantly from those of adults due to their unique anatomy, growth potential, and the dynamic nature of bone remodeling which influence the presentation, treatment, and prognosis of fractures in this population.

UNIQUE ANATOMICAL AND PHYSIOLOGICAL FACTORS

Growth Plates (Physis)

The most significant difference between pediatric and adult bones is the presence of growth plates, or physes, which are zones of cartilage near the ends of long bones responsible for growth. In children, these growth plates are the weakest part of the bone and are susceptible to injury. Physeal injuries are most commonly classified using the Salter–Harris classification, which helps to guide treatment and predict long-term outcome.

Early and accurate identification of growth plate injuries is critical because mismanagement can result in complications such as growth arrest, leading to angular deformities or limb length discrepancies.

Open Physes and Long-term Growth Implications

Fractures involving the physis carry the risk of growth disturbances. Growth plate injuries, particularly Salter–Harris types III, IV, and V, can lead to premature closure of the physis, resulting in limb length discrepancies or angular deformities. This risk underscores the importance of proper diagnosis and follow-up for fractures involving the physis. Long-term monitoring is often necessary to assess for growth disturbances. In cases where growth arrest occurs, surgical options such as epiphysiodesis or limb-lengthening procedures may be required to address discrepancies.

Periosteum and Healing Potential

The periosteum, a dense membrane that covers bones, is more robust and active in children. This thick periosteum contributes to the rapid healing potential of pediatric fractures by forming a stabilizing sleeve around the injury and providing a scaffold for new bone formation. The active periosteum allows for quicker callus formation and, often, a faster return to function. In many cases, the periosteum remains intact on the concave side of incomplete fractures, such as greenstick or torus fractures, which helps to maintain stability and aids in easier reductions compared to adults.

Bone Plasticity and Unique Fracture Patterns

Children's bones are less brittle and more flexible than adult bones, a property that leads to distinctive fracture patterns not commonly seen in adults. These unique fracture types are due to the elasticity of pediatric bone and may not always be easily visible on X-rays, requiring a high level of suspicion for proper diagnosis. Common pediatric fracture types include:

- *Greenstick fractures:* Incomplete fractures where the bone bends on one side and breaks on the opposite side.
- *Torus (Buckle) fractures:* Compression injuries where the bone buckles but does not completely break.
- *Plastic deformation:* A phenomenon in which bones bend without fracturing, often seen in long bones such as the forearm and fibula.

Remodeling Potential

Younger children, particularly those with fractures near growth plates, have a remarkable capacity for correcting deformities over time. However, the degree of remodeling depends on:

- *Age of the child:* Younger children have greater remodeling potential.
- *Proximity to a growth plate:* Fractures closer to active growth plates remodel better.
- *Plane of deformity:* Deformities in the plane of motion of a joint are more likely to remodel.

Nonetheless, certain fracture locations, such as midshaft fractures or fractures in older children nearing skeletal maturity, have less remodeling capacity, and these may require more precise reduction and stabilization.

COMPLICATIONS IN PEDIATRIC FRACTURES

- *Premature physeal closure/growth arrest:* This is particularly a concern with *Salter-Harris types III, IV, and V fractures,* where the fracture line extends through the physis or crushes it.
- *Limb length discrepancy*: There can be shortening or lengthening.
- *Angular deformities:* If one part of the growth plate closes prematurely while the rest continues to grow, the bone may grow abnormally, resulting in an angular deformity.

  A serious complication of supracondylar fractures, Volkmann's ischemic contracture, occurs when increased pressure in the forearm due to swelling (compartment syndrome) leads to ischemia and muscle necrosis.
- *Refracture:* Children who return to activity too quickly after fracture healing are at risk of refracture, especially in cases of incomplete bone healing. Proper rehabilitation and a gradual return to activity are necessary to prevent reinjury.
- *Nonaccidental trauma (NAT):* Fractures in nonambulatory children or fractures in unusual locations should raise suspicion for NAT. Certain fracture patterns, such as posterior rib fractures or metaphyseal corner fractures, and multiple fractures in different healing stages are highly specific for child abuse and warrant further investigation, including skeletal surveys and involvement of child protective services.

INTERPRETATION OF PEDIATRIC X-RAYS

Challenges in Pediatric Radiography

Interpreting pediatric X-rays can be more challenging than adult radiographs due to the evolving nature of a child's bones. Growth plates, secondary ossification centers, and developing bone structures must be considered when evaluating X-rays for fractures or other pathologies.

Normal Developmental Variations

In children, it is essential to differentiate normal developmental anatomy from fractures. Common developmental features include:

- *Ossification centers:* Appear at predictable ages but may mimic fractures. For example, the elbow has multiple ossification centers (CRITOE: *C*apitellum, *R*adial head, *I*nternal epicondyle, *T*rochlea, *O*lecranon, and *E*xternal epicondyle), which ossify at different stages.
- *Accessory ossicles:* Small bones that develop near joints and can be confused with fracture fragments.
- *Growth plates:* These should not be mistaken for fracture lines. They are smooth, well-circumscribed, and symmetric.

Systematic Approach to X-ray Interpretation

A systematic approach is key to ensuring that subtle findings are not missed. The following steps are recommended:

- *Patient's identification:* Ensure the X-ray corresponds to the correct patient and anatomical region.
- *Bone alignment:* Assess the alignment of bones, looking for any displacement or angulation that could indicate a fracture.
- *Growth plate evaluation:* Examine growth plates for any disruption that may suggest a Salter–Harris fracture.
- *Bone contour:* Trace the contour of the bone to identify any cortical disruptions or fractures.
- *Soft-tissue assessment:* Look for signs of soft-tissue swelling or joint effusions, which can indicate underlying fractures.
- *Comparison with opposite side:* In unclear cases, a comparison view of the opposite limb may help to identify subtle fractures or variations in anatomy.

BIBLIOGRAPHY

1. Harris WH. Radiology of infancy and childhood, 5th edition. Philadelphia: Saunders; 2011.
2. Krug RE. Pediatric radiology: The Essentials, 2nd edition. Philadelphia: Lippincott Williams & Wilkins; 2013.
3. Teichman JJ. Interpreting pediatric X-rays: a practical guide. London: Springer; 2018.
4. Tempkin DP, Reilly BD. Essentials of pediatric radiology, 3rd edition. New York: Springer; 2015.

Growth Plate Injuries

Zubair Ahmad Lone, John Mohd, Naresh Rana

Growth plate injuries, also known as physeal injuries, are a significant concern in pediatric orthopedics as they can have long-term consequences on bone growth and development. The growth plate (physis) is a cartilaginous region located between the metaphysis and epiphysis of long bones. It is responsible for longitudinal growth and remains open until skeletal maturity, making it particularly vulnerable to trauma. Understanding the nature of these injuries, their classification, treatment, and long-term outcomes is essential for clinicians managing pediatric patients.

ANATOMY OF THE GROWTH PLATE

The growth plate is composed of four zones, each with distinct cellular characteristics that contribute to bone growth **(Fig. 1)**:

- *Resting/germinal zone:* The zone closest to the epiphysis, consisting of resting chondrocytes.
- *Proliferative zone:* Chondrocytes divide and stack in columns, contributing to longitudinal bone growth.
- *Hypertrophic zone:* Chondrocytes increase in size, eventually undergoing apoptosis.
- *Calcification zone:* The matrix surrounding the chondrocytes calcifies, and new bone is laid down by osteoblasts.

Injury to any part of the growth plate can disrupt normal growth and may lead to complications such as growth arrest, deformity, or limb length discrepancies. Most growth plate injuries typically occur through the *hypertrophic zone* of the growth plate.

The hypertrophic zone is particularly vulnerable because the chondrocytes in this

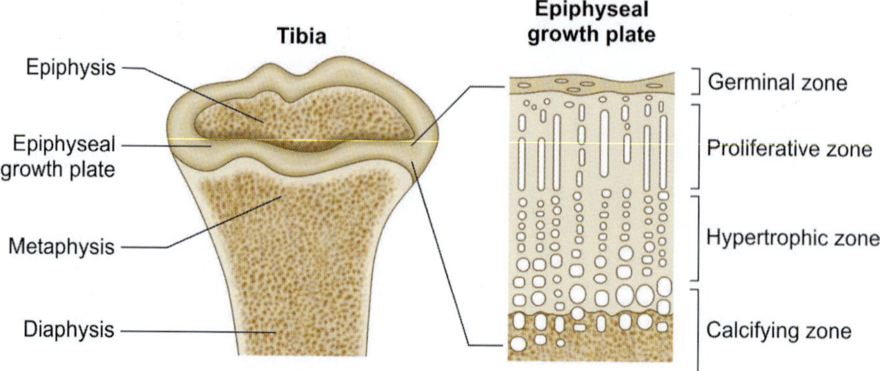

FIG. 1: Depicting various zones of growth plate.

region are large and undergoing changes before being replaced by bone, making the structure weaker compared to the other zones.

SALTER–HARRIS CLASSIFICATION OF GROWTH PLATE INJURIES

Growth plate fractures are classified using the Salter–Harris system, which is the most widely used and clinically relevant classification. This system categorizes fractures based on the involvement of the growth plate, metaphysis, and epiphysis **(Fig. 2)**:

- *Type I:* The fracture line runs through the physis without involving the bone. The prognosis is generally good, with minimal risk of growth disturbance **(Fig. 3)**.
- *Type II:* The most common type, this fracture extends through the physis and metaphysis but spares the epiphysis. The *Thurston-Holland sign* is typically seen in *Salter-Harris Type II fractures.* This sign refers to a triangular fragment of metaphyseal bone that remains attached to the epiphysis after a fracture has occurred. It is a characteristic radiographic finding and helps to confirm the diagnosis of a Type II growth plate The prognosis is generally favorable with proper management **(Fig. 4)**.

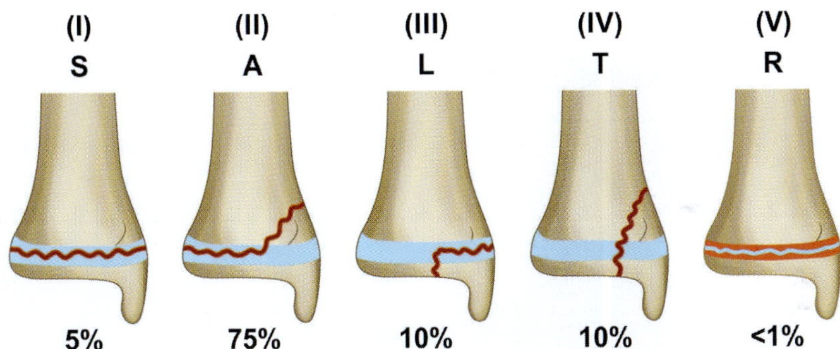

FIG. 2: Shows the Salter–Harris classification.

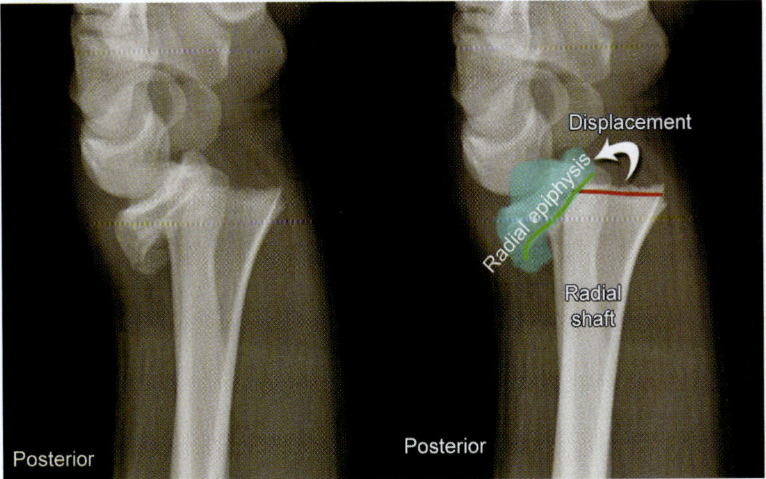

FIG. 3: Type I injury.

- *Type III:* The fracture involves the physis and epiphysis but spares the metaphysis. This type of fracture can disrupt the joint surface, leading to potential long-term complications if not treated properly **(Figs. 5A to F)**.
- *Type IV:* This fracture crosses the physis, metaphysis, and epiphysis, posing a high risk of growth arrest and deformity **(Figs. 6A to C)**.
- *Type V:* A compression injury to the physis, often difficult to diagnose on initial imaging. It carries the highest risk for growth disturbance and often results in premature closure of the growth plate.

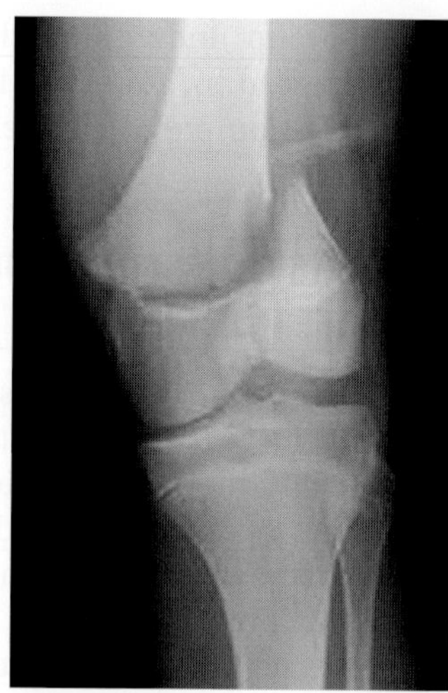

FIG. 4: Type II injury with Thurston Holland sign, needs anatomical reduction (close/open) and fixation.

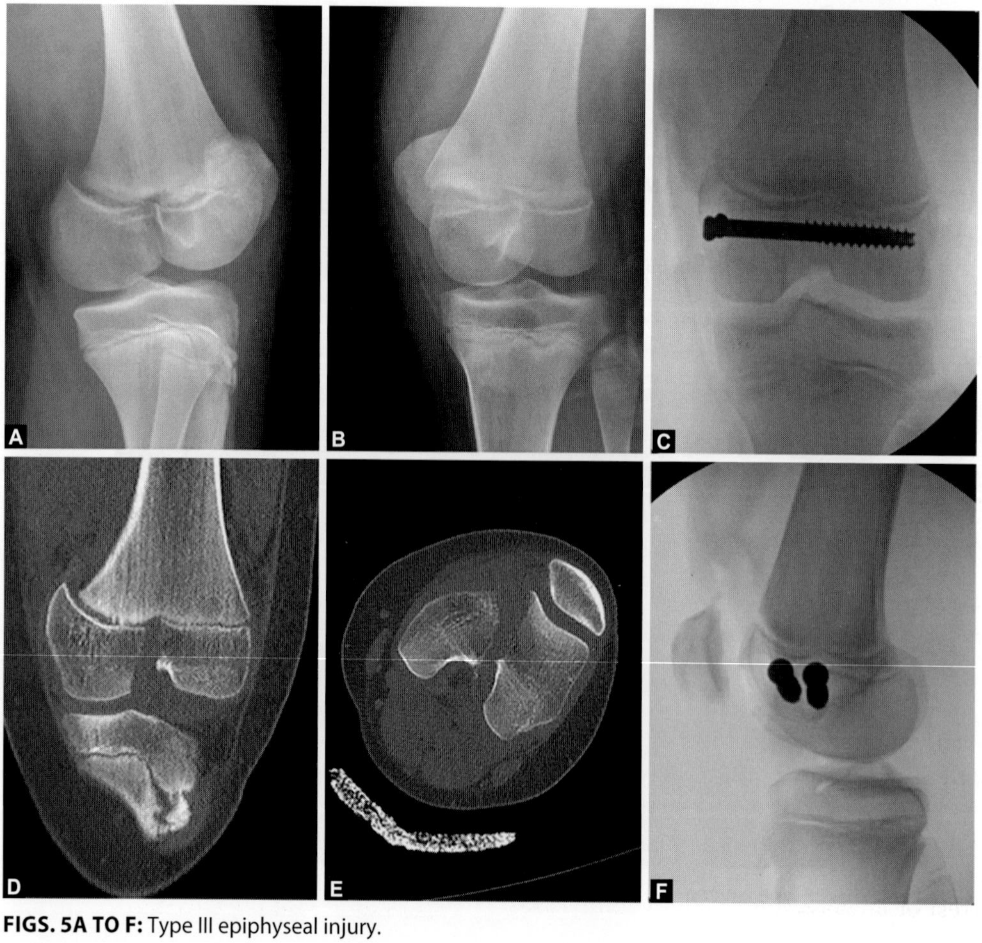

FIGS. 5A TO F: Type III epiphyseal injury.

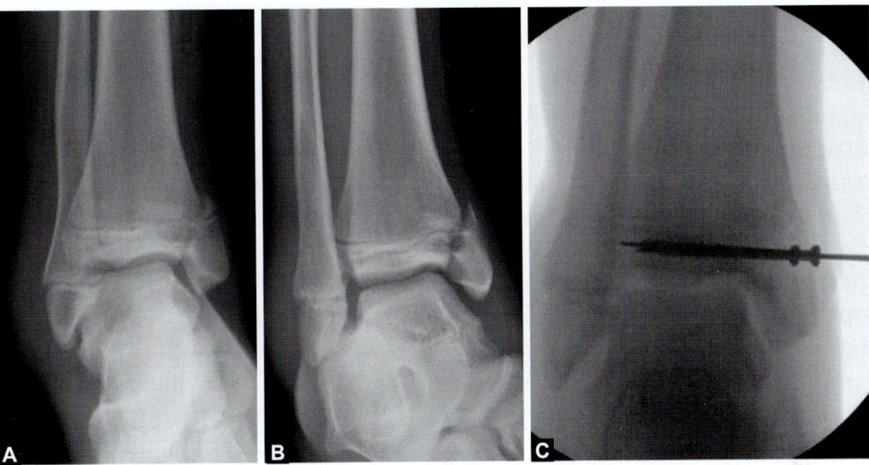

FIGS. 6A TO C: Type IV injury.

PRACTICAL CONSIDERATIONS IN CLINICAL MANAGEMENT

Imaging and Diagnosis

X-rays are the first-line imaging modality for suspected growth plate injuries. However, in cases of subtle fractures or suspected Type V injuries, MRI may be necessary for better visualization of the physis and surrounding soft tissues. Ultrasound can be useful in younger children where ossification is incomplete. At times CT scan may be needed to define fracture more clearly.

Timing of Intervention

Prompt intervention is critical in managing growth plate injuries to prevent growth disturbances. Delayed treatment or inadequate reduction of displaced fractures can lead to poor functional outcomes, including limb length discrepancies and joint deformities.

Long-term Follow-up

Given the potential for growth disturbance, patients with growth plate injuries should be followed until skeletal maturity. Serial radiographs and clinical examinations are necessary to monitor for signs of growth arrest or angular deformity. In some cases, corrective surgery may be required to address complications such as limb length discrepancy.

MANAGEMENT GUIDELINES FOR EACH TYPE OF INJURY

Salter–Harris Type I: Through the Physis

- X-rays may appear normal due to the fracture being solely through the cartilage. Clinical signs such as tenderness over the physis help to guide the diagnosis.
- *Treatment:*
  - *Nondisplaced fractures:* Immobilization in a cast or splint for 3–4 weeks. No reduction is typically required.
  - *Displaced fractures:* Gentle closed reduction (manipulation) under anesthesia may be necessary to realign the fracture.
- *Prognosis:* Excellent, with low risk of growth disturbance when properly managed.

Salter–Harris Type II: Through the Physis and Metaphysis

- X-ray usually shows the metaphyseal fragment, aiding in diagnosis.

- *Treatment:*
  - *Nondisplaced fractures:* Closed reduction is typically not required. Immobilization in a cast for 4–6 weeks is sufficient.
  - *Displaced fractures:* Closed reduction is required, followed by casting. Severe displacement may necessitate percutaneous pinning or, rarely, open reduction and internal fixation (ORIF).
- *Prognosis:* Generally favorable with a low risk of growth arrest if reduction is achieved early.

Salter–Harris Type III: Through the Physis and Epiphysis

- X-ray and MRI may be needed to assess joint involvement and the extent of epiphyseal damage.
- *Treatment:*
  - *Nondisplaced fractures:* Immobilization with a cast is sufficient.
  - *Displaced fractures:* Anatomical reduction is crucial to restore joint alignment and prevent long-term complications. ORIF is often required to ensure accurate reduction of the fracture.
- *Prognosis:* Risk of growth disturbances is higher than in Types I and II fractures due to joint involvement. Early and precise reduction improves the outcome.

Salter–Harris Type IV: Through the Metaphysis, Physis, and Epiphysis

- X-rays, often supplemented with MRI or CT scans, are used to assess the full extent of the fracture, especially regarding joint involvement.
- *Treatment:*
  - *Nondisplaced fractures:* Conservative management with immobilization may be attempted, though this type often requires surgery.
  - *Displaced fractures:* ORIF is typically necessary to ensure proper alignment of both the joint surface and growth plate. Failure to achieve accurate reduction increases the risk of growth arrest and deformity.
- *Prognosis:* Poorer than Type I–III fractures due to the high risk of growth disturbances. Careful long-term monitoring is required to assess for complications such as growth arrest and angular deformities.

Salter–Harris Type V: Crush Injury to the Physis

- Initial X-rays may appear normal with MRI or follow-up imaging being necessary to detect physeal damage. A high index of suspicion is required based on the mechanism of injury and clinical presentation (e.g., pain localized to the growth plate).
- *Treatment:*
  - *Nondisplaced injuries:* Immobilization and close monitoring are usually recommended.
  - *Surgical options:* If growth arrest occurs, surgical procedures such as guided growth (epiphysiodesis) or limb-lengthening surgeries may be required to correct deformities or limb length discrepancies.
- *Prognosis:* This type of injury has the worst prognosis due to the high likelihood of permanent growth arrest. Close follow-up with serial X-rays is essential to monitor for signs of growth disturbances.

BIBLIOGRAPHY

1. Ogden JA. Skeletal Injury in the Child, 3rd edition. Philadelphia: Saunders; 2000.
2. Peterson HA. Physeal fractures: Part 1. Classification, anatomy, and pathophysiology. J Pediatr Orthop. 2013;33 Suppl 1.
3. Salter RB, Harris WR. Injuries involving the epiphyseal plate. J Bone Joint Surg Am. 1963;45(3): 587-622.

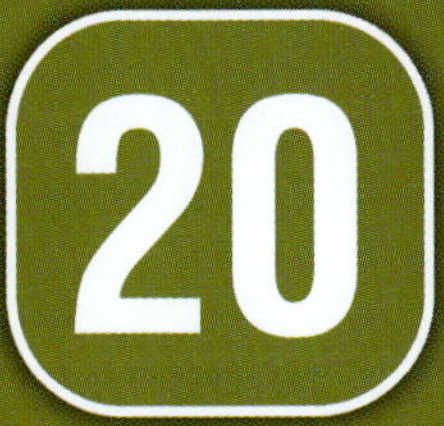

Common Pediatric Fractures of Upper Limb

Pediatric Shoulder Fractures

Harsh Chauhan, Yassar Arfat

CLAVICLE FRACTURES

The most common shoulder injuries in children, typically resulting from direct trauma or falls and birth-related injuries.

- The most common type of clavicle fracture in pediatric patients is midshaft fracture.
- Injury to the medial or lateral clavicle may lead to physeal disruption, which is commonly classified as Salter–Harris type 1 or 2 fractures.
- *Medial clavicle injury*: Dislocation of the sternoclavicular joint is rare but possible.
- *Lateral clavicle injury*: Metaphyseal fractures may occur, often leaving the ligaments intact.

Management

Most cases are managed conservatively with sling or shoulder immobilization or figure-of-eight brace immobilization, the duration of immobilization is generally 2–4 weeks, followed by progressive range of motion as tolerated.

Absolute indications for operative intervention in children and adolescents with clavicle fractures, including compound fractures, skin tenting/compromise, and major vascular injury. Refractures and rarely nonunion also need fixation.

- Closed reduction and internal fixation using TENS.
- Open reduction and internal fixation (ORIF) with plates and screws (extremely rare situations).

PROXIMAL HUMERAL FRACTURES

More common in the age group of 5–12 years, these fractures can involve the humeral head, neck, or tuberosities and are classified using the Salter–Harris system when the growth plate is involved. Physeal injuries and greenstick fractures of the proximal humerus metaphysis comprise the majority of fractures in this region.

About 80% of humeral growth occurs at the proximal physis, thereby providing excellent remodeling potential to this region and allowing for high tolerance to angulation and displacement.

Mechanism of injury

- Birth-related injuries seen in Breech presentation, shoulder presentation, and hyperextension injuries of the arm during delivery.
- *Direct injury*: fall onto the affected shoulder or arm.
- *Indirect injury*: common in sports-related injury.
- *Pathological fracture*: Benign lesions—unicameral bone cysts or aneurysmal bone cysts and less often malignant lesions (osteogenic sarcoma), commonly involve the proximal humerus and may first present with pathological fracture.

Evaluation

Apart from routine evaluation, a focused examination: Palpate for any chest tenderness and pulmonary status assessment should be performed to rule out any underlying thorax injury, especially in direct trauma cases.

Classification (Table 1)

The *Salter–Harris classification* is used to categorize fractures involving the growth plate (physis) in children and adolescents, as these fractures can impact future bone growth and development. The humeral physis is extracapsular and thus more susceptible to injury **(Figs. 1A to D)**.

Acceptable Alignment of Proximal Humerus Fractures (Table 2)

Conservative management of proximal humerus fractures: Mostly patients managed with sling or shoulder immobilization for 3–4 weeks.

TABLE 1: Neer–Horowitz classification of proximal humerus fractures.

Grade I	<5 mm displacement (Minimally displaced)
Grade II	Dispalcement less than one-third of the shaft width
Grade III	Displacement more than one-third and less than two-thirds of the shaft width
Grade IV	Dispalcement more than two-thirds of the shaft width

Indications for Operative Management

- Compound fractures
- Fractures with neurovascular or severe soft-tissue injury
- significantly displaced fracture with intra-articular extension
- Displaced tuberosity fractures
- Irreducible or unstable fractures in older adolescents with unacceptable alignment

Methods for operative intervention are closed/open reduction and fixation with K-wires or TENS. Postprocedure sling-and-swathe immobilization is needed for 2–4 weeks.

SHAFT FRACTURE OF THE HUMERUS

- Humeral shaft fractures usually occur due to birth injuries during breech presentation and difficult deliveries.
- Other common causes are battered baby syndrome, direct impact onto the arm,

TABLE 2: The acceptable alignment of proximal humerus fractures.

Age	Angulation	Displacement
<5 years	70°	100%
5–11 years	40–70°	50–100%
>12 years	<40°	<50%

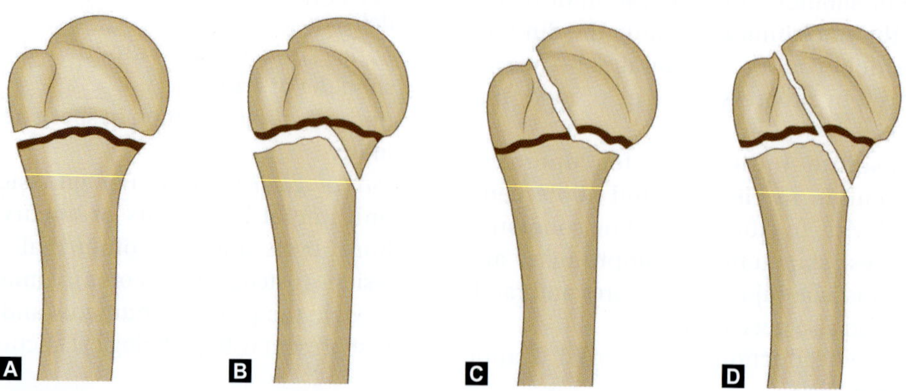

FIGS. 1A TO D: Physeal injury of the proximal humerus. (A) Salter–Harris type I; (B) Salter–Harris type II; (C) Salter–Harris type III; and (D) Salter–Harris type IV.

hyperextension/hyperrotational injury, and pathological fracture.

- Radial nerve palsy is commonly associated with shaft of humerus fracture. Therefore, neurological assessment is critical, particularly for assessing radial nerve function.

Acceptable alignment:

- In younger children:
  - <35–45° angulation
- In older children:
  - <20° varus or valgus
  - <20° Procurvatum
  - <15° rotational malalignment
  - A shortening of <2 cm

Management is mostly conservative with a sling or shoulder immobilization. Coaptation splinting (also referred to as U-slab **Fig. 2**), hanging cast (in case of overriding and shortening), and functional bracing have been advocated for the treatment of humeral shaft fractures.

Indications for the operative treatment of humeral shaft fractures include open fractures, fractures with neurovascular injury, floating elbow injuries, and failure to achieve adequate reduction with conservative methods. Methods for surgical fracture fixation, including ORIF using plate-and-screw constructs, intramedullary nailing, and external fixation.

SCAPULAR FRACTURES

Scapular fractures are relatively rare in children and are usually associated with high-energy trauma. They can involve the body, acromion, or glenoid and are often confused with the numerous secondary ossification centers in the immature scapula.

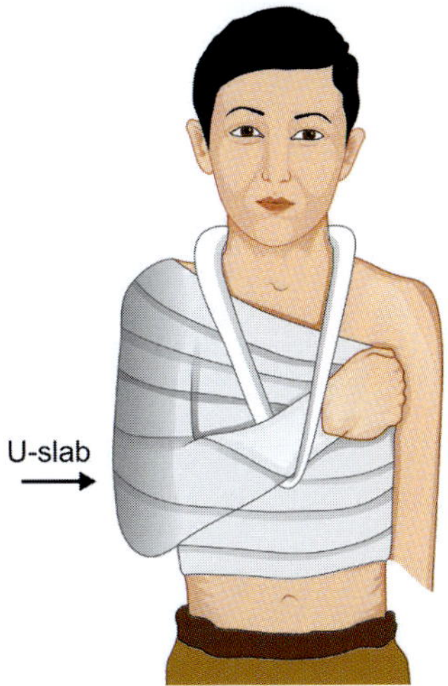

FIG. 2: Shows a U-slab and sling.

Most scapular fractures are treated nonoperatively.

Complications and Follow-up

- *Malunion or rarely nonunion*: This can occur if alignment or fixation is inadequate, potentially requiring further intervention.
- *Growth plate injury*: Fractures involving the growth plates can affect normal bone development, necessitating close monitoring.
- *Rotator cuff injury*: Although rare, rotator cuff injuries can occur in severe fractures and require additional treatment.

Regular follow-up visits are necessary to monitor healing, address complications, and adjust treatment as needed.

BIBLIOGRAPHY

1. Gagnon D, Dyer GS, MacKenzie W. Outcomes of surgical intervention for pediatric scapular fractures: a review of 15 cases. J Orthop Trauma. 2024;38(2):89-95.
2. Pritchett JW. Pediatric shoulder injuries: the growing child. Clin Orthop Relat Res. 2022;480(1):88-98.
3. Sulaiman AR, Sabir AB, Awan SI. Management of pediatric shoulder girdle fractures: a review. J Child Orthop. 2021;15(2):112-9.

Pediatric Elbow Fractures

Suraydev Aman Singh, Saravjeet Kour

- Elbow fractures are one of the most frequently occurring fractures encountered in the pediatric population, accounting for 10–15% of all childhood fractures.
- Falling onto an outstretched hand forms the common mechanism in these injuries.
- Diagnostic imaging of pediatric elbow fractures is challenging due to the relative radiolucency of cartilaginous bones, in addition to the sequential appearance of secondary ossification centers around elbow.

APPLIED ANATOMY

- Ossification centers around elbow can be remembered by the mnemonic *CRITOE* **(Figs. 1A and B)**.
    - Ossification begins with *C*apitellum around 1 year followed by *R*adial head and *I*nternal (Medial) epicondyle at 3 and 5 years respectively. *T*rochlea starts ossifying around 7 years followed by *O*lecranon at 9 years, and finally *E*xternal (Lateral) epicondyle appears by 11 years of age.

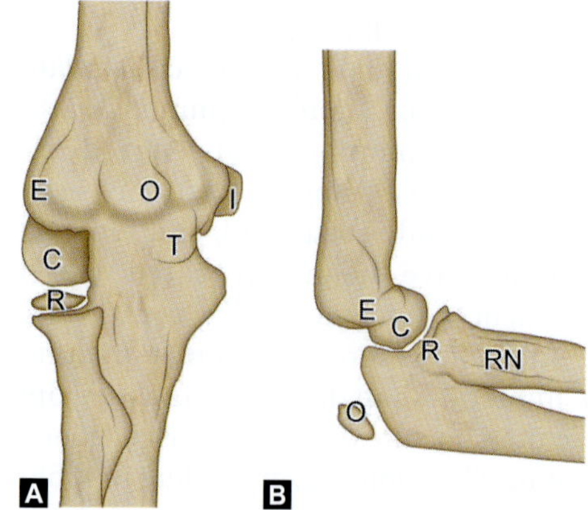

FIGS. 1A AND B: Depicting ossification centers around elbow in anteroposterior (AP) and lateral views.

[C: capitellum; R: radial head: I: internal (medial) epicondyle; T: trochlea O: olecranon; E: external (lateral) epicondyle; RN: radial neck]

ANATOMIC ALIGNMENT

Anterior Humeral Line

- In a normal elbow, a line drawn along the anterior humeral cortex should intersect the middle third of capitellum on a lateral radiographic projection.
- However, anterior humeral line (AHL) should cross the capitellum and not necessarily the middle third only, as was earlier believed.
- The most reliable factor in detecting the presence of minimally displaced supracondylar humerus (SCH) fractures **(Fig. 2)**

Baumann Angle

- On a standard anteroposterior (AP) view, it is the angle formed between physeal line of lateral condyle intersecting with

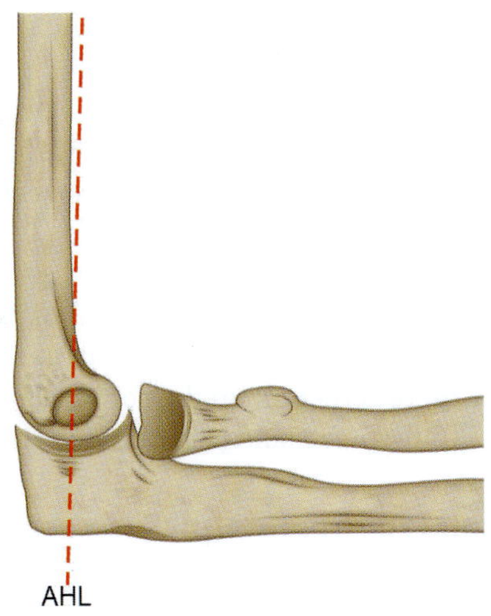

FIG. 2: Showing the passage of anterior humeral line (AHL) through capitellum on a true lateral projection.

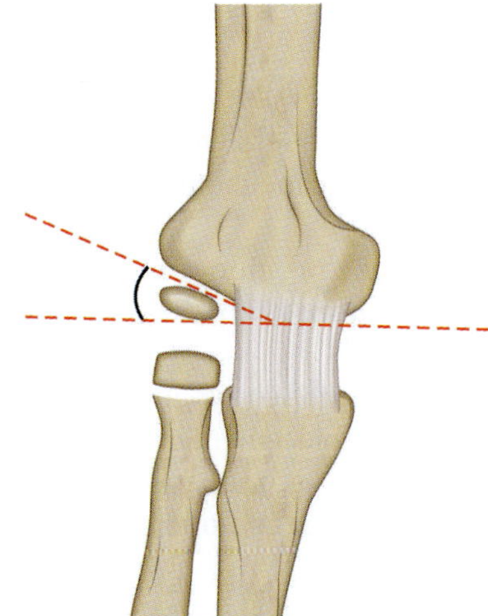

FIG. 3: Illustrating Baumann's angle.

a line perpendicular to the long axis of humeral shaft.

- *Normal values*: 9–26°.
- Inappropriate restoration (<10°) is a reliable predictor of varus angulation of distal humerus **(Fig. 3)**.

Radiocapitellar Line

- A line parallel to and bisecting the radial head and neck should intersect through the capitellum in all radiographic planes.
- *Presence of either of the lines, i.e., AHL, radial head-capitellar line, denotes the presence of a fracture or dislocation or both.*

Fat Pad

- Displacement of fat pads, especially posterior, is a helpful aid in identifying minimally displaced fractures.
- Similarly, the anterior fat pad or sail sign being a more sensitive indicator of small joint effusions, if displaced indicates the likelihood of an occult fracture.

CLINICAL EVALUATION

- Examination of neurovascular status is critical, especially in cases of SCH fractures, where there is a significant risk of brachial artery and median nerve injury (anterior interosseous nerve).

IMAGING MODALITIES

Radiographs

- Standard projections include AP and lateral views.
- Additional views include oblique views (internal and external) to delineate the entire extent of fracture and to quantify displacement.
- A radiograph of the contralateral extremity is of utmost importance in cases to diagnose undisplaced or minimally displaced fractures.
- Ossification centers and temporal alignment landmarks such as AHL, Baumann's angle, etc., are critical in diagnosis.

Computed Tomography

- Useful for evaluating complex fractures or when detailed bone structure visualization is needed.

Magnetic Resonance Imaging

- Rarely employed to assess soft-tissue damage or intra-articular involvement not captured by X-rays or to assess viability of fragments in cases of neglected fractures.

Most common fractures around the pediatric elbow innclude with are as below:

SUPRACONDYLAR FRACTURES

- These injuries predominantly occur in children aged 5–8 years.
- *Mechanism of injury:* typically resulting from a fall onto an outstretched hand putting the elbow in hyperextension.
- The majority (95%) of them are extension-type injuries in which the distal fragment is angulated/displaced posteriorly, marked by the AHL passing anterior to the capitellum on a lateral radiograph.
- The remaining 5% are flexion-type injuries that involve anterior displacement of the distal fragment and are often caused by a direct anterior force against a flexed elbow.
- The Gartland classification is most widely used to classify extension type supracondylar fractures and guide treatment:
    - *Type I:* Nondisplaced or minimally displaced fractures. Sometimes, the posterior fat pad may be the only evidence of such fractures **(Figs. 4A and B)**.
    - *Type II:* Displaced fractures with a presumably intact, yet hinged posterior cortex. The AHL passes anterior to the capitellum or in minimally displaced fractures may intersect the capitellum **(Figs. 5A and B)**.
    - *Type III:* Completely displaced fractures with disruption of both cortices. In addition to extension, there is rotation in the coronal and/or transverse plane **(Figs. 6A and B)**.

Flexion Type Supracondylar Humerus Fracture

Flexion type of supracondylar fractures are less common compared to extension type, please refer to **Figures 7A and B**.

Management

Conservative

Type I SCH and less commonly stable type II injuries can usually be managed conservatively.

- Immobilize the elbow in a *long arm posterior splint* with the elbow at 90° flexion.
- Follow-up with X-rays in 1–2 weeks to ensure no displacement occurs.
- After 3–4 weeks, transition to physical therapy for range of motion.

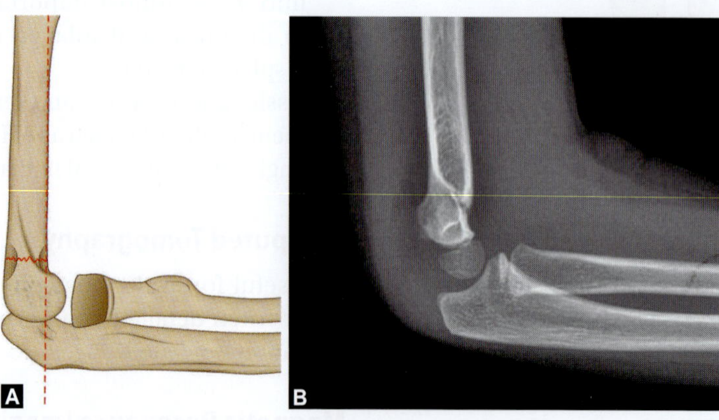

FIGS. 4A AND B: Illustration (left) and lateral radiograph (right) of Type I supracondylar humerus (SCH) fracture.

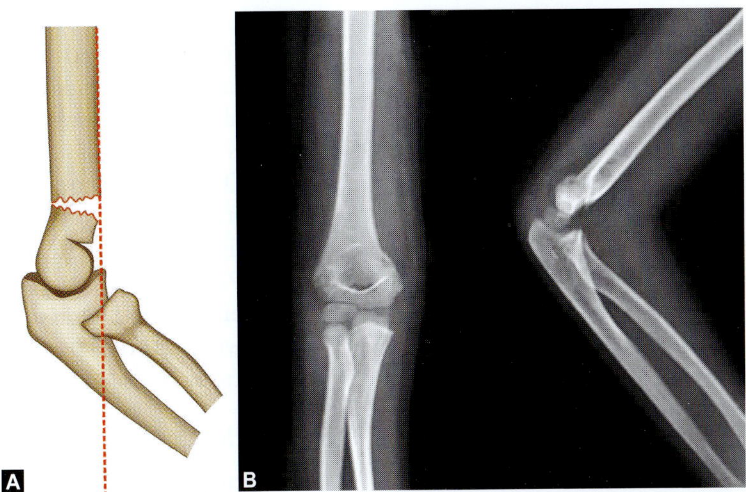

FIGS. 5A AND B: Illustration (left) and radiographs (right) of Type II supracondylar humerus (SCH) fracture.

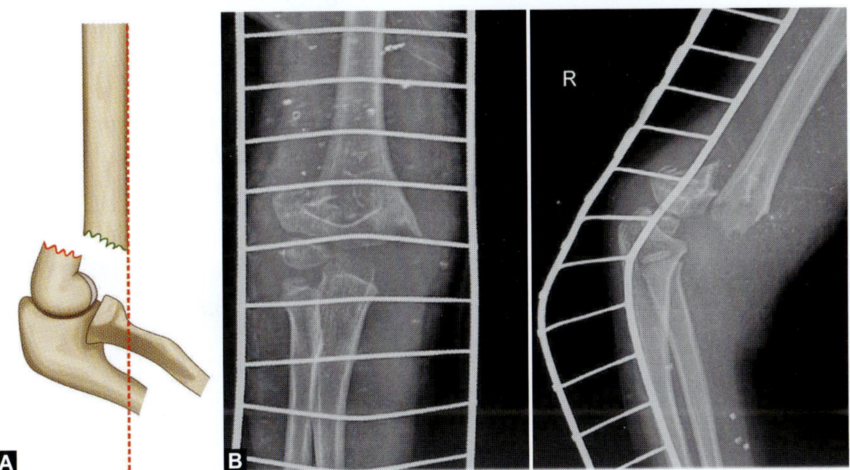

FIGS. 6A AND B: Illustration (left) and radiographs (right) of Type III supracondylar humerus (SCH) fracture.

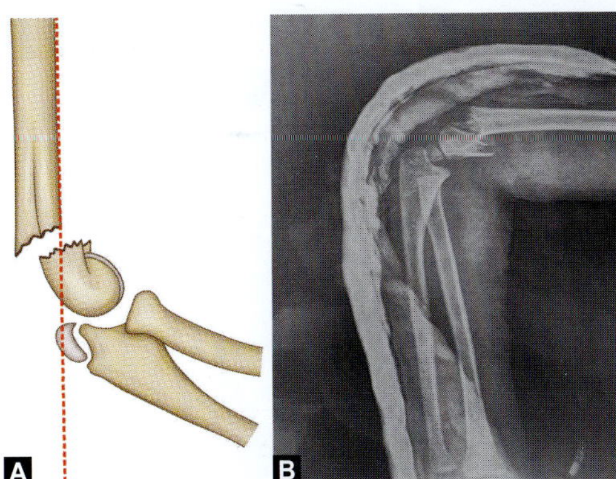

FIGS. 7A AND B: Illustration and lateral radiograph depicting flexion type supracondylar humerus (SCH) fracture.

Surgical Management

- *Types II and III fractures* being unstable, generally require surgical intervention.
- *Emerging trends for optimal outcome for type II SCH fractures conjure closed reduction and percutaneous pinning rather than cast immobilization.*
- *Closed reduction and percutaneous pinning (CRPP) technique:*
  - Perform reduction under fluoroscopy (in an operating room).
  - Stabilize the fracture with *Kirschner wires (K-wires).*

  - Typically, two to three pins are used, crossing the fracture in different configuration
- *Open reduction:* reserved for cases where closed reduction fails or when there is a need to address neurovascular compromise. The best approach to open reduction depends on several factors, including the degree of fracture displacement, associated neurovascular injuries, and the location of the fracture. The anteromedial and anterolateral approaches are most commonly used for open reduction of supracondylar fractures, with the anteromedial approach being ideal for cases involving vascular injury. Two to three Kirschner wires (K-wires) are commonly used depending on the fracture type and surgeon's preference.
- *Configuration of K-wires:*
  - *Two K-wires:*
    - Usually for less complex fractures (Gartland type 2 or stable fractures)
    - Inserted in a crossed configuration (one medial and one lateral) or two lateral K-wires if there is concern about ulnar nerve injury.
  - *Three K-wires:*
    - Often used for more unstable fractures (Gartland type 3 or displaced fractures).
    - Provides added stability, with either two lateral and one medial wire or three lateral wires in some cases **(Figs. 8A to E)**.

Postoperative Care

- After pinning, the elbow is immobilized in a *splint* or *cast* for 3–4 weeks.
- Regular follow-up with X-rays to monitor healing and pin placement.
- Pins are usually removed in the clinic after 3–4 weeks.

Complications to monitor for:

- *Neurovascular injury:* Monitor for median, ulnar, or radial nerve injuries.

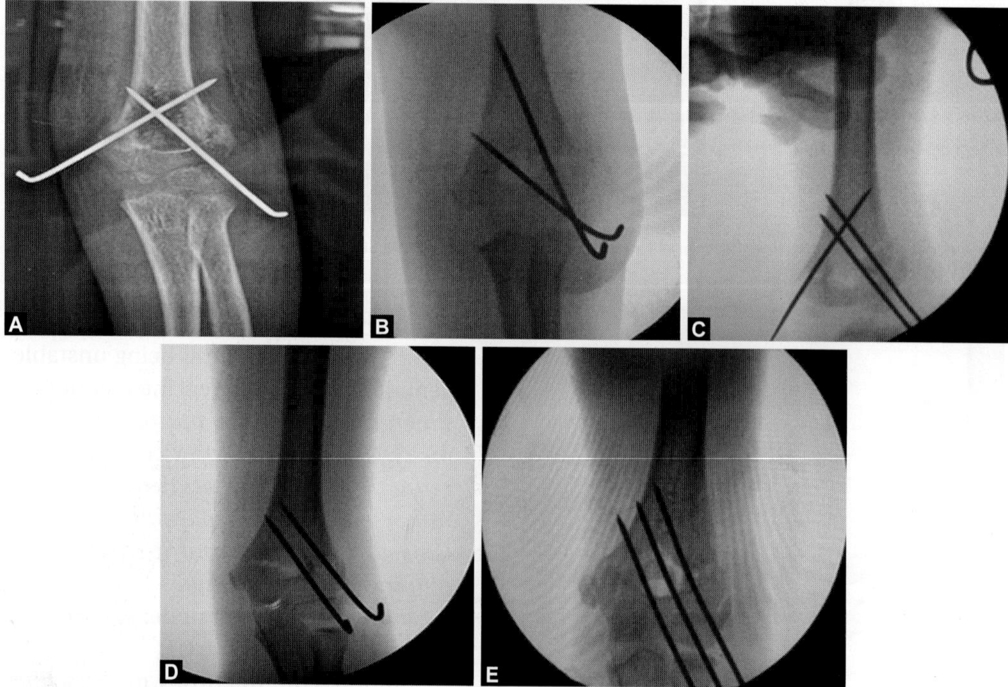

FIGS. 8A TO E: Radiographs showing different configuration of K-wires used for fixation of supracondylar humerus (SCH) fractures.

- *Compartment syndrome:* This can be limb threatening and hence have a low threshold to suspect and treat this complication.
- *Malunion or cubitus varus (Gunstock deformity):* More common in Type III fractures.
- *Infection (with pinning):* Pin site infection is a possible complication.

Management of Vascular Injuries Associated with Supracondylar Fractures of the Elbow

It can be serious and requires urgent intervention to prevent ischemia and limb loss. The *brachial artery* is particularly at risk, especially in *completely displaced (Gartland Type III)* fractures, where bone fragments can impinge on or tear the artery.

- *Initial assessment and diagnosis:*
    - Evaluate for signs of *vascular compromise:*
        - Absent or weak radial pulse
        - Cold, pale, or cyanotic hand
        - Capillary refill time >3 seconds

  Doppler ultrasound may be used in the emergency room to assess the *brachial artery* and confirm flow to the hand.
- *Immediate reduction* (if not yet attempted) can sometimes restore blood flow by releasing pressure on the artery.
- *Closed reduction and monitoring:*
    - If there is a vascular injury but the hand remains viable (i.e., no signs of irreversible ischemia also called as *pulseless pink hand*), attempt *closed reduction.*
    - After reduction, *reassess the vascular status:*
        - If the pulse returns and the hand becomes warm, continue with nonsurgical management and monitor closely.
        - If the pulse remains absent but the hand is *well perfused* (warm with good capillary refill), you may opt to *monitor the patient carefully.* In this scenario, a Doppler can confirm flow despite an absent palpable pulse, indicating possible arterial spasm.
        - If the hand remains *cold or cyanotic,* urgent surgical exploration is needed.
- *Indications for open vascular exploration:*
    - *Absent pulse* and *poor perfusion* (cold and pale hand) despite closed reduction.
    - *Doppler ultrasound* shows absent flow in the brachial artery, and the hand shows signs of ischemia.
    - *Progressive ischemia* after reduction, indicating vascular injury despite initial improvement.
- *Surgical exploration and management of vascular injury:*
    - *The anteromedial approach* is the preferred incision for exposing the brachial artery in cases where vascular injury is suspected. Always reduce the fracture through the same approach and fix and then deal with vascular injury with various options available:
        - *Exploration and direct arterial repair:*
            - If the artery is *contused* or *partially torn,* it may be repaired with fine vascular sutures.
            - For a *complete transection* of the brachial artery, options include *end-to-end anastomosis* or *interposition grafting* (often using the saphenous vein).
            - *Fasciotomy* may be necessary if there is concern for *compartment syndrome,* which can occur due to prolonged ischemia and reperfusion injury.
            - *Intraoperative Doppler ultrasound* can be used to confirm restoration of blood flow through the repaired artery.

- *Postoperative care:*
  - *Monitor vascular status* closely after surgery, checking pulses, capillary refill, and temperature of the hand regularly.
  - *Anticoagulation:* Some surgeons may use a *heparin* infusion or other anticoagulation to prevent thrombosis in the repaired artery, but this should be done with caution due to the risk of bleeding from the fracture site.
  - Immobilize the arm in a *long arm splint* after surgery.
  - *Physical therapy* begins once the vascular injury is resolved and fracture healing is sufficient to tolerate gentle motion.
  - Continue monitoring for *complications* such as re-occlusion of the artery, infection, or compartment syndrome and *nerve injury:*
    - The *median nerve* runs adjacent to the brachial artery and may be damaged during the fracture or during surgical exploration. Postoperative nerve function should be closely monitored.

LATERAL CONDYLE FRACTURES

- The mechanism of injury is a fall on the outstretched hand with varus force being transmitted to the distal humerus.
- Utilize internal oblique view in addition to conventional Ap and lateral radiographs to delineate the fracture displacement.
- *Song et al.* classification is recently the most preferred system for pediatric lateral condyle humerus fractures, based on displacement along with rotation of fracture fragment.
  - *Type 1:* Displacement ≤ 2 mm with fracture limited to metaphysis only.
  - *Type II:* Displacement ≤ 2 mm with fracture extending to epiphyseal articular cartilage.
  - *Type III:* Displacement ≤ 2 mm with medial and lateral displacement of fragment, unstable fractures.
  - *Type IV:* Displacement > 2 mm without rotation of fragment.
  - *Type V:* Displacement > 2 mm with fragment malrotation **(Fig. 9)**.

Other Classification

- *Milch classification* (used to assess the extent of the fracture):
  - *Milch type I:* Fracture through the ossification center, less serious.
  - *Milch type II:* Fracture extends into the trochlear groove, potentially more unstable.
- *Displacement:*
  - *Nondisplaced:* <2 mm displacement.
  - *Displaced:* ≥2 mm displacement.

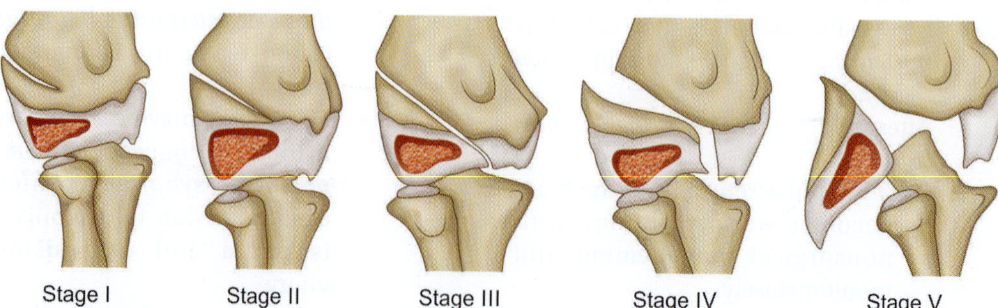

FIG. 9: Sketch illustration of Song et al. classification of pediatric lateral condyle humerus fracture.

Treatment Guidelines based on Displacement

- *Nondisplaced fracture (<2 mm displacement)*
  - *Conservative treatment:*
    - Immobilization in a long-arm cast with the elbow flexed at about 90°.
    - Follow-up X-rays are taken after 7–10 days to ensure the fracture remains nondisplaced.
    - Immobilization is typically maintained for 4–6 weeks.
    - After cast removal, physical therapy may be required to regain motion and strength.
- *Minimally displaced fracture (2–4 mm displacement)*
  - Closed reduction and percutaneous fixation.
- *Displaced fracture (>4 mm displacement)*
  - *Surgical treatment:*
    - The fracture is reduced surgically, and fixation is performed using screws or pins (typically Kirschner wires) to stabilize the fragment **(Figs. 10A to D)**.
    - Immobilization in a cast or splint follows surgery for 4–6 weeks.
    - Physical therapy postsurgery is important to restore motion and prevent stiffness.

Complications to look for:

- Nonunion or malunion
- Stiffness or loss of motion
- Lateral condyle overgrowth
- Cubitus valgus

MEDIAL EPICONDYLE FRACTURES

- Mechanism of injury involves a fall on an outstretched hand with valgus stress across the elbow, sometimes leading to a condition known as "Little Leaguer's elbow" as traction from medial collateral ligament and flexor mass leading to avulsion of the medial epicondylar apophysis.
- Associated with posterior elbow dislocation in about 50% of cases.
- These fractures occur primarily in adolescent boys involved in sports like baseball or gymnastics.
- These fractures are broadly classified on the basis of displacement of fracture with >5 mm displacement of the fragment, ulnar nerve entrapment symptoms, and incarceration of the fragment within the joint warranting surgical intervention otherwise conservative treatment in a pop cast for 3–4 weeks is acceptable **(Fig. 11)**.

Classification

- *Nondisplaced:* Minimal or no gap between the bone fragments.
- *Displaced:* A gap > 5 mm between fragments.
- *Associated with elbow dislocation:* This is often more complex due to joint instability.

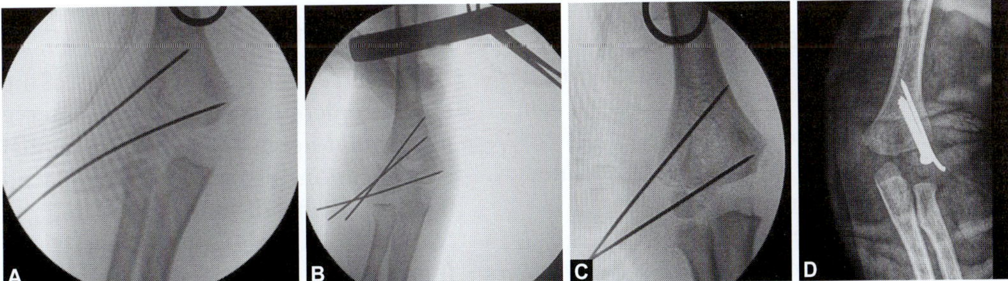

FIGS. 10A TO D: Radiographs showing different configuration of fixation for lateral condyle humerus fracture.

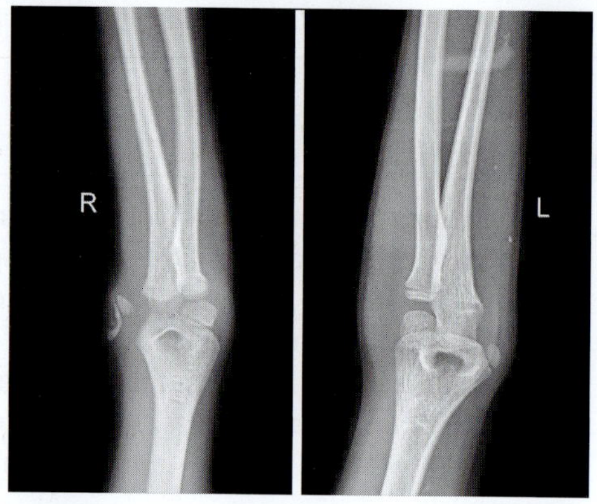

FIG. 11: Radiographs showing displaced fracture medial epicondyle.

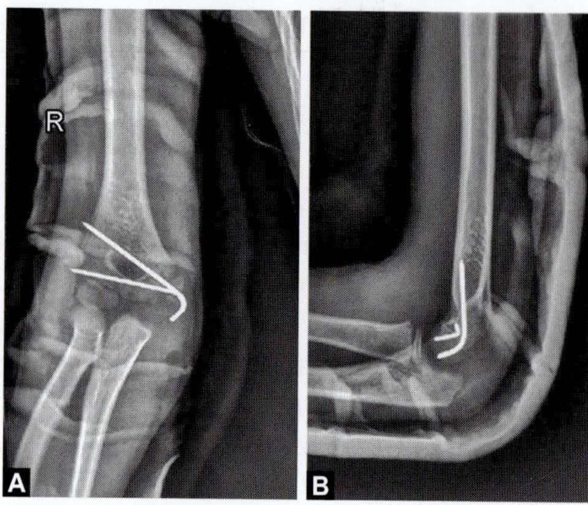

FIGS. 12A AND B: Radiographs showing fixation of medial condyle fracture.

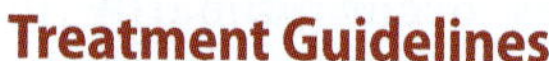

Treatment Guidelines

- *Nondisplaced or minimally displaced fracture (<5 mm displacement)*
  - *Conservative management:*
    - Immobilization in a long-arm cast or splint, with the elbow flexed to about 90°.
    - *Immobilization period:* 3–4 weeks (varies depending on healing rate).
    - Follow-up X-rays to ensure the fracture remains nondisplaced.
    - Physical therapy after cast removal to restore motion and strength.
  - *Rehabilitation:*
    - Gentle range-of-motion exercises usually begin after 3–4 weeks of immobilization.
    - Gradual strengthening once full motion is achieved.

Surgical Indications

- Displacement > 5 mm
- Elbow dislocation with associated instability
- Entrapment of the ulnar nerve
- Open fractures or fractures associated with soft-tissue injury
- *Surgical treatment:*
  - *Open reduction and internal fixation:*
    - Fixation typically involves using screws or Kirschner wires (K-wires) to hold the fragment in place.
    - Postsurgical immobilization is typically required for 3–4 weeks, followed by gradual range-of-motion exercises **(Figs. 12A and B)**.

Fractures Associated with Elbow Dislocation

These cases are more complex and often require surgery because the dislocation can make the fracture more unstable.

- *The management involves*:
  - Reduction of the elbow dislocation.
  - Open reduction and internal fixation to stabilize the medial epicondyle fragment.
  - Immobilization for 3–4 weeks post-operatively.
  - Follow-up for signs of instability or nerve damage.

Complications to Monitor

- *Ulnar nerve injury:* The proximity of the medial epicondyle to the ulnar nerve means that nerve damage is a potential complication, especially in displaced fractures or after dislocation.
- *Nonunion or malunion:* Failure of the fracture to heal properly may require surgical intervention.
- *Chronic elbow instability:* Especially with associated elbow dislocations.

- *Loss of range of motion:* Particularly loss of full extension is a common issue if physical therapy is not started early.

PROXIMAL RADIUS FRACTURES

- These fractures usually occur in children aged 9–10 years.
- Often results from fall on an outstretched hand with valgus stress causing the capitellum to strike the proximal radius.
- Majority of these fractures can be managed nonoperatively with immobilization alone or closed reduction followed by immobilization while ones with >45° angulation may preferably be managed with closed reduction or open reduction followed by internal fixation once satisfactory reduction is achieved **(Fig. 13)**.
- Open reduction and internal fixation is often associated with greater loss of range of motion and osteonecrosis of the radial head and should be reserved for cases with higher degrees of displacement with concomitant injuries.
- Another technique commonly used is the *Metaizeau technique* **(Figs. 14A to C)** for the fixation of radial neck fracture. This technique is minimally invasive and typically involves using an elastic intramedullary nail to realign and stabilize the fracture of the radial neck, commonly in pediatric patients **(Figs. 14A to C)**.

OLECRANON FRACTURES

- Olecranon fractures are rare pediatric injuries usually resulting from a fall onto an outstretched hand with an elbow in flexion **(Fig. 15)**.
- These fractures can be classified depending on the mechanism of injury: Fall with elbow in flexion causes transverse fracture of olecranon; longitudinal fracture lines due to varus or valgus stresses with elbow in extension and anterior tension failure due to direct trauma **(Fig. 16)**.

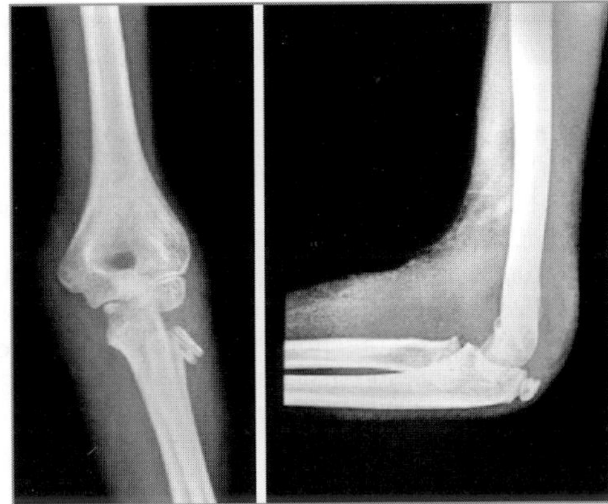

FIG. 13: Radiographs showing fracture radial neck.

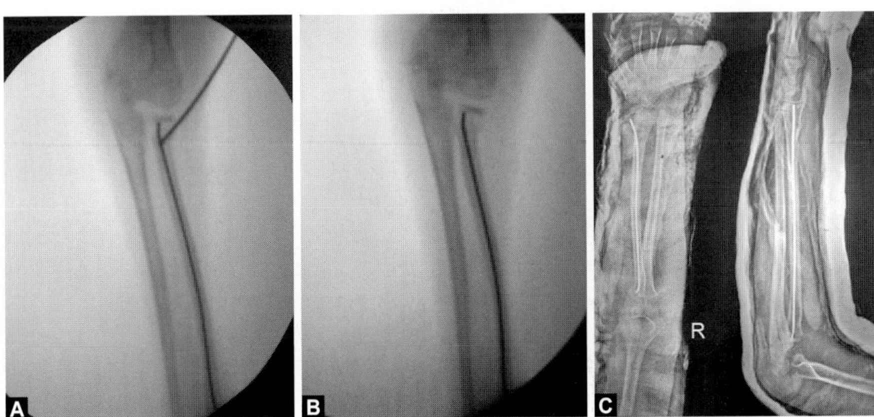

FIGS. 14A TO C: Metaizeau technique for fixation of radial neck fracture.

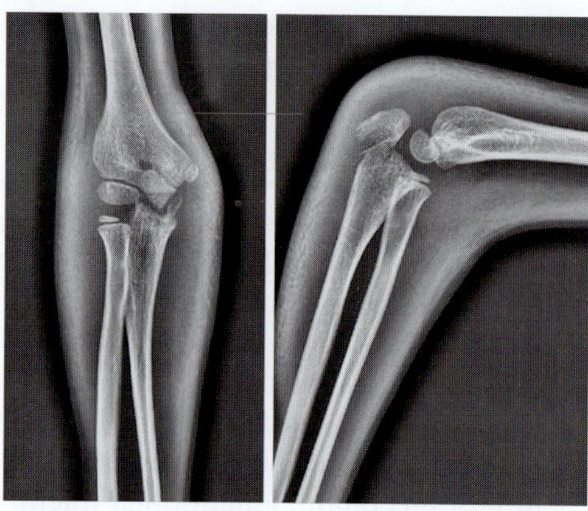

FIG. 15: Radiographs showing fracture of olecranon.

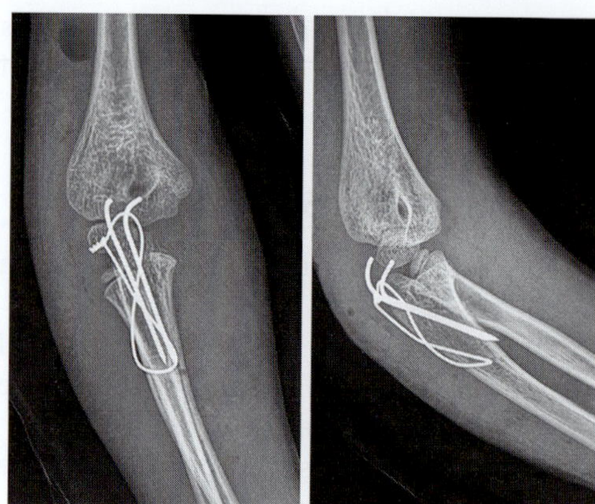

FIG. 16: Radiographs showing fracture.

- Undisplaced fractures are managed conservatively while displaced, intra-articular fractures require surgical intervention.

BIBLIOGRAPHY

1. Gartland JJ. Management of supracondylar fractures of the humerus in children. Surg Gynecol Obstet. 1959;109(2):145-54.
2. Hill CE, Cooke S. Common Paediatric Elbow Injuries. Open Orthop J. 2017;11:1380-93.
3. Skaggs DL, Hale JM, Bassett J, Kaminsky C, Kay RM, Tolo VT. Operative treatment of supracondylar fractures of the humerus in children. The consequences of pin placement. J Bone Joint Surg Am. 2001;83(5):735-40.
4. Song KS, Kang CH, Min BW, Bae KC, Cho CH. Internal oblique radiographs for diagnosis of nondisplaced or minimally displaced lateral condylar fractures of the humerus in children. J Bone Joint Surg Am. 2007;89(1):58-63.
5. Tornetta P, III, Ricci WM, Ostrum RF, McQueen MM, McKee MD, Court-Brown CM. Rockwood and green's fractures in adults, 9th edition. United States: Lippincott Williams & Wilkins; 2019.

Pediatric Forearm Fracture

Sakib Arfee

Forearm fractures are one of the most common skeletal injuries in children.

The majority of forearm fractures result from falls on an outstretched hand (FOOSH) and road traffic accidents. Other commonly encountered mechanisms encompass direct blows, sports-associated injuries, and vehicular injuries. The incidence of these fractures peaks at around school-going age, particularly during increased playful activities.

ANATOMY AND BIOMECHANICS

Pediatric bones are more elastic and much less dense. This flexibility in comparison to adult bones results in typical fracture patterns like greenstick or buckle fractures. The presence of growth plates (physis) in children influences fracture management **(Figs. 1A to C)**.

CLASSIFICATION

No established classification for pediatric forearm fractures is available. In the pediatric age group, fracture forearms are categorized based on, which includes the involvement of one or both bones, the type of fracture and the degree of displacement. Commonly used related classification systems are:

- *AO/OTA classification:* This classification provides a comprehensive categorization of fractures based totally on their vicinity and complexity, inclusive of the ones of the forearm.

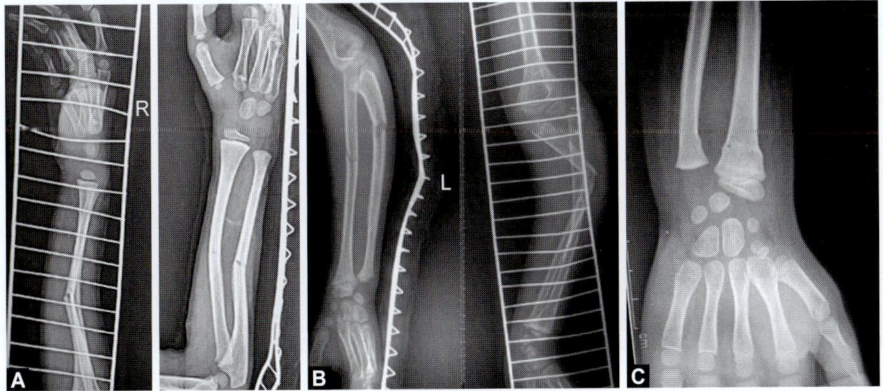

FIGS. 1A TO C: Showing displaced fracture mid-third forearm, displaced fracture proximal third of forearm and torus fracture of distal radius and buckling of distal ulna.

- *Common fracture types*:
    - *Greenstick fractures:* Incomplete fractures wherein the bone bends and only one cortex breaks.
    - *Buckle (Torus) fractures:* Compression fractures that cause bulging of the cortical bone without a cortical break.
    - Complete fractures
    - Compound fractures

MANAGEMENT

Both nonsurgical and surgical interventions, depending on the fracture type and severity.

Nonsurgical Management

- *Immobilization:* Most of the pediatric forearm fractures are treated with immobilization using a cast or splint. The choice between a cast and a splint depends on the fracture type and location and the amount of soft-tissue swelling and skin condition. Initially, at times better to apply slab after provisional reduction and then convert to cast once swelling settles down. Casting provides more definitive rigid support, while splinting is a temporary/definitive support allowing for some swelling and adjustment.

For displaced fractures, a closed reduction may be performed to realign the bone fragments before casting or slab application. This is usually done under sedation or anesthesia to ensure proper alignment and to make the reduction painfree. The patient should have a regular follow-up with weekly X-rays for the initial few weeks to detect any redisplacement.

Surgical Management

Indications: Open fractures, failed closed reduction, and fractures that fail to heal with conservative treatment.

- *Surgical technique:* Surgical options include internal fixation with plates and screws, flexible intramedullary nailing, single bone fixation, and external fixation devices. The choice of technique depends on the fracture pattern, age, and surgeon's preference **(Figs. 2A to C)**.

At times fixation of only one bone (more displaced one) is sufficient if other bone is less displaced and within acceptable limits.

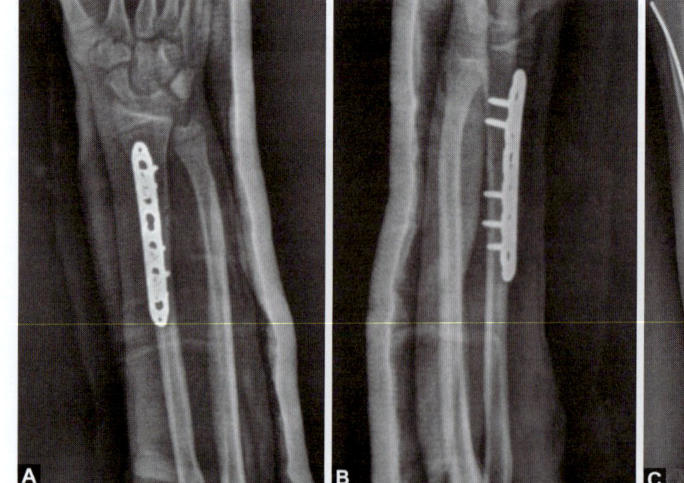

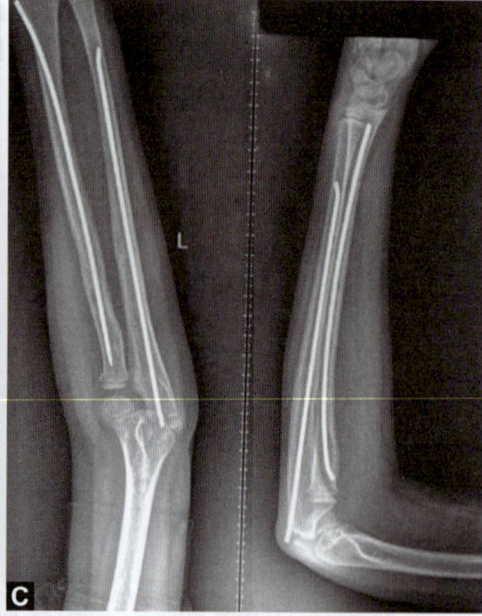

FIGS. 2A TO C: Showing fractured radius in a child fixed with plate anteroposterior (AP) and lateral view and fracture of radius and ulna fixed with titanium elastic nail system (TENS) nail ap and lateral view.

The entry point of titanium elastic nail system (TENS) in managing forearm fractures—attempt should be made to strict avoid injury to the growth plate while doing so.

For the Radius

The TENS nail is usually inserted through the *dorsal aspect of the distal radius*, proximal to the radial styloid. This is approximately 2 cm proximal to the growth plate in pediatric cases or near the distal metaphysis in adults.

For the Ulna

The TENS nail is inserted through the *posterior aspect of the distal ulna,* typically near the *olecranon*. Some surgeons may choose to insert it through the proximal part of the ulna just below the olecranon process.

Postoperative Management

- *Monitoring:* Regular follow-up is essential to monitor fracture healing and check for potential complications. Repeat X-rays may be needed.
- *Rehabilitation:* In the pediatric age group because of lack of compliance and not being able to follow the surgeon's advice, physical therapy may be recommended to restore range of motion, strength, and function following the removal of a cast or after surgical intervention.

Complications

Most pediatric forearm fractures heal well with appropriate treatment, however, complications can arise. These include:

- *Refracture:* Occurs in about 5% of patients of pediatric age group. It is most likely to occur after open fractures and greenstick fractures.
- Delayed union or nonunion
- Malunion
- *Infection:* Open fractures or surgical procedures carry a risk of infection in all patients of all age groups. However, pediatric age group has to be closely monitored for this because of decreased immunity and subtle signs of infection. which requires prompt management with antibiotics and possibly intervention.
- *Growth disturbances:* Fractures involving the physeal plate can affect future bone growth, potentially leading to limb length discrepancies or angular deformities.
- *Compartment syndrome:* Forearm fractures are the second leading cause of compartment syndrome in the pediatric age group after supracondylar fracture.
- *Synostosis:* it is uncommon and reported more often after high-energy trauma, surgical intervention, associated head injuries, and repeated manipulations.

BIBLIOGRAPHY

1. Chia B, Kozin SH, Herman MJ, Safier S, Abzug JM. Complications of pediatric distal radius and forearm fractures. Instr Course Lect. 2015;64: 499-507.
2. Noonan KJ, Price CT. Forearm and distal radius fractures in children. J Am Acad Orthop Surg.1998;6(3):146-56.
3. Pace JL. Pediatric and adolescent forearm fractures: current controversies and treatment recommendations. J Am Acad Orthop Surg. 2016;24(11):780-8.

CHAPTER 20.4

Pediatric Wrist and Hand Fractures

Sakib Arfee

Wrist and hand in children are protected against fracture by the cushioning effect of cartilaginous carpals which remain so till late childhood. Hence, carpal fractures in children are a result of massive trauma and are almost always associated with other fractures like forearm fractures.

CLASSIFICATION

Wrist Fractures

- Greenstick fractures
- *Buckle (Torus) fractures:* Compression fractures that cause bulging of the cortical bone without a cortical break.
- Complete fractures
- Compound fractures
- Most commonly, epiphyseal injuries

Distal Ulna Fractures

Rarely occur in association with distal radius fractures. They may be isolated or part of an injury pattern that includes both bones.

Hand Fractures

- *Carpal fractures:* Ossification of carpals begins at 2–3 months in capitate and proceeds clockwise direction and continues to do so till 9th or 10th year of life. Scaphoid fracture is most common carpal fracture in adults and in children. Distal pole avulsion is most common in children. It can occur in association with ligamentous injury. Adolescent athletes contribute in majority to this fracture.
- *Metacarpal fractures:* Often the result of direct trauma or punching. They can be classified into:
    - *Boxer's fracture:* Involves the fifth metacarpal neck and is commonly seen in adolescents.
    - *Thumb metacarpal fractures:* Typically result from trauma and can involve the base of the first metacarpal, e.g., Bennett and Rolando fracture.
- *Phalangeal fractures:* These can occur in any of the phalanges and are often the result of direct blows or crushing injuries. They may involve:
    - *Distal phalanx fractures:* Commonly associated with nail bed injuries. Mallet fracture is particular to adolescent patients than soft-tissue mallet because of maturing physis.
    - *Middle phalanx fractures:* Often result from sports or trauma.
    - *Proximal phalanx fractures:* Can affect joint function and require careful management.

Pediatric wrist fractures are classified as **(Fig. 1)** Salter–Harris classification—

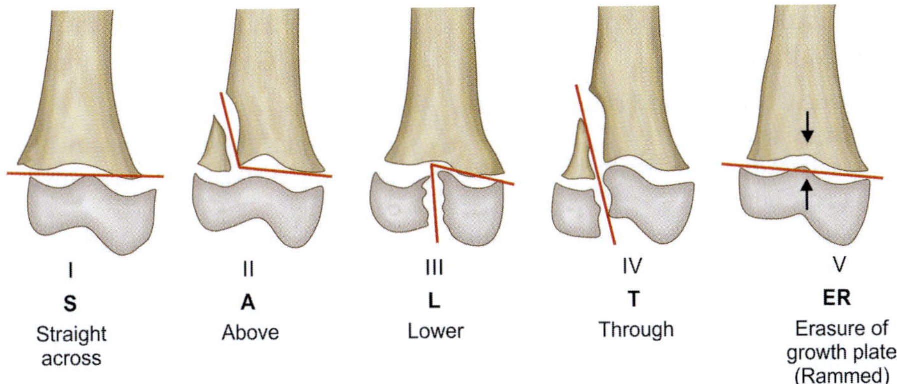

FIG. 1: Classification of pediatric wrist fractures.

used for fractures involving physis. It is categorized into five types, ranging from simple separation through the physeal plate to greater complex injuries involving the metaphysis and epiphysis.

DIAGNOSIS

Clinical evaluation: Detailed history and examination are critical. Key elements include:

- *Mechanism of injury:* Understanding how the injury occurred helps in predicting the type of fracture.

MANAGEMENT

Nonsurgical Treatment

- *Casting:* Primary method for managing stable fractures. Options include:
    - *Short-arm casts:* Typically used for distal radius and ulna fractures.
    - *Long-arm casts:* Sometimes required for more severe or unstable fractures.
- *Splinting:* For less severe injuries or as an initial treatment before casting.
- *Adequate pain management:* Nonsteroidal anti-inflammatory drugs (NSAIDs) (e.g., ibuprofen) and acetaminophen are commonly used for pain relief.

Surgical Treatment

- *Indications for surgery:* Include displaced, unstable fractures, or when reduction is not achieved or maintained.
- *Procedures:*
    1. *Closed reduction/open reduction and internal fixation (ORIF):* For complex fractures, especially when alignment cannot be maintained with casting alone. K-wires are most commonly used implant.
    2. *External fixation:* Sometimes used in cases with severe soft-tissue injury.

GENERAL TREATMENT APPROACH FOR EPIPHYSEAL INJURIES OF THE WRIST

Type I (Fracture Through the Growth Plate Only)

- *Treatment:* These are usually stable and can be treated nonsurgically. Management involves:
    - Immobilization with a cast or splint for 3–6 weeks
    - Monitoring through X-rays to ensure proper healing
- *Outcome:* Generally, excellent, as there is no disruption to the growth zone.

Type II (Fracture Through the Growth Plate and Metaphysis)

- *Treatment:* Often the most common type. Typically treated with:
    - Closed reduction (if necessary) to align the bone
    - Casting for 4–6 weeks to maintain proper alignment
- *Outcome:* Generally, good with proper alignment; occasional follow-ups to ensure normal growth plate function.

Type III (Fracture Through the Growth Plate and Epiphysis)

- *Treatment:* This involves the articular surface, so:
    - Precise reduction is critical to avoid joint deformity.
    - Closed or open reduction may be necessary to ensure the joint is properly aligned.
    - Cast immobilization or sometimes surgical fixation if the reduction is not stable.
- *Outcome:* The prognosis is good if well-aligned, but complications like growth disturbances can occur.

Type IV (Fracture Through the Metaphysis, Growth Plate, and Epiphysis)

- *Treatment:* These injuries involve both the joint surface and the growth plate, requiring:
    - Open reduction (surgical) with internal fixation to ensure precise alignment of all components.
    - Postsurgical immobilization for healing.
- *Outcome:* Higher risk for growth arrest or deformity due to damage to the growth plate.

Type V (Crush Injury to the Growth Plate)

- *Treatment:* These are the most severe and often difficult to detect initially:
    - Immobilization and close observation, though surgical intervention might not correct the injury.
    - Frequent monitoring with X-rays to assess growth plate function.
- *Outcome:* Poorer prognosis due to the potential for growth arrest or deformity.

BIBLIOGRAPHY

1. Choi PD, Herring JA. Evaluation and management of paediatric hand and wrist fractures. Orthopaed Traumatol Surg Res. 2018;104(2):155-64.
2. Hresko MT. Paediatric wrist fractures: an overview. J Paediatr Orthopaed. 2014;34(3):237-44.
3. McCarthy JC, Hennrikus WL. Paediatric hand and wrist fractures: treatment and outcomes. Curr Opin Pediatr. 2016;28(1):39-44.

SECTION

21

Pediatric Spine Fractures

CHAPTER 21.1

Pediatric Spinal Fracture

Nishank Mehta, Prashant Tank

- Spinal fractures and spinal injuries in children are rare—patients aged <15 years account for <10% of overall burden of spinal trauma.
- Apart from the most prevalent causes seen in young adults—motor vehicle accidents and fall from height—other causes of pediatric spinal trauma are sporting injuries, birth injuries, and non-accidental injuries/child abuse.
- As opposed to adults where thoracolumbar spine injuries account for 80% of cases—in children, injuries are more common in the cervical spine and account for 80% of cases (reasons detailed in subsequent sections).

ANATOMY AND BIOMECHANICS

- The paraspinal musculature as well as the ligamentous structures are relatively underdeveloped.
- Cartilaginous spine and relatively lax ligaments in younger children lend more elasticity, flexibility, and deformability to the spine when compared to adults.
- Vertebral fractures are less frequent in children—instead, epiphyseal detachments, joint dislocations/subluxations, ligamentous injuries, and lesions of ossification centers are more common.
- *Pediatric spinal trauma is most often seen in the cervical spine (80%)—due to the following reasons:*
  - *Increased head:* Trunk ratio—younger children have a relatively larger and heavier head and, hence, the junction between the head and the trunk (the upper cervical spine) represents a sudden transition in anatomical and biomechanical terms. As the child grows, the head: trunk ratio of size and weight gradually decreases.
  - *Weak neck musculature:* The neck muscles in children are not as well-developed as in adults and, hence, are unable to withstand the forces of sudden trauma. Children typically do not have the reflexes of adults as well.
  - *Increased mobility at the cervical spine:* The facet joints in the upper cervical spine are more horizontally oriented in children (25–30°) as compared to adults (60–70°). In addition, children also have shallow occipital condyles and underdeveloped uncovertebral joints, decreasing the overall stability in this part of the spine. Both transverse (flexion-extension) and rotational mobility in children is substantially higher when compared to adults, making the cervical spine more prone to sudden acceleration and deceleration injuries.

- In younger children (<8 years of age), spinal injuries most commonly involve the upper cervical spine (first three segments) and the craniovertebral junction. Between the age of 8–12 years, the location of injury shifts from the upper cervical spine to the lower cervical spine. Beyond the age of 12 years, the adult distribution of injury is noted with thoracolumbar injuries and injuries in the cervicothoracic region becoming more common.
- With age, the enlargement of the ossification centers and fusion of the cartilaginous joints (synchondroses) increases the stiffness of the pediatric spine, making fractures more common than joint dislocations and ligamentous injuries.

EVALUATION

- The evaluation must follow advanced trauma life support (ATLS) protocols. Children with spinal injuries usually have one or more associated injuries.
- Localized pain and inability to move the injured portion of the spine is the most common presenting symptom. Other symptoms are headache and subjective feeling of instability and neurological symptoms.
- In infancy, spinal trauma may present as unexplained respiratory distress, hypotonia, or weakness of specific muscle groups.
- Children with head injuries who have altered level of consciousness are at high risk of an additional spinal injury being missed. In particular, the possibility of SCIWORA (Spinal Cord Injury Without Radiographic Abnormality) (detailed in the subsequent portion) should be kept in mind.

IMAGING

- Conventional radiographs are the first line of investigation for children suspected to have spinal injury.
- However, children with a high velocity injury, who have suffered from an unwitnessed traumatic injury, those who are unconscious or those with focal neurological deficit require a head and spine CT.
- Whole body CT is recommended if additional injuries to chest and abdomen are present or suspected.
- MRI has limited role in adult spinal trauma—however, in children the possibility of a spinal cord injury remains in spite of a CT scan not showing any vertebral fracture or joint subluxation—hence, MRI should be strongly considered if radiograph or CT findings do not explain the clinical/neurological symptoms adequately.
- Dynamic radiographs (flexion-extension views) are important adjuncts as children with spinal injuries often exhibit late instability. Paraspinal spasm and guarding present in the emergency department confounds the diagnosis of instability in the acute setting—hence, when suspected delayed dynamic radiography should be performed to rule out subtle instability patterns and clear the child for unrestricted sporting or physical activities.
- Synchondroses of C2 (the apical odontoid synchondrosis) may appear separate in children aged between 6 and 12 years and may be mistaken for a type II dens fracture. Dorsal tilting of the dens is normal, but ventral tilting is not.
- Atlas may appear to be "spread" on the axis in open-mouth views in children up to 7 years of age due to the discrepancy of growth between these two bones. This has been referred to as a "Pseudo-Jefferson" fracture.
- *SCIWORA:*
    - The term "SCIWORA (Spinal Cord Injury Without Radiographic Abnormality)" was first used by Pang and Wilberger in 1982.

- SCIWORA may be seen in as much as one-third of all injuries in younger children—it is more common in the cervical spine and very often presents with severe neurological compromise.
- It is also seen in the thoracic spine—in association with severe injuries and prolonged hypotension.
- Injury occurs due to sudden and severe flexion and distraction of the cervical spine—primarily attributed to the increased elasticity of the pediatric spine which allows it to deform excessively without disruption of bony or ligamentous elements.
- Another possibility is an epiphyseal separation of the vertebral end plate which reduces spontaneously, but the initial displacement has caused the spinal cord injury.

- *Pseudosubluxation:*
  - Children aged <8 years may show abnormal translation of one vertebra over the other in the upper cervical spine—this is most often noted as an anterior displacement between C2 and C3, and less commonly between C3 and C4. The incidence of this finding is around 20% and is referred to as "pseudosubluxation". To differentiate pseudosubluxation which is a normal phenomenon from pathological subluxation after trauma, the posterior cervical spinolaminar line (Swischuk line) is used. A line joining the anterior cortical borders of the spinous processes of the atlas (C1) and C3 should be no >2 mm away from the anterior cortical border of the spinous process of C2.
  - The cervical spine may be kyphotic in children as a normal finding. Anterior wedging of immature vertebral bodies is also common and may be confused with compression fractures.
  - While in adults, a limit of 3 mm is used to define a normal Atlanto-dens interval (ADI)—in children, this may be considered to be normal up to 5 mm.

SPECIFIC INJURIES

- *Cervical spine:*
  - Atlanto-occipital dislocation:
    - Primary stabilizers are the alar ligament, joint capsule, and tectorial membrane.
    - Can be diagnosed using Powers ratio and C1–C2 to C2–C3 ratio (a ratio > 2.5 is suggestive of injury).
    - Associated with high rates of mortality
    - Initial treatment comprises halo immobilization without traction; definitive treatment is surgical fusion.
  - Atlanto-axial injury (AAI):
    - Failure of apical and alar ligaments results in AAI and poses a risk of spinal cord compression.
    - This can be diagnosed as ADI > 10–12 mm (note that as mentioned above, the normal ADI in children is up to 5 mm).
    - Initial management is closed reduction in extension followed by halo immobilization; definitive treatment is by posterior C1–C2 fusion which is also mandated if closed reduction is unsuccessful.
  - Rotary subluxation of the atlantoaxial joint:
    - Should be suspected in a child presenting with painful torticollis, involving lateral neck flexion and rotation of the head in the opposite direction.
    - Can be categorized as follows: Type I—rotation without significant subluxation (MC type); Type

2—rotation combined with 3-5 mm of anterior displacement; Type 3—more than 5 mm anterior displacement resulting in decreased space for the spinal cord and associated with bilateral anterior facet dislocations; and Type 4—posterior displacement of axis over atlas.
    - Initial management is with 2 weeks of cervical traction followed by 4 weeks of halo immobilization. Delays in diagnosis and inadequate treatment may mandate surgical stabilization.
- ○ Odontoid fracture:
    - Relatively common—occurs at the level of synchondrosis located at the base of the odontoid.
    - Patients are typically neurologically intact—successful reduction is common and can be followed by a brief period of immobilization.
- ○ Subaxial cervical spine injury:
    - Uncommon in younger children, incidence rises in children aged >9 years.
    - Depending on the morphology of the injury, it may require surgery.
- ○ Os odontoideum:
    - The well-corticated odontoid process with no continuity with the C2 body.
    - May be associated with atlantoaxial instability and resultant myelopathy.

- *Thoracic and lumbar spine:*
    - ○ Thoracolumbar spine injuries become more common as children get older.
    - ○ The fracture pattern depends on the mechanism of injury and its severity, and this has important implications of spinal stability.
    - ○ Moderate loading in flexion leads to compression fractures.
    - ○ Axial loading as seen in fall from height leads to a burst fracture with failure of the "middle" column (posterior vertebral wall) as well.
    - ○ Flexion-distraction injury refers to the simultaneous application of a flexion moment with posterior distractive force and can lead to the so-called "Chance" fracture.
    - ○ Translational injuries are extremely rare in children due to the inherent elasticity of the spinal column.

BIBLIOGRAPHY

1. Kewalramani LS, Tori JA. Spinal cord trauma in children. Neurologic patterns, radiologic features, and pathomechanics of injury. Spine. 1980;5(1):11-8.
2. Pang D, Wilberger JE. Spinal cord injury without radiographic abnormalities in children. J Neurosurg. 1982;57(1):114-29.
3. Swischuk LE. Anterior Displacement of C2 in Children: Physiologic or Pathologic: A Helpful Differentiating Line. Radiology. 1977;122(3):759-63.
4. Taylor AR. The mechanism of injury to the spinal cord in the neck without damage to the vertebral column. J Bone Joint Surg Br. 1951;33-B(4):543-7.
5. Vanderhave KL, Chiravuri S, Caird MS, Farley FA, Graziano GP, Hensinger RN, et al. Cervical spine trauma in children and adults: perioperative considerations. JAAOS: J Am Acad Orthop Surg. 2011;19(6):319-27.
6. Viccellio P, Simon H, Pressman BD, Shah MN, Mower WR, Hoffman JR, et al. A prospective multicenter study of cervical spine injury in children. Pediatrics. 2001;108(2):e20.

SECTION

22

Common Pediatric Fractures of Lower Limb

Pediatric Hip Fractures and Dislocations

Shubam Surmal

Pediatric hip dislocations occur less frequently than in adults but present with unique challenges due to the growing anatomy of children.

EPIDEMIOLOGY

Boys are more frequently affected, particularly in the adolescent age group, where increased physical activity and participation in sports contribute to a higher risk.

MECHANISM OF INJURY

The typical mechanism involves a high-energy impact that causes axial loading on a flexed, adducted hip. A dashboard injury during a car crash is a classic example. Anterior dislocations, though less common, are typically caused by force applied to an extended and externally rotated hip. These mechanisms differ slightly from those in adults due to the increased elasticity and plasticity of pediatric bones.

CLASSIFICATION

- *Posterior dislocation:* The most common type, where the femoral head is displaced posteriorly, is often associated with a shortened, internally rotated limb **(Fig. 1)**.
- *Anterior dislocation:* Less common, with the femoral head displaced anteriorly, presenting with an externally rotated and abducted limb **(Figs. 2A and B)**.

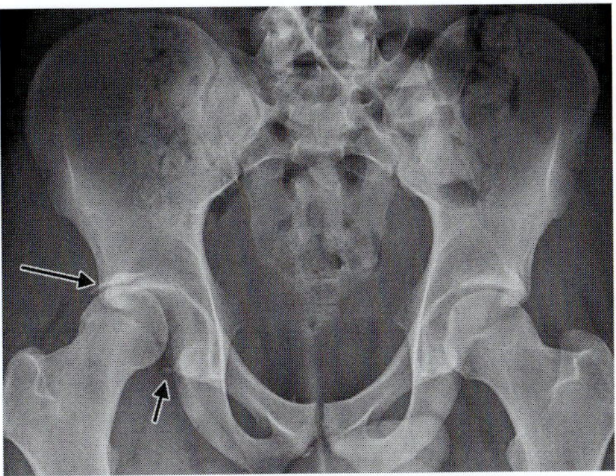

FIG. 1: Shows a fracture of the posterior wall of the acetabulum and a small intra-articular fragment (arrows).

- *Central dislocation:* Rare, often associated with acetabular fractures due to significant trauma.

IMAGING

- *X-rays:* Apart from confirming the diagnosis, it also helps to rule out associated fractures.
- *CT scan:* Used when fractures are suspected or after reduction to confirm the alignment of the joint.

MANAGEMENT

Emergency Reduction

Pediatric hip dislocations require prompt reduction to minimize the risk of complications such as avascular necrosis (AVN).

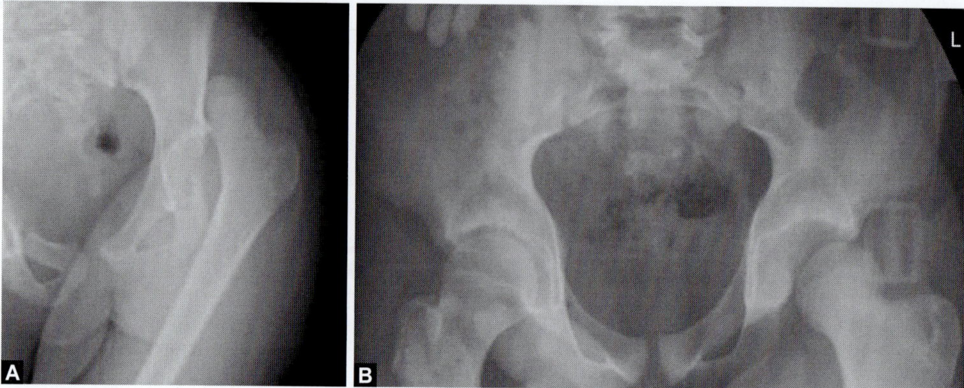

FIGS. 2A AND B: Showing posterior dislocation of hip joint.

Closed reduction under sedation or general anesthesia is the preferred initial treatment.

- *Closed reduction:* Typically performed using techniques like the Allis or Bigelow maneuver, depending on the type of dislocation.
- *Open reduction:* Required in cases where closed reduction is unsuccessful or if there is an associated fracture, particularly of the acetabulum.

Postreduction Care

- Postreduction imaging is necessary to confirm proper alignment and to assess for fractures or soft-tissue damage.
- Immobilization is typically done with a spica cast or traction, depending on the age of the patient and the severity of the injury.
- Restricted weight-bearing for several weeks is essential, followed by a gradual return to activity under the guidance of physical therapy.

Complications

Avascular Necrosis

Avascular necrosis remains the most feared complication, with an incidence of 8–20% in pediatric hip dislocations. Early detection via MRI is key to managing this condition, and timely reduction can reduce the risk.

Recurrent Dislocation

Although rare in children, recurrence can occur, especially if the initial reduction was not optimal or if there were associated fractures. Careful monitoring and follow-up are crucial.

Post-traumatic Arthritis

It is more common in case of high velocity injury associated with chondral damage or in cases with late treatment and incongruent joint.

PEDIATRIC HIP FRACTURES

These fractures occur as a result of very high-energy trauma with exceptions being some underlying metabolic bone disease or tumors, which occur due to minor trauma.

Imaging and Diagnosis

- Anteroposterior radiograph in extension and internal rotation and a cross-table lateral view is advised. Frog leg view is not promoted as it can cause fracture displacement.
- Any breach in bony trabeculae near the ward triangle is an impacted or undisplaced fracture.
- A hip fracture can be difficult to diagnose on X-rays due to limited ossification of

the proximal femur. Stress fractures are not picked on routine radiographs, MRI, CT scan, or technetium bone scan can demonstrate increased uptake at the fracture site. In infants, ultrasound can pick up epiphyseal separation.

Classification: Delbet classification **(Figs. 3A to D)** is most widely used to classify pediatric hip fractures as it is also having prognostic importance.

Type 1: These are transphyseal fractures of the femoral head, these fractures can also occur along with dislocation. These are rare fractures and constitute about 8% of femoral neck fractures in children. Unstable slipped capital femoral epiphysis (SCFE) of preadolescence can be differentiated from traumatic separation as the former follows a prior period of activity-related hip or knee pain, and can occur with minor trauma and the presence of multiple comorbid factors.

The fractures associated with dislocation have got bad prognosis as compared to fractures without dislocation, as premature physeal closure and osteonecrosis can occur in about 100% of cases.

Type 2: These are the most common fractures and are actually transcervical type and constitute about 45–50% of all femoral neck fractures. *Type 2 fractures* have having 28% incidence of developing osteonecrosis.

Type 3: Also known as cervicotrochanteric fractures. These constitute about 34% of pediatric hip fractures and are the second most common type. These fractures occur at or just above the anterior intertrochanteric line. Due to differences in the anatomy of capsule insertion, these fractures can be intra- or extracapsular. The incidence

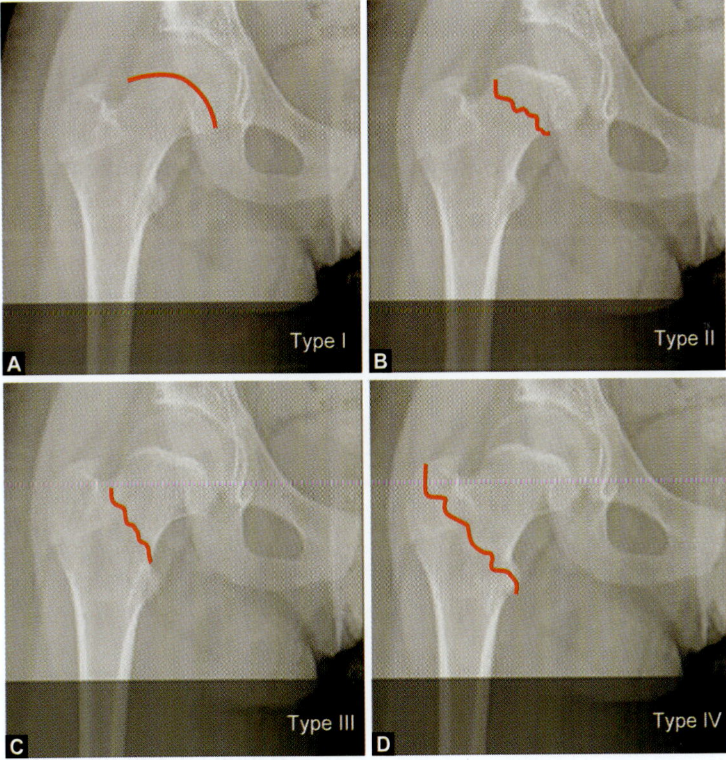

FIGS. 3A TO D: Various Delbet types of femoral neck fractures in children.

of osteonecrosis is about 18%. Premature physeal closure and coxa vara are known complications.

Type 4: These are intertrochanteric fractures and constitute about 12% of total pediatric hip fractures. These fractures have having least complications as compared to types 1, 2, and 3.

Treatment

The complication rates like nonunion, coxa vara, and delayed union unite high in conservative treatment like hip spica as compared to internal fixation. The recommended treatment is the early anatomic reduction and internal fixation whether open or closed whenever possible *nonoperative treatment.*

HIP FRACTURES

Nonoperative Treatment (Table 1)

Various indications and relative contraindications of conservative treatment are described in **Table 1**.

Operative Treatment

Internal fixation is recommended for displaced femoral neck fractures; if the fracture is not reduced closely, open reduction is indicated.

TABLE 1: Shows indications of conservative treatment in pediatric fracture neck of the femur.

Indications	Relative contraindications
• Infants and toddlers 0–2 years with stable minimally displaced type 1 fractures • Nondisplaced types 2 and 3 fractures in younger children (0–5 years) • Nondisplaced stress fractures	• Type 1 fractures >2 years • Displaced fractures • Older children (>5 years with types 2 and 3) fractures

Percutaneous fixation with pinning or screws is recommended in undisplaced fractures. Open reduction is done by Watson-Jones (anterolateral approach) or the Smith-Peterson approach (anterior approach). Also, younger children have better prognoses than older ones.

Type 1

Undisplaced and minimally displaced fractures up to 2 years of age can be treated in spica casting for 6 weeks, in abduction and neutral rotation. If the fracture seems displaced at any moment during casting, open reduction internal fixation with 2 mm smooth K wires crossing the physis is recommended. The K wires should be buried underneath the skin and retrieved once the fracture is healed.

In older and adolescent children 4–7 mm cannulated screws crossing physis are considered.

Types 2 and 3

Anatomic reduction is mandatory and if fractures are not reduced in close reduction, open reduction is done.

Up to 8 years of age, the fractures are stabilized with 4–4.5 mm cannulated screws and after 8 years 6.5 mm cannulated screws are used. The physis penetration generally is not recommended but when the fixation is unstable, the physis must be penetrated. Usually, most fractures are united stable with screws without physis penetration. Two to three screws are used depending on the size of the femoral neck.

Some studies suggest that if physis is not crossed with an implant, spica casting is given as an additional protection, to prevent complications.

Type 4

Both displaced and undisplaced fractures are treated in spica casting for 12 weeks. Displaced fractures in age >3 years are treated with a pediatric dynamic hip screw, if not reduced closely a lateral approach with anterior extension is advised. Serial radiographs are required to check for union status, if fracture on the radiograph is obscured with spica casting, a CT scan is advised.

In all type 1 fractures, spica casting is mandatory except in adolescents where larger screws are sufficient to hold the reduction. In types 2 and 3, spica casting is recommended where screws do not cross physis, in type 4 fractures managed with dynamic hip screws, no spica casting is recommended.

The common complications after pediatric hip fractures are osteonecrosis, malunion (coxa vara), nonunion, and physeal arrest.

Osteonecrosis is the most serious complication related to pediatric hip fracture. It is as prevalent as 30%. The risk is more in 1B Delbet type and displaced ones and old age.

The incidence of osteonecrosis on basis of Delbet classification is 38% in type 1, 28% in type 2, 18% in type 3, and 5% in type 4, respectively.

Some studies have revealed that patients treated in <24 hours and patients who have undergone hip aspiration have got comparatively better results.

Coxa Vara and Premature Physeal Closure

The risk of premature physis closure is increased with the used implant perforates physis. It is prevalent in about 28% of fractures, mostly seen in Delbet type 2 or type 3 fractures.

Nonunion: The incidence of nonunion is seen in about 7% of patients with pediatric hip fractures, mostly seen in delbet type 2 and 3. It occurs due to nonanatomic reduction.

One very rare complication is chondrolysis. It is seen when the implant penetrates a joint like SCFE fixation.

BIBLIOGRAPHY

1. Agarwala S, Jain D, Joshi VR, Sule A. Efficacy of alendronate, a bisphosphonate, in the treatment of AVN of the hip. A prospective open-label study. Rheumatology (Oxford). 2005;44(3):352-9.
2. Alho A. Concurrent ipsilateral fractures of the hip and femoral shaft. Acta Orthop Scand. 1996;67: 19-28.
3. Ashwood N, Wojcik AS. Traumatic separation of the upper femoral epiphysis in a 15 month old girl: An unusual mechanism of injury. Injury. 1995;26:695-6.
4. Ayadi K, Trigui M, Gdoura F, Elleuch B, Zribi M, Keskes H. Traumatic hip dislocations in children. Rev Chir Orthop Reparatrice Appar Mot. 2008; 94(1):19-25.
5. Bagatur AE, Zorer G. Complications associated with surgically treated hip fractures in children. J Pediatr Orthop B. 2002;11:219-28.
6. Bali K, Sudesh P, Patel S, Kumar V, Saini U, Dhillon MS. Pediatric femoral neck fractures: Our 10 years of experience. Clin Orthop Surg. 2011;3(4):302-8.

Pediatric Femoral Shaft Fractures

Zubair Ahmad Lone, Irfan Malik, John Mohd, Amit Thakur

Pediatric femoral shaft fractures are among the common injuries in children and invariably occur due to high-velocity trauma.

CLASSIFICATION

Pediatric femoral fractures may anatomically be classified as subtrochanteric fractures, shaft fractures, and supracondylar fractures.

RADIOGRAPHIC EVALUATION

It is essential to include the hip and the knee joints in the radiograph to rule out associated injuries of the ipsilateral hip and knee. Very rarely advanced radiological tools like CT and MRI are needed to rule out a stress fracture or any associated ligamentous injuries.

MANAGEMENT

The treatment is individualized and the decision is taken based on the patient's age, whether the fracture is open or closed, the pattern of the fracture, the weight of the child, the anatomical location of the fracture, and whether the fracture is length stable or not. The ideal treatment method for a pediatric femoral shaft fracture, according to Staheli, should be comfortable and convenient for the child and must maintain length as well as alignment. Evidence-based management options for these fractures according to the child's age are summarized in **Table 1**.

Most children with closed femur fractures below the age of 5 years are managed conservatively. Infants below the age of 6 months have good results with the Pavlik harness. However, posterior splintage is another option in case of nonavailability of the Pavlik harness.

Hip spica casting is the preferred treatment method for children over 6 months and up to 5 years. Hip spica may be applied either immediately post-trauma or after a brief period of traction till the time the fracture

TABLE 1: Management options for pediatric femoral shaft fractures based on age of the child.

Age of child	<6 months	6 months to 5 years	5–11 years	>11 years
Recommended treatment	Pavlik harness	Primary hip spica cast	Elastic intramedullary nailing	Locked intramedullary nailing
Alternative treatment	Posterior splintage	• Delayed spica casting after initial traction • Elastic intramedullary nailing	• Submuscular bridge plating • External fixation • Locked intramedullary nailing	• Submuscular bridge plating • External fixation

becomes sticky and length stable. Previously, Gallow's traction was another popular method of conservative management in children below 2 years of age, however, it is not used nowadays due to the chances of neurovascular compromise. The acceptability criteria for closed reduction in children being managed conservatively are summarized in **Table 2**.

Children aged 5 years or more with femoral shaft fractures are managed operatively. Elastic intramedullary nailing gives predictably good results in the age group of 5–11 years, in children weighing < 45 kg. Titanium elastic nails (TENS) are commonly used and are inserted in a retrograde manner, starting proximal to the distal femoral physis **(Fig. 1)**. Elastic intramedullary nailing should be avoided in length unstable fractures in which there is comminution and have a long spiral or oblige patterns, as shortening may ensue postfixation. In such cases, submuscular bridge plating and external fixation are better options.

Rigid trochanteric entry nails, avoiding the classical entry sites, are used in children beyond 11 years. The nails are designed in such a fashion that the entry is made in a trochanteric or extratrochanteric area, so as to avoid the physes of the proximal femur. However, in our country, these are not available in all orthopedic trauma set-ups. Hence, flexible intramedullary nails and submuscular plating may also be utilized in this age group. Submuscular bridge plating is a good option for subtrochanteric and supracondylar femur fractures **(Figs. 2 and 3)**. External fixators may be used for open injuries in most patients with good results, however, pin site infection and refractures have been observed, limiting its use for closed fractures.

TABLE 2: Acceptable reduction criteria for pediatric shaft femur fractures.

Age	Coronal malalignment	Sagittal malalignment	Shortening
<2 years	30°	30°	15 mm
2–5 years	15°	20°	20 mm
6–10 years	10°	15°	15 mm
≥11 years	5°	10°	10 mm

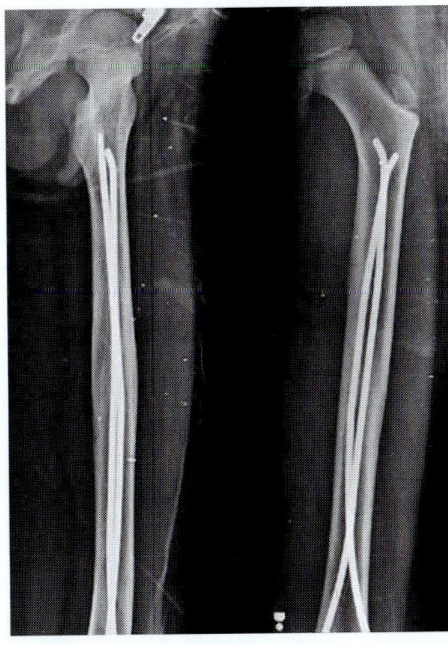

FIG. 1: Plain radiograph of a pediatric femoral shaft fracture, managed with titanium elastic nails (TENS).

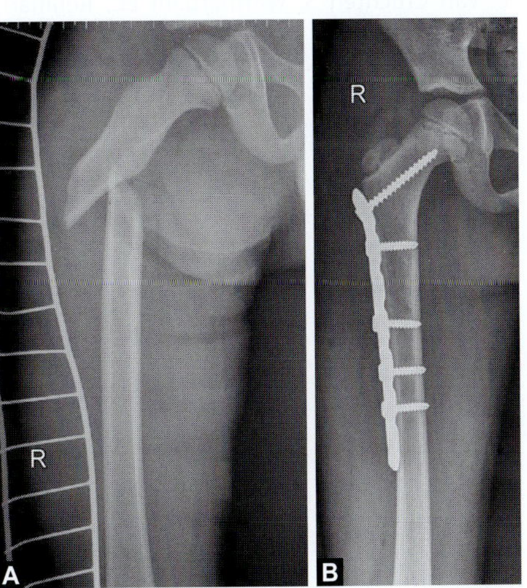

FIGS. 2A AND B: Pediatric subtrochanteric femur fracture managed with plating.

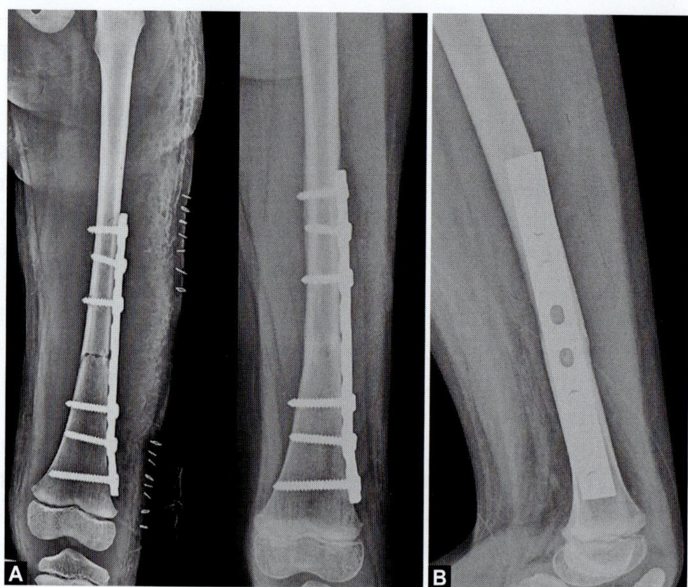

FIGS. 3A AND B: Fracture distal third of the femur in a child managed with submuscular plating. (A) immediate postoperative X-rays; (B) Anteroposterior (AP) and lateral X-rays after 6 months.

BIBLIOGRAPHY

1. Hidalgo Perea S, Loyst RA, Botros D, Barsi JM. Outcomes in early versus delayed management of pediatric femoral shaft fractures. J Pediatr Orthop. 2024;44(3):e238-41.
2. Kakakhel MMG, Rauf N, Khattak SA, Adhikari P, Askar Z. Femoral shaft fractures in children: Exploring treatment outcomes and implications. Cureus. 2023;15(10):e46336.
3. van Cruchten S, Warmerdam EC, Reijman M, Kempink DR, de Ridder VA. Current practices in the management of closed femoral shaft fractures in children: A nationwide survey among Dutch orthopaedic surgeons. J Orthop. 2023;45:1-5.
4. Zamzam M, Bopari N, Arapovic A, Kamel-ElSayed S, Saleh ES. Comparing the outcomes of titanium and stainless steel flexible nails in repairing pediatric long bone fractures. Orthop Rev (Pavia). 2024;16:116898.

CHAPTER 22.3

Pediatric Knee Fractures

Aditya Chaubey, Manish Singh, Pankaj Vir Singh

Pediatric knee injuries can be both soft tissue as well as bony injuries.

ANTERIOR CRUCIATE LIGAMENT INJURIES

Anterior cruciate ligament (ACL) injuries in pediatric patients have been increasing due to greater participation in high-level sports. Unlike in adults, the concern in pediatric patients is not just restoring knee stability but also preserving the growth plate.

NONOPERATIVE VERSUS OPERATIVE MANAGEMENT

- *Nonoperative treatment:* Historically recommended in skeletally immature patients to avoid growth plate damage. However, recent studies suggest that nonoperative management can lead to secondary meniscal and chondral injuries due to chronic instability.
- *Operative treatment:* Physeal-sparing ACL reconstruction techniques are now preferred for many pediatric patients. These include:
    - *Extraphyseal techniques:* Such as iliotibial band (ITB) reconstruction.
    - *All-epiphyseal techniques:* In skeletally immature patients, tunnels are drilled entirely within the epiphysis to avoid growth plate disturbance.
    - *Partial transphyseal techniques:* In older adolescents closer to skeletal maturity, these techniques involve small tunnels that pass through the physis, minimizing damage while restoring stability.

PATELLAR DISLOCATION

Patellar instability is another common injury in the pediatric population, often associated with an immature skeletal system and ligamentous laxity. First-time dislocations can typically be managed nonoperatively, but recurrent dislocations may require surgical intervention.

Nonoperative Management

Initial dislocations are often treated with:

- *Immobilization:* Short-term immobilization followed by rehabilitation focusing on quadriceps strengthening.
- *Rehabilitation:* Emphasis on strengthening the vastus medialis obliquus (VMO) to stabilize the patella and improve tracking

Operative Management

In cases of recurrent dislocation or associated osteochondral injuries, surgery may be necessary:

- *Medial patellofemoral ligament (MPFL) reconstruction:* The MPFL is commonly reconstructed using autografts or allografts. Techniques should consider the patellar growth plate to avoid injury.

- *Tibial tubercle osteotomy:* In skeletally mature adolescents with significant malalignment or high Q-angles, this procedure is sometimes warranted.
- *Trochleoplasty:* Rarely indicated in pediatric patients but may be considered in cases of severe trochlear dysplasia.

MENISCAL INJURIES

Meniscal tears in children can occur due to traumatic injuries, often associated with ACL tears, or in the setting of discoid menisci, which are more prone to tears. The goal of treatment is to preserve the meniscus whenever possible, given its vital role in knee joint biomechanics and long-term joint health.

Conservative versus Surgical Management

- *Conservative treatment:* Small stable tears, particularly those located in the peripheral (vascular) zone, can be treated with immobilization and rehabilitation.
- *Surgical treatment:* Repair is preferred over meniscectomy, especially in traumatic tears. Techniques include:
  - *All-inside, inside-out, or outside-in repairs:* Depending on the location and extent of the tear.
  - *Discoid meniscus:* Partial meniscectomy is often necessary to contour the meniscus, preserving as much tissue as possible while restoring normal biomechanics.

TIBIAL SPINE AVULSION FRACTURES

Tibial spine avulsion fractures are functionally similar to ACL injuries in children. These fractures occur at the attachment of the ACL to the tibial eminence and are more common in pediatric patients due to the relative weakness of the bone compared to the ligament.

Classification and Treatment

Meyers and McKeever Classification (Figs. 1 and 2)

- *Type 1 fractures:* Nondisplaced fractures are typically managed with immobilization in extension.
- *Types 2 and 3 fractures:* These involve partial or complete displacement of the tibial spine. Reduction and fixation are generally required, and arthroscopic techniques are favored.
  - *Suture fixation:* Using fiber wires or other suture materials to secure the avulsed fragment.
  - *Screw fixation:* Can be considered but must be used cautiously in younger patients to avoid physeal injury.
  - They can be treated by open as well as arthroscopic assisted (preferred).

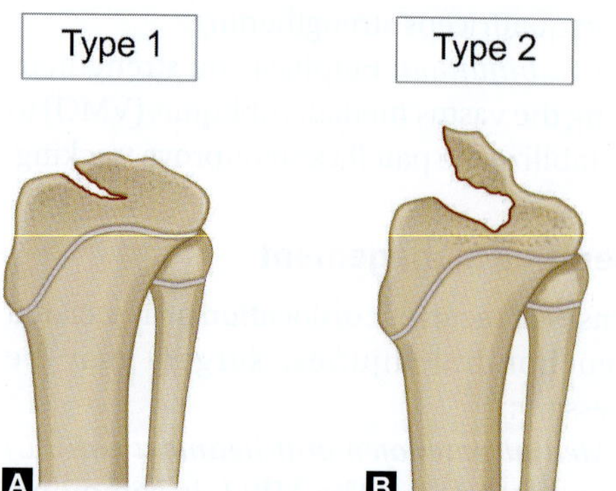

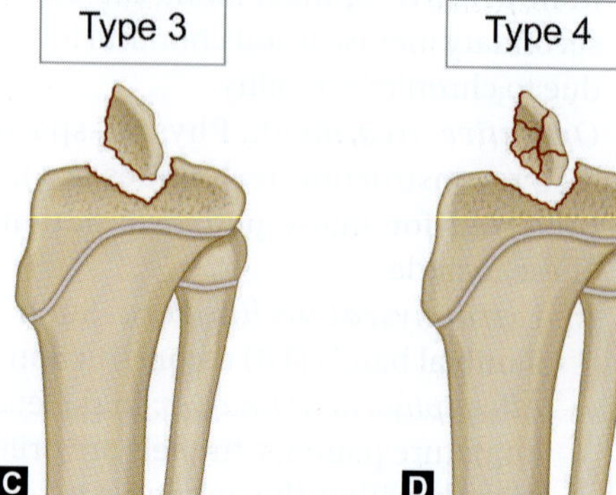

FIGS. 1A TO D: Meyers and McKeever classification.

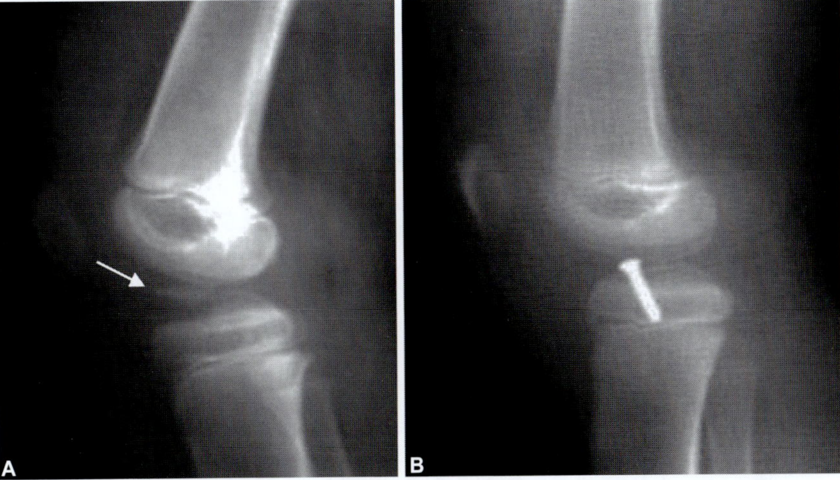

FIGS. 2A AND B: Fixation of the tibial spine with screw.

OSTEOCHONDRAL FRACTURE

Osteochondral fracture of the knee, particularly involving the lateral aspect of the medial femoral condyle, is common in children and adolescents. The condition involves subchondral bone necrosis with overlying cartilage damage, and its treatment depends on lesion stability **(Fig. 3)**.

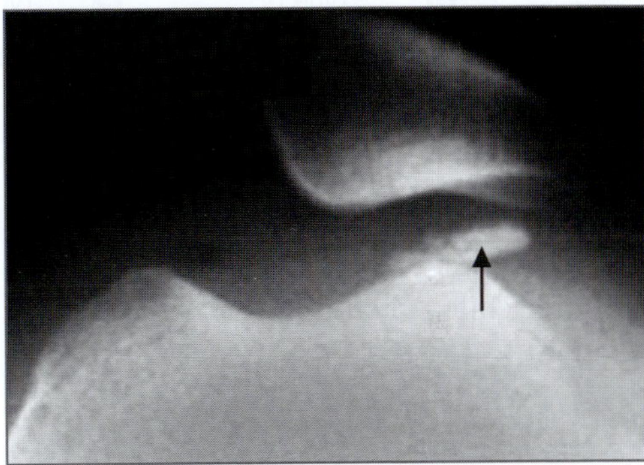

FIG. 3: Osteochondral fracture of femoral condyle.

Nonoperative versus Operative Management

- *Nonoperative treatment:* Stable lesions without loose fragments may respond to activity modification and bracing.
- *Operative treatment:* Unstable lesions or those with loose fragments require surgical intervention. Techniques include:
    - *Drilling:* To promote revascularization in stable but symptomatic lesions.
    - *Fixation:* For unstable lesions, fixation using bioabsorbable pins or screws is performed to restore the cartilage surface.
    - *Cartilage restoration procedures:* In cases of significant cartilage damage, procedures such as microfracture, autologous chondrocyte implantation (ACI), or osteochondral autograft transplantation (OATS) may be necessary.

DISTAL FEMUR FRACTURES IN CHILDREN

The distal femoral physis is one of the most active growth plates in the body, contributing significantly to longitudinal bone growth.

Classification

Distal femur fractures in children can be classified based on their anatomical location

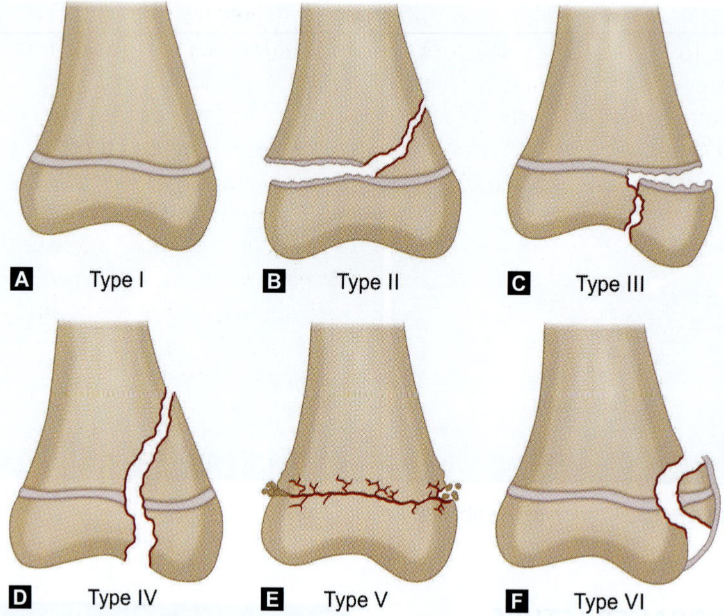

FIGS. 4A TO F: Salter–Harris fractures: Classification of distal femur classification.

and whether the physis is involved. Classified using the Salter–Harris system **(Figs. 4A to F)**:

- *Supracondylar fractures:* These occur above the growth plate, typically in older children who are nearing skeletal maturity **(Fig. 5)**.

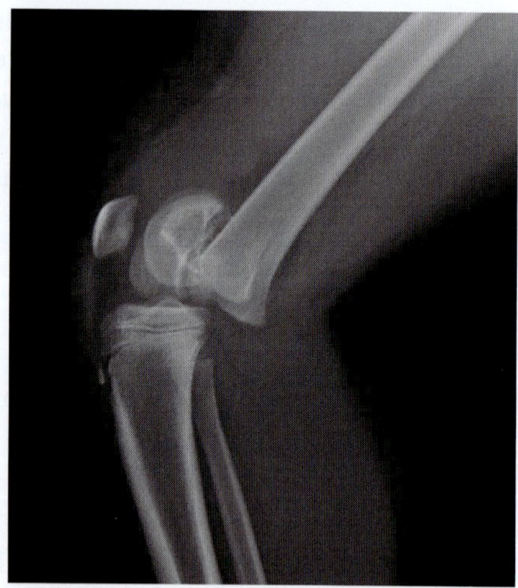

FIG. 5: Type 1 epiphyseal injury distal femur.

Treatment

Nonoperative Treatment

Nonoperative management is generally reserved for:

- *Minimally displaced fractures:* These can be managed with closed reduction and casting.
  - *Long-leg casting* is typically employed for 4–6 weeks, followed by a period of functional rehabilitation.
  - Frequent follow-up is necessary to monitor for loss of reduction or angular deformities **(Figs. 6A and B)**.

Operative Treatment

Most displaced distal femur fractures in children require surgical intervention, especially when the physis is involved or there is significant displacement. Surgical techniques aim to restore alignment while minimizing damage to the growth plate.

- *Physeal-sparing fixation:* In younger children with significant remaining growth potential, care is taken to avoid crossing the growth plate with fixation devices.
  - *Smooth Kirschner wires (K-wires)* or *screws* are often used to avoid disrupting the physis **(Figs. 7A and B)**.

Plates and screws: In older children or adolescents closer to skeletal maturity, locking plates and screws may be used for better stabilization. Intra-articular fractures (Salter–Harris III or IV) often require open reduction and internal fixation (ORIF) to ensure proper joint alignment and avoid future degenerative changes **(Figs. 8 and 9)**.

- *External fixation:* Used in high-energy, comminuted fractures or when there is significant soft-tissue damage or risk of compartment syndrome.
- *Flexible intramedullary nails:* These can be considered in older children or adolescents for supracondylar fractures, especially in fractures with significant comminution.

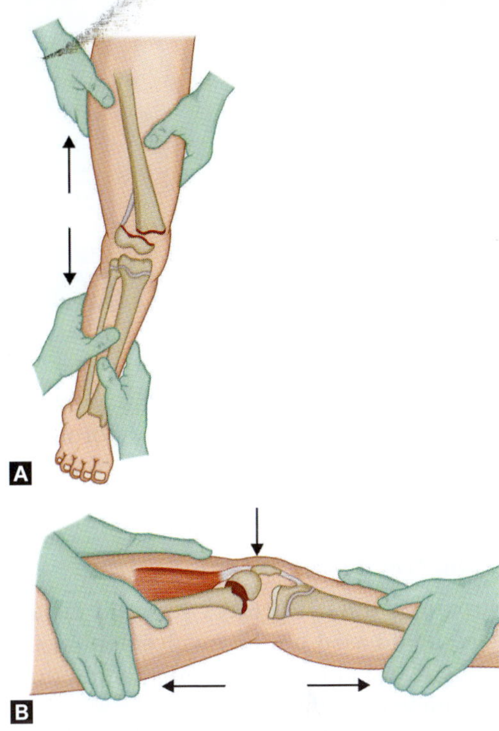

FIGS. 6A AND B: Reduction maneuver for displaced type 1 epiphyseal injury.

GROWTH ARREST AND PHYSEAL BAR FORMATION

The risk of growth arrest is a significant concern in fractures involving the distal femoral physis. Growth plate injuries, particularly Salter–Harris types III, IV, and V, carry a high risk of growth disturbances, which may lead to limb length discrepancies or angular deformities.

- *Physeal bar resection:* If a growth arrest is identified early (within 6–12 months), surgical resection of the physeal bar may restore growth. This is typically done in combination with interposition materials to prevent recurrence of the bar.

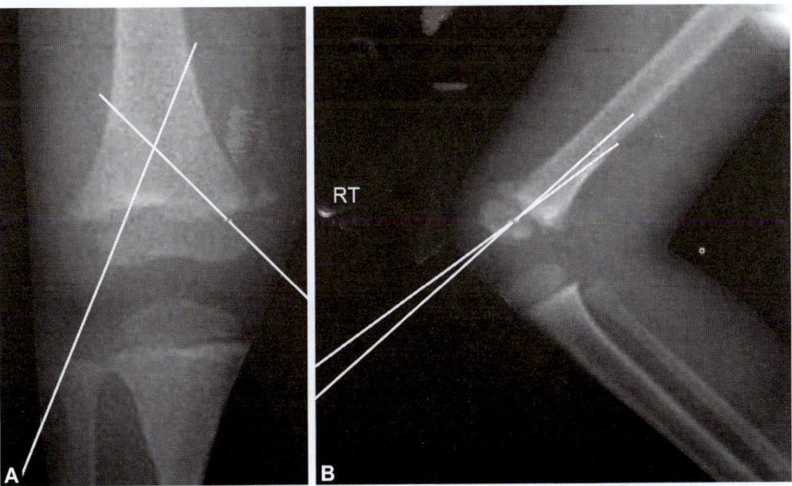

FIGS. 7A AND B: *Cross-pinning* for Salter–Harris type I or II fractures, smooth pins can be used for fixation across the physis in a way that minimizes physeal damage.

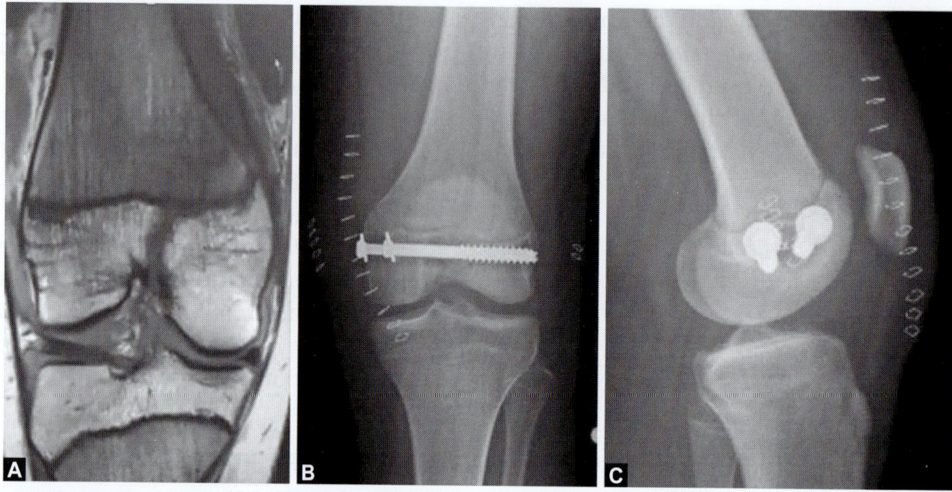

FIGS. 8A TO C: Type 3 epiphyseal injury fixed with a screw.

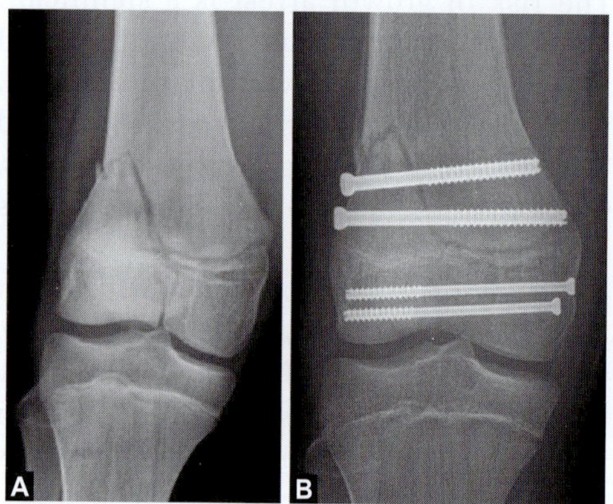

FIGS. 9A AND B: Type 4 epiphyseal injury fixed with screws.

- *Epiphysiodesis:* In cases where the child is nearing skeletal maturity and there is a significant limb length discrepancy, epiphysiodesis of the contralateral growth plate may be performed to equalize limb lengths.

PROXIMAL TIBIA FRACTURES IN CHILDREN

The proximity of neurovascular structures like the popliteal artery, as well as the potential for growth disturbances, requires careful evaluation and treatment. Proximal tibial fractures can lead to significant complications, including growth arrest, leg length discrepancies, angular deformities, and compartment syndrome.

Classification of Proximal Tibia Fractures

Proximal tibial fractures in children are classified based on the involvement of the physis and the location of the fracture. Common types include:

- For physeal fractures refer to Salter–Harris classification
- *Metaphyseal fractures:* Refer to **Figures 10A and B.**
- *Tibial tubercle fractures:*
  - These fractures involve the tibial tubercle, the site of attachment for the patellar tendon. They are typically seen in adolescents engaged in sports or during periods of rapid growth **(Fig. 11)**.

PROXIMAL TIBIAL SHAFT FRACTURES

These fractures occur below the physis in the shaft and are often the result of high-energy trauma. Physical examination should assess for neurovascular compromise due to the proximity of the palpation for compartment syndrome, which can be a complication in these fractures, is also critical.

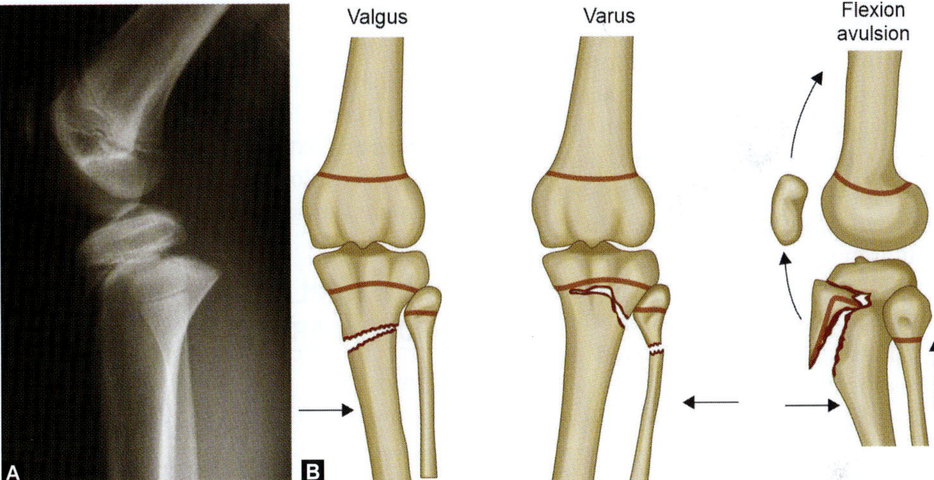

FIGS. 10A AND B: Metaphyseal fractures.

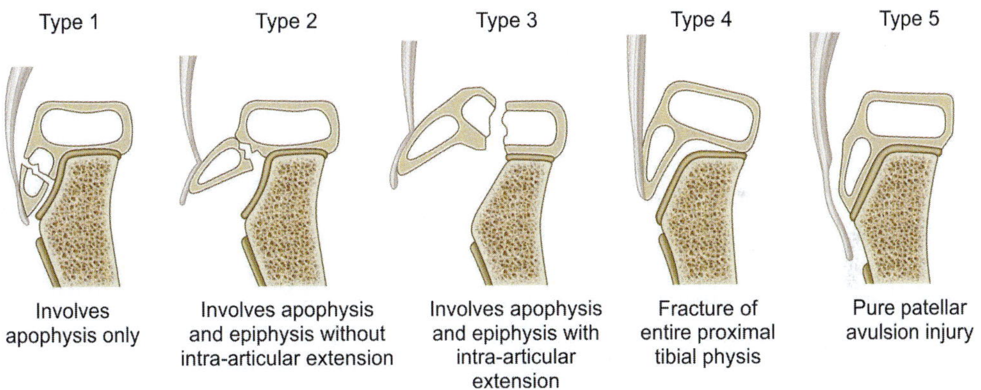

FIG. 11: Ogden classification.

Source: Images from R&W: Fractures in the Children, 9th edition (Fig. 26.11).

Treatment of Proximal Tibial Fractures

The treatment of proximal tibial fractures in children depends on the type of fracture, degree of displacement, and patient's skeletal maturity.

Nonoperative Treatment

Nonoperative management is typically reserved for fractures that are:

- *Minimally displaced:* Fractures with no or minimal displacement (e.g., Salter-Harris I or II fractures) can be treated conservatively.
- *Stable fractures:* These fractures are stable upon imaging and do not require surgical fixation.

Management includes:

- *Casting/Bracing:* Closed reduction, if necessary, followed by immobilization with a long-leg cast for 4–6 weeks. Casting is typically employed for nondisplaced or minimally displaced metaphyseal or Salter-Harris type I and II fractures.
- *Close follow-up:* Regular radiographic monitoring is essential to ensure that there is no loss of reduction or progressive deformity during healing.

Operative Treatment

Surgical intervention is required for displaced fractures, unstable fractures, or fractures with intra-articular involvement (Salter–Harris III or IV). Surgical techniques vary depending on the type of fracture and patient's age.

- *Physeal–Sparing techniques:* In younger children with significant growth remaining, physeal-sparing fixation is paramount to avoid growth arrest. Smooth pins or small screws are often used to avoid crossing the physis.
- *Closed or open reduction with internal fixation:*
    - For *Salter–Harris III or IV fractures,* anatomical reduction of the articular surface is critical to prevent post-traumatic arthritis and long-term joint dysfunction. ORIF is typically performed using screws placed parallel to the physis.
    - *Tibial tubercle fractures:* Often require ORIF to reattach the avulsed fragment to the tibia, typically using screws or tension band wiring **(Figs. 12A and B)**.
- *Flexible intramedullary nails:* In cases of displaced proximal tibial shaft fractures, flexible intramedullary nailing may be employed, particularly in older children with near-skeletal maturity. This technique provides stabilization while promoting early mobilization.
- *External fixation:* It is used in severe open fractures, comminuted fractures, or when there is extensive soft-tissue injury. It is also employed in cases where compartment syndrome is a concern.

GROWTH PLATE INJURIES AND GROWTH ARREST

Injuries to the proximal tibial physis can lead to growth disturbances.

Management of Growth Arrest

- *Physeal bar resection:* Early resection of physeal bars can restore growth in some cases, particularly if <50% of the physis is involved.
- *Epiphysiodesis:* In children nearing skeletal maturity, epiphysiodesis (intentional closure of the contralateral growth plate) may be performed to equalize leg lengths.

Management of Angular Deformities

Osteotomy: Corrective osteotomies may be necessary for significant angular deformities. This is more likely to be required in older

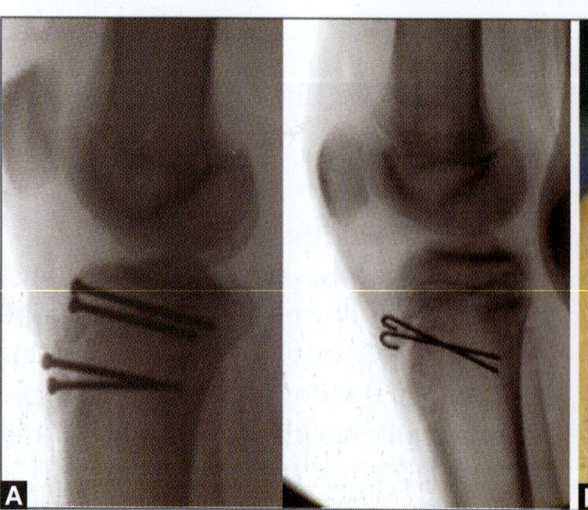

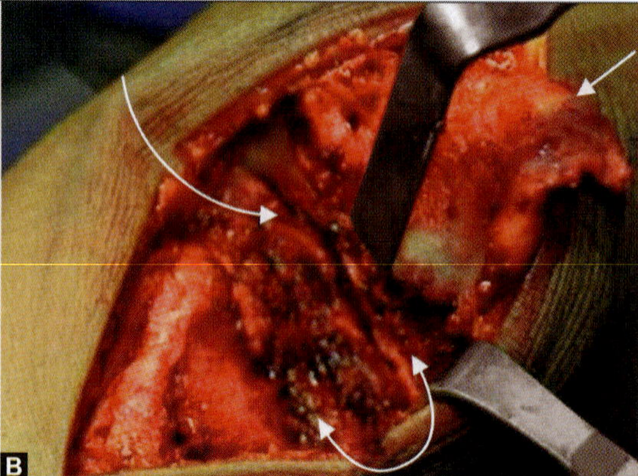

FIGS. 12A AND B: Fixation of tibial tubercle fixation with screws and wires.

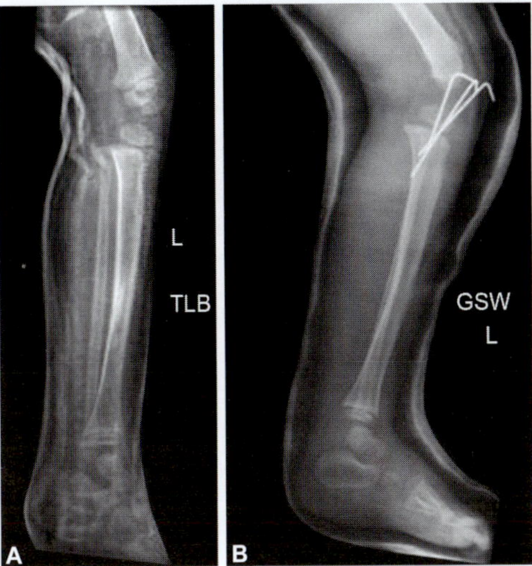

FIGS. 13A AND B: Fixation of type 1 proximal tibial epiphysis with K-wires.

children who have completed most of their growth **(Figs. 13A and B)**.

PEDIATRIC PATELLAR FRACTURE

Classification of Patella Fractures

- Undisplaced or minimally displaced fractures
- Displaced fractures
- Comminuted fractures
- Osteochondral fractures

Conservative Management (for Undisplaced or Minimally Displaced Fractures)

Immobilization: The knee is immobilized in full extension using a cast or knee brace for 4–6 weeks.

- *Weight-bearing:* Depending on the stability of the fracture, weight-bearing may be allowed with crutches.
- *Physical therapy:* Once healing is confirmed (after 4–6 weeks), gradual strengthening and range of motion exercises are introduced to regain function.
- *Follow-up X-rays:* Periodic imaging is done to monitor healing.

Surgical Management (for Displaced, Comminuted, or Complex Fractures)

- *Open reduction and internal fixation:* With wires, screws, or tension band wiring techniques to hold the bone fragments together shown in **Figures 14A and B**.
- *Excision of fragments:* In cases where small fragments cannot be fixed, they might be excised, especially in osteochondral fractures.
- *Postoperative care:* Immobilization followed by physical therapy is crucial after surgery.

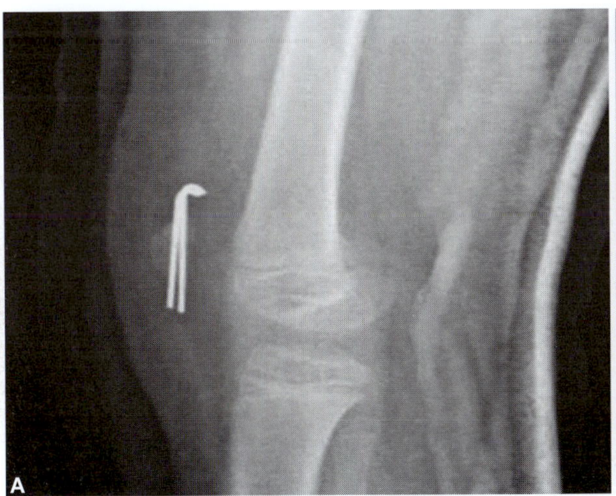

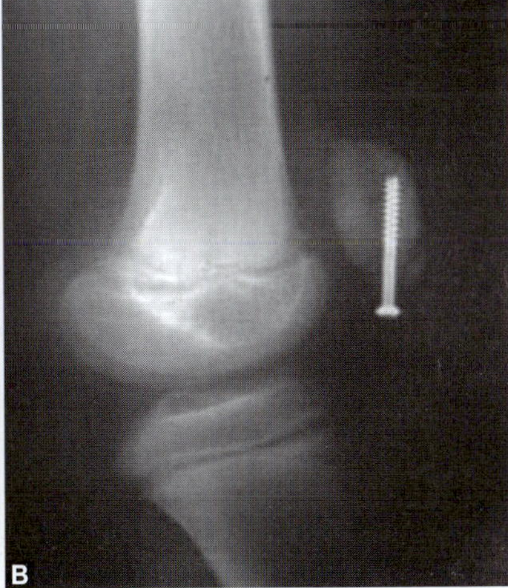

FIGS. 14A AND B: Fracture patella fixed with wires and screw.

BIBLIOGRAPHY

1. Chambers C. MRI findings in pediatric physeal fractures of the knee. Springer J Pediatr Radiol. 2023. (This study examines the diagnostic value of MRI in identifying growth plate fractures in pediatric knees)
2. Bonasia DE, Amendola A, Rosso F, Rossi R. Pediatric anterior cruciate ligament reconstruction with over-the-top femoral position and all-epiphyseal tibial tunnel. Arthrosc Tech. 2024;13(4):102903.
3. Li C, Huang X, Yang Q, Luo Y, Li J, Ye S. Arthroscopic fixation techniques for tibial eminence fractures in pediatric patients: a review. Front Surg. 2023. (This paper reviews the latest arthroscopic techniques for tibial eminence fractures, a common pediatric knee injury, and highlights best practices for treatment outcomes)
4. Pediatric Knee Trauma Radiographic Evaluation. A guide on radiographic techniques for evaluating fractures of the femur, patella, and tibia in pediatric knee trauma. Orthobullets. 2023.

CHAPTER 22.4

Pediatric Tibia and Fibula Fracture

Mohamad Waseem Dar

The tibia fractures are classified on the basis of fracture location and pattern of fracture. The main types are:

- *Diaphyseal fractures:* Involving shaft.
- *Metaphyseal fractures:* Involving area between epiphyseal and diaphyseal area.
- *Physeal (growth plate) fractures:* Classified using the Salter-Harris system—
  - *Types I and II:* Usually managed nonoperatively.
  - *Types III, IV, and V:* Involve the epiphysis and/or metaphysis and may require surgical intervention to prevent growth disturbance.
- *Toddler's fracture:* A minimally or nondisplaced spiral fracture of the tibia without fibular involvement, often in children younger than 3 years.
- *Buckle (Torus) fractures:* These fractures are quite common.
- *Incomplete fracture:* Greenstick fracture of tibia and fibula. Usually, they are unicortical fracture.
- *Complete fracture:* Here, fracture involves both cortices.

PRINCIPLES OF MANAGEMENT

Management depends on the type of fracture, patient's age, and the potential for bone remodeling and growth.

Nonoperative Management

Nonoperative management is preferred in the majority of pediatric tibia and fibula fractures due to the inherent potential for remodeling. Key approaches include:

- *Casting and immobilization:*
  - *Buckle (Torus) fractures:* Managed with a removable splint or above knee leg cast for 4–6 weeks. Followed by patellar tendon bearing cast for 4–6 weeks. Early mobilization is encouraged.
  - *Toddler's fracture:* Typically treated with above knee leg cast for 4–6 weeks, allowing weight-bearing as tolerated.
  - *Nondisplaced and minimally displaced diaphyseal fractures:* Managed with a long leg cast for 4–6 weeks, with nonweight bearing initially, followed by gradual weight-bearing as the fracture stabilizes.
  - *Isolated fibular fractures:* Often do not require specific treatment beyond pain management unless associated with a tibial fracture.
- *Close monitoring:* Regular follow-up radiographs every 1–2 weeks initially to ensure that the alignment is maintained. Follow-up intervals can be extended as

TABLE 1: Alignment and its accepted parameters

Alignment	Accepted parameter
Angulation in sagittal plane	≤5–10°
Angulation in coronal plane	≤5–10°
Rotation	5°
Cortical apposition	50%

TABLE 2: Indication for operative treatment.

Absolute indication	Relative indication
Unacceptable reduction	Multiple long bone fracture
Fracture instability	Floating knee
Compartment syndrome	Spastic syndrome
Compound fracture	Bleeding diathesis
Significant soft-tissue coverage loss	Neurovascular injury

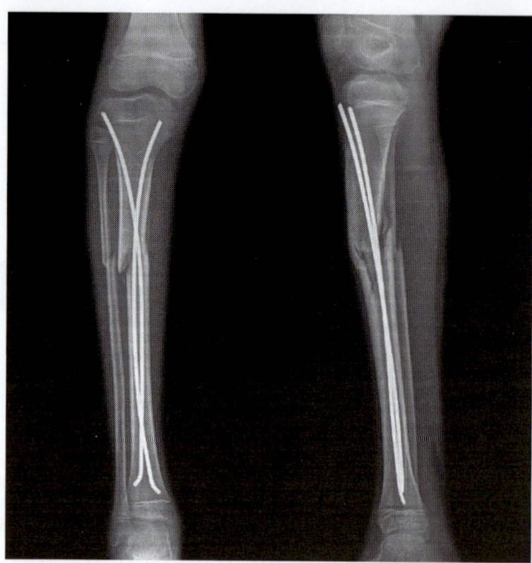

FIG. 1: Shows fractured tibia and fibula with titanium elastic nails (TENS) nailing of tibia.

the fracture heals. *The time of fracture healing varies as per age:*

- 2–3 weeks for neonates
- 4–6 weeks for children
- 10–14 weeks for adolescents

Acceptable criteria for tibial shaft fracture reduction **(Table 1)**.

Children <8 years of age can accept 100% translation and up to 10% sagittal and coronal angulation.

Operative Management

Surgical intervention is considered in specific circumstances:

- *Indications for surgery* **(Table 2)***:*
  - *Open fractures:* Immediate surgical debridement and stabilization are required. Treatment options include flexible intramedullary nailing, external fixation, or plating.
  - *Displaced or unstable fractures:* Closed reduction and percutaneous pinning or elastic stable intramedullary nailing (ESIN) are often employed, especially for fractures that cannot be adequately aligned by closed means.
  - *Physeal fractures (Salter-Harris types III, IV, and V):* Require anatomical reduction, often achieved via open or closed reduction with internal fixation, to minimize growth disturbances.
  - *Polytrauma or compartment syndrome:* Emergent intervention with possible fasciotomy and external fixation for stabilization.
- *Surgical techniques:*
  - *Elastic stable intramedullary nailing:* Preferred for diaphyseal fractures, providing flexible stability and allowing early mobilization **(Fig. 1)**.
  - *External fixation:* Used in open fractures, polytrauma, or fractures with significant soft-tissue damage.

INDICATION FOR OPERATIVE TREATMENT

Refer to **Table 2**.

BIBLIOGRAPHY

1. American Academy of Orthopaedic Surgeons (AAOS). Pediatric Tibia and Fibula Fractures Clinical Practice Guidelines. 2023.
2. Herring JA. Tachdjian's Pediatric Orthopaedics: From the Texas Scottish Rite Hospital for Children, 6th edition. Philadelphia, PA: Elsevier; 2021.
3. Scherl SA, Miller L. Tibial Shaft Fractures in Children. J Am Acad Orthop Surg. 2020;28(12): 485-96.
4. Shannak AO, Bou-Said DS. Pediatric Tibial Fractures. Clin Orthop Relat Res. 2019;477(6): 1457-66.

CHAPTER 22.5

Pediatric Ankle and Foot Fracture

Aman Koul

- The residual deformities in the ankle and foot are less tolerated because of their weight-bearing nature compared to the upper limb.
- Syndesmotic injuries, often ligamentous, can occur with tibial or fibular fractures, especially in sports involving cutting or pivoting movements.

ASPECTS OF DEVELOPMENT

- At birth, there occurs primary ossification of the tibia and fibula.
- About 6 months of age is when the distal tibial ossification center first emerges.
- Between 1 and 3 years, the distal fibular center emerges.
- Distal tibial physeal closure starts centrally and closes last on the lateral side in females between the ages of 12 and 15 and in boys between the ages of 14 and 18.
- In adolescents, growth shifts from the ankle to the knee, and the distal fibular physis becomes more undulated, increasing stability as the fibula undergoes lateral translation and reduced external rotation.
- The leg grows 3–6 mm/year, with the distal tibia contributing 40% of tibial growth and 17% of overall lower extremity growth.

TIBIOFIBULAR SYNDESMOSIS

- Unlike adults, children and adolescents do not have well-established radiographic criteria for syndesmotic dysfunction.
- Skeletally immature patients are not eligible for adult criteria, such as increased clean space beyond 6 mm or elimination of tibiofibular overlap.
- Syndesmotic integrity is important for treatment decisions, with the need for surgery being significantly higher in children with ankle fractures, a medial clear space over 5 mm, or fused physes.
- In children, a widened medial clear space > 5 mm on the mortise view is a strong predictor for surgical fixation.

FRACTURES AROUND ANKLE

- Ankle joint fractures are often classified as physeal and avulsion fractures.
- The distinctions in the damage received by juvenile and adult skeletons are explained by physis patency.
- An open physis guards against damage to the syndesmosis and ligaments.
- Open physes are far more susceptible to shear and rotational pressures than the stronger surrounding ligaments.
- Children may get physeal or avulsion fractures from injury mechanisms that cause adult ankle sprains.

- When avulsion fractures are treated effectively, they heal well and do not require further care.

CLASSIFIED AS PER THE SALTER–HARRIS FRACTURE TYPES

For epiphyseal injuries refer to Salter-Harris fracture classification as given in **Figures 1A to F**.

DIAS–TACHDJIAN CLASSIFICATION

- Combines adult ankle fracture models like Lauge-Hansen with Salter-Harris classifications to describe pediatric ankle fractures based on foot position and direction of force during trauma **(Fig. 2)**.
- Four injury mechanisms are described in the Dias-Tachdjian system, which helps to guide treatment by indicating the direction of injury and suggesting how to immobilize the ankle for closed reduction.
- Understanding these mechanisms aids in closed reduction by immobilizing the ankle in the direction opposite to the injury's force trajectory.
- *Supination—inversion*:
  - The most typical kind of fracture
  - Distal fibula nondisplaced Salter-Harris type I or II fracture.
  - May proceed to a medial malleolus Salter-Harris type III or IV fracture.
  - Affects less than one-third of the mediolateral epiphysis.
- *Supination—external rotation:*
  - This condition starts with a distal tibia physeal fracture that includes a big medial or posteromedial Thurston-Holland fragment.
  - It may also have an associated fibular fracture that is unrelated to the physis.
- *Pronation—external rotation:*
  - This condition presents with a transverse fracture of the fibular diaphysis, lateral translation at the

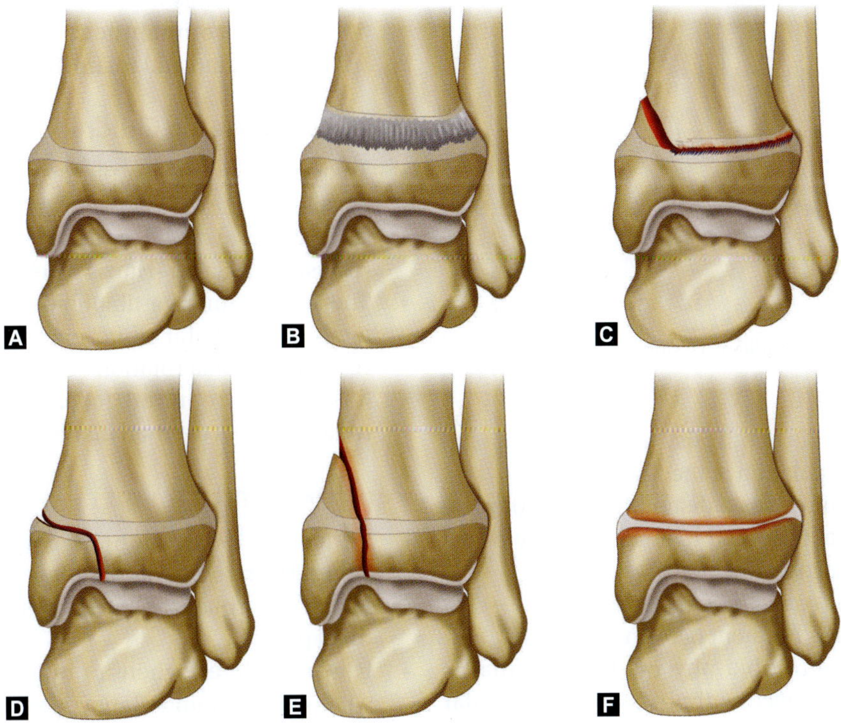

FIGS. 1A TO F: Classified as per the Salter–Harris fracture types.

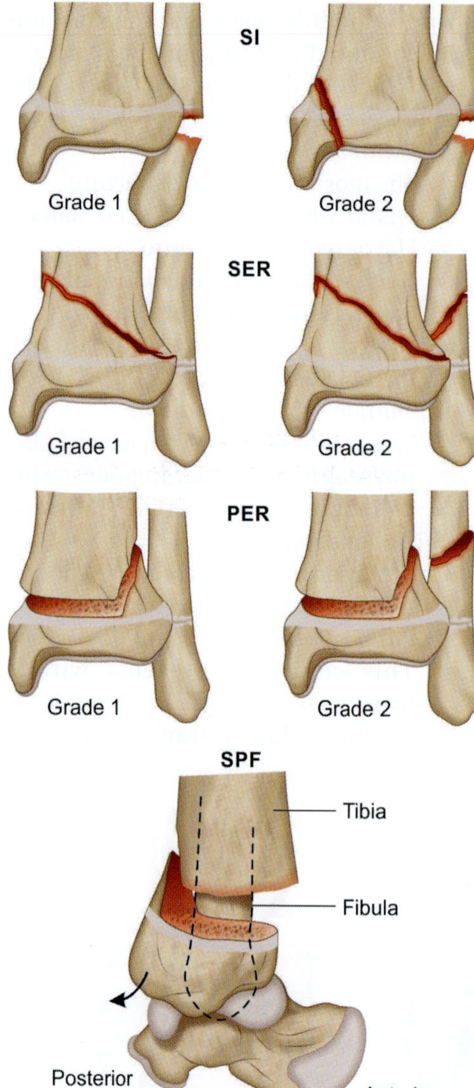

FIG. 2: Dias–Tachdjian classification.

tibial epiphysis, and apical medial angulation at the fibular shaft.
    - It involves a distal tibial growth plate fracture with a small laterally based fracture fragment.
- *Supination—plantar flexion:*
    - Less frequent pattern of fracture.
    - Distal tibia physeal fracture that is displaced without associated fibular fracture.
    - The majority of the tibial Thurston-Holland fragment is posterior, and the displacement is usually mild.

TRANSITIONAL FRACTURES

Arise in girls aged 12–15 years and males aged 14–18 years during the 18-month developmental window of distal tibial physeal closure.

- *Triplane fractures:*
    - Occur in the early phases of physeal closure.
    - Represents 5–10% of pediatric intra-articular ankle injuries.
        - A multiplanar subset of Salter-Harris type IV fractures.
    - Involves fracture lines through coronal, sagittal, and transverse planes.
    - Typically results from supination—external rotation, but other mechanisms exist.
    - Classified by the number of fragments (two-, three-, or four-part fractures) **(Figs. 3A to F)**
    - CT is recommended for accurate classification and treatment planning.

Tillaux Fractures in Children

- Take place in the last phases of physeal closure.
- Anterolateral tibial epiphysis fracture (transitional Salter-Harris type III).
- The anterior-inferior tibiofibular ligament avulses the distal tibial epiphysis as a result of external rotation of the foot.
- CT may be required for evaluation if radiography is deemed inadequate.

Periosteal Entrapment

- Periosteal entrapment is common in Salter-Harris type II and triplane fractures in the anterolateral corner of the distal tibial physis.
- It is considered when a physeal gap or widening of 3 mm or larger is evident at a distal tibial physeal fracture site.

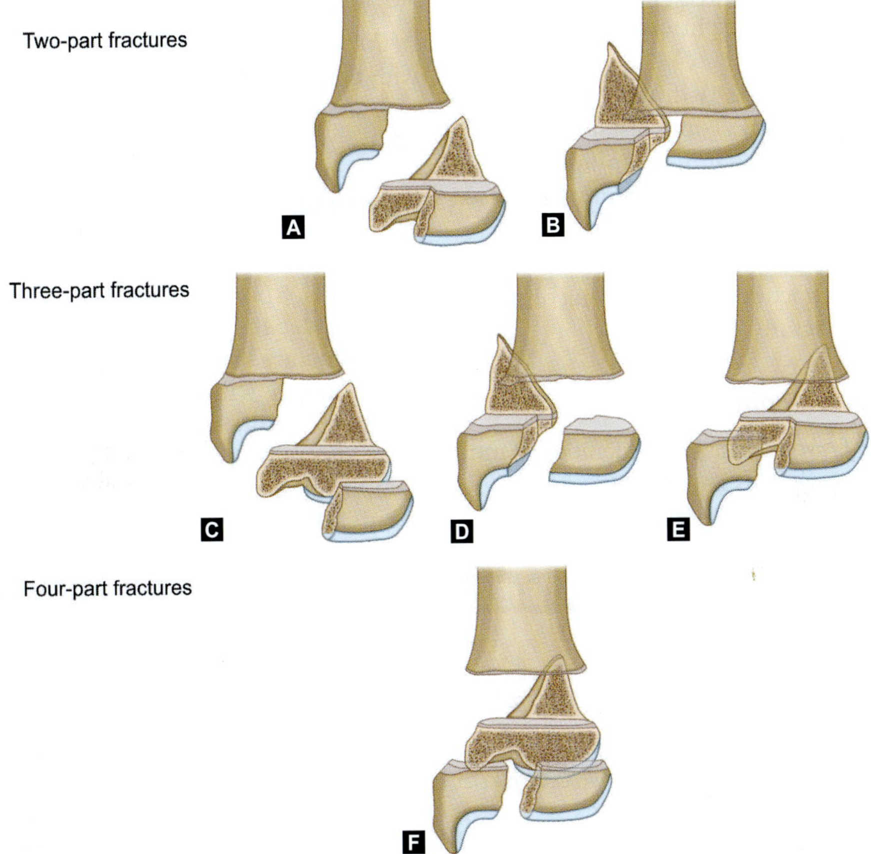

FIGS. 3A TO F: Classified by the number of fragments (two-, three-, or four-part fractures).

Tibiotalar Dislocation

- Owing to physeal fragility, rare in youngsters with underdeveloped skeletons.
- *Mechanism:* Inversion and plantar flexion, which frequently results in posteromedial dislocation.
- May entail fibular physis and rupture of the lateral capsular ligamentous complexes.
- It may be closed or open, and neurovascular impairment may be present.
- Generally, tibiofibular syndesmotic integrity is preserved.
- Arranged according to the direction of displacement.

Ankle Fractures having the Highest Complication Risk

- Fractures involving high-energy mechanism of injury
- Fractures involving >2-mm articular displacement.
- Fractures involving >3-mm physeal widening.

TREATMENT APPROACHES

Fractures Amenable to Conservative Treatment

- All nondisplaced fractures
- Isolated fibular fractures

Indications for Surgical Management of Fractures

- Less than 3 years of growth remaining and persistent malalignment after closed reduction.
- More than 3 years of growth remaining and persistent physeal widening > 3 mm.

- Intra-articular fractures with >2-mm displacement at weight-bearing surface after reduction
- SH-III and SH-IV fractures of medial malleolus with >1-mm displacement
- More than 2-mm displacement in patients with Tillaux fracture after closed reduction
- Triplane fractures
- Fibular fractures accompanying displaced tibial fractures

Physeal Widening

- *Significance:* Persistent widening (>3 mm) indicates periosteal entrapment.
- *Required action:* Surgical treatment

Additional Considerations

Arthrodesis: Contraindicated in children with open physes, though it may be used for Lisfranc fractures in older adolescents and adults.

PEDIATRIC FOOT FRACTURES

These are common injuries, often resulting from falls, sports, or trauma. Treatment typically depends on the type and location of the fracture. Nondisplaced fractures may be managed with immobilization using a cast or splint, allowing natural healing. More severe fractures, such as displaced or complex fractures, might require reduction or surgical intervention.

BIBLIOGRAPHY

1. Cepela DJ, Tartaglione JP, Dooley TP, Patel PN. Classifications In Brief: Salter-Harris Classification of Pediatric Physeal Fractures. Clin Orthop Relat Res. 2016;474(11):2531-7.
2. Dias LS, Tachdjian MO. Physeal injuries of the ankle in children: classification. Clin Orthop Relat Res. 1978;(136):230-3.
3. Mencio GA, Swiontkowski MF. Green's Skeletal Trauma in Children, 5th edition. Philadelphia, PA: Elsevier/Saunders; 2014.
4. Podeszwa DA, Mubarak SJ. Physeal fractures of the distal tibia and fibula (Salter-Harris Type I, II, III, and IV fractures). J Pediatr Orthop. 2012; 32(suppl 1):S62-8.
5. Rapariz JM, Ocete G, González-Herranz P, López-Mondejar JA, Domenech J, Burgos J, et al. Distal tibial triplane fractures: long-term follow-up. J Pediatr Orthop. 1996;16(1):113-8.
6. Wuerz TH, Gurd DP. Pediatric physeal ankle fracture. J Am Acad Orthop Surg. 2013;21(4):234-44.

SECTION

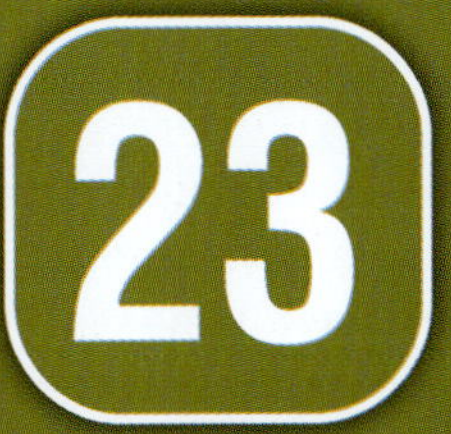

Problem Solving and Decision-making in Fracture Management

CHAPTER 23.1

How Not to Miss Commonly Missed in Fractures

John Mohd, Farid Hussain Malik

Fractures can sometimes be subtle or atypical, leading to misdiagnosis or delayed treatment.

COMMONLY MISSED FRACTURES AND STRATEGIES FOR DETECTION

Scaphoid Fracture

Clinical presentation: Patients typically present with wrist pain following a fall on an outstretched hand, often with tenderness in the anatomic snuffbox.

Reasons for Missed Diagnosis

- Normal initial X-rays (up to 20% may be missed)
- Insufficient attention to subtle signs of injury

Tips and Tricks

- *Palpation technique:* Always palpate the entire wrist, emphasizing the snuffbox. Note any tenderness as a critical indicator.
- *Compression test:* Apply gentle compression to the scaphoid to reproduce pain.
- *Use of scaphoid views:* Incorporate scaphoid-specific views [e.g., posteroanterior (PA), lateral, and oblique views] in your X-ray protocol.
- *MRI or CT for high suspicion:* If initial X-rays are inconclusive and suspicion is high, consider MRI or CT, especially in young athletes or high-risk individuals.

Femoral Neck Fracture, Especially with Ipsilateral Femoral Shaft Fracture

Reasons for Missed Diagnosis

- Subtle nondisplaced fractures can be overlooked on standard views.
- Misdiagnosis due to pre-existing degenerative changes.

Tips and Tricks

- *Detailed examination:* Always assess for leg position, especially in elderly patients; note any signs of hip fracture.
- *Obtain lateral views:* Always include lateral and cross-table views in your imaging to capture missed fractures.
- Use of *thin-cut CT section* whenever there is a suspicion.
- *Use MRI for nondisplaced fractures:* Consider MRI if suspicion persists despite normal X-rays, as it can reveal stress fractures and marrow edema.

Tibial Plateau Fracture

Clinical presentation: Often due to falls or high-energy trauma, patients present with knee swelling and pain, possibly with instability.

Reasons for Missed Diagnosis

- Subtle fractures might not be visible on standard views.
- Misinterpretation of knee swelling as a soft-tissue injury.

Tips and Tricks

- *Joint line tenderness:* Pay close attention to joint line tenderness; it is a key indicator of possible fracture.
- *Stress views and CT scans:* Use stress views or a CT scan if suspicion remains high.
- *Evaluate associated injuries:* Always assess for associated ligamentous injuries that can accompany plateau fractures, which may indicate fracture presence.

Osteoporotic Vertebral Fractures

Clinical presentation: Older adults present with back pain, which may be mistaken for muscle strain or degenerative changes.

Reasons for Missed Diagnosis

- Inattention to clinical signs like kyphosis or height loss
- Failure to perform appropriate imaging studies

Tips and Tricks

- *Assess risk factors:* Identify patients with risk factors for osteoporosis (e.g., age, history of fractures, and steroid use).
- *Utilize vertebral imaging:* Employ lateral X-rays or MRI to evaluate for subtle compression fractures.

Fifth Metatarsal Fracture (Jones Fracture)

It often occurs after an inversion injury, with lateral foot pain and swelling.

Reasons for Missed Diagnosis

- Commonly misdiagnosed as a sprain due to similar presentations.

Tips and Tricks

- *Focus on tenderness and function:* Assess for localized tenderness over the base of the fifth metatarsal and check for functional limitations.
- *Specialized views:* Include specific views for the foot, especially in cases of high suspicion.
- *Utilize MRI for inconclusive cases:* Consider MRI if initial imaging fails to confirm the diagnosis but symptoms persist.

Pediatric Fractures, Especially Around the Physeal Line

Here again, focus examination, different views of X-rays like internal oblique view in suspected lateral condyle fracture and having a comparative X-ray view of the opposite side in identical position.

Humeral Head Fracture

- Often occurs in elderly patients after falls.
- This can be mistaken for soft-tissue injuries or shoulder dislocations; careful imaging and assessment are needed.

Calcaneal Fracture

Risk of missed diagnosis: Often overlooked in cases of ankle injuries or sprains; requires dedicated imaging of the heel.

Radial Head Fracture

- Frequently associated with elbow injuries after falls.
- This can be subtle on initial X-rays; the "fat pad sign" or additional views may be necessary for diagnosis.

Stress Fractures

- Can occur in various bones (e.g., femur, tibia, and metatarsals) due to repetitive stress.
- Often present with gradual pain that may be mistaken for other conditions; may not show up on initial imaging.

Acetabular Fractures

- Often a result of high-energy trauma, such as motor vehicle accidents.
- Subtle fractures can be missed on standard X-rays, necessitating CT for proper assessment.

Sacroiliac/Lumbosacral Fractures

- Can occur during high-energy trauma or falls.
- May be confused with the lumbar spine or hip injuries; require specific imaging for confirmation.

Cervico-dorsal Fractures

Plan X-rays can easily miss subtle fractures, and in such a situation, a CT scan is a must if there is any suspicion.

GENERAL STRATEGIES FOR ENHANCING DIAGNOSTIC ACCURACY

Comprehensive History and Examination

- *Detailed mechanism of injury:* Gather comprehensive details regarding the injury mechanism; understanding the forces at play can guide your assessment.
- *Focused physical examination:* Systematically assess the entire affected region, checking for tenderness, deformity, and functional impairment.

Imaging Protocols

- *Advanced imaging:* Always consider the use of advanced imaging (MRI/CT) when the diagnosis is unclear or when clinical suspicion remains high despite negative X-rays.
- *Reassess imaging:* If initial X-rays do not show a fracture, but clinical suspicion is strong, do not hesitate to repeat imaging after a short interval or additional view like oblique views. Comparative views of the opposite (normal) side in cases of children if there is any confusion between fracture and growth plate line.

Follow-up and Patient's Education

- *Routine follow-ups:* Implement protocols for follow-up appointments in patients with high suspicion of fractures.
- *Educate patients:* Provide clear guidance on warning signs (e.g., increasing pain, and inability to bear weight) that should prompt immediate re-evaluation.

Clinical Decision-making Tools

- *Develop clinical pathways:* Establish guidelines for evaluating specific injuries to standardize the assessment and management process.
- *Utilize scoring systems:* Consider using decision-making tools or scoring systems to stratify risk and guide imaging decisions.

SUMMARY

To avoid missing these fractures, one should maintain a high index of suspicion, especially in patients with risk factors, utilize appropriate imaging, and ensure thorough clinical evaluations. Being aware of these commonly missed fractures can significantly improve diagnostic accuracy and patient's outcomes.

BIBLIOGRAPHY

1. Link TM, Guglielmi G, van Kuijk C, Adams JE. Radiologic assessment of osteoporotic vertebral fractures: diagnostic and prognostic implications. Eur Radiol. 2005;15(8).
2. Buijze GA, Doornberg JN, Ham JS, Ring D, Bhandari M, Poolman RW. Surgical compared with conservative treatment for acute nondisplaced or minimally displaced scaphoid fractures: a systematic review and meta-analysis of randomized controlled trials. J Bone Joint Surg Am. 2010;92(6):1534-44.
3. Reiman MP, Thorborg K, Goode AP, Cook CE, Weir A, Hölmich P. Diagnostic accuracy of imaging modalities and injection techniques for the diagnosis of femoroacetabular impingement/labral tear: A systematic review with meta-analysis. Am J Sports Med. 2017;45(11):2665-77.

CHAPTER 23.2

Decision-making and Planning the Treatment of Fractures

Shabir A Dhar

Effective decision-making in fracture management is at the core of achieving successful patient's outcomes. It involves more than just selecting a fixation method—it requires a systematic evaluation of the patient, the fracture, and the surgical environment to make informed and evidence-based choices. This chapter focuses on how decision-making, backed by comprehensive treatment planning, can ensure optimal surgical outcomes. By integrating both clinical judgment and the latest scientific advancements, decision-making in fracture management becomes a dynamic process that enhances patient's safety, minimizes complications, and promotes faster recovery.

DECISION-MAKING IN FRACTURE MANAGEMENT

Decision-making in fracture care follows a structured approach where multiple factors converge to inform the best course of action. Key components of this decision-making process include:

- *Patient-specific factors:* Age, comorbidities, bone quality, activity level, and individual needs.
- *Fracture-specific considerations:* Type, location, complexity, and associated soft-tissue damage.
- *Available resources and expertise:* Surgical techniques, implants, and healthcare infrastructure.
- *Anticipation of risks and complications:* Proactively addressing potential challenges such as infection, nonunion, and nerve injury.

The interplay between these elements guides every step of fracture management, ensuring a tailored approach to each patient's unique situation.

PREOPERATIVE PLANNING

Patient's Evaluation and Risk Stratification

The first critical decision point in fracture management is the thorough evaluation of the patient which involves:

- *Patient's general health:* Pre-existing conditions such as diabetes, osteoporosis, or cardiovascular disease can affect healing and surgical risks. For instance, an elderly patient with osteoporotic bone will require a different fixation strategy compared to a young and healthy individual.
- *Functional demands:* The patient's occupation, lifestyle, and expectations will influence the choice of treatment. For example, athletes or laborers may prioritize rapid return to full function, prompting more aggressive surgical approaches, while elderly patients may prioritize stability and pain-free mobility.
- *Bone quality:* Patients with poor bone quality due to age or osteoporosis may

require specific implants such as locking plates or intramedullary nails to ensure sufficient fixation strength.

Decision point: Should conservative management be considered, or is surgical intervention necessary? *At this stage more important decision is when not to operate.*

Accurate Fracture Assessment and Classification

Accurate classification and understanding of the fracture are essential for making informed decisions about the surgical approach. This involves:

- *Fracture classification systems:* Utilizing standardized systems like the *AO/OTA classification* helps to categorize the fracture and predict outcomes. The classification assists in selecting the appropriate fixation method, anticipating healing challenges, and guiding intraoperative decision-making.
- *Imaging decisions:* Advanced imaging modalities such as *CT* and *MRI* are often necessary in complex fractures. For example, CT scans with three-dimensional (3D) reconstruction are invaluable in understanding multifragmentary fractures or intra-articular injuries, where anatomic restoration is critical.

Selecting the Right Fixation Strategy

The fixation method is another key decision point that must be tailored to the fracture type and patient's factors:

- *Fixation devices:* The choice among *locking plates, intramedullary nails,* and *external fixation* depends on fracture stability, bone quality, and the patient's activity level. For instance, locking plates are preferred in osteoporotic fractures due to their ability to secure fixation in weak bones.

Decision point: What fixation method offers the best balance between stability and biological preservation? In elderly patients or those with osteoporosis, locking plates provide greater fixation strength. However, in healthy patients with good bone stock, intramedullary nailing may be preferred for its less invasive approach.

Preoperative Timing Decisions

The timing of surgery is another critical element. For certain fractures, immediate intervention is crucial, such as in:

Should surgery be immediate or delayed? Open fractures or those associated with vascular compromise demand urgent intervention, while others may benefit from delayed definitive fixation to allow for patient's stabilization.

INTRAOPERATIVE DECISION-MAKING

Choosing the Surgical Approach

Factors influencing this decision include:

- *Decision point:* Is the primary goal anatomical reduction, or is biological preservation more important? For intra-articular fractures, anatomic reduction is essential, whereas in long bone fractures, biological healing with minimal soft-tissue disruption is often prioritized. However, MIPPO should not be at the cost of quality reduction and fixation.

Make sure the availability of image intensifier if and when needed and there should not be any compromise regarding this.

Intraoperative Flexibility/Backup Alternative Option

Despite meticulous preoperative planning, intraoperative decisions often need to adapt to unexpected challenges, such as:

- *Bone quality issues:* If poor bone quality is encountered intraoperatively, the fixation method may need to be adjusted. For example, changing from standard screws to locking screws if the bone is osteoporotic.

- *Fracture extension or comminution:* Discovering additional fracture fragments or comminuted areas may necessitate altering the planned fixation strategy, possibly adding supplementary fixation (e.g., additional plates or screws).

Decision point: How to adapt the plan intraoperatively to changing conditions? Surgeons must be prepared to modify the surgical plan based on real-time findings to ensure optimal fixation and patient's safety.

POSTOPERATIVE DECISION-MAKING

Rehabilitation Protocols

Postoperative decision-making continues into rehabilitation, where early mobilization and weight-bearing decisions significantly impact recovery:

When should weight-bearing be initiated? For fractures with stable fixation, early mobilization promotes better outcomes, but in fractures with more complex fixation or poor bone quality, delayed weight-bearing may be necessary to prevent complications.

Monitoring and Addressing Complications

Decision-making in the postoperative phase involves ongoing assessment of healing progress:

When to intervene in delayed or complicated healing? Early detection of nonunion or infection allows for prompt intervention, such as revision surgery or bone grafting, to ensure better long-term outcomes.

CONCLUSION

Decision-making in fracture management is a dynamic and multiphased process that requires a combination of clinical expertise, careful planning, and adaptability. From the initial evaluation to intraoperative adjustments and postoperative management, each decision point significantly impacts patient's outcomes. By following a structured, evidence-based approach, surgeons can enhance their ability to anticipate challenges, minimize complications, and ultimately deliver optimal surgical results tailored to the needs of each patient.

BIBLIOGRAPHY

1. Spronk I, Loggers SAI, Joosse P, Willems HC, van Balen R, Gosens T, et al. Shared decision-making for the treatment of proximal femoral fractures in frail institutionalised older patients: healthcare providers' perceived barriers and facilitators. Age Ageing. 2022;51(8):afac174.
2. Barbilian AG, Sporea C, Ferechide D. Transforming the management of articular fractures in the foot: a critical examination of current methods and future directions. J Pers Med. 2024;14(5):525.

Index

Page numbers followed by *f* refer to figure, *fc* refer to flowchart, and *t* refer to table.

A

B

C

D

E

F

G

H

J

K

L

M

N

Q

R

S

T

U

V

W

X

Y

Z